FUNDAMENTALS OF EEG TECHNOLOGY

Volume 1
Basic Concepts and Methods

Fundamentals of EEG Technology

Volume 1: Basic Concepts and Methods

Fay S. Tyner, R. EEG T.
Consulting EEG Technologist
Atlanta Neurological Clinic

John R. Knott, Ph.D.
Emeritus Professor (Neurology and Psychiatry)
University of Iowa
Clinical Professor of Neurology
Tufts University School of Medicine
Lecturer in Neurology
Boston University School of Medicine

W. Brem Mayer, Jr., M.D.
Atlanta Neurological Clinic
Clinical Associate Professor of Neurology
Emory University School of Medicine

LIPPINCOTT WILLIAMS & WILKINS
A **Wolters Kluwer** Company
Philadelphia • Baltimore • New York • London
Buenos Aires • Hong Kong • Sydney • Tokyo

Lippincott Williams & Wilkins, 227 East Washington Square, Philadelphia, PA 19106-3780.

Printed in the United States of America

Great care has been taken to maintain the accuracy of the information contained in the volume. However, Raven Press cannot be held responsible for errors or for any consequences arising from the use of the information contained herein.

Library of Congress Cataloging in Publication Data

Tyner, Fay S.
Fundamentals of EEG technology.

Includes index.
Contents: v. 1. Basic concepts and methods.
1. Electroencephalography. 2. Brain—Diseases—Diagnosis. I. Knott, John R. (John Russell), 1911– II. Mayer, W. Brem. III. Title. IV. Title: Fundamentals of EEG technology. [DNLM: 1. Electroencephalography. WL 150 T988f]
RC386.6.E43T95 1983 616.1'207547 82-42548
ISBN 13: 978-0-89004-385-1
ISBN 10: 0-89004-385-X (v.1)

18

To our students—
from whom we continue to learn

Preface

The purposes of this book can be better understood if we distinguish *technology* from *technique*. The latter is a collection of technical methods. The former is concerned with scientific knowledge applied to the solution of problems in a specific, practical field. An EEG technician is taught to carry out routine procedures, in a semi-automatic manner, without necessarily understanding the reasons for doing so. An EEG technologist, however, must acquire not only technical skills but also develop a firm understanding of basic principles in a variety of scientific areas, all of which contribute to the practice of clinical electroencephalography.

As clinical EEG has developed, continued reliance upon seemingly simple, rule-of-thumb techniques to secure adequate clinical records has become progressively self-defeating. As instrumentation becomes more reliable and operationally less complex, methods and procedures should advance in order to use the new instrumentation effectively. Those who are technologists must keep abreast of continuing developments or risk reverting to the level of technicians.

This book has been written because we felt that no suitable textbook was available for beginning students that would provide a sufficiently broad base of information in the relevant areas. Our plan has been to start with relatively simple introductory material and build a set of steps by which the student may reach the levels of knowledge required to successfully carry out the duties of a clinical EEG technologist.

There also has been need for a textbook that can be efficiently used by those who have had some prior exposure to electroencephalographic techniques and who desire an introduction to the principles upon which EEG technology is based. These readers may begin at levels appropriate to their experience and knowledge, exploring onward for new information and looking back when necessary for review.

As work on this book progressed, we became aware of the fact that the material being covered was more massive than had been anticipated, if adequate coverage was to be given to all topics. Not only should the principles and methods be discussed, but the clinical applications should receive much-needed attention. If an EEG technologist is to adequately carry out assignments involving sick people, then he/she should understand the types of sicknesses encountered in the daily practice of EEG technology, as well as the EEG characteristics associated with various diseases. For these reasons we have divided the book into two volumes. Volume 1 deals with *Basic Principles and Methods*. Volume 2 deals with *Clinical Correlations* and will include an elementary outline of those features of neuroanatomy and neurophysiology that are of concern to technologists. Each volume has been designed to stand on its own, although the information developed in Volume 1 has direct application in Volume 2, and information contained in Volume 2 will sometimes fill in further details alluded to in Volume 1.

The present volume is aimed not only at the beginning and advanced student of EEG technology but also at students of clinical electroencephalography who are entering the field from medical areas such as neurology or pediatrics. Those who interpret EEG records must comprehend the role of EEG technology, as well as the role of the technologist, in the production of the EEG record. Without such a basic understanding, no EEG can be interpreted reliably.

Chapter 5, "Some Principles of Electricity and Electronics," has been developed to provide basic material with direct applications to EEG technology. Other chapters, particularly the chapter on the EEG amplifier, will refer, directly or indirectly, to this basic chapter. It is our belief that both the technologist and the electroencephalographer must relate operational procedures in the clinical laboratory to basic scientific principles.

The chapters dealing with electrodes, polarity and localization, and the design and use of montages also make reference to material included in earlier chapters. The intent has been to accustom the technologist and the electroencephalographer to approach recording problems in a flexible rather than a stereotyped manner.

The chapter dealing with the description and classification of electroencephalographic activity is designed to bring together those basic concepts and data that make electroencephalography a useful clinical procedure. The technologist who collects the information that becomes "the EEG record" must be able to comprehend, moment by moment, all of the information accumulating at the output of the multiple channel instrument. The EEG record is the common meeting ground where the combined skills of the technologist and the interpreter are utilized to solve a medical problem. The final, joint solution is the product of EEG technology.

Fay S. Tyner
John R. Knott
W. Brem Mayer, Jr.

Acknowledgments

Our task in assembling this volume has been aided by many technologists and electroencephalographers. Space does not allow us to name them all, although most are listed in the references following each chapter. Each will recognize his or her place in shaping our thoughts about EEG technology. We must, however, acknowledge some of those who, at critical moments, rendered direct assistance to us in our labors: Dr. Albert M. Grass, Mr. George Klem, Dr. Virginia B. Knott, Dr. Cesare T. Lombroso, Dr. Timothy A. Pedley and Mr. Peter J. Seaba. We also are indebted to the Grass Instrument Company for permission to use, with modifications, materials from its instrument manuals. All of these shall be held blameless for errors we may, in spite of their efforts, have committed.

Contents

Chapter 1

The Electroencephalogram

An electroencephalogram, abbreviated EEG,[1] is a visible record of the amplified electrical activity generated by the nerve cells of the brain. In literal translation from ancient Greek roots (1), the word means:

electro—electrical
encephalo—brain
gram(ma)—picture

By placing electrodes on the scalp and amplifying the electrical activity that they pick up, an "electrical brain picture" can be recorded through the skull and made to appear in written form, seen as rising and falling electrical potentials called brain waves.

Our knowledge and understanding of how the potentials responsible for these wavy lines are generated is incomplete. However, the sources of electrical activity are in the millions of nerve cells that compose the brain substance. What is recorded from the scalp electrodes is probably the collective activity of many nerve cells in a small area under each electrode. This area is on the *cortex,* the outer surface of the brain. The nerve cells, called *neurons,* in this small area of the cortex generate changing electrical potentials. When the potentials in many neurons are changing synchronously (at the same time or in an orderly sequence), they create rhythms of various types. The synchrony and resulting rhythms of cortical neurons may be influenced by local changes and by changes in nerve cells in other parts of the brain.

As first discovered in man by Hans Berger in 1924 and reported by him in 1929 (1,3), a pair of electrodes can be placed on the front and back of the head and connected to a sensitive recording device that displays the potential differences between the two points. Figure 1.1 schematically illustrates amplification and recording of brain activity from a pair of electrodes on the scalp. It is obvious that there is variability from moment to moment (seen as the up and down movements of the pen) and that this variability occurs in two dimensions. One is *time* and the other is *amplitude*.

The variability in time is expressed as frequency (cycles per second or *hertz,* abbreviated *Hz*). In Fig. 1.2, a 1-sec block of time is marked by the horizontal bar. Within this second, the pen moves up and down ten and one-half times. Thus, during this particular time, the electrical activity being generated by the brain has a frequency of 10.5 Hz. There are slight changes in the frequency of the EEG from moment to moment; absolutely unvarying frequencies are rare.

As one glances across the six seconds of record, it is also obvious that the waves are changing in height or amplitude. Amplitude is an index of voltage. The larger the amplitude, the higher the voltage. The voltages in the EEG are extremely small and are measured in millionths of a volt, called *microvolts* (μV). The vertical bar in Fig. 1.2 represents an amplitude of 50 μV.

From the electrical activity shown in Fig. 1.2 we can see that four general frequencies are occurring in the EEG. The most prominent is approximately 10.5 Hz. This frequency most often is recorded in the back of the head, and was first described by Berger (2), who called it the *alpha* rhythm (Fig. 1.2A). This activity may vary from person to person and ranges from 8 to 13 Hz.

Low voltage waves at approximately 20 Hz also were observed by Berger (2). He named these *beta* waves. The term beta is now used to describe activity faster than 13 Hz. Activity at 15 Hz can be seen in Fig. 1.2B.

Although alpha and beta waves were the first to be defined, other types of activity were later described. Waves in the frequency range from 4 to 7 Hz are called *theta* waves, the name applied by a pioneering English

[1] The abbreviation EEG is used in different ways at different times. An *electroencephalogram* is a completed record or recording; EEG is a noun in this context. An *electroencephalograph* is the instrument used to produce the record; EEG in this case may be used as a noun for the entire term or as an adjective, as in "EEG instrument." Another usage comes in "EEG technologist," in which case EEG stands for *electroencephalographic*, an adjective. *Electroencephalography,* a noun meaning a field of study, is also abbreviated EEG. The use of the abbreviation should not cause confusion if it is read in context.

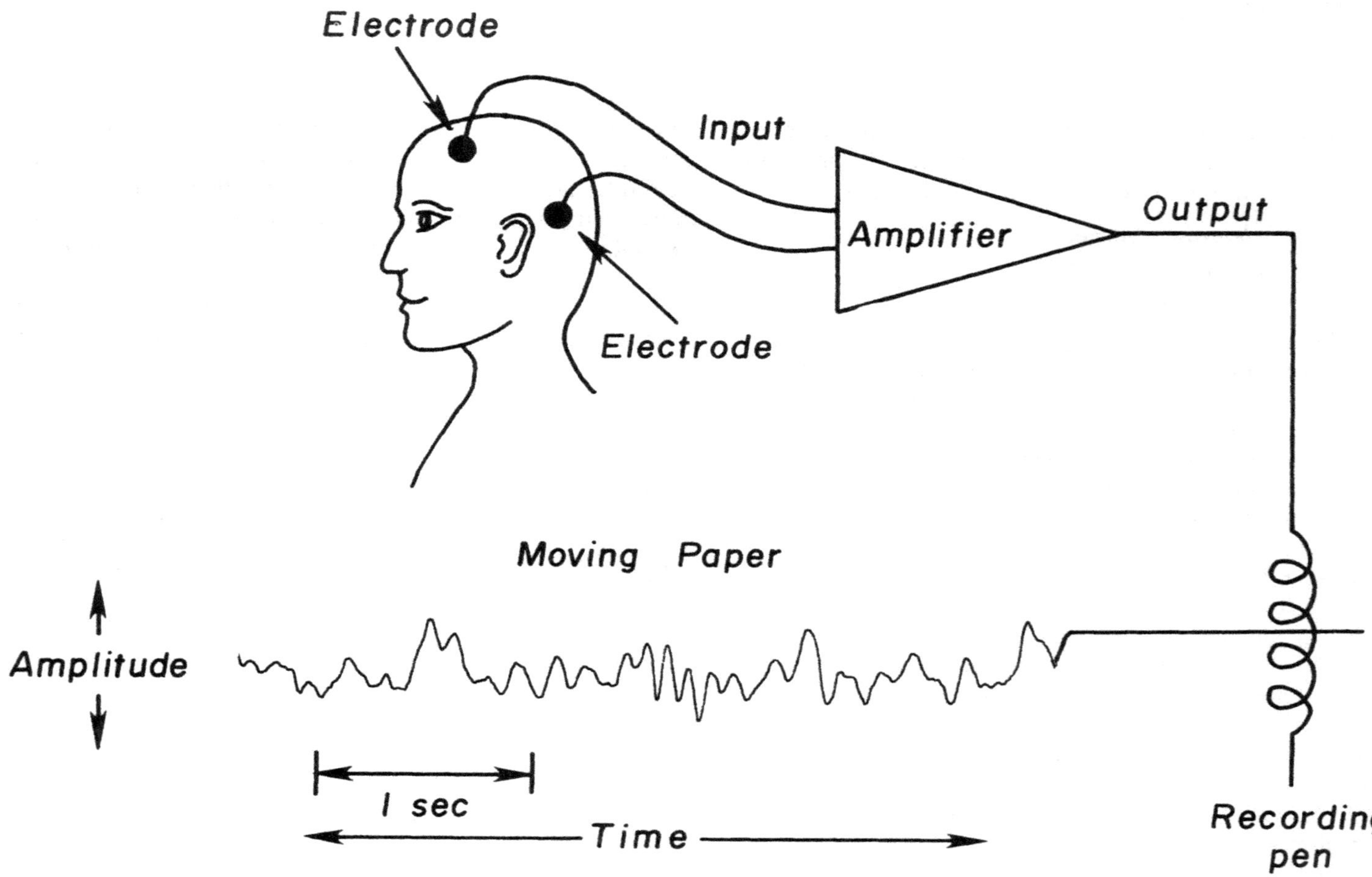

FIG. 1.1. Electrodes attached to the scalp detect electrical activity of the brain that travels to the inputs of the amplifier. The voltage at the output of the amplifier is greatly amplified (up to one million times). The output voltage drives a recording pen that writes on moving paper.

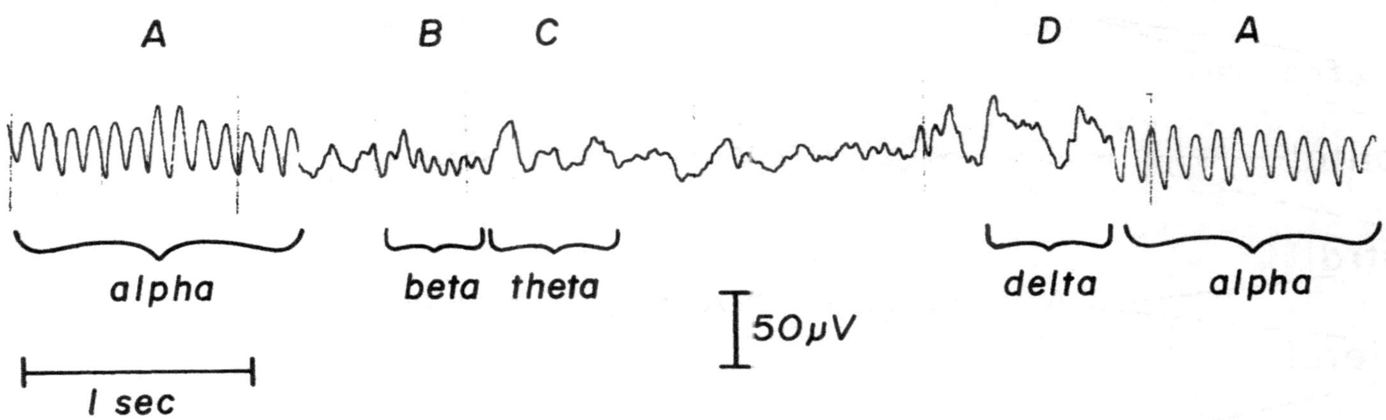

FIG. 1.2. Examples of different types of activity in a short sample of EEG. (See text for discussion.)

electroencephalographer, W. Grey Walter and his colleague Vivian Dovey (4). An example of such activity can be seen in Fig. 1.2C.

In the normal waking adult, activity below 4 Hz is relatively rare. However, waves in this range are seen in Fig. 1.2D. These particular waves are nearly 0.33 sec in duration, which is equivalent to a frequency of approximately 3 Hz. In this instance, beta waves are superimposed. The extremely slow waves are called *delta* waves. This name also was introduced by Walter and Dovey (4) and is used to classify any wave with a frequency of less than 4 Hz.

Thus, in one brief sample of EEG activity from an awake adult, we see some of the varieties of frequencies that occur in the EEG, their moment-to-moment variability, and their classification.

This one-channel recording is elementary. Modern EEGs never have less than 8 channels, and most have 16 or more channels. Fig. 1.3 shows an 8-channel record and indicates the areas of the brain that are being recorded and the abbreviations used to refer to these electrode derivations.

In healthy persons, changes in EEG activity regularly occur during changes in levels of consciousness. (By a healthy person, we mean one with no complaints, no symptoms, and no history of neurological or other significant disease.) The changes may be more prominent in some areas of the brain than in others and may be related to different states of reactivity. The healthy adult, relaxed and awake with eyes closed, usually will show alpha activity in the posterior areas of the head. If he is instructed to open his eyes, alpha will show a decrease in voltage (attenuation) in the posterior areas, as a consequence of visual stimulation (Fig. 1.4). If he engages in simple mental activity such as solving an arithmetic problem (e.g., being asked to multiply 23 × 4 and giving the answer as soon as possible), a change quite similar to that seen with the eyes open will occur. The posterior alpha rhythm loses voltage (is attenuated) and is reestablished after the answer is given.

There are a number of interesting EEG changes that occur in sleep. Sleep is not a steady state that remains at a fixed level from beginning to end. From the characteristics of the EEG, one can discriminate wakefulness, drowsiness, and light and deeper sleep. These will be discussed in detail in Chapter 14.

Not all EEGs are "normal." If they were, EEG would not have clinical applications and there would be no profession of EEG technology. Electroencephalography has many medical and scientific applications that are continually increasing in scope. When the brain is significantly involved in an illness, there may be correlated changes in its electrical activity. For example, a brain tumor may be revealed by *delta* (slow) activity in the

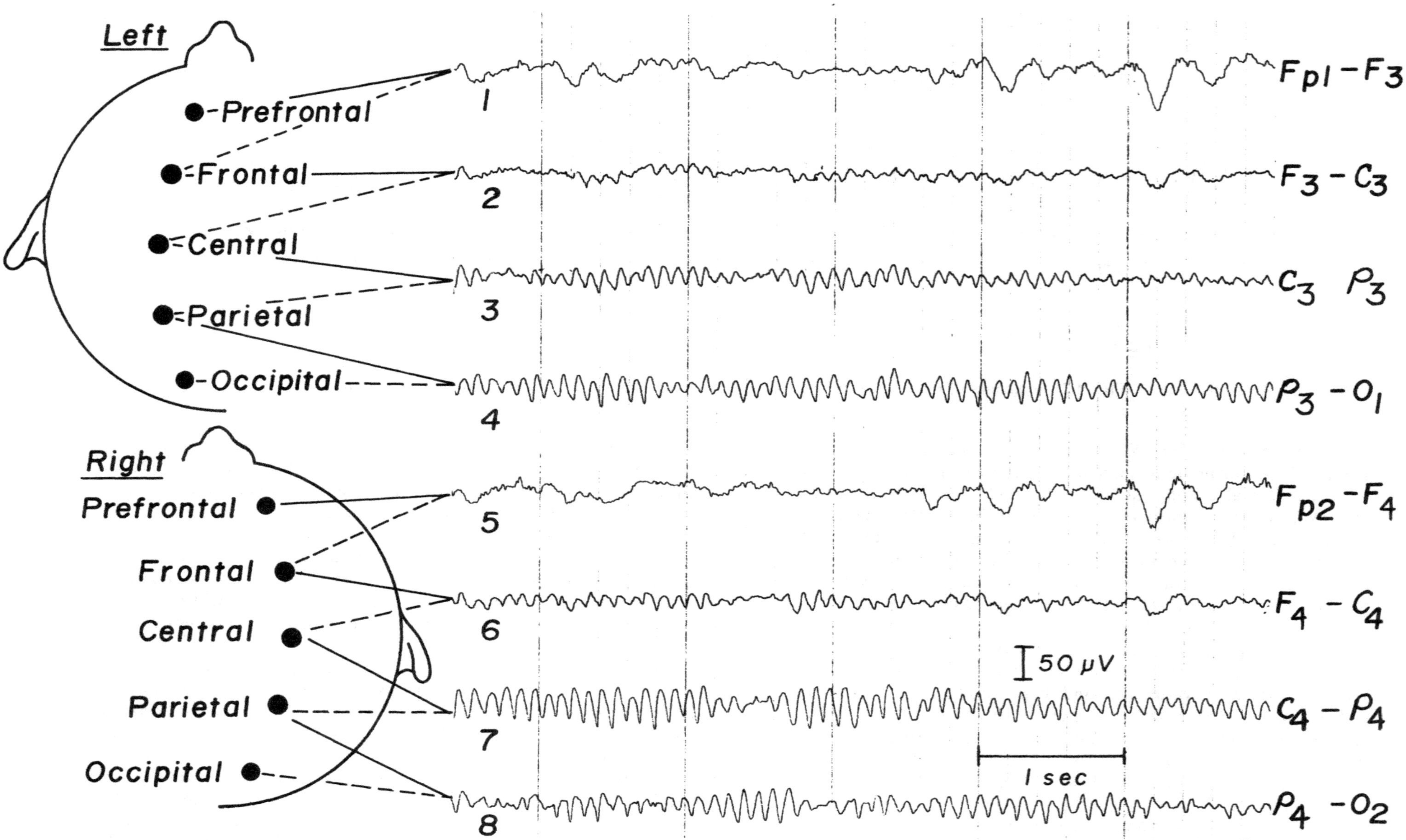

FIG. 1.3. Eight channels of recording from a 20-year-old subject with closed eyes.

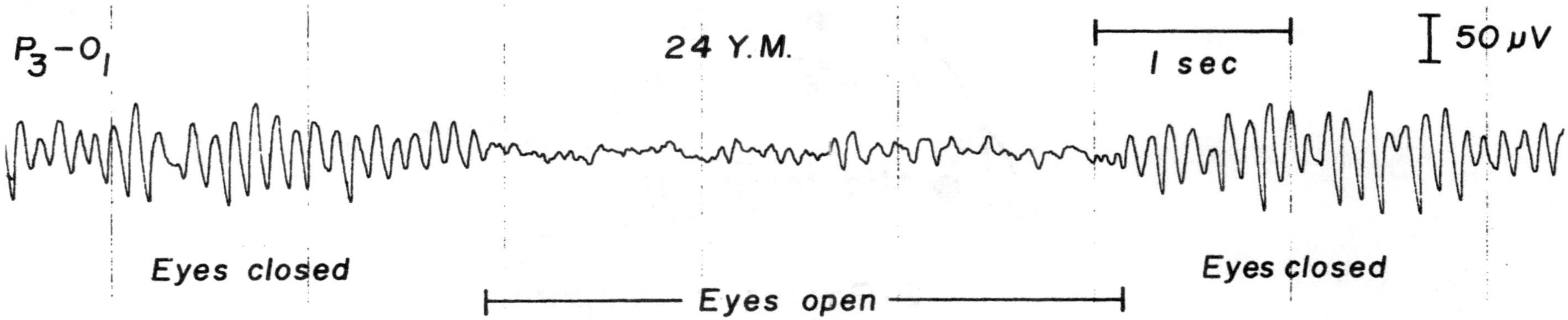

FIG. 1.4. Reactivity of alpha rhythm to eye opening.

region where the tumor is located (Fig. 1.5). Individuals with epilepsy may have distinctive types of EEG abnormalities, not only during their attacks but, more importantly, between clinically detectable seizures. These may appear as single or multiple high voltage, very fast waves, called *spikes,* appearing frequently or infrequently (Fig. 1.6). The high voltage, fast waves (spikes) may be associated with a slow wave, and such discharges are sometimes called *spike-and-wave discharges* (Fig. 1.7).

Changes in the electrical activity of the brain associated with disease make EEG an important, but not an infallible, diagnostic procedure. The major contribution of EEG lies in its ability to evaluate physiological disturbances of brain function not associated with structural lesions.

The EEG examination is carried out by placing a number of electrodes on the head (usually at least 21). These are securely attached in predetermined locations (see Chapter 11). The patient is placed in a relaxed position. The technologist instructs the patient to keep his eyes closed, although he may be requested to open and close them briefly at intervals in order to evaluate reactivity of the brain to visual stimuli. Drowsiness and sleep are usually encouraged to increase the range of activity under examination (see Chapter 15).

Electrical activity other than that generated by the patient's brain may be recorded. This activity is called *artifact* (see Chapter 16). Artifacts often are so similar to the real EEG activity in voltage and frequency that they seriously blur or even obscure the record. The exact origin of such activity must be determined by observation or by monitoring procedures. The origin may be physiological, but not of brain origin (e.g., electrical activity from muscles of the face and scalp). The origin may be external (e.g., radiated currents from nearby electrical equipment).

Recording in the resting and sleeping states should be made for a minimum of 20 to 30 min. In addition, some *activation procedures* may be carried out (see Chapter 15). These include *hyperventilation* (rapid, deep breathing) and *photic stimulation* (rhythmic flashes of bright light). These additional procedures create physiological conditions that may evoke abnormalities that may not otherwise occur in the EEG. The entire procedure, from applying electrodes, to the end of the recording, usually will require one hour or more.

Maximal information from the EEG is dependent upon the EEG technologist's knowledge of the particular neurological disease for which the patient is referred, full understanding of the capabilities of the EEG instrument, and its skillful use.

A well-recorded EEG can provide the neurologist with a continuous record of functional changes in activity in many areas of the living, reacting brain. This information can be correlated with the neurological examination and other special examination procedures (e.g., X-ray, CT scan). The synthesis of these data is necessary for the diagnosis, prognosis, and

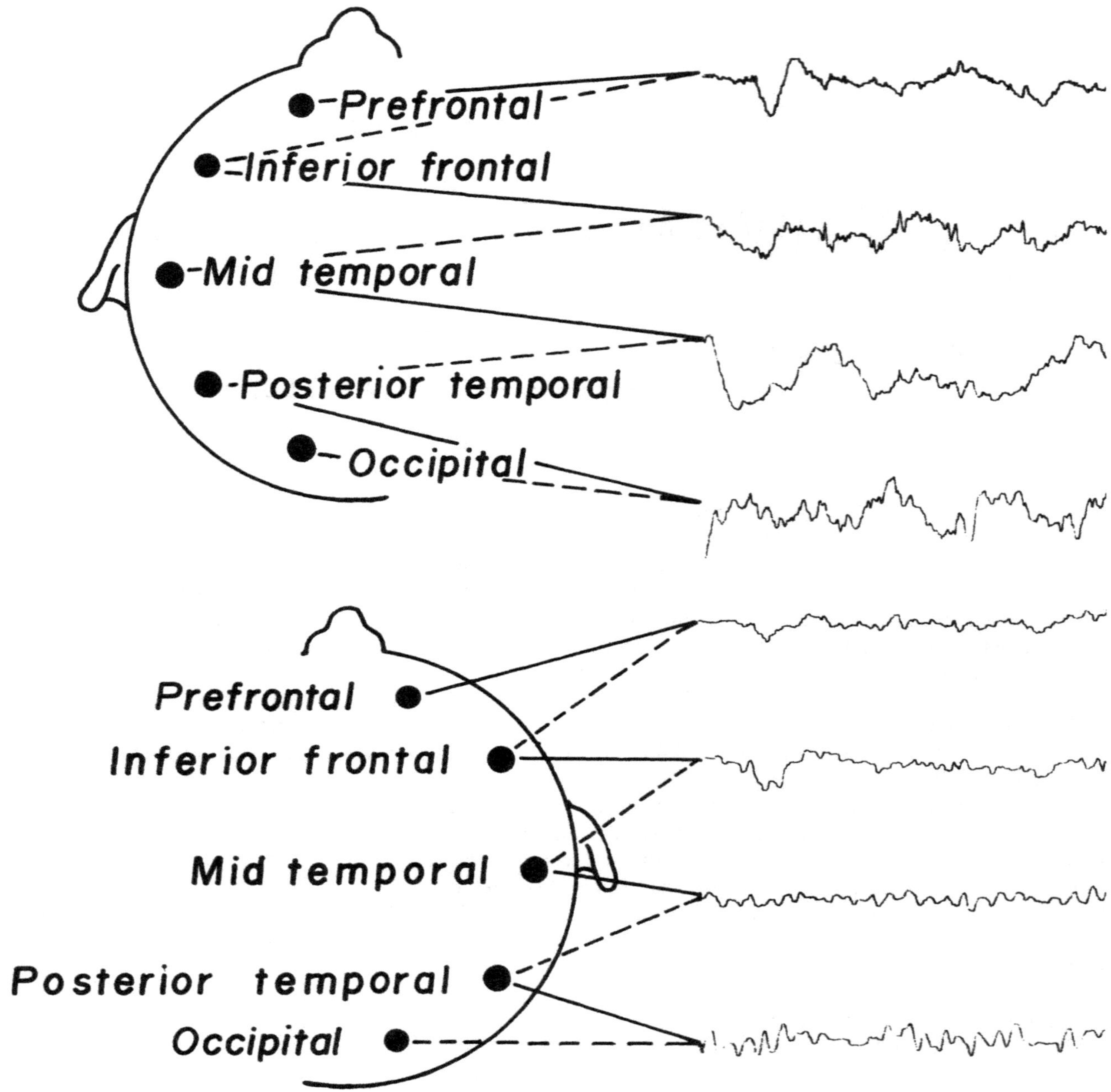

FIG. 1.5. Example of localized EEG abnormality showing excessive slow activity over the left hemisphere, greatest in the left frontotemporal areas. The right hemisphere is essentially normal.

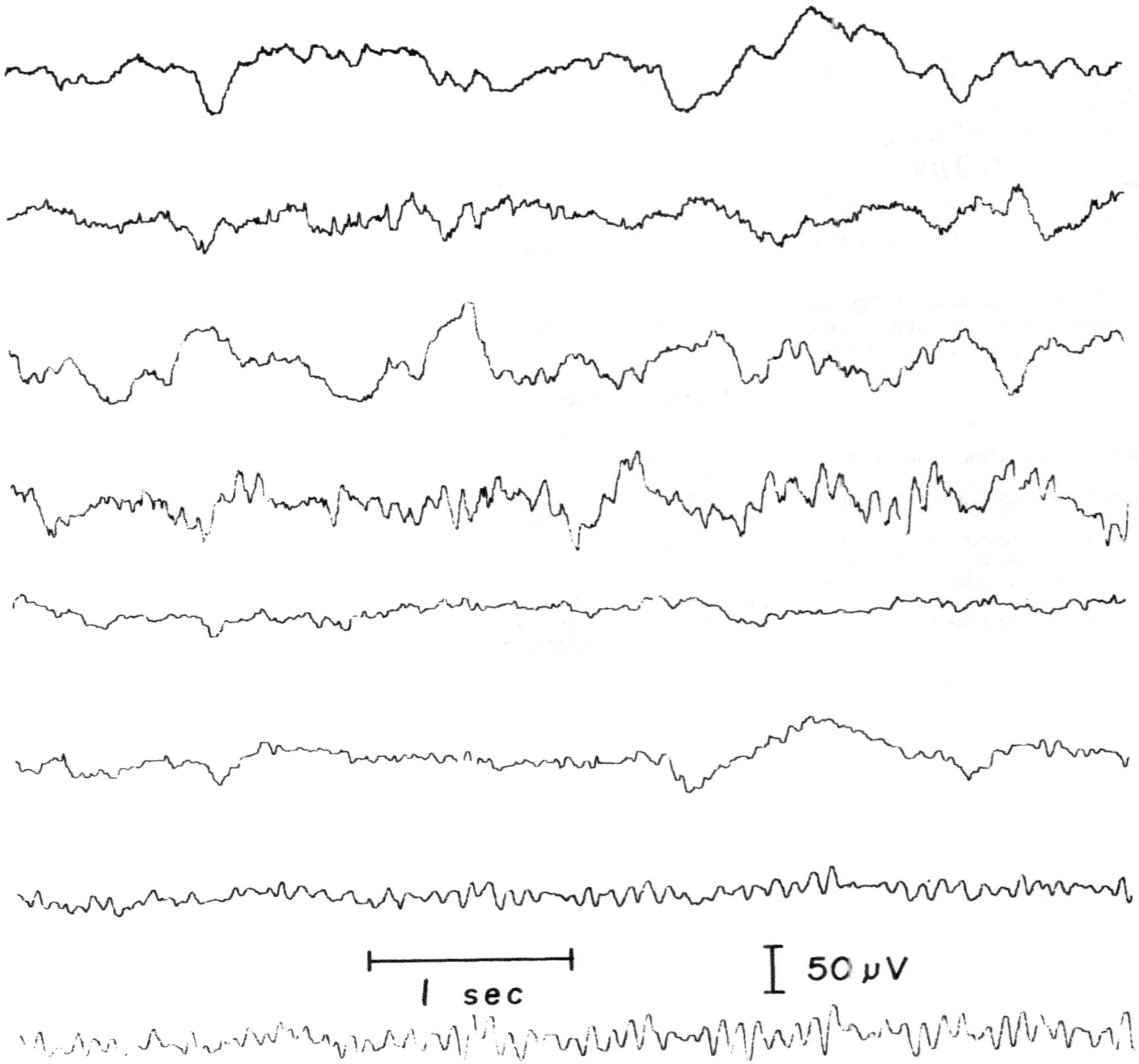

1 sec
50 μV

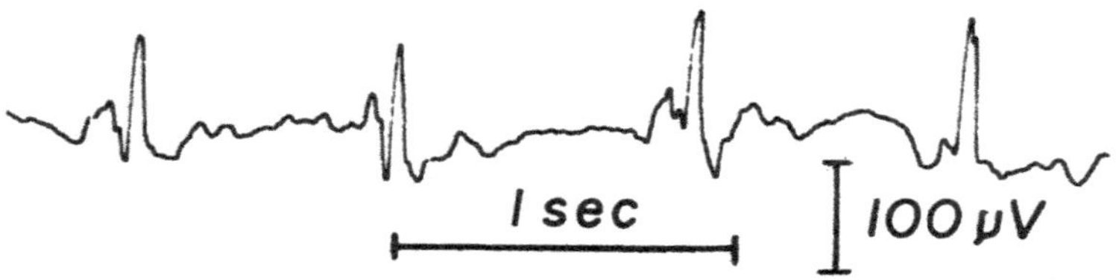

FIG. 1.6. Abnormal EEG with spike and sharp activity. (See text for discussion.)

therapy of patients who are suspected of having a wide range of neurological problems: seizures; brain tumors; cerebrovascular, metabolic, or toxic disorders; infectious or degenerative diseases of the brain.

REFERENCES

1. Berger, H. (1929): Über das Elektrenkephalogramm des Menschen. *Arch. Psychiatr. Nervenkr.*, 87:527–570.
2. Berger, H. (1930): Über das Elektrenkephalogramm des Menschen. Zweite Mitteilung. *J. Psychol. Neurol.*, 40:160–179.
3. Gloor, P. (1969): Hans Berger and the discovery of the electroencephalogram. Introduction to Hans Berger on the electroencephalogram of man. The fourteen original reports, translated and edited by P. Gloor. *Electroencephalogr. Clin. Neurophysiol.*, Suppl. 28:1–36.
4. Walter, W. G., and Dovey, V. J. (1944): Electroencephalography in cases of subcortical tumor. *J. Neurol. Neurosurg. Psychiatry*, 7:57–65.

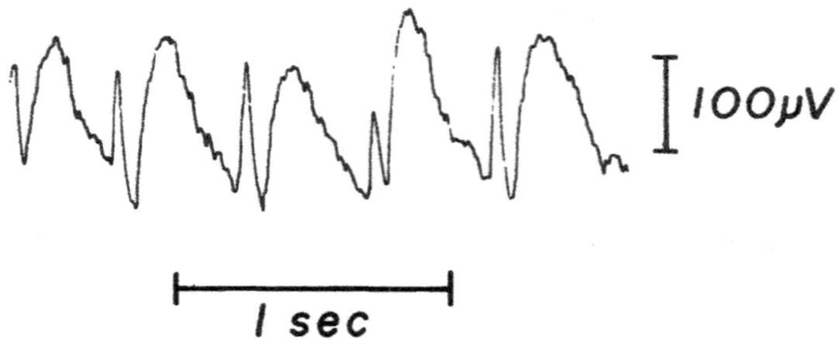

FIG. 1.7. Spike-and-wave discharge. (See text for discussion.)

Additional Sources

Adrian, E. D. (1971): The discovery of Berger. In: *Handbook of Electroencephalography and Clinical Neurophysiology, Vol. 1,* edited by W. A. Cobb, pp. 5–10. Elsevier, Amsterdam.

Brazier, M. A. B. (1961): *A History of the Electrical Activity of the Brain—The First Half-Century,* Macmillan, New York.

Cobb, W. (1971): The past forty years of EEG. In: *Handbook of Electroencephalography and Clinical Neurophysiology, Vol. 1,* edited by W. A. Cobb, pp. 25–50. Elsevier, Amsterdam.

Oldendorf, W. H. (1980): *The Quest for an Image of Brain.* Raven Press, New York, (see esp. pp vii–viii, 113–114).

O'Leary, J. L., and Goldring, S. (1976): *Science and Epilepsy,* Raven Press, New York.

Chapter 2

The EEG Instrument

Equipment for recording the EEG is produced by a number of manufacturers. Each electroencephalograph may have its own distinctive appearance, but underneath their "skins" the various instruments are remarkably similar. The accompanying diagrams dissect electroencephalographs as a class so that their common features can be discussed. With this chapter at hand, the reader can follow the functions of any instrument from the input (the point at which the voltage at the scalp enters the equipment) to the output (the permanent, visible EEG record).[1]

The chain of events involved in recording begins with the *electrodes* (Fig. 2.1), although they are not a structural part of the equipment. A specific and detailed discussion of this critical part of the input system is given in Chapter 10.

The first part of the actual instrument is called the *electrode board,* sometimes referred to as the jackbox (Fig. 2.2). The electrodes are plugged into small receptacles in the electrode board. These receptacles are called *jacks*. The wire from the electrode has a terminal *pin*. The jacks into which the pins are inserted have either numerical or anatomical identifications. Numbered jacks are usually used in research, and anatomical descriptors (see Chapter 11) should be, and usually are, used for clinical recording.

The electrode board is connected to the instrument by a long, shielded, multiple-conductor *input cable* (Fig. 2.3). Through this cable, each electrode is connected to a specific point on a multiple contact switch known as the *electrode selector* (Fig. 2.4). This selector is composed of rows of pushbutton, slide, rotary, or other switching devices that connect the electrodes to the amplifiers. These *switches* are arranged in pairs corresponding to the two inputs of each amplifier. The top switch of the pair is designated *Input Terminal 1*. The lower switch of the pair is designated *Input Terminal 2*. For purposes of simplicity, we have shortened this to "Input 1" and "Input 2". (In the United States, Input 1 often is designated G1, and Input 2, as G2.) By using the electrode selector, the technologist can select manually any pair of electrodes and connect them to the input terminals of any amplifier. In order to accommodate all of the electrode positions recommended by the International EEG Federation (1), at least 23 selector points are necessary. Provision for more is desirable, and most modern instruments include several additional electrode locations.

The selection of a pair of electrodes for Inputs 1 and 2 is called a *derivation* (2). The order in which the derivations are selected will determine the electroanatomical picture of the brain that will be displayed by the EEG instrument. Such an arrangement of derivations is called a *montage* (2). The design of montages is discussed in detail in Chapter 13.

To simplify the task of the EEG technologist, who must periodically during the recording arrange as many as 16—frequently 32 or more—amplifier inputs whenever a montage is changed, a *master electrode selector* switch (Fig. 2.5) may be used. This switch enables the tech-

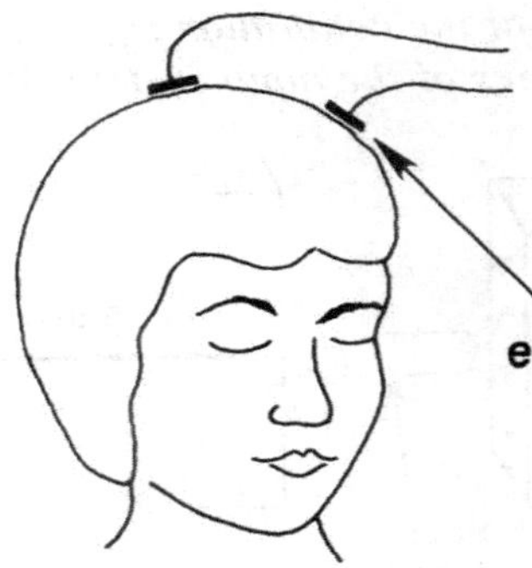

FIG. 2.1. EEG electrodes.

[1] The present analysis of Any EEG Instrument originally was developed by JRK between 1965 and 1972 in collaboration with Lila Snodgrass Banks, R. EEG T., and Peter J. Seaba, M.S. It has been widely used in teaching (cf., Knott, J. R., EEG Instrumentation—An Introduction, Department of Continuing Education, Boston University School of Medicine, May 12–13, 1979). The present version is an evolutionary offshoot of earlier models.

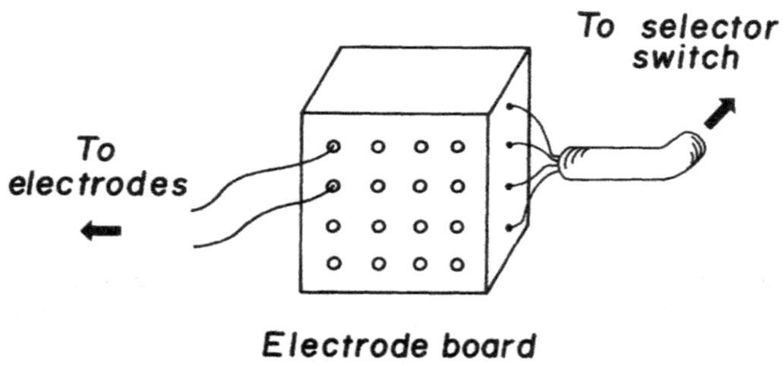

FIG. 2.2. Electrode board.

nologist to change an entire montage with only one adjustment. Master electrode selectors are available for all instruments, usually as an option (although they are regarded by many electroencephalographers and technologists as a basic necessity).

Another critical part of the input system is the *calibrator* (Fig. 2.6). This device is switched selectively in or out of the input circuit so that a precise, preselected voltage within the range of EEG activity (recommended range to include 2 μV and 1 mV) (1) can be applied simultaneously to the inputs of all amplifiers and the output of each amplifier will be displayed by the corresponding ink-writing mechanism. By examining the simultaneous display of the calibration pulses on all channels, the technologist and interpreter of the EEG can be certain that all channels are performing identically and that all instrument control settings are properly adjusted.

It should be emphasized that the calibration signal should go through all electronically active sections of the input system. If there are electrically active circuits in the electrode board, they also should be calibrated (1).

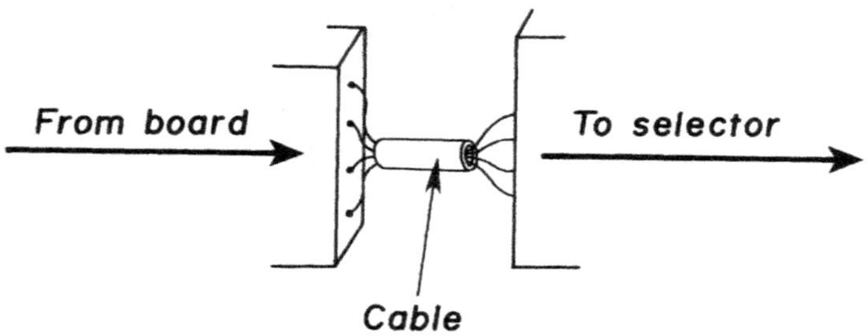

FIG. 2.3. Input cable.

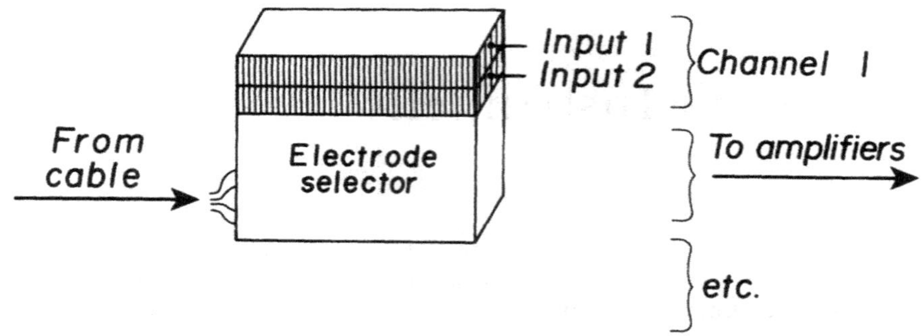

FIG. 2.4. Electrode selector.

Modern EEG instruments provide for on-line checks of the resistance of electrodes selected for input to any given channel (1). This *electrode test* measures the total resistance of the two electrodes under test. (Fig. 2.7). (Some instruments indicate the difference in resistance between pairs of electrodes; this is not a comparable procedure.)

The *amplifier* (Fig. 2.8) is a carefully designed electronic magnifying glass. It enables the technologist to process the extremely small signals from the brain (at the microvolt level) so that the voltage changes can be given sufficient power for graphic recording directly on moving paper. The maximum available amplification is approximately one million times.

All EEG amplifiers should have the following controls available on each channel (1):

1. sensitivity (multiplier; step; equalizer) (Fig. 2.8A)
2. low frequency filter (Fig. 2.8B)

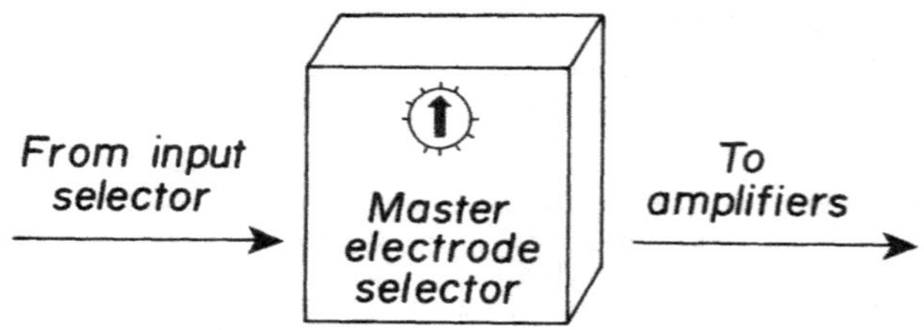

FIG. 2.5. Master electrode selector switch.

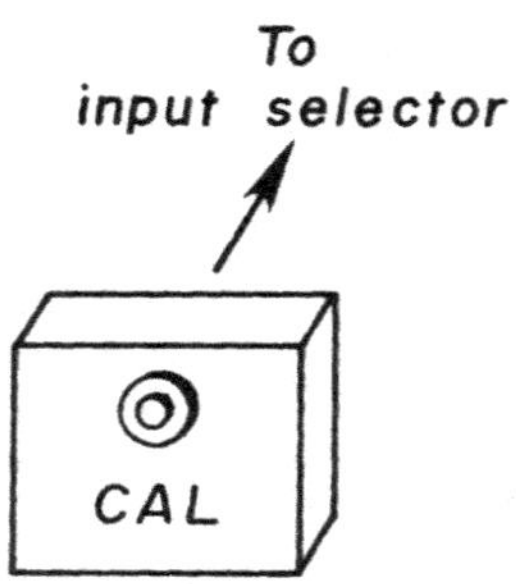

FIG. 2.6. Calibrator.

3. high frequency filter (Fig. 2.8C)
4. 60-Hz rejection filter (Fig. 2.8E)
5. electrical baseline adjustment (Fig. 2.8D)

In addition, there should be an OFF-STANDBY-ON switch (Fig. 2.8F).

Sensitivity is defined as microvolts (μV) of input required to produce 1 millimeter (mm) of pen deflection at the output. If 1 μV of input produces 1 mm at the output, the sensitivity is 1 μV/mm. If 10 μV produces 1 mm of deflection, the sensitivity is 10 μV/mm. A sensitivity of 1 μV/mm is 10 times the sensitivity of 10 μV/mm, since one-tenth of the input voltage produces the same output (1 mm).

An EEG amplifier has three controls that regulate sensitivity. The *main sensitivity control* has step settings (Fig. 2.8Aa) that may range from 1 μV/mm to 70 mV/cm (or, on some instruments, 150 mV/cm). These settings are in fixed steps. An adjunct control, the *sensitivity equalizer* (Fig.

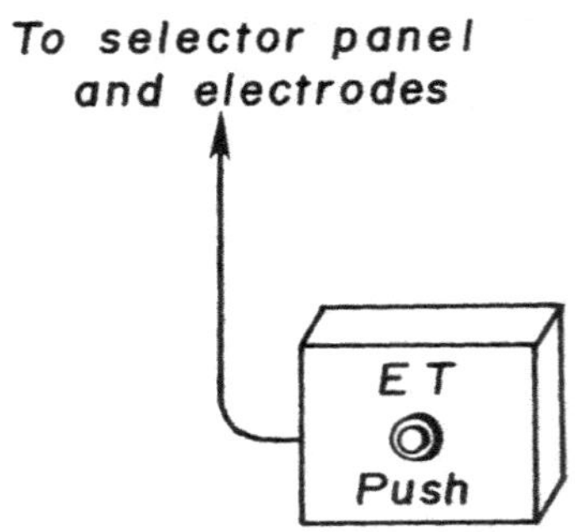

FIG. 2.7. Electrode test.

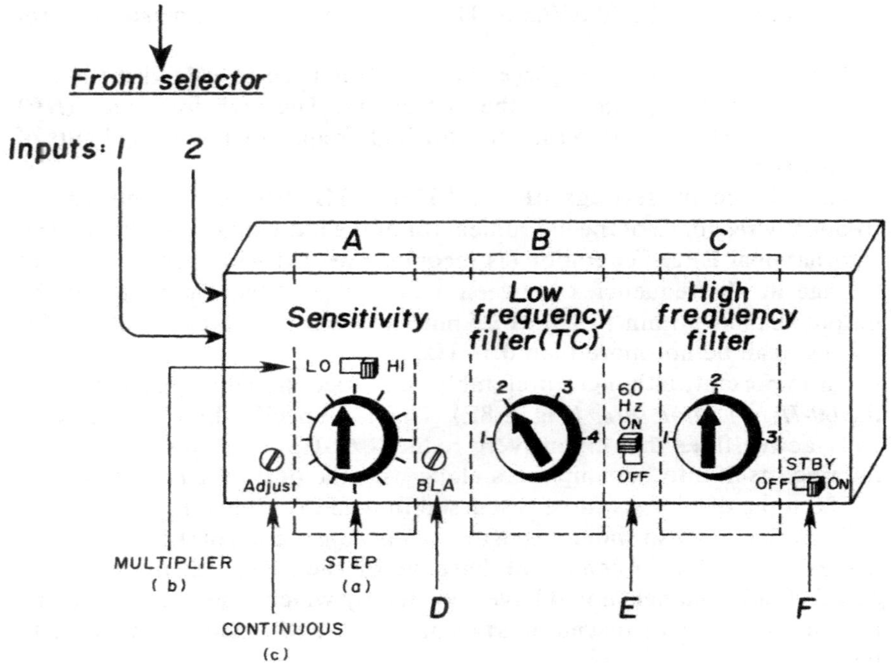

FIG. 2.8. Amplifier, with sensitivity control (A), low frequency filter (B), high frequency filter (C), electrical baseline adjustment (D), 60-Hz rejection filter (E), and OFF-STANDBY-ON switch (F).

2.8Ac, "adjust"), is a continuous control that enables the technologist to set precisely the sensitivity in each channel. The maximum sensitivity of an EEG amplifier should be not less than 1 μV/mm (1). The third sensitivity control, called a *multiplier* (Fig. 2.8Ab), enables the technologist to change the overall sensitivity of any individual channel by a constant factor. For example, if the multiplier shifts the scale from microvolts per millimeter to millivolts per centimeter, the sensitivity will be reduced by a factor of 100. There are 1,000 microvolts in a millivolt, and there are 10 millimeters in a centimeter; the ratio is $1{,}000 \div 10 = 100$.

Some instruments use multipliers for individual channels only, with a multiplication range from 20 to 0.25. In this case, the sensitivity (μV/mm or mV/cm) cannot be read directly from the master dial when the multiplier is any number other than 1. If the master sensitivity is set on 10 μV/mm and the channel multiplier is set on 4, for example, the sensitivity of the channel will be 40 μV/mm. This setting is not on the master control dial.

The *low frequency* (*LF*) *filter* (Fig. 2.8B) is used to establish the low frequency recording limits of the instrument. The *high frequency* (*HF*) *filter* (Fig. 2.8C) is used to establish the high frequency recording limits of the instrument.

The choice of settings of the LF and HF filters determines the frequency response of the instrument (or of the individual amplifiers). The International EEG Federation (1) recommends that with a constant input voltage at all frequencies between 1 and 60 Hz, the amplitude at the output shall be within 10% (or 0.25 mm) and that the lowest available LF setting shall be not more than 0.16 Hz.

An important, although (preferably) only occasionally used control is the *60-Hz rejection filter* (Fig. 2.8E). This is a specifically tuned, electrically active filter that extensively reduces 60-Hz interference that may interject itself into the amplifiers along with the desired EEG activity.

The topic of filters will be discussed in detail in Chapter 8.

Each channel also should have a *baseline adjust* control (Fig. 2.8D) that makes it possible to center the baseline of each channel at "electrical zero." Each channel should have a switch by which it separately may be turned ON or OFF or placed on STANDBY (Fig. 2.8F) when no data are to be displayed.

All clinical EEG instruments have *master channel controls* (Fig. 2.9) that enable the technologist to change any of the principal control functions simultaneously in all channels. These include sensitivity (Fig. 2.9A), low frequency (Fig. 2.9B), high frequency (Fig. 2.9C), and 60-Hz (Fig. 2.8E).

There is yet another control on the EEG instrument, known as the *chart drive* (Fig. 2.10), that enables the technologist to adjust the speed of the recording paper beneath the pens. The standard chart speed for clinical EEGs is 30 mm/sec, but this may be increased (usually to 60 mm/sec) or decreased (usually to 15 mm/sec). Some instruments now provide six chart speeds. Other chart speeds are usually available for special use. There also is an ON/OFF switch for the chart drive, and incorporated in this switch is a master ON/OFF switch for the ink-writing galvanometers.

The *ink-writing galvanometers* (Fig. 2.11) provide an instant write-out of the EEG record. These galvanometers function as recording voltmeters. A moving coil, placed inside a strong magnetic field, has an ink-writing pen mounted on the coil, just as a pointer is mounted on a meter.

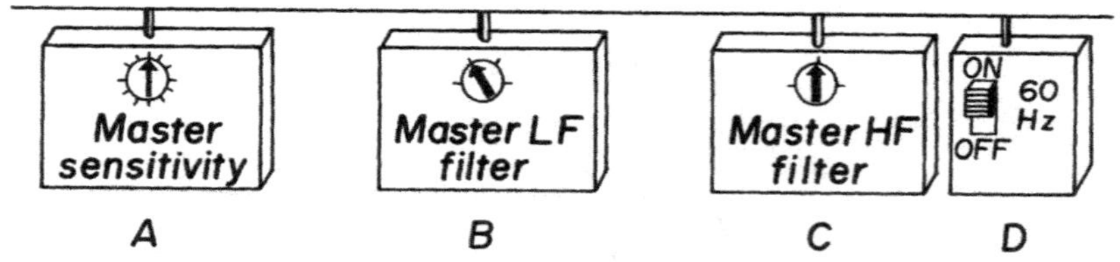

FIG. 2.9. Master channel controls for sensitivity (A), low frequency (B), high frequency (C), and 60 Hz (D).

The magnitude of the deflection of the pen should be directly proportional to the input voltage. Because the signal is made up of voltages of different polarities (negative and positive), the pens of the galvanometers are adjusted so that zero (no voltage) is at the center point or *baseline*. Any applied voltage will move the pen from zero (see Chapter 5 for more details). The direction of the movement of the pens and its relation to negative and positive electrical processes in the brain are discussed in Chapter 12.

The *power supply* (Fig. 2.12) is a critical part of the entire EEG instrument; it transforms *alternating current* drawn from the domestic power mains (nominally 120 V) to lower voltage *direct current* (usually in the 1–24 V range). These voltages must be maintained at their stated value at all times. The power supply is designed so that *leakage currents* (see Chapters 5 and 6) are held to specified minimal levels to insure patient and operator safety. There should be an easily accessible ON/OFF switch, and

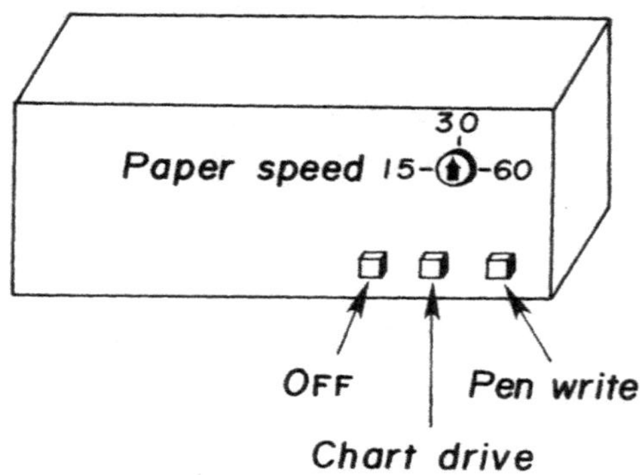

FIG. 2.10. Chart drive.

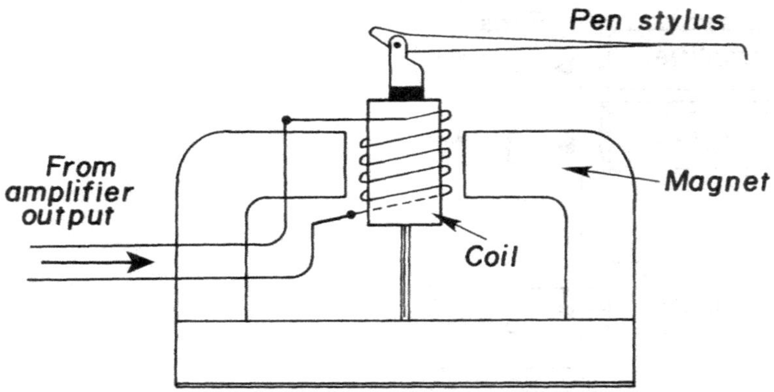

FIG. 2.11. Ink-writing galvanometers.

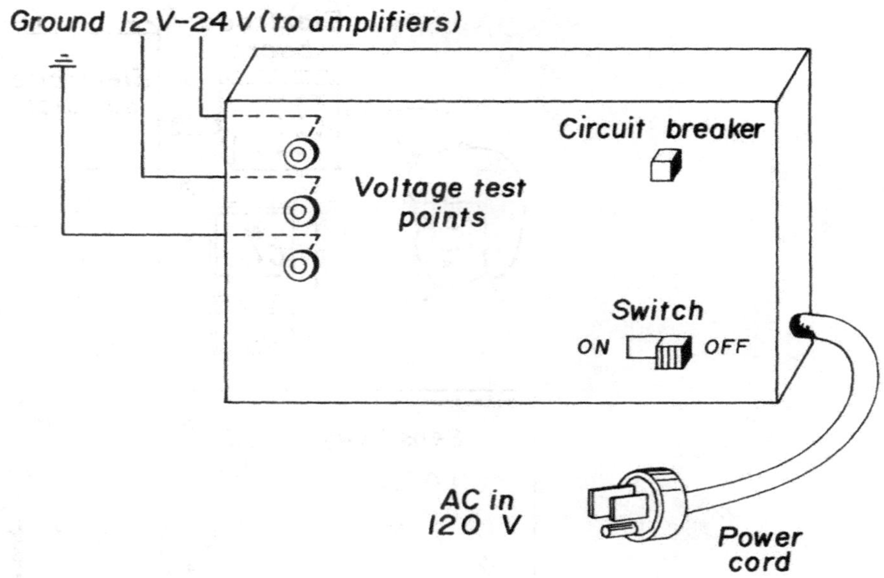

FIG. 2.12. Power supply.

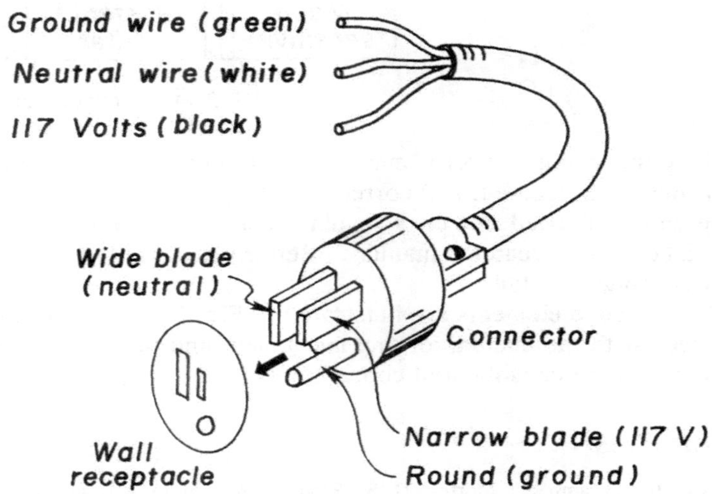

FIG. 2.13. Power cord.

the power supply should be properly fused or protected with a circuit breaker so that, in case of component failure, the instrument will not be damaged nor a hazard created for the patient or technologist.

There also should be easily accessible and clearly labeled *voltage test points* on the instrument so that the EEG technologist can locate sources of instrument faults should they develop (1).

An integral, although often overlooked, part of the instrument is the *power cord* and its male connector (Fig. 2.13). This is a three-conductor cord with color-coded wires. It must be constructed to specifications that will limit leakage current. The three-prong connector plug must be hospital grade (see Chapter 6). This plug is inserted into a three-prong hospital grade wall receptacle that must be properly wired to provide specified voltage to the instrument.

The EEG instrument is grounded through the third (green) wire of the power cord. It is essential that the ground wire has no interruption in it between the instrument and the ground connection in the wall receptacle, and that the green wire in the wall receptacle be correctly connected to the building ground. The safety of the patient and the technologist depends on this.

The instrument manual provided by the manufacturer should be considered a part of the instrument. A well-motivated technologist will read the manual with the instrument at hand. In this way it will be possible to follow all operational directions and to understand the functions of the instrument controls. By studying "trouble shooting" procedures as de-

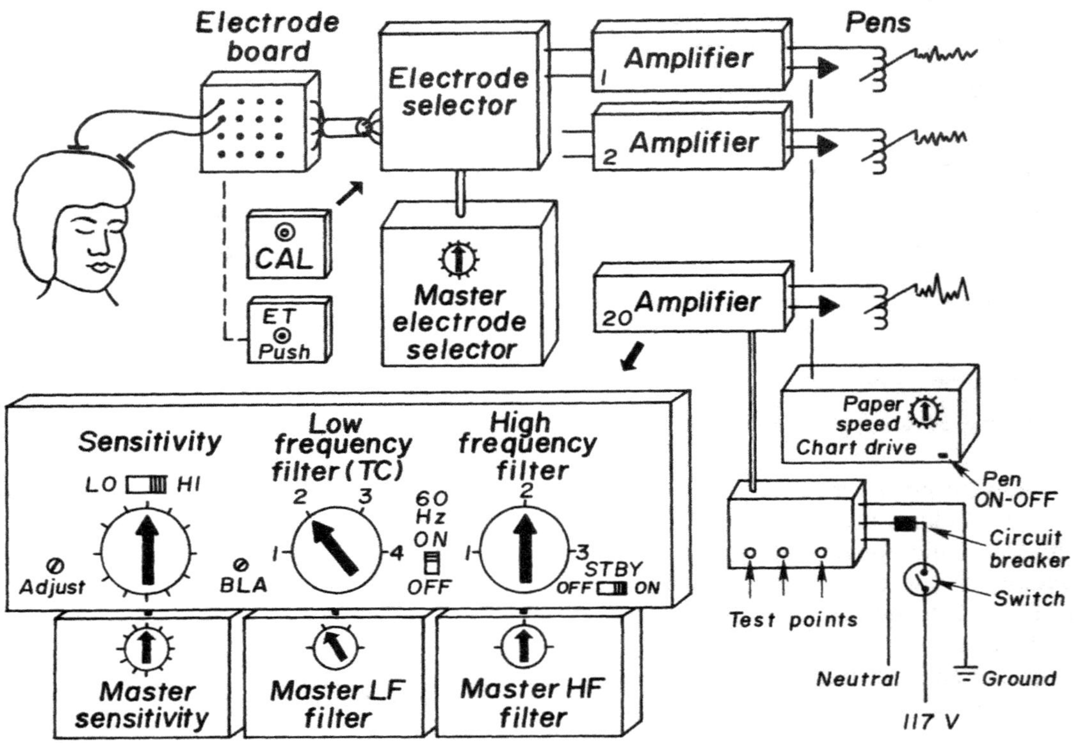

FIG. 2.14. Common components of a typical electroencephalograph.

scribed in the manufacturer's manual, instrument faults can be more quickly identified, located, and corrected if they occur. Preventive maintenance can be carried out on a regular basis. There is an old saying: "When all else fails, read the manual." Better yet: Read the manual first, and fewer things will fail.

All of the above elements are illustrated in Fig. 2.14. The diagram can be followed with the manual for any instrument and the total function of the system can be consolidated conceptually.

REFERENCES

1. Barlow, J. S., Kamp, A., Morton, H. B., Ripoche, A., Shipton, H., and Tchavdarov, D. B. (1978): EEG instrumentation standards (revised 1977): Report of the Committee on EEG Instrumentation Standards of the International Federation of Societies for Electroencephalography and Clinical Neurophysiology. *Electroencephalogr. Clin. Neurophysiol.*, 45:144–147.
2. Chatrian, G. E., Bergamini, L., Dondey, M., Klass, D. W., Lennox-Buchthal, M., and Petersén, I. (1974): A glossary of terms most commonly used by clinical electroencephalographers. *Electroencephalogr. Clin. Neurophysiol.*, 37:538–548.

Additional Sources

Beckman Instruments, Inc. (1974): *Accutrace Electroencephalograph Instrument Manual.* Schiller Park, Illinois.

Cooper, R., Osselton, J. W., and Shaw, J. C. (1980): *EEG Technology,* 3rd ed. Butterworths, London.

Grass Instrument Company (1973): *Grass Model 8 Instruction Manual. Part II: Theory and Application.* Grass Instrument Co., Quincy, Massachusetts.

Chapter 3

The EEG Technologist

Electroencephalographic technologists usually are classified on the basis of their training and work experience. At the first level, that of technologist-trainee, the student is involved in clinical practice under close supervision. As learning increases, supervision decreases. At the completion of training, the individual should be qualified to carry out EEG examinations under the supervision of experienced technologists. After a year of experience and having successfully taken the examinations of the American Board of Electroencephalographic Technologists, Inc., the new technologist qualifies for higher levels of classification. Responsibilities now go beyond relatively routine recording, and may include supervision of students and junior staff. Five years of experience and Board registry qualifies the technologist as a "Technologist III," the classification from which chief technologists are drawn. The chief technologist is the laboratory supervisor and administrator and often has full responsibility for managing the technical aspects of the EEG service (1–3).

Regardless of the level at which an EEG technologist is employed, he or she is the critical link in the chain between the referring physician and the EEG interpretation. An EEG recorded without satisfactory attention to clinical and technical detail may prove to be of little value, while a record obtained under optimal conditions, in which EEG technique is adapted to the clinical problems, can contribute significantly to the diagnosis and treatment of the patient.

The EEG technologist deals with a succession of patients who are literally more or less sick. Some are in terminal agony. Some are not very ill in a physical sense. Some are apparently healthy. All, however, have complaints and have sought the assistance of, or have been brought to, a physician for diagnosis and treatment.

Usually the physician is, or seeks the advice of, a qualified neurologist, who specializes in diseases of the nervous system. Ideally, the neurologist will examine the patient and determine whether an EEG is a necessary part of the series of diagnostic tests to be used in evaluating the patient's difficulties. A referral for an EEG is then prepared; this is a statement that usually outlines the patient's symptoms and may indicate the physician's diagnostic hypothesis. An appointment for the EEG examination is made. The patient appears at the laboratory. At this point, the EEG technologist takes over.

On the basis of the information supplied by the referring physician, a broad outline of the examination plan is formed. If the background information is not sufficiently explicit, the technologist may need to inquire discreetly of the patient about the complaints that led him to the neurologist. This information is needed because the characteristics of electrical activity of the brain may differ in various neurological diseases, and different recording strategies are needed for different problems.

The technologist should explain to the patient the procedures to be carried out so that good rapport will be established and the patient will be put at ease. The application of the electrodes should be done with such thoroughly practiced skill that the record will be of high technical quality. After the instrument is calibrated, the examination begins.

The technologist is in complete charge of the examination. On the basis of the facts given in the referral and the medical history gleaned from the patient, the choices of electrode combinations and the examination strategy will be formulated by the technologist. This requires sufficient knowledge of neurological disorders for an understanding of the patient's medical history. It requires knowledge of the best way to display the EEG information, which depends on the choice and order of using montages (see Chapter 13) and the choice and use of the instrument controls (see Chapter 8).

The technologist must thoroughly understand the information being poured out continuously by the EEG instrument. This information must be correlated with the patient's medical history and with all behavioral changes of the patient during the examination. Thus, a continuously updated descriptive report of the EEG must be formulated by the technologist throughout the examination. Further changes in the strategy then can be made.

At the conclusion of the examination, the electrodes are removed and the patient is assured that a report of the examination will be sent promptly to the referring physician. Technologists must never tell the patient that a record is normal or abnormal. It is easy to explain to the patient that two kinds of expertise are involved in the process of EEG: technical and medical. Recording the EEG is the responsibility of the technologist. The interpretation of the EEG is the responsibility of an electroencephalographer, who has medical expertise and can provide correlations between the EEG and the patient's illness.

However, the responsibilities of the technologist do not end at this point. A terminal set of calibrations must be recorded. A description of any unusual behavior of the patient during the recording must be attached to the record. A descriptive report of the EEG findings also may be attached. Certain bookkeeping and clerical functions may be required of the technologist. A complete identification of the record must be prepared. The electrodes must be cleaned and the laboratory made ready for examining the next patient.

Under the best conditions, the electroencephalographer will frequently consult the recording technologist about many of the records. Whether consulted or not, the technologist should read the reports on all patients recorded under his or her direction. If there is any significant difference between the technologist's descriptive report and the interpreter's report, there should be a consultation to resolve areas of unclarity or disagreement. *It is important to remember that the technologist was there and saw and heard what occurred throughout the recording*. On the other hand, the interpreter is often in possession of other facts. Interchange between technologist and interpreter can produce a more comprehensive report as well as provide a continuing educational process for both. When the final report goes back to the referring physician, the technologist can have the satisfaction of knowing that the attentive application of his or her knowledge and skills has contributed to the resolution of a diagnostic problem.

REFERENCES

1. American EEG Society (1980): 1. Standards of practice in clinical electroencephalography. In: *Guidelines in EEG—1980*. American EEG Society, Tucker, Georgia.
2. American EEG Society (1980): 2. Recommended job descriptions for electroencephalographic technologists. In: *Guidelines in EEG—1980*. American EEG Society, Tucker, Georgia.
3. American EEG Society (1980): 3. Minimum technical requirements for performing clinical electroencephalography. In: *Guidelines in EEG—1980*. American EEG Society, Tucker, Georgia.

Additional Sources

Hector, M. L. (1980): *EEG Recording*, 2nd ed. Butterworths, London.[1]

MacGillivray, B. B., Binnie, C. D., and Osselton, J. W. (1974): Section III. Recording the EEG. In: *Handbook of Electroencephalography and Clinical Neurophysiology, Vol. 3, Part C: Traditional Methods of Examination in Clinical EEG*, edited by B. B. MacGillivray, pp. 3C-58–3C-87. Elsevier, Amsterdam.

[1] This is an account of the practice of EEG technology in Europe, particularly in France, and offers an interesting contrast to the current American outlook.

Chapter 4

Dealing with Numbers

In the daily practice of EEG technology, it is necessary to deal with numbers. For example, the technologist must be familiar with numbers in order to 1) calibrate the EEG instrument accurately, 2) determine the frequencies present in the EEG, 3) measure the voltages of the activity, and 4) understand the amounts of medication a patient receives. The numbers involve measurements and computations based on units of distance, weight, and time. Distance and weight are expressed in metric units and are based on the decimal system. Time is not based on a decimal system; we have a 24 hr day, with 60 min to the hour and 60 sec to the minute. However, subdivisions of seconds are in decimal terms.

THE METRIC SYSTEM

The metric system is easy to handle because it operates on a base of 10—exactly as do most monetary systems. There are 100 pennies in a U.S. dollar. In Great Britain, there are 100 pence in a pound. A system based on the number 10 is a decimal system. For example, 10 is ten times larger than 1. The number 100 is ten times larger than the number 10. In the other direction (making numbers smaller, or dividing), the value 0.1 is one-tenth as large as 1.0. The number 0.01 is one-hundredth as large as 1.0. It is one-tenth as large as 0.1.

The metric unit of *distance* commonly used in EEG is the *centimeter* (*cm*). The unit of *weight* is the *gram* (*g*). The unit of *time* in EEG is the *second* (*sec*). These three units form the *centimeter—gram—second* (*CGS*) system of measurement. The metric system is used by most countries of the world. It is slowly being adopted in the United States, Canada, and the United Kingdom.

These units have standard multiples and fractions. Conversions into larger (multiple) and smaller (fractional) units are merely a matter of moving the decimal point the required number of places in the proper direction. When we move decimals, we are either multiplying or dividing by a factor of 10.

Distance

Multiples of distance, beginning with 1 cm, are:

100 cm = 1 meter (m) (39.4 inches)
1,000 m = 1 kilometer (km) (0.62 miles)

Metric fractions of distance (more often used in EEG and the biological sciences) are:

1 millimeter (mm) = 0.1 cm (one-tenth of a cm, or one-thousandth of a m)
1 micrometer or micron (μm) = 0.001 mm (one-thousandth of a mm, or one millionth of a m)

EEG technologists deal with millimeters and centimeters on a daily basis when measuring the frequencies and voltages displayed in EEG records (see Chapter 7). They deal with measurements of the patient's head in centimeters and millimeters to determine the placements of electrodes (see Chapter 11). Also, medical charts usually give the height and weight of patients in metric terms. A 6-foot 7-inch basketball player would be described as being 200.7 cm tall (79 inches multiplied by 2.54).

Weight

The most frequently used multiple of weight is the kilogram (kg).

1,000 g = 1 kg (2.205 lb)

If the basketball player weighed 224 pounds, his weight would be given in the medical chart as 101.6 kg. (224 divided by 2.205).

Fractional units of weight in the metric system are:

1,000 milligrams (mg) = 1 g
1 mg = 0.001 g
0.1 mg = 0.0001 g
1 microgram (μg) = 0.000001 g

Time

Time is given in terms of minutes, hours, and seconds. Divisions of time of less than 1 sec are expressed in the decimal system as milliseconds and microseconds. Thus:

1,000 milliseconds (msec) = 1 sec
1,000 microseconds (μsec) = 1 msec.

Volume

It also is necessary to have units of volume, used in fluid measurement. Units of volume are derived from units of distance.

The basic unit of volume is the *cubic centimeter* (*cc*). Figure 4.1 shows a cube, 1 cm in length on each of its sides. The volume within the cube is a cubic centimeter.

Conversion to the most used multiple of 1 cc introduces a new measure, the *liter*.

1 liter = 1,000 cc

In liquid measurement, 1 cc is referred to as 1 *milliliter* (*ml*). The units of cc and ml are equivalent in the measurement of liquids. In hospital practice, liquid drugs are prescribed in milliliter doses, but measurement may be made in cubic centimeters or fractions of cubic centimeters.

From units of volume, we also define the units of weight. One gram is the weight of 1 cc of water at a temperature of 4° C.[1] Most medications are prescribed in milligram or milliliter doses. Sometimes these may be prescribed in tenths of a milliliter (i.e., 0.1 ml).

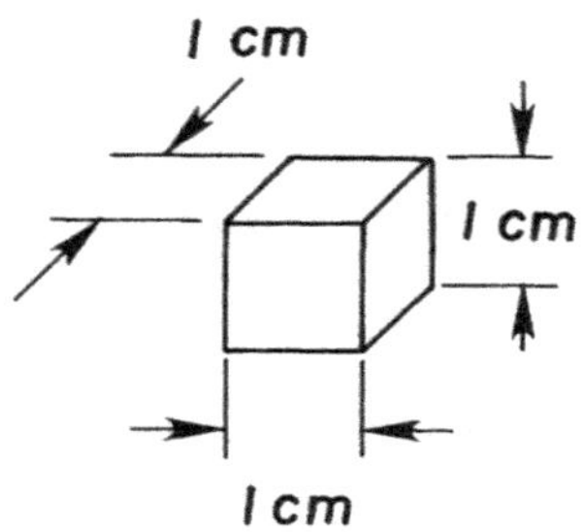

FIG. 4.1. One cubic centimeter (schema).

[1] Temperature can be converted from Fahrenheit to Celsius as follows: C° = 5/9 (F° − 32). Celsius can be converted to Fahrenheit: F° = 9/5 C° + 32.

The dose given often is dependent upon the patient's body weight and is administered as a certain number of *milligrams per kilogram* of body weight. A 125-pound woman has a metric weight of 56.7 kg. If this woman is given a drug at a prescribed dose of 20 mg/kg, she would receive 1,134 mg. Conservatively, this might be rounded off to 1 g (1,000 mg) per dose.

Metric System Prefixes and Symbols

The metric system prefixes and symbols for multiples and fractions in the decimal system used in EEG are summarized below:

Multiples

mega (M)	= 1 million (1,000,000)
kilo (k)	= 1 thousand (1,000)

Fractions

deci (d)	= 1 tenth (0.1)
centi (c)	= 1 hundredth (0.01)
milli (m)	= 1 thousandth (0.001)
micro (μ)	= 1 millionth (0.000001)
nano (n)	= 1 billionth (0.000000001)
pico (p)	= 1 trillionth (0.000000000001)

The prefixes *mega* and *pico* will be encountered in Chapter 5; *nano* appears in scientific literature related to EEG (e.g., nanosec).

Fractions are numerical expressions, such as 2/3 or 3/4. The number above the line is the *dividend*. The number below the line is the *divisor*. The dividend is divided by the divisor, yielding the *quotient*. The quotient of 2/3 is 0.667 and of 3/4 is 0.750.

FORMULAS

When using numbers, we frequently use formulas. A formula is a mathematical equation that expresses a general fact or principle. For example, the formula D = R × T gives distance traveled (D) in terms of constant rate of speed (R) and time (T). Shorthand symbols are used so that formulas do not need to be spelled out in words. These should be recalled from primary and secondary arithmetic:

The symbol "×" means multiply, as $2 \times 4 = 8$.
The symbol "·" also means multiply, as $2 \cdot 4 = 8$.

Another way to indicate that two quantities are to be multiplied is to put each in parentheses next to each other, as:

$$(2)(4) = 8.$$

If there is a number in front of the first parenthesis, such as $9(10 \times 2)$, the quantity 20 is multiplied by 9, and the total equals 180. If, however, a "+" sign separates the 9 and the (10×2), i.e., $9 + (10 \times 2)$, then the 9 is added to the quantity 20 and the total is 29. Another example:

$$x = 9 + (2 \times 2) + (4 \times 4)$$
$$x = 9 + (4) + (16)$$
$$x = 29.$$

However, if:

$$x = 9 + (2 \times 2)(4 \times 4)$$

then,

$$x = 9 + (4)(16)$$
$$x = 9 + 64$$
$$x = 73.$$

Another example:

$$x = 9 + (2 \times 2)(4 - 2)$$
$$x = 9 + (4)(2)$$
$$x = 9 + 8 = 17.$$

The shorthand symbol for "divide by" is ÷. The first number is divided by the second number, as in

$$9 \div 3 = 3$$

This can also be written as

$$\frac{9}{3} = 3$$

or, as

$$9/3 = 3.$$

(Notice that the symbol "/" sometimes can mean something else, as in "30 mm/sec" and μV/mm." Here, it means "per", i.e., 30 mm per sec or 10 μV per mm.)

Returning to the matter of formulas, suppose it is necessary to solve the equation:

$$x = \frac{1}{1/2 + 1/3 + 1/4}$$

The fractions first are converted to their decimal equivalents:

$$x = \frac{1}{0.500 + 0.333 + 0.250.}$$

The numbers in the denominator then are added:

$$x = \frac{1}{1.083}$$

The final division is carried out:

$$x = 0.923.$$

The answer is usually "rounded off" to the nearest two-place number. In this case, since the third decimal is less than 5, the answer is 0.92. If the third decimal had been 5 or higher, the "rounded" value would have been 0.93.

One further example of multiplication and division and the use of fractions:

$$x = \frac{3(9 \times 2)}{3 + (9 + 2) + (3 \times 3)(4 + 6)}$$
$$x = \frac{3 \times 18}{3 + 11 + (9)(10)}$$
$$x = \frac{54}{104}$$
$$x = 0.519$$
$$x = 0.52$$

(In this instance, the answer was rounded off to give a two-place figure.)

Problems requiring these simple manipulations of numbers will be encountered later in this text, especially in Chapters 5 and 8. All practical problems involving time, frequency, and voltage use the same procedures.

DECIMALS

There are orderly relationships between all numbers in the decimal system. All multiples of units of 10 have zeros added to the decimal place moved to the right for each step. There are six steps from 1 to 1,000,000. From one to one million, the decimal moves six places, as shown in Table 4.1.

As units are divided, decreasing from 1.0 to 0.000001, each step moves the decimal one or more places to the left. From one to one-millionth, the decimal moves six places (Table 4.2). Note from Table 4.2 that 1,000 millionths (0.001000) equals one one-thousandth (0.001). Note also from Table 4.1 that 1,000 one thousands (1,000 × 1,000) equals one million (1,000,000).

The usual system of manual multiplication can be awkward and inconvenient when the numbers are very large or very small. Suppose it is necessary to multiply one one-millionth by one thousand. In the usual form the process would be:

```
   0.000001
    × 1000
 ----------
    000000
   000000
  000000
 000001
 ----------
 000.001000
```

TABLE 4.1 *Decimal multiples*

One	1.0 (the unit)
Ten	10.0 (one place to the right)
One hundred	100.0 (two places to the right)
One thousand	1000.0 (three places to the right)
Ten thousand	10,000.0 (four places to the right)
One hundred thousand	100,000.0 (five places to the right)
One million	1,000,000.0 (six places to the right)

TABLE 4.2. *Decimal fractions*

One	1.0 (the unit)
One-tenth	0.1 (one place to the left)
One one-hundredth	0.01 (two places to the left)
One one-thousandth	0.001 (three places to the left)
One one-millionth	0.000001 (six places to the left)

Division also can be awkward, as in the following example:

Divide 0.003 by 240.

In the usual process:

0.003/240

or

```
     0.0000125
240 |0.0030000
       240
      ----
       6000
       4800
      ----
       1200
       1200
      ----
```

SCIENTIFIC NOTATION

Instead of these lengthy procedures, it is possible to employ scientific notation to multiply or divide. Scientific notation is an exponential system that says that 1,000 can be written as:

$$1 \times 10^3$$

or

$$1 \times (10)(10)(10)$$

The number written above the 10 (in this example, 3) is called the exponent. If the number is a whole number, the exponent is positive. If the number is a fraction, the exponent is negative. The exponent tells how many times 1 is to be multiplied by 10, or how many places the decimal point is to be moved.

1×10^3 is a whole number: 1,000
4.2×10^2 is a whole number: 420
1×10^{-3} is a fraction: 0.001
2.1×10^{-4} is a fraction: 0.00021

If the exponent is a zero, there is no change in the position of the decimal point. For example, the whole number 9, is expressed as 9×10^0 (or 9×1).

Table 4.3 combines Tables 4.1 and 4.2 and gives the exponential form of each number as used in scientific notation together with the common names and arithmetical values. Note that a positive exponent indicates the number of places the decimal is moved to the right. A negative exponent indicates the number of places the decimal is moved to the left. Thus: $2.23 \times 10^3 = 2{,}230$. And: $1.41 \times 10^{-3} = 0.00141$.

Scientific notation makes multiplication and division less complex. For example, to multiply 1×10^3 by 1×10^{-6}, all that is required is to add the exponents. A positive 3 and a negative 6 equals negative 3. The final exponent of the multiplication is $^{-3}$, or 10^{-3}, which is one one-thousandth (0.001).

Suppose it is necessary to multiply 2,320,000 by 0.0002. The first number can be expressed as 2.32×10^6. The second number is 2×10^{-4}. Then:

$$(2.32 \times 10^6)(2 \times 10^{-4}) = (4.64 \times 10^2) = 464.$$

The 2.32 is first multiplied by 2, which is equal to 4.64. Then the exponents are added:

TABLE 4.3. *Relationships of units by ten or tenths and their equivalents in scientific notation*

One million	1,000,000.0	(100,000 ×10)	1×10^6
One hundred thousand	100,000.0	(10,000 ×10)	1×10^5
Ten thousand	10,000.0	(1,000 ×10)	1×10^4
One thousand	1,000.0	(100 ×10)	1×10^3
One hundred	100.0	(10 ×10)	1×10^2
Ten	10.0	(1 ×10)	1×10^1
One (the unit)	1.0	(10 ÷10)	1×10^0
One-tenth	0.1	(1 ÷10)	1×10^{-1}
One-hundredth	0.01	(0.1 ÷10)	1×10^{-2}
One-thousandth	0.001	(0.01 ÷10)	1×10^{-3}
One ten-thousandth	0.0001	(0.001 ÷10)	1×10^{-4}
One one-hundred-thousandth	0.00001	(0.0001 ÷10)	1×10^{-5}
One-millionth	0.000001	(0.00001 ÷10)	1×10^{-6}

$$(+6) + (-4) = 2$$

thus

$$4.64 \times 10^2 = 464.$$

Another solution to the same problem would express 2,320,000 as 232×10^4. The value 0.0002 is 2×10^{-4}, as before. Then:

$$(232 \times 10^4)(2 \times 10^{-4})$$

The exponents, when added, equal zero, so the total is

$$464 \times 10^0 = 464.$$

Division is accomplished by subtracting exponents. The problem: 1,000 divided by 100 becomes:

$$(1 \times 10^3) \div (1 \times 10^2) = (1 \times 10^{3-2}) = (1 \times 10^1) = 10.$$

If we wish to solve the problem 27,000 divided by 3,000, it can be written as:

$$(27 \times 10^3) \div (3 \times 10^3) = \frac{27}{3}(10^3 - 10^3) = 9(10^0) = 9.$$

Suppose the problem is: 27,000/0.003. Then:

$$(27 \times 10^3) \div (3 \times 10^{-3}) = 9(10^6) = 9{,}000{,}000.$$

When subtracting a negative, it is changed to a positive. Thus:

$$(+3) - (-3) = 6.$$

This problem, if solved by long division, would appear:

$$0.003 \overline{)27{,}000} \text{ or } 3\overline{)27{,}000{,}000}^{\;9{,}000{,}000}$$

PRESENTATION OF NUMERICAL INFORMATION

Numbers are tools that are used by EEG technologists in their role as applied scientists. Through the proper use of numbers, problems can be solved and meaningful answers to various questions can be summarized. There are two basic methods of summarizing numerical information. One is through the use of a table, and the other is through the use of a graph.

These will be encountered not only in this book, but in virtually all of the EEG literature.

Tables

A table is a systematic arrangement of items of information, usually in columns and rows, so that there is a cross-indexing of the items of information. There have been several examples of tabular presentation in this chapter (Tables 4.1 to 4.3).

Graphs

Graphs are used to demonstrate relationships between two variables. A graph has two axes: the horizontal axis, called the X axis, and the vertical axis, called the Y axis. Figure 4.2 illustrates the graphic display of information. The solid dots and solid line show a 1:1 relationship between measures of X and measures of Y. This is a linear relationship: Every time X is increased by 1, Y also is increased by 1. This can be expressed as X = Y.

The dashed line with open circles in Fig. 4.2 also shows a linear relationship. However, in this case, whenever X is increased by 1, Y increases by 2. The relationship is expressed as X = 2Y.

Figure 4.3 illustrates another relationship between X and Y. This is a nonlinear relationship because the points on the X-axis and the Y-axis cannot be connected by a straight line. This is a curvilinear plot. In the example shown, Y increases as the square of X. That is, when X = 1,

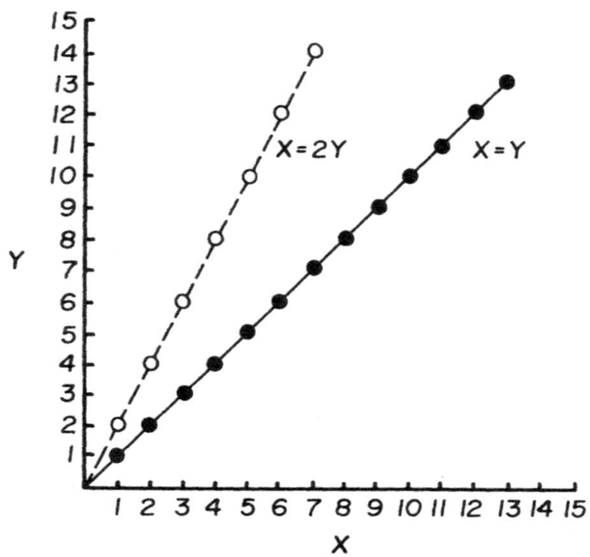

FIG. 4.2. Graphic representation of linear relationships (see text).

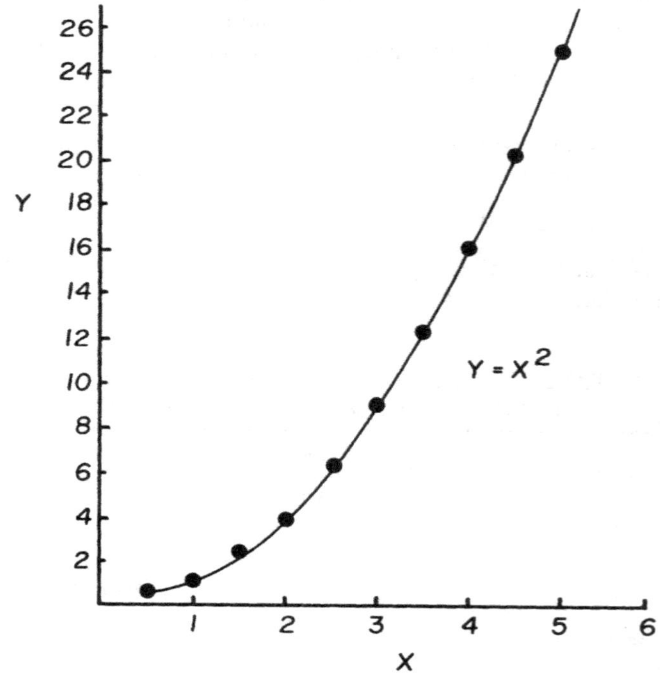

FIG. 4.3. Graphic representation of a curvilinear relationship: Y increases as the square of X (see text).

Y = 1; when X = 2, Y = 2^2 (or 4); when X = 3, Y = 9, and so on. The relationship is $Y = X^2$.

Figure 4.4 illustrates still another curvilinear relationship between X and Y. In this case, as X becomes larger, Y becomes smaller, and the relationship is inverse and nonlinear. The relationship is given by the formula:

$$Y = \frac{1}{X} \text{ or, } XY = 1.$$

Practical Use of Tables and Graphs in EEG

One important item of information with which EEG technologists deal is head size. Measurements are made for each patient's head to determine the location of the recording electrodes. One of the measurements is the head circumference (see Chapter 11). Suppose that we want to know the changes in head circumference that occur with age in boys and girls. Such information has been published. Meredith (2), for example, has assembled findings from nearly 150 studies on human head circumference from age 2 years to adulthood, on males and females, for various racial and regional groups. Each mean in Table 4.4 is based on roughly 1,000 subjects. From this table it is apparent that a) head circumference increases from age 2 to age 18; b) boys, on the average, have larger head circumferences at all ages than girls; c) the actual mean increase from 2 to 18 appears to be about the same (approximately 7 cm) for boys and girls; and d) the increase in average size after age 16 is greater in males than in females.

The same information can be displayed in a graph (Fig. 4.5). To compare the mean head growth of boys and girls in relation to age, age is plotted on the X-axis and head circumference on the Y-axis of the graph. This shows that the mean head circumferences increase steadily throughout the 2- to 18-year age range and also that at all ages the average head circumference of boys is greater than that of girls. Although the 7-cm increase from 2 to 18 years for both boys and girls is readily apparent from either the table or the graph, the graph more easily conveys the point that the differences between boys and girls are not constant at all ages and that there is not a strictly linear relationship between the two variables.

Another example of graphic display depicts the range of the average frequency of the alpha rhythm in normal adult subjects (Fig. 4.6). Measurements were made of the occipital alpha rhythms in 200 symptom-free adults (1). The range was observed to be from 8 to 12 Hz. The subjects were grouped on the basis of frequency, from 8.5 to 11.5 Hz in steps of 0.5 Hz. All subjects whose alpha rhythm was 9.76 to 10.25 Hz were grouped as "10 Hz," and so on. The percentage of the total group (200) that fell at each designated frequency was then computed. The data were plotted

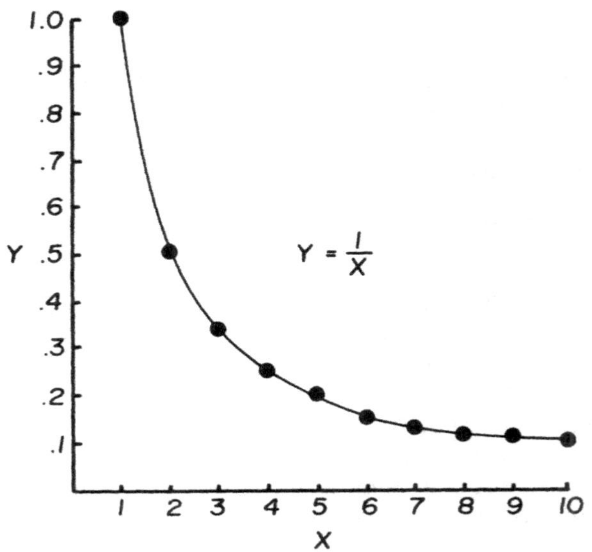

FIG. 4.4. Graphic representation of a curvilinear relationship: Y decreases as the reciprocal of X (see text).

TABLE 4.4. *Mean head circumference (cm) for caucasoid individuals of Europe and the United States**

	Mean age (years)									
	2	4	6	8	10	12	14	16	18	"Adult"
Males	49.1	50.7	51.7	52.3	52.8	53.4	54.2	55.2	56.2	56.8
Females	48.0	49.6	50.6	51.3	52.0	53.0	53.9	54.7	55.0	55.0

* Modified from Meredith (2).

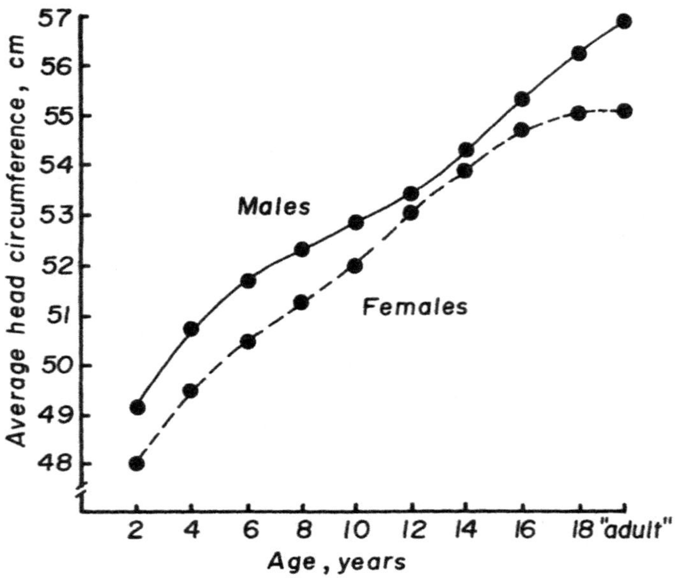

FIG. 4.5. Mean (average) head circumference as a function of age in children 2 to 18 years of age and adulthood.

so that alpha frequency is on the X-axis. The percent of total numbers of subjects at each alpha frequency is on the Y-axis.

This graph, called a bar graph, presents the distribution of alpha frequencies. The most commonly observed frequency (10 Hz) occurs in 35% of the cases. This is the mode. It also shows that the extreme ranges of alpha frequency (8.75 Hz or below, and 11.25 Hz or above) occurred in less than 10% of the subjects. About 40% had frequencies of 9.5 or 10.5 Hz, and about 15% had frequencies at 9 or 11 Hz. The distribution of frequencies around the mode is therefore readily grasped.

SIMPLE STATISTICAL CONCEPTS

If such characteristics as head size and alpha frequency are measured in a large group, keeping age (and gender) constant and choosing the subjects at random, it will be found that the distribution of individual measurements tends to form a bell-shaped curve, known as a normal curve, as shown in Fig. 4.7. The average (mean) is the sum of the measures divided by the number of measures.

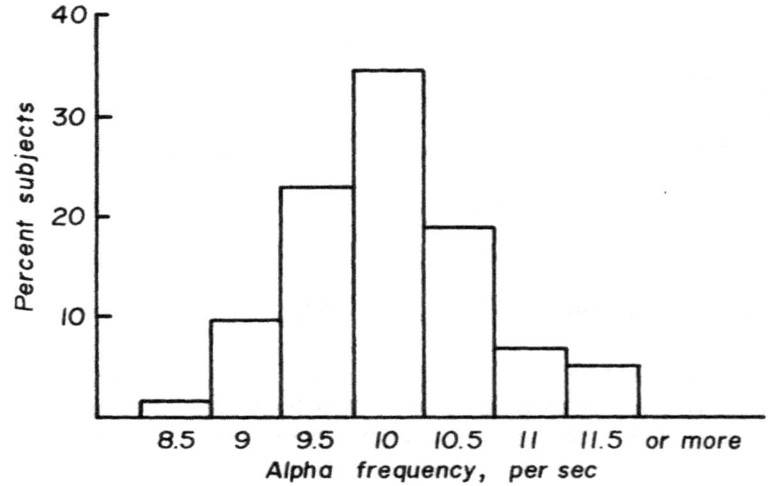

FIG. 4.6. Distribution of average frequency of alpha rhythm in a group of 200 subjects. [Redrawn from Kellaway (1).]

Standard Deviation

The variability of a distribution can be expressed in terms of a statistical measure known as the standard deviation (SD). The SD is an index of the differences between the group average and the individual scores or measures in a normal distribution. About 68% of all measures will be within 1 SD of the mean. About 5% will be either 2 SDs above or 2 SDs below the mean, and 0.2% will be beyond 3 SDs.[2]

Individual deviation is not particularly meaningful if it is less than 2 SDs from the average, but if an individual deviates by 2.5 or 3 SDs, it is possible to regard this as quite clearly unusual and perhaps abnormal.

[2] Another measure is the percentile, which tells what percentage of a large group falls below a given score. A measure that is at the 99th percentile is larger than 99% of the other scores; it is 2.33 SDs above the average. The 50th percentile is the same as the median.

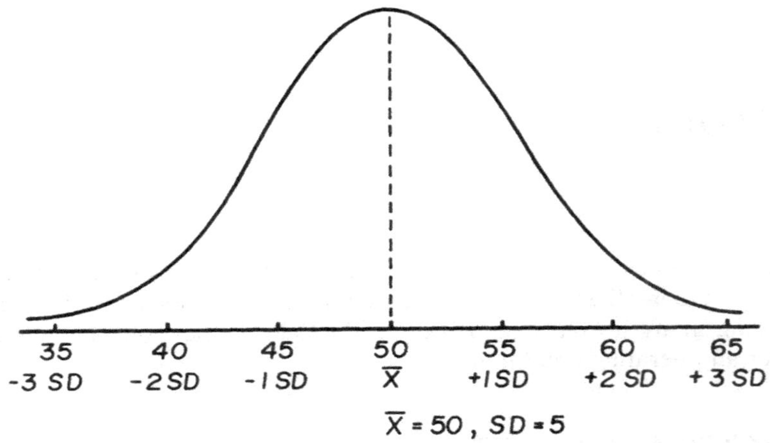

FIG. 4.7. Hypothetical bell-shaped curve representing the normal distribution of a randomly distributed variable. The mean (average) is 50 and the standard deviation is 5.

Groups may be compared by examining the overlap of their distributions. There are statistical methods by which their means may be compared. Unless the proper statistical test has been applied, even if the difference in the means is large, it cannot be considered statistically significant.

Means, SDs, and other statistical measures must be based on sufficiently large samples to attain suitable reliability. Further information about statistical techniques can be found in textbooks in this branch of science (see Additional Sources).

SUMMARY

In this chapter, we have learned that the decimal system and the metric system have a common feature: Measures are based on the number 10.

In the metric system, distance, volume, and weight are interrelated. The decimal system provides orderly relationships between very large numbers (thousands, millions, thousands of millions, and millions of millions) and very small numbers (thousandths, millionths, and trillionths). By using scientific notation, large numbers can be expressed more easily. Formulas are used to present the numerical relationships between variables. Tabular and graphic displays of numerical information are methods of summarizing data that make it possible to establish relationships or to judge the variability of any measure within a group.

REFERENCES

1. Kellaway, P. (1979): An orderly approach to visual analysis: The parameters of the normal EEG in adults and children. *In: Current Practice of Clinical Electroencephalography*, edited by: D. W. Klass and D. D. Daly, pp. 69–147. Raven Press, New York.
2. Meredith, H. V. (1971): Human head circumference from birth to early adulthood: Racial, regional and sex comparisons. *Growth*, 35:233–251.

Additional Sources

Heathkit Learning Publications. (1978): *D.C. Electronics*. (Appendix A: Scientific Notation). Heath Co., Benton Harbor, Michigan.

Kimble, G. A. (1978): *How to Use (and Misuse) Statistics*. Prentice-Hall, Englewood Cliffs, New Jersey.

Oliva, R. A., LaMont, M. D., and Fowler, L. (1978): *Understanding Calculator Math*, 3rd ed. Texas Instruments Learning Center, Dallas, Texas.

Swinscow, T. D. V. (1978). *Statistics at Square One*, 4th ed. British Medical Association, London.

Chapter 5

Some Principles of Electricity and Electronics

Electricity is a word that has several meanings, but its definition is entirely theoretical. No one can point to electricity, only to its effects. Classically, electricity was studied through its natural effects, such as lightning, or through creating static charges that can be generated in certain materials by rubbing them with cloth or fur. Two types of static charges were thus demonstrated: "positive" and "negative." Much later, electric currents were created by chemical means. These currents could be conducted by wires from the point of generation to some other location. Still later, electromagnetic generators were invented, which opened up a new world of science and technology.

In modern usage, the field of electrical engineering deals with heavy electrical machinery such as motors, generators, and transmission lines. Electronics, on the other hand, deals with the behavior of electrons and with devices that use electrons to perform their functions. The relationship between the two fields is defined by the fact that it is electrons that make up the flow of current used to operate heavy electrical machinery, and it is upon principles developed by electrical engineers and physicists that the modern field of electronics was nurtured and grew.

Electricity is defined as

> 1: a fundamental entity of nature consisting of negative and positive kinds of electricity composed respectively of electrons and protons or possibly of electrons and positrons, . . . observable in the attractions and repulsions of bodies electrified by friction and in certain natural phenomena (as lightning . . .), and usually utilized in the form of electric currents . . . 2: a science that deals with the phenomena and laws of electricity. (12)

Our knowledge of electricity has evolved over hundreds of years. In the last 50 years industrial and scientific applications have been expanding rapidly. Although developments in electronics have become increasingly complex and sophisticated, the principles are straightforward. A knowledge of basic electronics enables the EEG technologist to understand the fundamental design and operation of EEG equipment. This in turn makes possible the intelligent use of instrumentation, provides a base for understanding many artifacts, and insures the safe application of equipment under all operating conditions.

ELECTRICAL CIRCUITS

A practical electrical circuit is exemplified by a flashlight. A basic part of a flashlight is a source of electrical energy or force called a *battery*. In addition, there is a *switch,* which turns the flashlight ON, enabling electrical *current to flow* through a lamp or bulb. If current flows in the circuit, the lamp radiates light.

This verbal description is summarized in a schematic representation shown in Fig. 5.1A. Pictorial symbols are used to depict the battery, the lamp and the switch (shown in the OPEN position). The connecting lines represent the conducting pathway through which current flows when the switch is CLOSED—i.e., when its contact points touch, as shown in Fig. 5.1B. With the switch closed, the flow of current through the wire in the bulb raises the temperature of the wire (called a *filament*) and it glows, emitting rays of light.

Figure 5.1C is an equivalent of Fig. 5.1A, B. The lamp is symbolized by a *resistor* (*R*). This circuit shows the same three elements. These are: a source of *voltage* (*E*), a resistance (the lamp), and with the *switch* (*Sw*) in the closed position, a conducting path through which current can flow. This is further schematized in Fig. 5.2. The battery is labeled *E,* which stands for *electromotive force* (also called *EMF*). The resistor is labeled R, as before. The switch is closed. The arrows indicate that current (I) is flowing in the circuit, and that the current flows from the positive pole of the battery (marked +), to and through the resistor R, and returns to the battery at its negative pole (marked −).

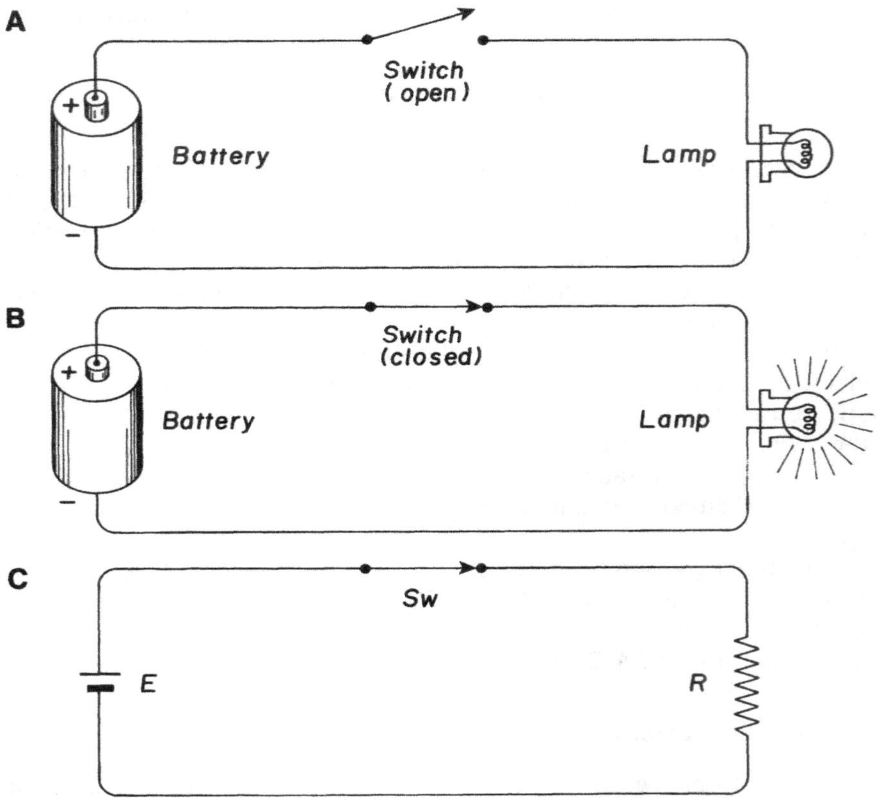

FIG. 5.1. **A:** Basic circuit of flashlight, switch 'open'. **B:** Basic circuit of flashlight, switch closed. **C:** Equivalent circuit of flashlight with switch closed. The resistor (R) is electrically equivalent to the lamp **(A, B)** and the schematic equivalent of the battery is substituted.

FORMS OF ELECTRICITY

Static Electricity

Electrical energy was first observed by man as static electricity. Lightning, which accompanies turbulent storms, is a type of static electricity. An electrical charge is built up between two clouds, caused by the rubbing together of air masses of different temperatures and humidities. When the charge becomes exceedingly large, it discharges to an area of lower charge, either the earth or another cloud. Another way to generate static electricity was known to Greek philosophers in pre-Christian times. Small static electrical charges were created by rubbing amber with fur. Interestingly, the Greek word for amber is *elektron*. Still another method of producing static electricity occurs commonly in northern latitudes in the winter time. When an individual walks across a rug, an electrical charge is built up in the person. Touching a metal object discharges the static charge, and a spark "jumps" to the object. Current flows and the individual feels a shock. When the electrical charge of the individual and the metal object is equalized, the spark stops and the sensation ends.

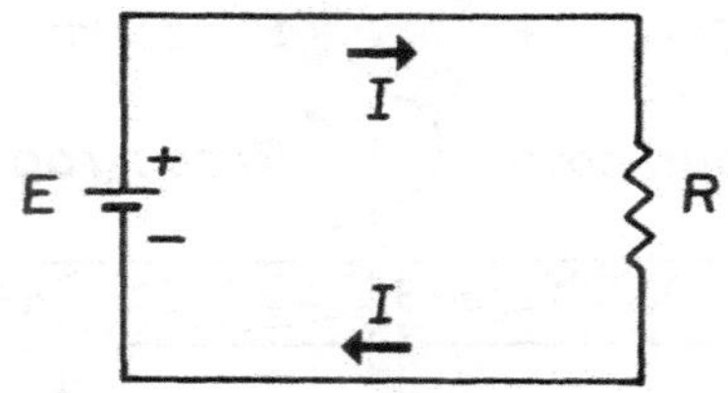

FIG. 5.2. Current flows from positive pole to and through resistor and returns to negative pole.

Static electricity also can be experimentally generated by rubbing a comb with a silk cloth. An electrical charge is built up in the comb. This charge can be transferred to another object such as small ball of crumpled tissue paper hung from a nonmetallic support by a string. If two paper balls are charged by contact with the same source, they will fly apart when placed next to each other. This illustrates a fundamental law of electricity: *Like charges repel.*

If a rod made of amber is rubbed with wool, and if two paper balls are charged by contact with the amber, the balls also will repel each other. However, if a ball charged by the amber–wool combination is placed close to a comb–silk charged ball, the two balls will swing toward each other. This illustrates the converse law: *Unlike charges attract.*

A glass jar can be prepared with a metal foil secured around both the outside and the inside of its walls. A connection to the inside foil can be made by means of a metal rod coming through the lid. This specially constructed jar is called a *Leyden jar,* because it was invented by early scientists at the University of Leyden in the Netherlands. Its construction is shown in Fig. 5.3. If a charged object is brought into contact with the

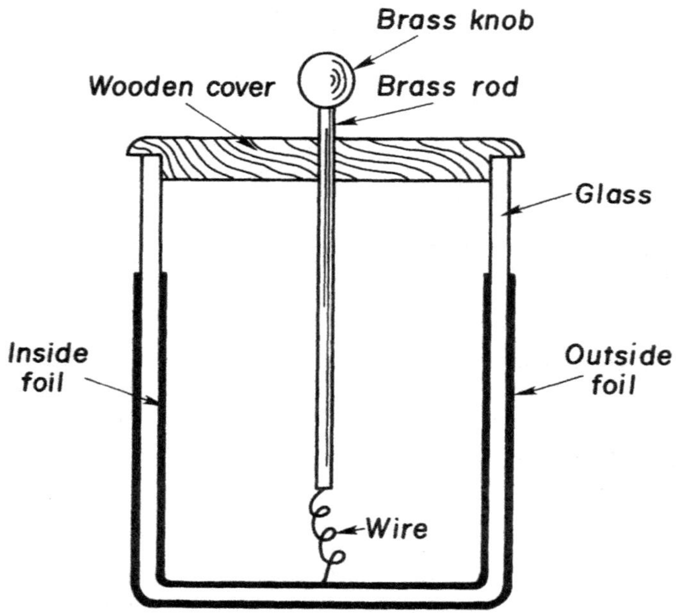

FIG. 5.3. Cross-sectional diagram of a Leyden jar.

external end of the rod, the charge is transferred to the inside foil and it can be stored. The Leyden jar was used in many early experiments on electricity. Benjamin Franklin is said to have demonstrated the presence of the electrical charge related to lightning by flying a kite in a thunder storm. The wet kite string served as a conductor. A metal key at the bottom of the string, when brought into contact with the rod of the Leyden jar, transferred the static charge of the atmosphere above the earth, through the string, to the jar. This charge could later be discharged by connecting the rod to the outside foil. When a conductor (metal wire) was connected to the top of the rod, and then brought close to the outside foil, a spark would jump to the outside. This made the charge on the outside and inside foils equal. [See Heathkit Learning Programs (5) for further discussion of static electricity and the Leyden jar.]

The Leyden jar was called a "condenser" because the electricity was "condensed" inside it. In present nomenclature, this is called a *capacitor*. A capacitor possesses the property of storing electrical energy. Capacitors are used in EEG equipment, and the effects of capacitance are frequently encountered.

Direct Current

In our introduction to the battery in the flashlight circuit, we have already met electricity in the form of direct current (DC). This type of electricity provides a steady source of current, flowing in one direction only. It was originally believed (100 years ago) that current flow proceeded from the positive to the negative pole. As we shall soon learn, this is not an accurate concept.

In a battery such as that used in a flashlight or a portable radio, the electrical energy is generated by chemical action. This energy is available and current flows whenever the switch of the circuit is closed. Opening the switch stops the current flow. Alternately closing and opening the switch creates a pulsating or discontinuous flow. This is illustrated in Fig. 5.4. [See Heathkit Learning Programs (5) for further discussion of direct current.]

The discharge of static electricity, stored in the capacitor formed by the Leyden jar, on the other hand, causes an abrupt and brief flow of current when a wire connected to the inside foil approaches the outside foil. This is shown in Fig. 5.5A,B.

Alternating Current

Another form of electricity is alternating current (AC). This is electrical energy that alternately flows in one direction and then the other. The everyday use of electricity in the home, in industry, in hospitals, and in laboratories involves 60-Hz AC. A 60-Hz alternating current completes one full cycle in 1/60 sec. It flows in a positive direction for half of the time

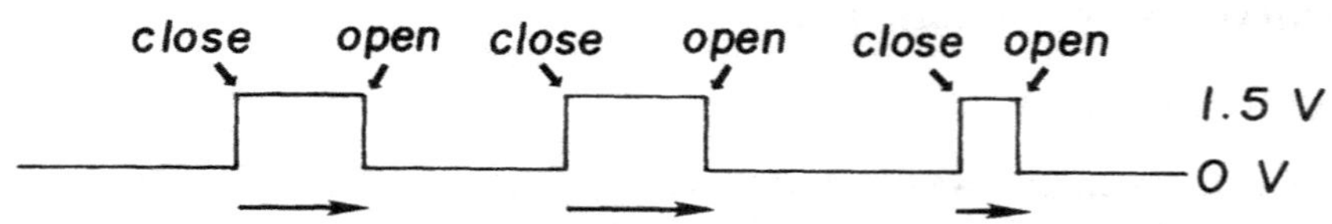

FIG. 5.4. Pulsating flow of DC current, that flows (→) when switch (Fig. 5.1) is closed.

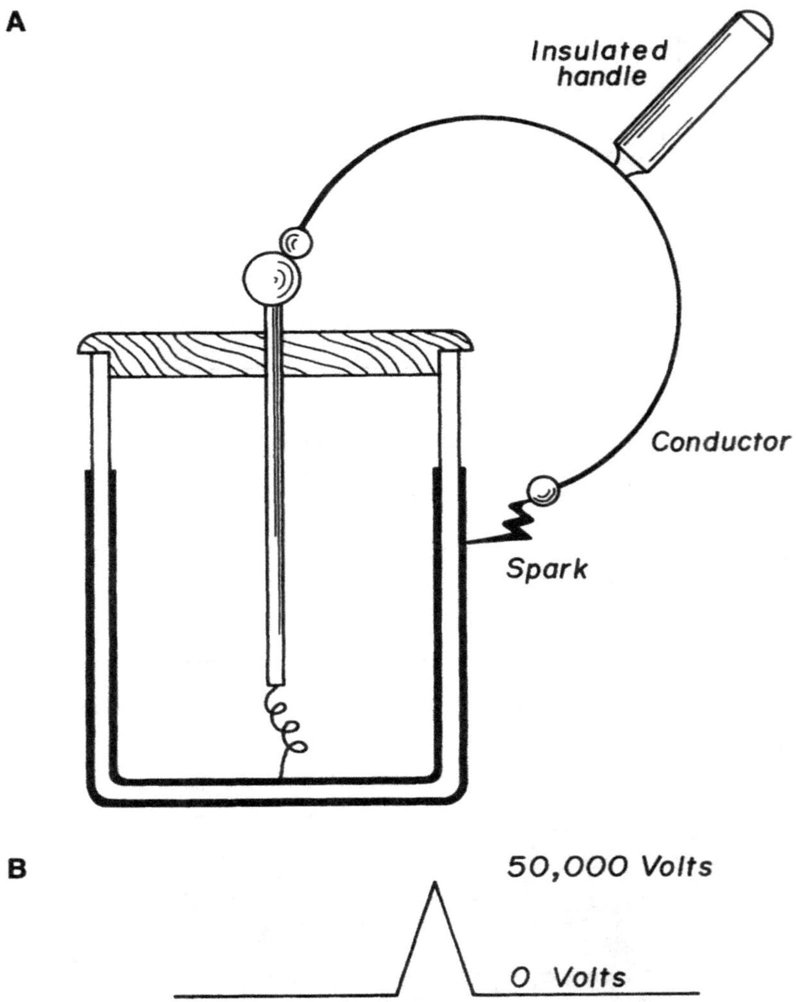

FIG. 5.5. A: Spark at discharge of Leyden jar. B: Current flow when Leyden jar is discharged by moving inside wire near outside foil. Peak voltage is shown.

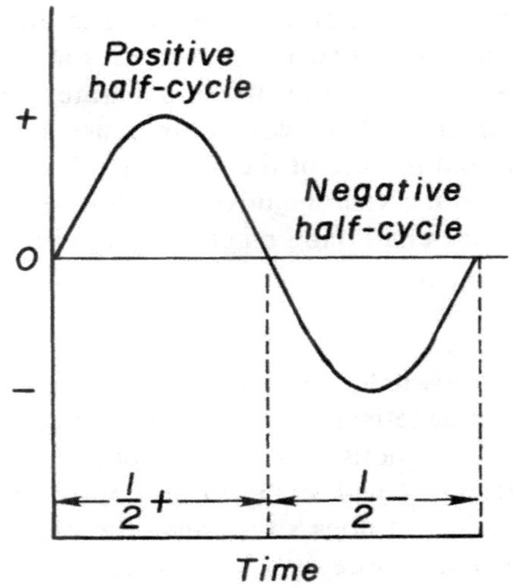

FIG. 5.6. Graphic presentation of alternating current flow. The current is assumed to begin to flow at time 0, with a value of 0 V. It rises to maximum during the first quarter of the cycle and returns to zero when half of the cycle is completed. It then reverses direction of flow, rising to maximum at three-quarters of the cycle, and returns to zero when the cycle is completed. The time necessary to complete the cycle is divided by the frequency of alternation. For example, a 60-cycle current completes one cycle in 1/60 sec. A 30-cycle wave completes one cycle in 1/30 (0.033) sec.

(i.e., 1/120 sec) and a negative direction for the remaining half cycle. This is illustrated in Fig. 5.6. [See Heathkit Learning Programs (7) for further discussion of alternating current.]

An elementary AC home or laboratory circuit is shown in Fig. 5.7A. This controls the ceiling lights in an EEG laboratory. This is the same circuit used to describe a flashlight, although the voltage involved is quite different, and the current is AC rather than DC. When the switch is closed, current flows and the light is "turned on." In the case of the flashlight, the current flow occurs in one direction continuously. In the case of the AC ceiling light, the current flows first in one direction and then in the other (Fig. 5.7B).

The DC provided by a battery is produced electrochemically. Two dissimilar metals, placed in an acid, develop a potential difference between them and, if a conducting path is provided, current will flow as long as the chemical reactions can be maintained. The life of the battery is a function of these reactions. If two such batteries are placed in series the voltage provided will be the sum of the separate voltages. If they are connected in parallel, the voltage will not increase but the current capacity will be doubled, and the life of the combined batteries will be longer. The AC that is used in the vast majority of industrial and domestic applications is generated by employing magnetic forces.[1]

MAGNETISM

Another area of knowledge involved in understanding principles of electricity concerns magnetism. [See Heathkit Learning Programs (5) for further discussion of magnetism.] If a magnetized iron bar (Fig. 5.8) is suspended by a thread, it will swing in an approximately north–south geographical orientation. It does so because the planet earth has a large magnetic field, exerting a force over small magnets. A common example of this effect is the familiar magnetic compass. The earth's north magnetic pole attracts one pole (one end) of the compass magnet.

If two bar magnets are brought together (Fig. 5.9), one of two things will occur. If two south or two north poles face each other, the bars will be forced apart. *Like forces repel.*

If the north pole of one bar is brought toward the south pole of the other, the two bars will snap together and it will require force to separate them. *Unlike forces attract.* These are the same general principles that apply to electrical charge.

ELECTROMAGNETIC FORCES

Magnetic force and current flow are related. Using one magnet, it is possible to generate an electrical current that will in turn have an effect on a second magnet. This is shown in the experiment schematized in Fig.

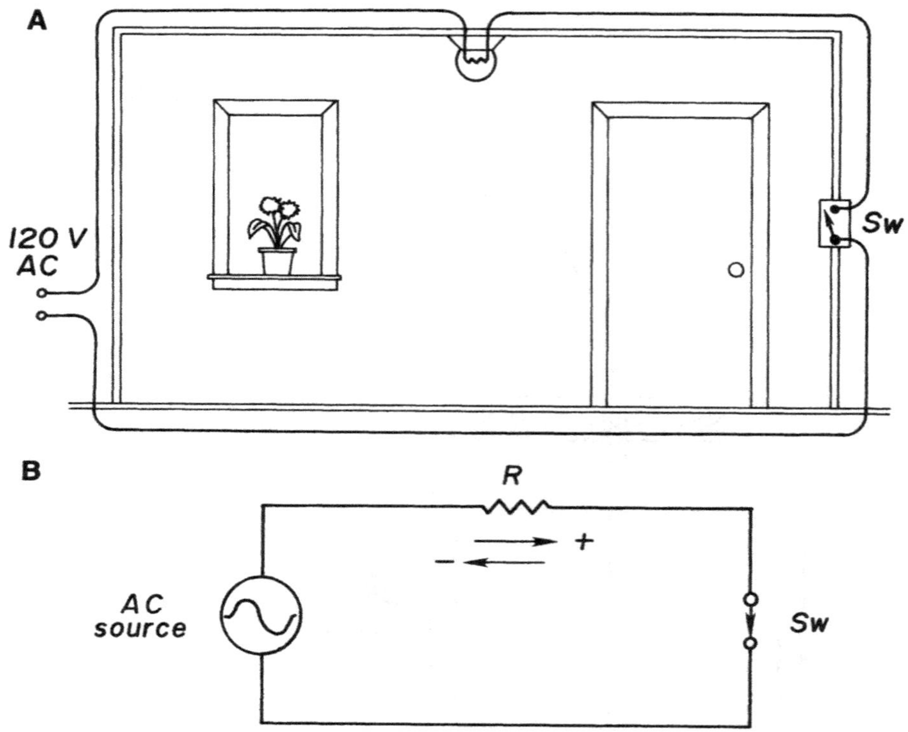

FIG. 5.7. **A.** Typical 120 V AC room light circuit (two-wire system). **B.** Equivalent circuit; when switch is closed, current alternately flows in one direction and then the other.

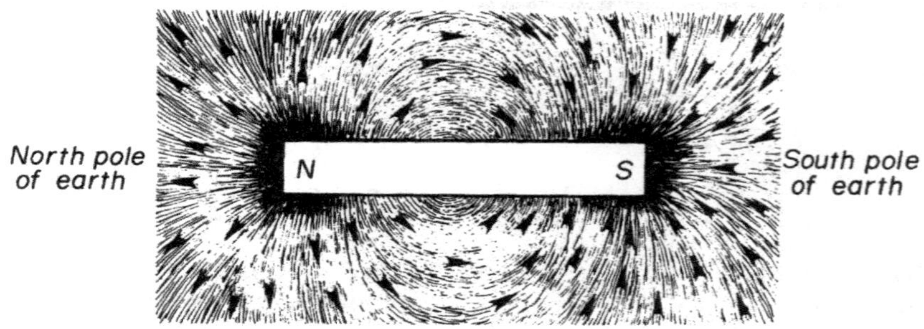

FIG. 5.8. A magnet and its magnetic field.

[1] There are other sources of EMF. Light may be converted to electrical energy by a photocell, made of material that emits electrons when placed in a lighted field. Pressure transducers convert movement to electrical energy. Some crystals develop a voltage across their structure when distorted by pressure. A thermocouple converts changes in temperature to electrical energy; if two wires, made of different metals, are twisted together a voltage difference develops between them when their temperature is changed. Devices using these sources often are used as monitoring equipment in EEG laboratories.

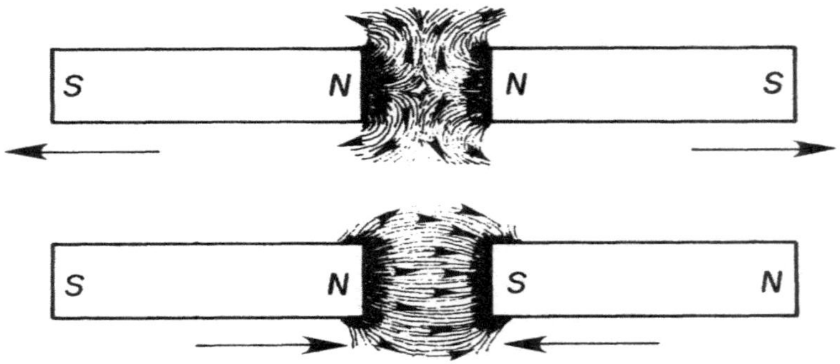

FIG. 5.9. Magnetic forces. Like forces repel (upper); unlike forces attract (lower).

5.10. A coil of wire is formed at each end of a continuous wire. A bar magnet is moved in and out through the coil of wire at one end. The coil at the other end surrounds a magnetic compass.

As the bar magnet is thrust to and fro within coil A, the compass needle inside the coil B moves to and fro. This occurs because as the magnet is thrust in and out of the loop of wire, the lines of force around the magnet "cut" across the coil of wire. This causes current to flow in the wire, first in one direction and then in the other. The current flowing in the wire around the compass needle creates an electromagnetic field. The polarity of the electromagnetic field reverses as the direction of movement of the bar reverses in the first loop. Because like forces attract and unlike forces repel, the to and fro movement of the compass needle occurs. If the bar is thrust in and held in a fixed position, the needle of the compass will give one swing and return to zero. Current does not flow when the magnetic field is no longer moving across, i.e., "cutting," coil A. This is an example of the electromagnetic effect and will be discussed again under the topic of inductance. [See Heathkit Learning Programs (5) for further discussion of electromagnetic forces.]

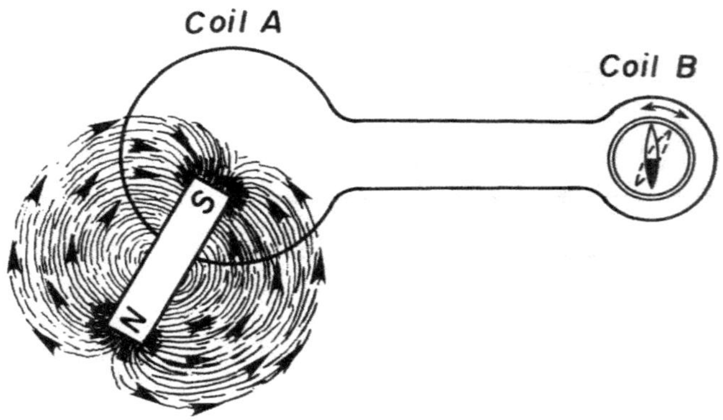

FIG. 5.10. As bar magnet is thrust in and out of large loop of wire (coil A), compass needle inside center of small loop (coil B) moves to and fro. Magnetic lines of force "cut" coil A at each passage of the magnet inducing field in small loop (see text).

An AC generator typically employs a coil of wire, rotating in a magnetic field. As the coil rotates within the field, the magnetic lines of force "cut" the wire, causing current to flow. As the coil rotates through one cycle, the voltage at the ends of the coil first increases then decreases to zero, increases again, and returns to zero [See Heathkit Learning Programs (5,6) for further discussion of AC generator.] The relation between the rotation and the output voltage appears in Figure 5.11. The rotation of the coil can be given in *degrees,* from 0° to 360°, then repeating. The voltage generated in the AC cycle can be referred to, then, as occurring at a particular number of degrees of phase. This concept also will be referred to later when the phase between two signals is compared.

ATOMIC THEORY

In the early days before the existence and structure of atoms was deduced, it was supposed that current flowed from a point of higher electromotive force to a lower point. Thus, it was assumed that current flowed from positive to negative. This assumption was to be modified by atomic theory [See Heathkit Learning Programs (5) for further discussion of atomic theory.]

The basic building blocks of the world around us are *elements.* There are 92 natural elements. An *atom* is the smallest piece of an element. Each atom has a *nucleus* made up of *protons* and *neutrons,* surrounded by numerous orbiting *electrons.* The number of electrons equals the number of protons. Hydrogen is the lightest of the elements. The symbol for hydrogen is H. Hydrogen has one proton and one electron in orbit (it is the only element without neutrons). Another element is oxygen. The symbol for oxygen is O. Oxygen has 8 electrons. The heaviest element is

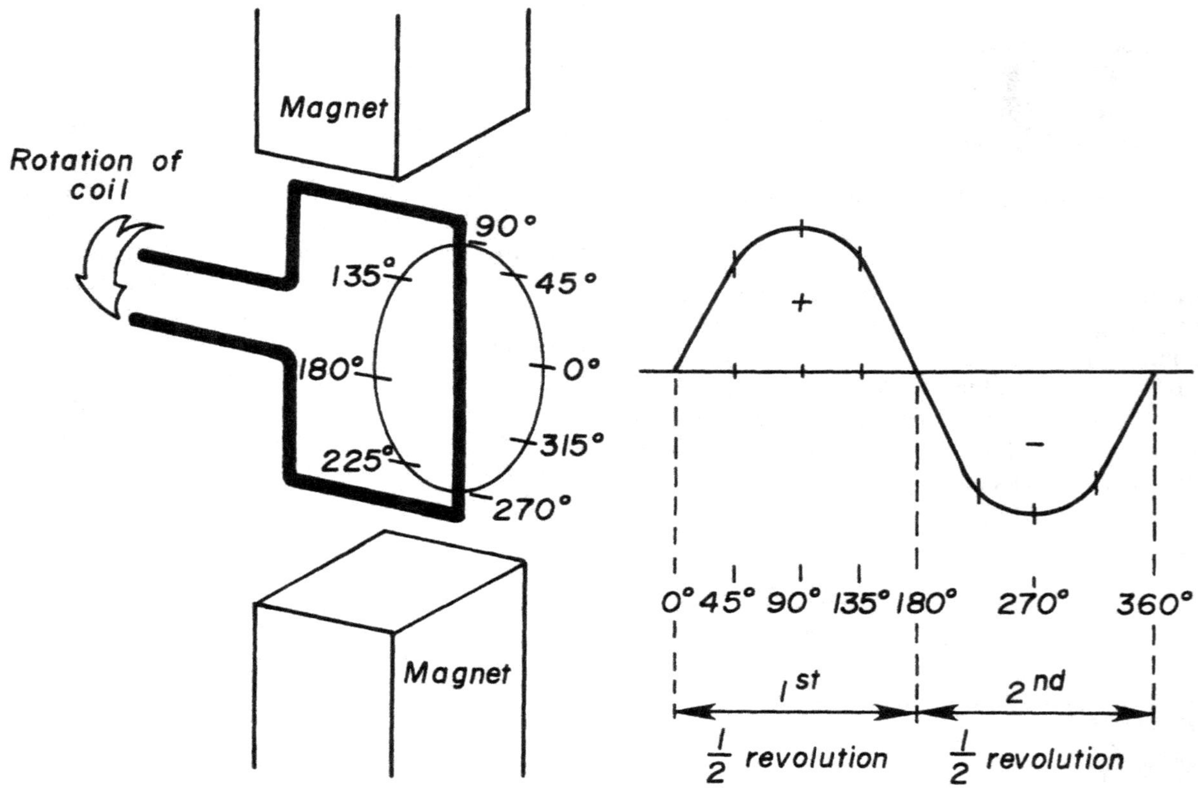

FIG. 5.11. Alternating current (see text).

uranium (U), with 92 electrons. Lead (Pb), which is a commonplace "standard of heaviness," has 82 electrons.

A *compound* is formed when two or more elements combine. When hydrogen and oxygen combine, for example, the compound water is formed. Water has two H atoms and one O atom. Its chemical formula is H_2O. Another common compound is table salt, which is made up of sodium (Na) and chlorine (Cl). When they combine, the compound is sodium chloride (NaCl). Water requires two hydrogen atoms and one oxygen atom whereas sodium chloride requires only one atom of each element. Sulfuric acid is composed of hydrogen, sulfur (S), and oxygen. Its formula is H_2SO_4.

Compounds always are made up of at least two elements; they may be very complex. They have indivisible units called *molecules*. The smallest piece of sodium chloride is a single molecule of NaCl. Compounds can be separated into the elements that form them, but the elements themselves cannot be subdivided.

Copper (Cu) is an element that is used to make wire. Let us suppose that the wire used in the experiment in Fig. 5.10 is pure copper. The smallest single bit of copper is an atom. The central nucleus of an atom is made up of positive charges called *protons*. The nucleus is surrounded by negative charges called *electrons*. The electrons orbit around the nucleus, much as the planets of the solar system revolve around the sun. The electrons are arranged in "shells" so that some electrons orbit in tracks nearer the nucleus and others in tracks farther away (Fig. 5.12).

The negative charge of the electrons balances the positive charge of the protons (the neutrons need not concern us in this discussion). In some atoms, it is possible to more easily dislodge electrons in the outermost shell than in other atoms. Electrons that have left their orbit become "free" and are able to move about.

Hydrogen, with one proton and one electron, has a hypothetical structure shown in Fig. 5.12A. The orbiting electron (−) forms a shell. In any element, the shell closest to the nucleus (N) and its proton (+) never contains more than two electrons. There is an orderly organization of electrons in shells. When more than two electrons revolve around an atom's nucleus, more shells are formed. The number of electrons in each shell is limited. A second shell may hold up to 8 electrons. A third may hold up to 18 electrons. A fourth shell may contain up to 32. Still more shells are formed for the heaviest atoms.

The number of electrons in the outermost shell is limited to a maximum of 8, although there may be fewer. This outer shell is called the *valence shell*. The electrons in the valence shell are farthest away from the protons in the atom's nucleus. The force of the attraction between unlike charged particles decreases with distance (Coulomb's law). It is therefore these valence electrons that can be freed from orbit most easily. When they are free, they can be moved in a wire as current.

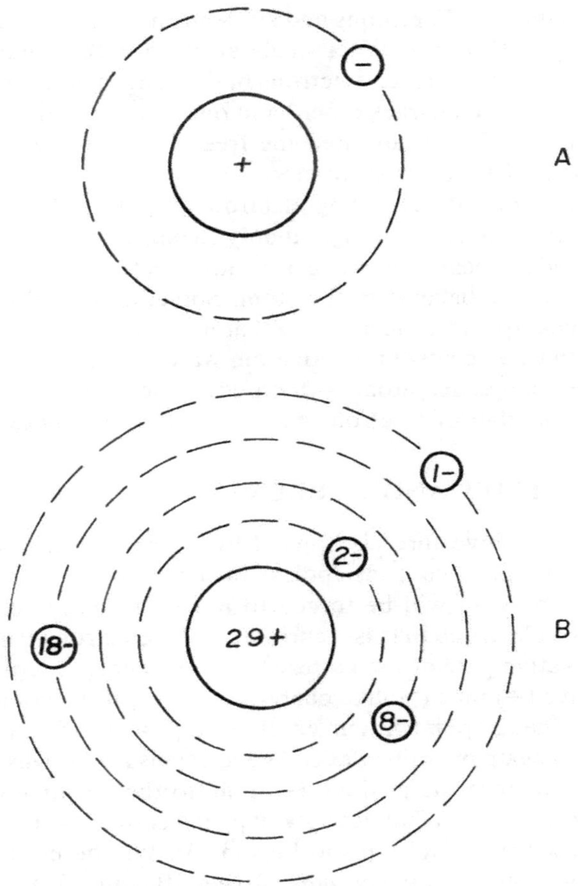

FIG. 5.12. Structures of hydrogen (H) atom (A) and copper (Cu) atom (B). Central nucleus is shown as inner circle. Number of protons (+) is indicated. Electrons are shown in orbit (see text).

A copper atom has 29 protons and 29 electrons. There are four shells, as shown in Fig. 5.12B. There is a single electron in the outer, or valence, shell. If two orbiting valence electrons of Cu come near each other, repulsion will occur ('like charges repel') and one or both of the electrons may be knocked out of orbit and become free. The free electrons then can wander around the atomic structure.

The nucleus and its remaining electrons now form a positive ion because it has 29 protons (positive) but only 28 negative electrons. If the free electron wanders near a positive ion, the electron may be pulled into orbit, restoring the balance of the atom. Sometimes an already balanced atom may pick up a free electron, so that it has an extra electron in orbit. It then becomes a negative ion. An atom which has lost an electron has a net positive charge. An atom with an extra electron has a net negative charge. The number of electrons gained or lost determines the charge.

ELECTRON FLOW AND CURRENT

If an electromotive force is applied by connecting the two ends of a copper wire to the two ends (poles) of a battery (Fig. 5.13), the free electrons in the wire will be forced to move in one direction. It is the movement of electrons that is "current." The electrons will move away from the negative pole of the battery (−) ('like charges repel') and travel to the positive (+) pole ('unlike charges attract'). If the connection to the battery is opened at point X, current flow stops and random movement of free electrons again prevails. Several generations ago, it was assumed that current flowed from the positive (+) pole to the negative (−) pole of a battery as in Fig. 5.2. What actually happens is that electrons, which are negative, flow from − to + (as in Figs. 5.13). We therefore have to deal with the concepts of *conventional current* (flowing from + to −) and *electron current* (flowing from − to +). [See Cannon and Luecke (1) and Heathkit Learning Programs (5) for further discussion of electron flow and current.] From this point on, unless otherwise stated, the word "current" will refer to electron current.

The magnitude of current is determined by the rate, in time, of electron flow past a given point. The unit of current is the *ampere* (A). One ampere equals a rate of electron movement past a given point, defined as one coulomb per second. A coulomb is equal to a charge of 6.25×10^{18} electrons. A calibrated meter, called an *ammeter*, can be used to determine the current flowing in the circuit, measured in amperes or in fractions of amperes (Fig. 5.14).

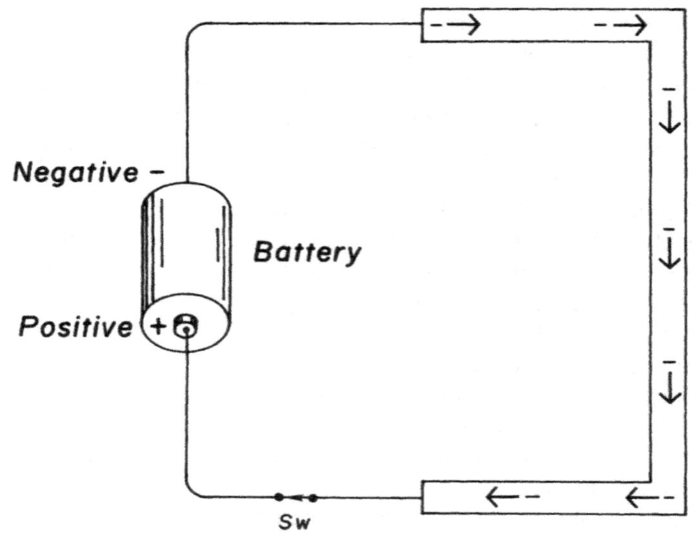

FIG. 5.13. Movement of electrons in electrical circuit.

Conductors

Materials that easily give up electrons are called conductors. Their free electrons are readily moved by an electromotive force. Current can flow through such materials with little resistance. Metals are good conductors.

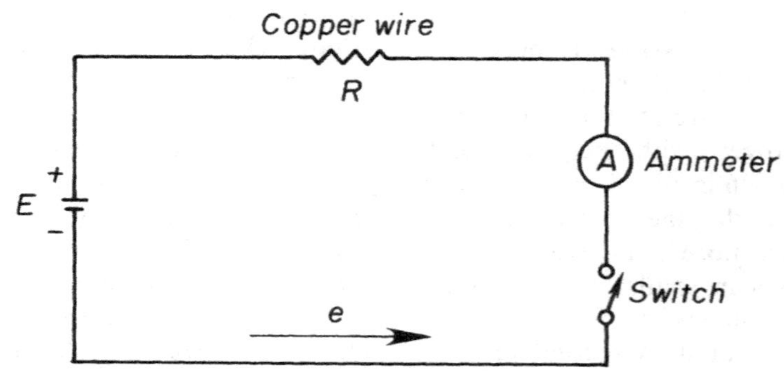

FIG. 5.14. When switch is closed, an electromotive force is applied and electrons (E) flow through the copper wire. This electron flow is current. There is some resistance (R) to the electron flow. The amount of current flowing is determined by an appropriate meter (A).

Typical conductors are silver (Ag), copper (Cu), gold (Au), platinum (Pt), tin (Sn), and iron (Fe).

Resistors

Not all elements give up electrons with equal ease. Iron (Fe) is a poorer conductor than silver (Ag) or copper (Cu) because its electrons are more closely bound to its nucleus. Therefore, iron has a higher resistance than silver or copper. The unit of resistance is the *ohm,* symbolized by the Greek letter omega (Ω).

Insulators

Insulators are materials which, even when subjected to strong electrical forces, will not readily give up electrons. Glass, porcelain, rubber, and many forms of plastic compounds are insulators. Air also is an insulator, but if the electrical force is very strong, current will flow through it and a spark will occur. A common example of such a spark is lightning. In this case, the insulator (air) does give up electrons and current flows through it. Solid insulators, for example plastics or some natural compounds such as mica, will be destroyed if subjected to excessive electromotive forces or voltages that break them down. [See Heathkit Learning Programs (5) and Rusgrove and Woodward (11) for further discussion of insulators.]

Semiconductors

Another group of elements belongs to a class of materials known as semiconductors. They are neither good conductors nor especially good insulators. Three of these elements are silicon (Si), germanium (Ge), and gallium (Ga). Their valence shells and valence electrons have special properties. The characteristics of semiconductors will be discussed in detail later in this chapter. It is through the understanding of the capabilities of semiconductors that modern electronics has developed and will continue to expand its applications in the future.

BASIC UNITS IN ELECTRICITY

The basic unit of electromotive force (E) is the volt (V). The basic unit of current (I) is the ampere (A). The basic unit of resistance is the ohm (R).

VOLTAGE

The battery in the schematic circuit of the flashlight provides the pressure that forces electrons to flow through the conductor. The flashlight bulb is a load that presents a resistance to flow of electrons or current. When the switch is closed and the circuit is completed, *electrons flow from the negative pole of the battery through the wire and bulb and return to the positive pole.*

The material used for the filament of the bulb is a conductor, but it is one that resists electron flow. If enough voltage is used to force enough electrons through this conductor, energy is given off, since both light and heat are produced. The resistance in the circuit is analogous to friction in a mechanical sense. To overcome the resistance, work must be done (i.e., energy is expended).

The pictorial symbols for battery, switch, conductor, resistor, and lamp were introduced in Figs. 5.1A–C and 5.2. Symbols for those and other common circuit elements are shown in Fig. 5.15.

OHM'S LAW

The basic principle by which voltage, current, and resistance are related is Ohm's law, which was formulated by the 19th century German physicist George Simon Ohm. As illustrated by the circuit model in Fig. 5.16, Ohm's law states that: Voltage (E) is equal to current (I) flowing in the circuit multiplied by resistance (R) in the circuit.

$$E = I \times R. \qquad (1)$$

If any two of the three variables are known, the other can be determined.

$$I = E/R \qquad (2)$$

(The current flowing in the circuit equals the voltage divided by the resistance.)

$$R = E/I \qquad (3)$$

(The resistance equals the voltage applied divided by the current.)

If the circuit has a resistance of 1,000 Ω, and the current is 0.01 A, what is the value of E? From equation 1 above,

$$E = 0.01 \times 1{,}000$$

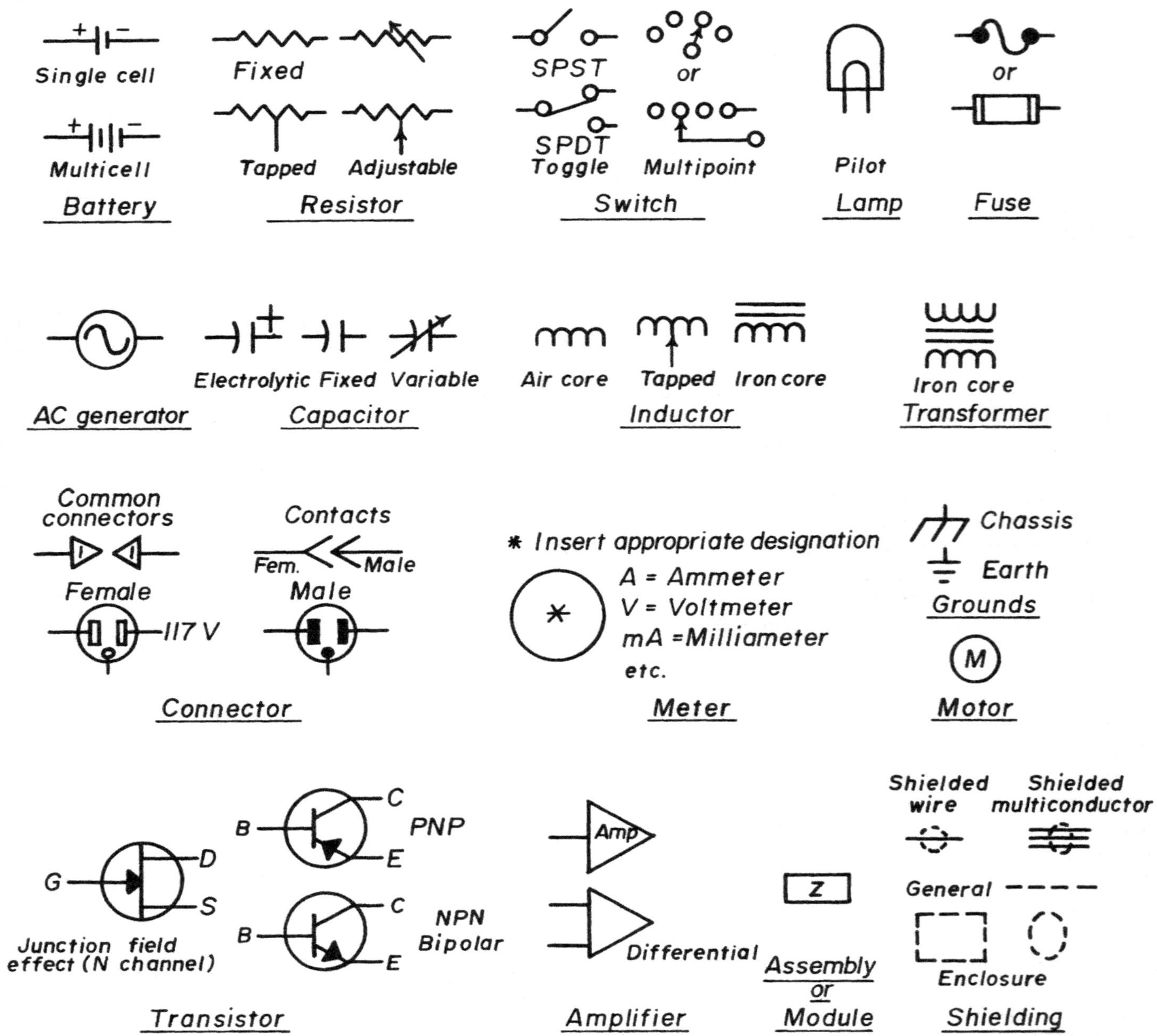

FIG. 5.15. Schematic symbols used in circuit diagrams. (Redrawn in part from ref. 10, frontispiece.)

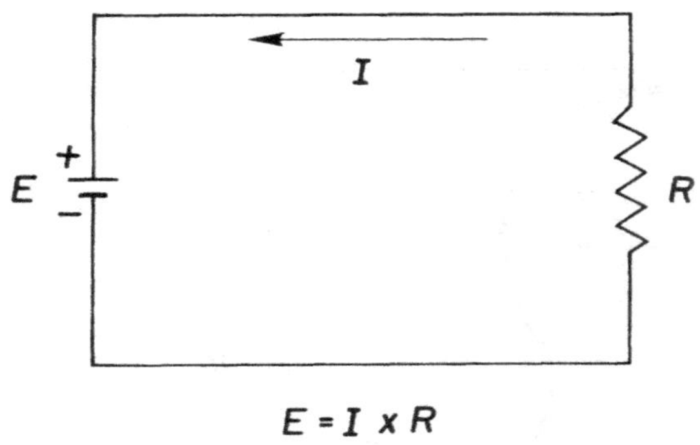

FIG. 5.16. Circuit model illustrating Ohm's law (see text).

or

$$E = 10\ V.$$

If the circuit has 20 V applied to it, and if the resistance in the circuit is 2,000 Ω, what is the current? From equation 2 above,

$$I = \frac{20}{2{,}000}.$$

$$I = 0.01\ A\ (10\ mA\ \text{or}\ 10^{-2}\ A).$$

If the current flowing in a circuit is 0.5 A and the voltage is 120 V, what is the resistance of the circuit? From equation 3 above,

$$R = \frac{120}{0.5}$$

$$R = 240\ \Omega.$$

ELECTRICAL PREFIXES

Subunits

The basic use of numbers has been presented in Chapter 4. Because these applications are relevant to EEG instrumentation and recording, let us consider the following:

A. Although the volt (V) is the basic unit of EMF, in practical EEG EMF is measured in μV.
   1. A millivolt (mV) is one one-thousandth of a volt (0.001 V or 1×10^{-3}). These units commonly are used in EKG, EMG, and sometimes in EEG.
   2. A microvolt (μV) is one one-millionth of a volt (0.000001 V or 1×10^{-6}). This is the commonest voltage measure in EEG.
   3. A nanovolt (nV) is one-thousandth of one-millionth of a volt (0.000000001 V or 1×10^{-9}). This measure is used in the special area of EEG dealing with evoked potentials.

B. Although the unit of current is the ampere (A), in practical EEG, smaller amounts are encountered.
   1. A milliampere (mA) is one one-thousandth of an ampere (0.001 A or 1×10^{-3}).
   2. A microampere (μA) is one one-millionth of an ampere (0.000001 A or 1×10^{-6}).

To review briefly, there are 1,000 mV in 1 V. There are 1,000 μV in 1 mV. One hundred microvolts is equivalent to 0.1 mV. A voltage of 500 μV is 0.5 mV.

A current of 0.1 A is 100 mA. A current of 0.1 mA is the same as a current of 100 μA.

Macrounits

When a prefix indicates a value of less than one, a lower case letter is used, for example, m = milli. When greater than one, an upper case letter is used, beginning with a million (mega = M), but a lower case letter is now used for a thousand (kilo = k). The voltages supplied by the power mains to EEG laboratories involve very large values of electromotive force, and may be expressed in thousands of volts of *kilovolts* (*kV*).

The unit of resistance is the ohm (Ω), but resistors used in the design, construction, and operation of EEG equipment usually have values measured in thousands of ohms. These are called *kilohms* (*k*Ω). Values of R measured in millions of ohms are called *megohms* (*M*Ω).

The following equivalents will provide examples from which the student can construct sample problems for solving Ohm's law, inserting micro and macro voltage and current values.

10,000 Ω equals 10 kΩ.
100,000 Ω equals 100 kΩ (and also equals 0.1 MΩ).
1,000,000 Ω equals 1 MΩ.

100 Ω equals 0.1 kΩ.
3,300,000 Ω equals 3.3 MΩ.
3,300 Ω equals 3.3 kΩ (and also equals 0.033 MΩ).
333,000 Ω equals 0.333 MΩ (and also equals 333 kΩ).

mega = M = 10^6	milli = m = 10^{-3}	nano = n = 10^{-9}
kilo = k = 10^3	micro = μ = 10^{-6}	pico = p = 10^{-12}

SOME SAMPLE PROBLEMS

1. How many volts are needed to cause 15 mA to flow in a circuit with a resistance of 1 MΩ? (15 kV)
2. If a circuit has a resistance of 3.3 kΩ, how much current will flow when a 10-V source is applied? (0.003 mA)
3. Twelve volts is applied to a circuit. By measurement with a milliameter, it is found that 0.5 mA flows. What is the resistance in the circuit? (24,000 Ω)

In clinical EEG practice, we deal with very low frequencies and the voltages are measured in microvolts. Ohm's law applies equally to DC and to AC. We might ask the question: How much current will pass through the input circuit of an EEG amplifier? A schematic diagram represents this circuit in Fig. 5.17. Assume that E is 20 μV. We know from the specifications of a modern instrument that the resistive impedance in the input circuit of the amplifier has a typical value of 20 MΩ. If we disregard the resistance of the electrodes, and the resistance through body tissue, we can compute the current in the input circuit from Ohm's law, I = E/R

$$I = \frac{0.000020}{20{,}000{,}000} = \frac{2 \times 10^{-5}}{2 \times 10^{7}}$$

$$I = 0.000{,}000{,}000{,}001 \text{ A} = 1 \times 10^{-12} \text{ A}.$$

This can be expressed as 1 pico ampere (pA).

RESISTANCE

Resistors in Series

If two or more resistors are connected in series, as in Fig. 5.18, the total resistance (R) in the circuit will be:

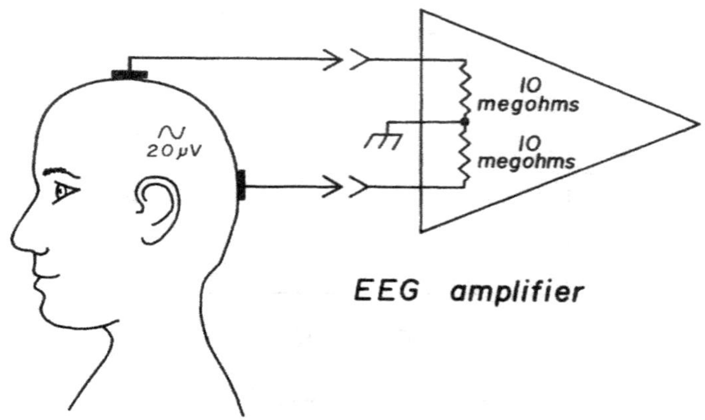

FIG. 5.17. Application of Ohm's law to input circuit of typical EEG amplifier. E = 20 uV; R = 20 MΩ. What is I? (see text).

$$R = R_1 + R_2 + \ldots + R_N$$

(where N is the total number of resistors).

If the values of R_1 = 5 kΩ and R_2 = 3 kΩ and R_3 = 2 kΩ, then the total resistance is 10 kΩ. If the voltage applied is 1 V, the total current in the circuit can be computed from the formula:

$$E = IR$$

or

$$I = E/R$$

thus,

$$I = 0.1 \text{ mA}.$$

The circuit also can be analyzed in the following manner. The total current in the circuit passes through each of the resistors. The voltage across each resistor is less than the total applied voltage. However, when the voltages are added, the total equals the applied voltage. This can be computed in the following manner. The resistance of R_1 equals 5,000 Ω and 0.1 mA flows through it; then E_{R_1} = IR or 5,000 × 0.0001 = 0.5 V from A to B. Then:

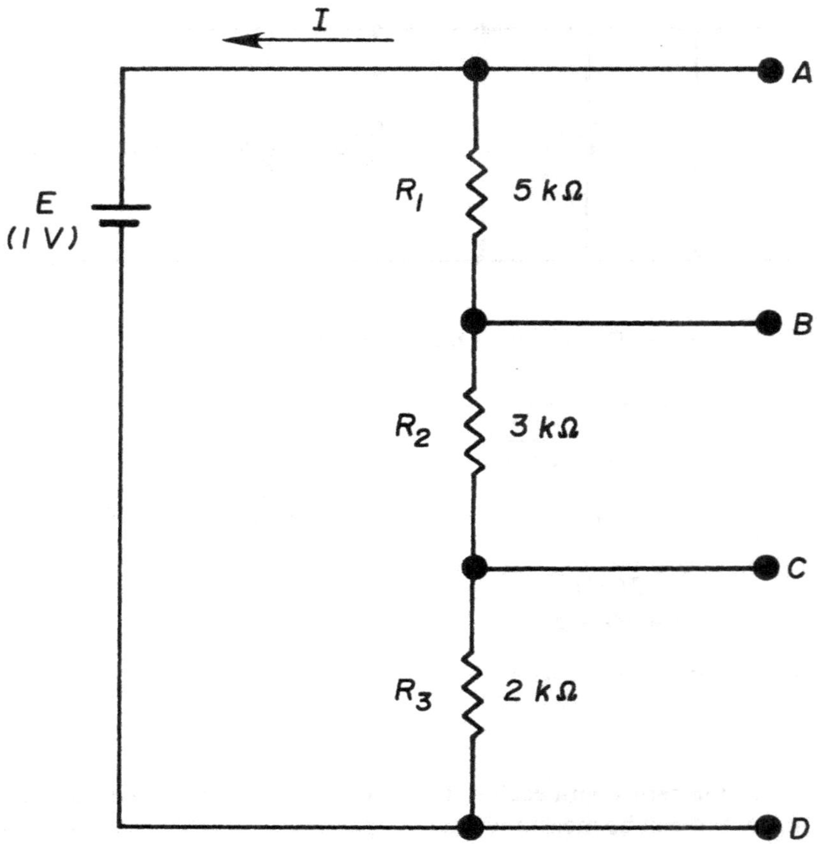

FIG. 5.18. Resistors in series.

$$E_{R_2} = 3{,}000 \times 0.0001 = 0.3 \text{ V from B to C}$$
$$E_{R_3} = 2{,}000 \times 0.0001 = 0.2 \text{ V from C to D.}$$
$$\text{Adding, } 0.5 \text{ V} + 0.3 \text{ V} + 0.2 \text{ V} = 1 \text{ V.}$$

This string of resistors (R_1, R_2, and R_3) forms a voltage divider. Between points A and B the voltage is 0.5 V. The voltage between B and D is 0.5 V. There is 0.2 V from C to D. If the total voltage was 10 V (instead of 1) it would be divided by the same proportions to 5, 3, and 2 V.

This is a practical control circuit. In an EEG instrument, it is called the sensitivity control. The sensitivity control of an EEG is a very precise voltage divider. By using the complete output, A to D in the example, maximum voltage (causing maximum pen deflection) is available at the output. This is the highest sensitivity of the particular circuit. The voltage between C and D is the lowest output available, which would correspond to the lowest sensitivity.

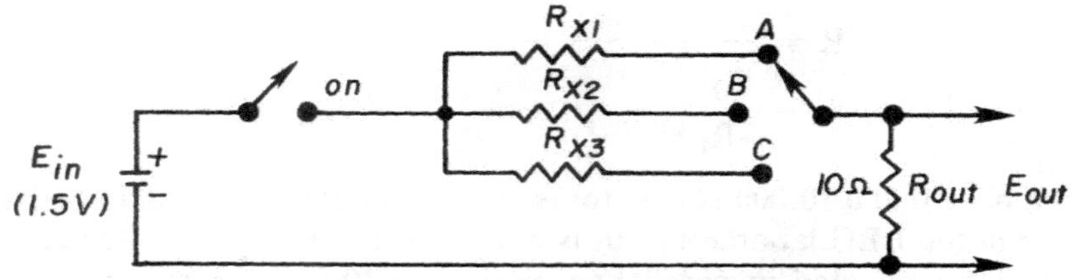

FIG. 5.19. Calibration circuit for EEG amplifier.

Another practical circuit using resistors in series is employed in the calibration circuit of a typical EEG instrument. Figure 5.19 schematically illustrates such a circuit.

When the switch is in position A, the $R_{\times 1}$ is 150,000 Ω, E_{out} will be 100 μV. When it is in position B, if $R_{\times 2}$ is 300 kΩ, E_{out} will be 50 μV. E_{out} will be 10 μV when the switch is in position C and $R_{\times 3}$ is 1.5 MΩ. The basic formula is:

$$E_{out} = E_{in}\left(\frac{R_{out}}{R_x + R_{out}}\right).$$

Since R_{out} (10 Ω) is negligible compared to R_x, it can be ignored in computing the divisor (e.g., $E_{out} = 10/150 \text{ k}\Omega \times 1.5 = 1 \times 10^{-4} = 100\ \mu\text{V}$).

Resistors in Parallel

When resistors are placed in parallel, as shown in Fig. 5.20, a different situation prevails. The voltage is constant across all resistors. The current now flows through resistors that are connected together at each end rather than being connected together end to end. Under these conditions, the total resistance of the circuit actually is less than the resistance of any individual resistor.

The formula for computing the total resistance of several resistors in parallel is:

$$R = \frac{1}{\frac{1}{R_1} + \frac{1}{R_2} + \frac{1}{R_3} + \ldots \frac{1}{R_N}}.$$

Suppose that a 10,000-Ω resistor is needed for calibrating an impedance meter in the EEG laboratory but is not available. Five 50,000-Ω resistors could be connected in parallel to produce a 10,000-Ω resistance in the circuit. This is shown together with the solution in Fig. 5.21.

The solution is simple if only two resistors are in parallel. The formula is:

$$R = \frac{R_1R_2}{R_1 + R_2}.$$

If a resistor with a value of 500 Ω is needed but is not available, such a resistance could be made by using two 1,000-Ω resistors in parallel. The solution by the formula yields a calculated resistance of 500 Ω.

$$R = \frac{1 \times 10^6}{2 \times 10^3} = 500$$

In the example of resistors in series, when a source of voltage is applied to the string of resistors, the current passing through the circuit is constant at all points and the current passing through each resistor is the same. This is not the case when resistors are in parallel. Using a 100-V source and a parallel resistive network with 1-kΩ, 2-kΩ, and 3-kΩ resistors (Fig. 5.22), the questions are: What is the current I_1 through the 1-kΩ resistor, I_2 through the 2-kΩ resistor, and I_3 through the 3-kΩ resistor? If a meter (M_1) is placed to measure current between the voltage source E and the three resistors in parallel, and if three other meters (M_2, M_3, and M_4) are placed in series with each of the resistors, the current in each branch of the circuit can be measured and compared with the total current in the circuit.

From Ohm's law, 100 mA current flows through the branch of the 1,000-Ω resistor (M_2); 50 mA flow through the 2,000-Ω branch (M_3); and 33 mA flow through the 3,000-Ω branch (M_4). The sum of the current flow in all branches is 183 mA, and M_1 will show the same value.

It is now possible, having determined the current flow in the individual branches, to cross-check the original computation of the value of three resistors in parallel. From Ohm's law, R = E/I, and inserting the values shown in the accompanying tabulation, R = 100 V/0.183 A, or R = 546.5 Ω. This is the same value obtained by going through the longer computation with the somewhat complex formula. From I = E/R, then 100/546.5 = 183 mA.

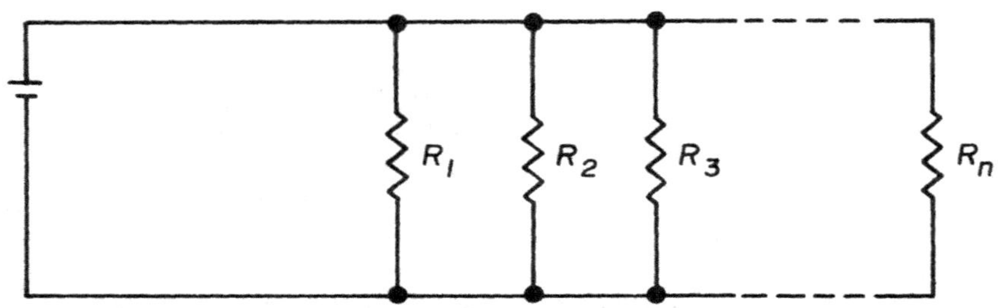

FIG. 5.20. Resistors in parallel.

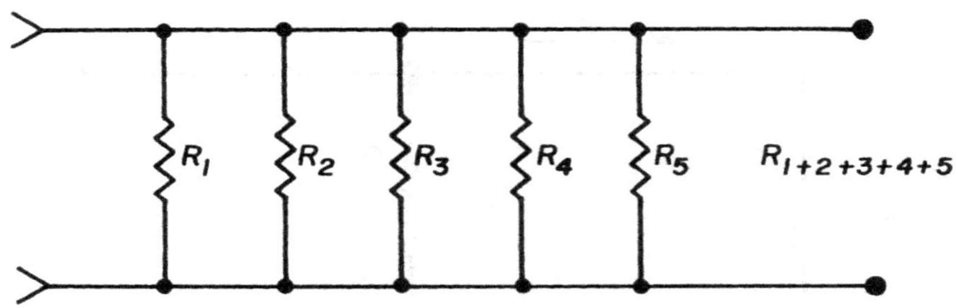

$R_1 - R_5$ each 50,000 ohms

$$R = \frac{1}{\frac{1}{50\,k\Omega} + \frac{1}{50\,k\Omega} + \frac{1}{50\,k\Omega} + \frac{1}{50\,k\Omega} + \frac{1}{50\,k\Omega}}$$

$$R = \frac{1}{.00002 + .00002 + .00002 + .00002 + .00002}$$

$$R = \frac{1}{.0001}$$

$$R = 10\ k\Omega$$

FIG. 5.21. Resistors in parallel. Schematic and solution of total resistance (see text).

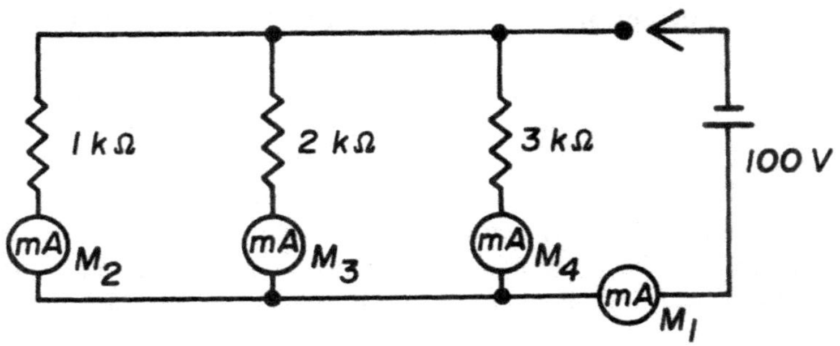

$$R = \frac{1}{\frac{1}{1\,k\Omega} + \frac{1}{2\,k\Omega} + \frac{1}{3\,k\Omega}}$$

$$R = \frac{1}{.001 + .0005 + .00033} = \frac{1}{.00183}$$

$$R = 546.5\,\Omega$$

$$\text{Total } I = \frac{E}{R}$$

$$= 183\text{ mA}$$

FIG. 5.22. Resistors in parallel. Schematic and solution of current flowing through each resistor (see text).

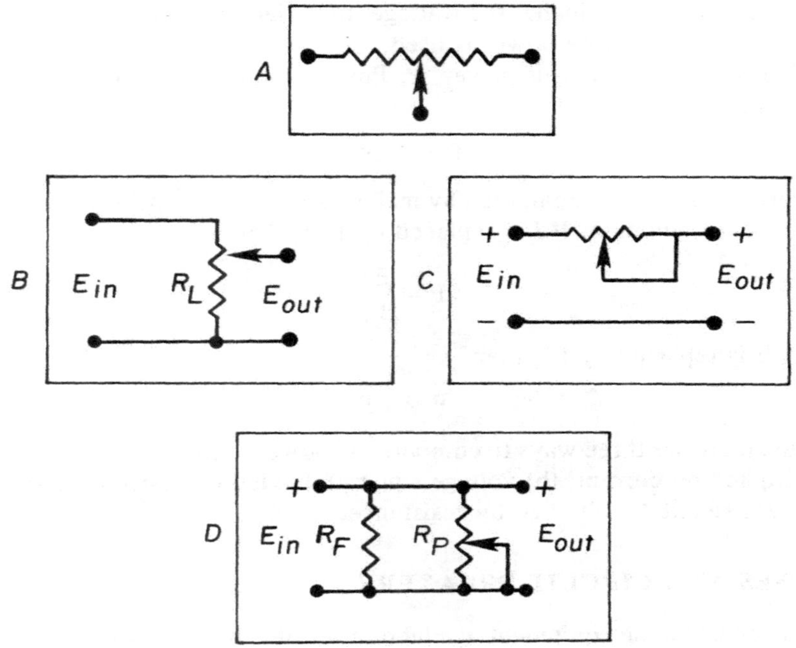

FIG. 5.23. **A:** Basic potentiometer symbol. **B:** Potentiometer as a fixed parallel load, E_{out} adjustable. **C:** Potentiometer in series circuit. **D:** Potentiometer in parallel with load to trim precisely total R.

Variable Resistors

All of the previous examples of the application of resistors have used a fixed resistor as the basic model. There are many applications that require resistance values that can be varied on a continuous scale. Figure 5.18 illustrates a circuit in which the total R could be varied in four steps from 0 Ω to 10 kΩ, with values available at 2 kΩ, 5 kΩ, and 10 kΩ. Suppose there is a need to adjust the value to be somewhere between 5 kΩ and 10 kΩ. A potentiometer would be used to carry out this function. A potentiometer is a wire-wound resistor (or, in some instances, a continuous carbon film) along which a slider can be moved to adjust the resistance to the desired value. The symbol for a potentiometer is shown in Fig. 5.23A and practical configurations are shown in Fig. 5.23B,C, and D (see figure legend).

Potentiometers are commonly used in EEG instruments. Some are used to make adjustments internally at the time of manufacture. Several are external controls used by the technologist. The sensitivity adjust and baseline adjust controls are potentiometers.

POWER

When the necessary voltage is applied across the terminals of a light bulb, electrical energy is converted to radiant energy in the visible spectrum. Household light bulbs come in various levels of brightness, usually expressed in terms of wattage, 40 watts, 75 watts, and 150 watts being fairly common. The higher the wattage, the brighter the lamp. The brighter the lamp, the more power is used.

The watt is the unit of power, P. Power equals voltage multiplied by current, or

$$P = E \times I.$$

Power also can be computed by making substitutions utilizing the basic Ohm's law equation. If I is replaced by E/R, then

$$P = \frac{E^2}{R}.$$

If E is replaced by IR, then

$$P = I^2R.$$

Thus, there are three ways to compute the power used in a circuit: voltage multiplied by current, (b) voltage squared divided by resistance, and (c) current squared multiplied by resistance.

FUSES AND CIRCUIT BREAKERS

When installing equipment in a laboratory, it is necessary to know how much power is required. Protective devices such as fuses (described below) will stop current flow when some critical power level is exceeded. An overloaded circuit is dangerous because increased power means increased heat. If 5 A current flows in a 120-V circuit, then P equals 600 watts (120 V × 5 A). If the circuit is fused for 1 kilowatt, it safely can provide 600 watts, but it cannot provide power for an instrument rated to use 1,500 watts. More current will flow than can be safely carried and the fuse will "blow." If the fuse did not blow, the wires in the circuit, which have resistance, would become hot. Such heating can cause fire. Overloaded circuits are a common cause of household and industrial fires.

If several appliances are placed on a single circuit, they must be considered as resistors in parallel. In a 120-V circuit, if one appliance has a resistance of 10 Ω, the current it draws will be 12 A. If a second appliance has a resistance of 20 Ω, the current it draws will be 6 A. If both are in the same circuit, R will be 6.66 Ω. The total current will be 18 A. The total power needed will be 2,160 watts and the circuit must be capable of carrying the current. When setting up EEG equipment, it always is necessary to add the watts required by the various instruments on a common circuit and to be certain that the circuit can handle the power requirements.

To avoid the dangers caused by overloading circuits, a special element, called a *fuse,* can be inserted between the voltage source and the appliance (see Fig. 5.15 for the schematic symbol). A fuse is a conducting element of short length designed to melt at a precomputed critical temperature that will be reached if the current is too large. When the current being drawn in a circuit is below this value, the fuse heats very little and will continue to carry current. If more current flows than the fuse is designed to carry, the metal will become hot and will exceed its melting temperature before current overload occurs. When it melts, it will open the circuit, effectively switching it off. Some fuses react rapidly. Others, called "slow blow" fuses, will temporarily carry a small overload.

Circuit breakers are commonly substituted for fuses in high power applications (e.g., the main power supply for an EEG instrument). Some circuit breakers, like a fuse, become hot when overloaded. Through expansion, a switch will be opened when excessive current flow causes the temperature to exceed the critical value. Other types are electromagnetic in function. [See Heathkit Learning Programs (8) for further discussion of circuit breakers.] The advantage of a circuit breaker is that it can be manually reset. A fuse, on the other hand, must be replaced before the instrument can be used again.

ELECTRICAL MEASUREMENTS AND METERS

Voltage, current, and resistance usually are measured with a meter. [See Heathkit Learning Programs (5) and Rusgrove and Woodward (11) for further discussion of meters.] A general purpose meter usually measures all three variables. Precision meters may be specialized to measure, for example, milliamperes, microamperes, or kilovolts.

The heart of a typical meter is a coil of wire suspended in bearings between the poles of a horseshoe magnet (Fig. 5.24). A needle is mounted on the coil, so that it moves from the left (zero) to extreme right (full-scale deflection). When current flows through the coil, the electromagnetic field causes it to move. The amount of movement is proportional to the amount of current.

Current is measured with an *ammeter*. Meters that measure small currents have milliampere scales. The basic circuit of a typical milliammeter is shown in Fig. 5.25. It will measure small currents typically in the 0 to 1

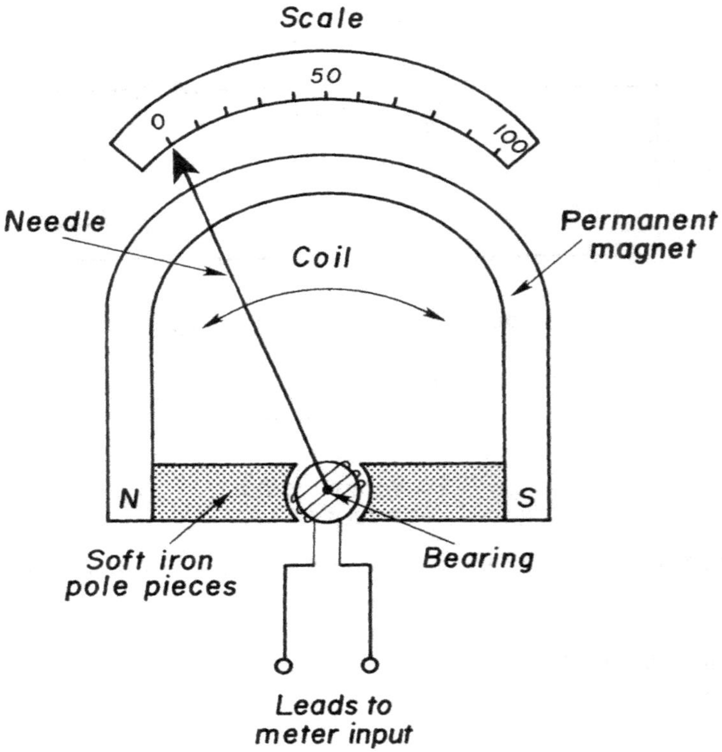

FIG. 5.24. Components of a typical meter.

mA range (the range of the basic movement). In actuality, meter measurements with 50 μA sensitivity often are used with *shunts* to extend their range.

The value R of the shunt resistor is chosen to permit current greater than 1 mA to flow through it, while current of up to 1 mA will flow through the resistance of the coil in the meter (R_m). This extends the range of the meter. If several shunt resistors are selectable by a switch, several current ranges can be measured (Fig. 5.26). The values of R_1 to R_4 can be calculated from the formula for resistors in parallel [$(R_m \times R_1)/(R_m + R_1)$] and then computing the branch currents.

The same basic meter movement can be used to measure voltage. However, it is necessary to insert a series resistor to act as a multiplier (Fig.

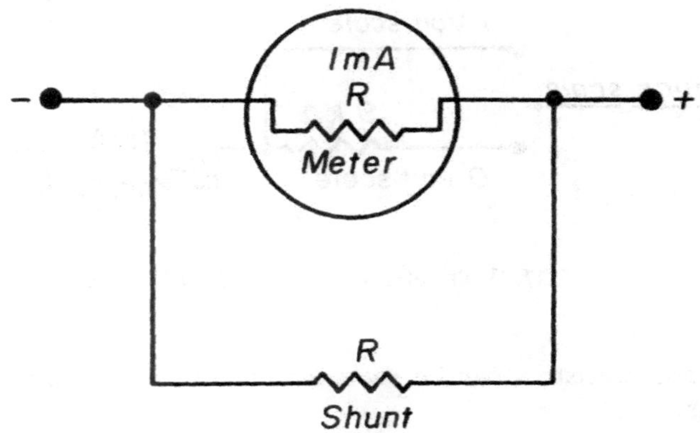

FIG. 5.25. Schematic circuit of milliammeter with shunt resistance.

5.27). If R_m is 1,000 ohms and full scale current is 1 mA, the basic movement can measure up to 1 V (E = I × R). To change the scale to 10 V, a 9,000-ohm series resistor can be added: E = I × R = 0.001 × (1 kΩ + 9 kΩ).

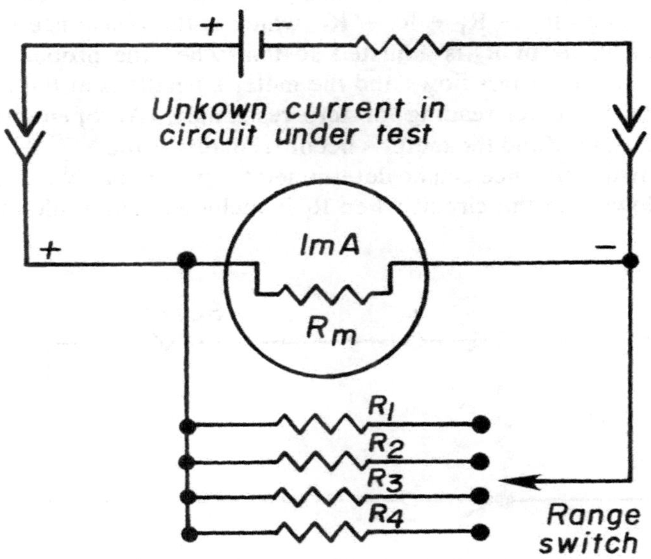

FIG. 5.26. Schematic circuit of ammeter with parallel resistors to change scale.

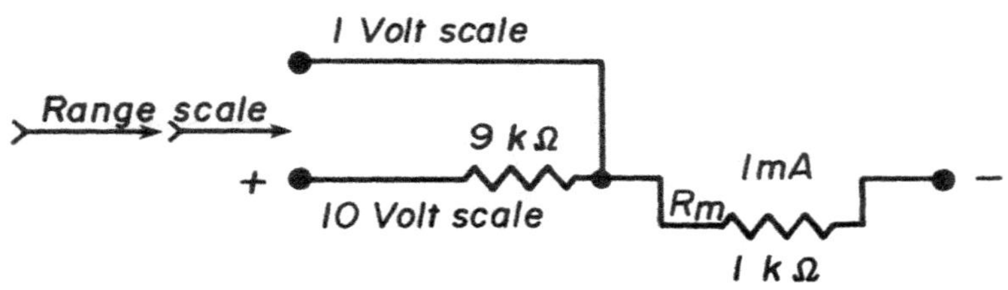

FIG. 5.27. Voltmeter with 1-V and 10-V scales.

Other series resistors can be switched in to provide ranges of 100 or 1,000 volts.

A *voltmeter* presents a resistance in parallel with the source when voltage measures are made (Fig. 5.28). The voltage across load R will therefore be affected by having meter R in parallel with load R. Consequently, it is desirable to have the value of the meter's R as large as possible. This increases the accuracy of measurement.

Resistance is measured with an *ohmmeter*. The basic circuit of such a meter is shown in Fig. 5.29. The battery, E, causes current to flow in the circuit, through $R_m + R_1 + R_2 + R_?$, which is the resistance to be measured. The value of R_2 is adjusted so that when the probes are short-circuited, exactly 1 mA flows and the meter's needle is at the right. This establishes the meter reading for zero resistance. (An open circuit is an infinite resistance and the meter's needle remains at the left.) The value of the unknown resistance can be determined from formula by measuring the current flowing in the circuit when $R_?$ is included. The scale of an ohmmeter is calibrated by the manufacturer. Usually several scales are selectable, indicated by multiplier values: R × 1; R × 10; R × 1,000.

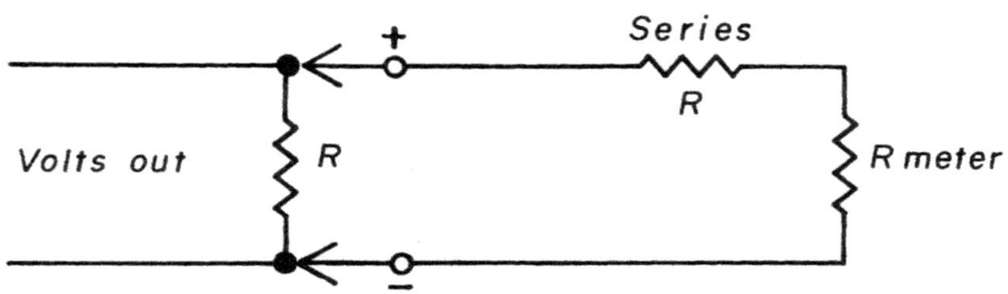

FIG. 5.28. Effect of internal resistance of voltmeter on measurement of voltage across a load. The two resistances are in parallel (see text).

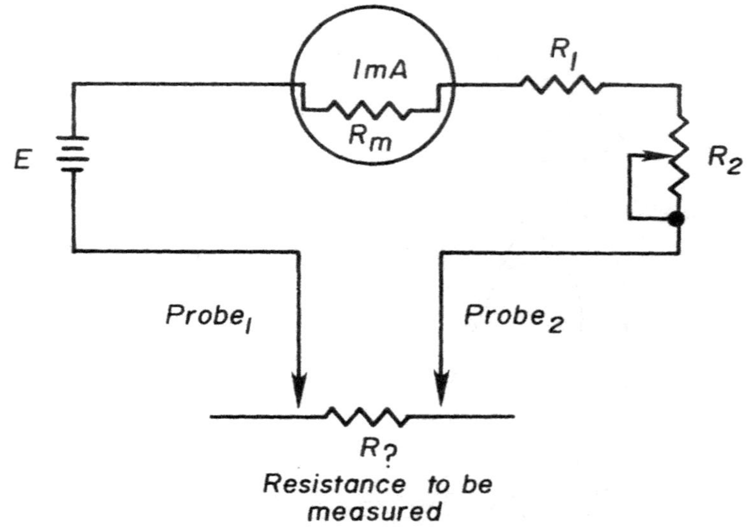

FIG. 5.29. Circuit of a typical ohmmeter. R? is the unknown resistance to be measured (see text).

CAPACITANCE

Electronic devices called capacitors are used to store electrical energy. [See Heathkit Learning Programs (5,6) and Rusgrove and Woodward (11) for further discussion of capacitors.] A *capacitor* is made up of two closely spaced flat metal plates separated by an insulating material called the dielectric. The dielectric of a capacitor may be air, glass, paper, mica, or any of several special plastics. If the two plates of a capacitor are connected to a battery, as shown in Fig. 5.30A, B, when the switch in the circuit is closed (A), free electrons (which are negative) will be attracted from the lower plate of the capacitor to the positive pole of the battery. This leaves a net positive charge on plate 1. An equal number of electrons will be repelled from the negative pole of the battery onto plate 2, leaving a net negative charge on plate 2. Consequently, the voltage (EMF) between the two plates becomes equal to the voltage of the battery. When

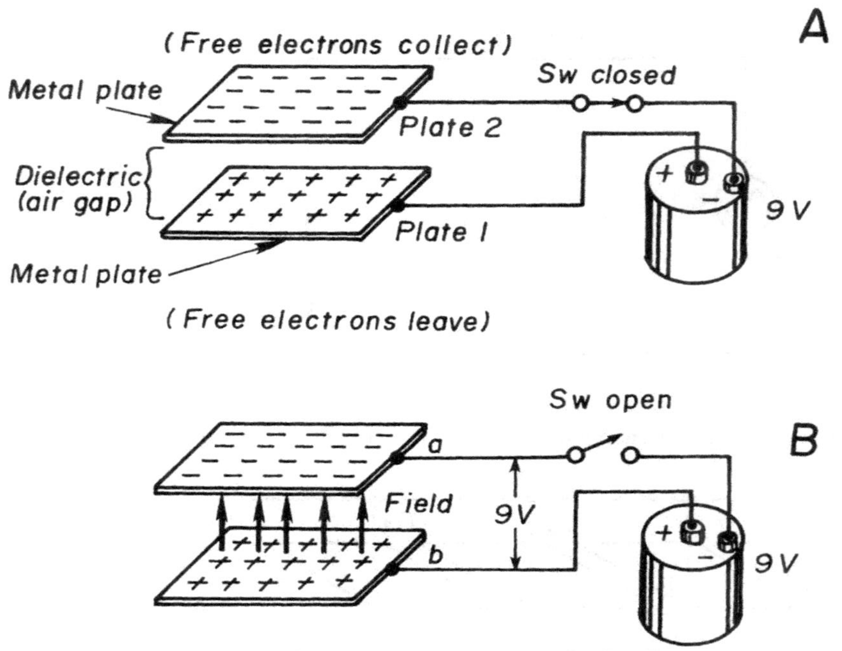

FIG. 5.30. Diagrammatic capacitor in a series with a 9-V battery.

the switch is opened, (B), the capacitor remains charged. If 9 V are used to charge the capacitor, there will be 9 V across the capacitor. This charge is maintained as an electrical field by the dielectric material that separates the positive and negative charges on the plates.

If a voltmeter with a very high resistance is inserted briefly at points *a* and *b* (Fig. 5.30B), the voltage measured between the plates of the charged capacitor will be equal to the battery voltage, i.e., 9 V in the example discussed.

Figure 5.31 shows, using the conventional schematic symbols, the equivalent circuit of the components in Fig. 5.30.

The electrical "size" of a capacitor (C) is an index of the number of electrons that it can store when a given voltage is applied. The unit of capacitance is the *farad* (F). The capacitance of any capacitor is determined by the surface area of the plates, the distance between the plates, and the dielectric.

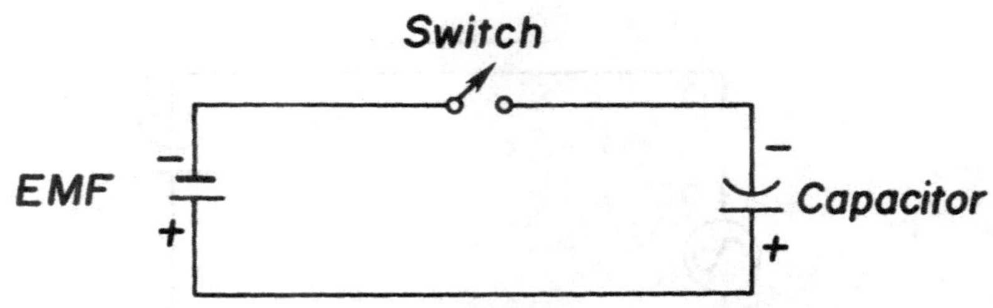

FIG. 5.31. Equivalent circuit of Fig. 5.30.

Because the farad is a large unit, in practical electrical circuits, it is necessary to deal with micro units of capacitance (millionths of farads) (10^{-6} F). The abbreviation is μF. There also are still smaller subunits, called picofarads (1×10^{-12} F), abbreviated pF; 1 pF is one millionth of 1 μF.

Direct current, which is unidirectional, does not "flow through" a capacitor. As described above, electrons flow onto one plate while electrons are removed from the other plate. Alternating current, however, flows first in one direction and then in the opposite direction. When a capacitor is connected in series with a source of AC and its load, one plate of the capacitor will be alternately positively charged (and the other alternatively negatively charged) as in Fig. 5.32 A, B. Although the AC does not "flow through" the capacitor, the circuit acts as though it does because of this continuous alternation of charge. The amount of flow will depend on the frequency of alternation of the current (in Hz) and upon the size of the capacitor and the voltage impressed from the generator. [See Heathkit Learning Programs (5,6) and Rusgrove and Woodward (11) for further discussion of AC current and capacitance.]

Capacitors in Parallel

When two or more capacitors are connected in parallel, the total plate area is increased and thus the capacitance is increased. Therefore, when 3 capacitors are in parallel, the total capacitance is the sum of C_1, C_2 and C_3, in μF. Figure 5.33A shows a schematic equivalent of parallel capacitors. Figure 5.33B diagramatically shows that the plate area is increased but the spacing is unchanged. Thus $C_{total} = C_1 + C_2 + C_3$. [See Heathkit Learning Programs (5) for further discussion of capacitors in parallel.]

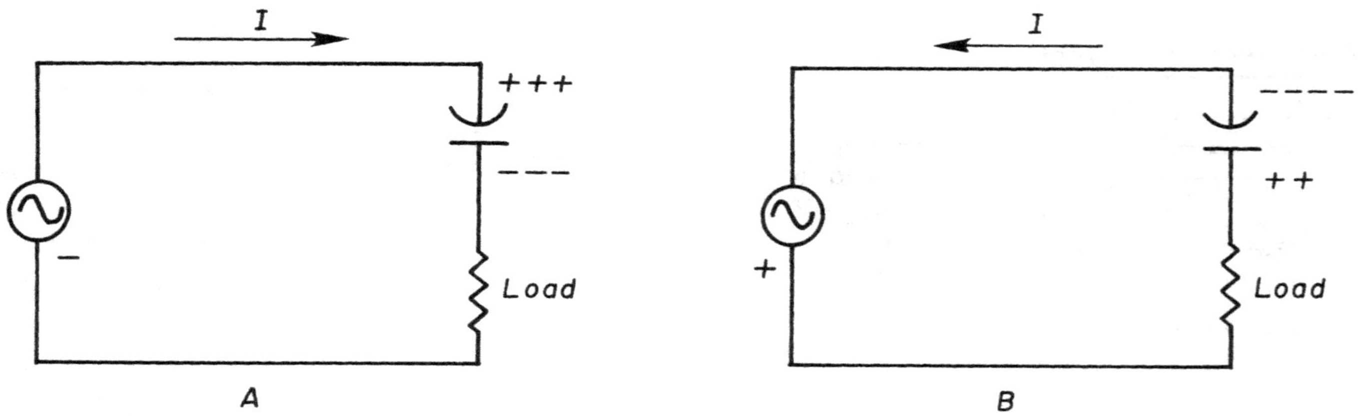

FIG. 5.32. **A:** Charge of capacitor on negative half-cycle of AC voltage. **B:** Reversal of charge on positive half-cycle of AC voltage.

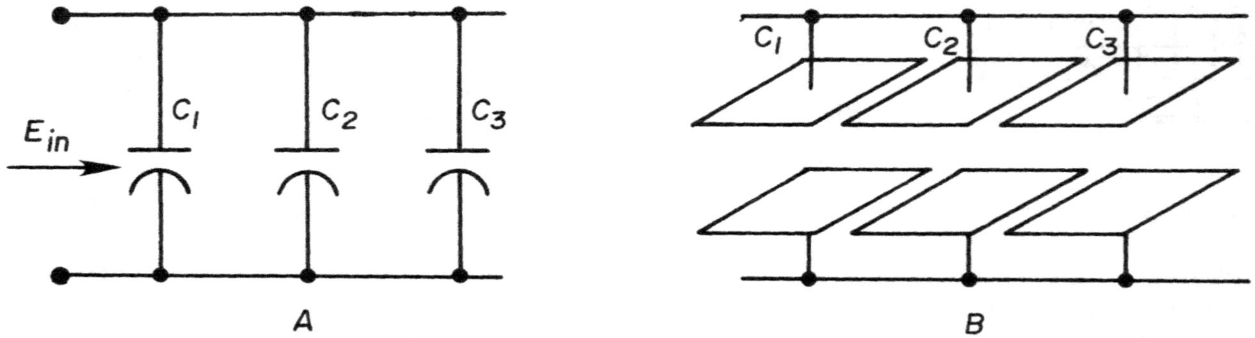

FIG. 5.33. **A:** Schematic diagram of capacitors in parallel. **B:** Pictorial diagram of **A** illustrating increase in equivalent size of plates.

Capacitors in Series

If capacitors are in series (Fig. 5.34A), the total capacitance is:

$$C_{total} = \frac{1}{\frac{1}{C_1} + \frac{1}{C_2} + \frac{1}{C_3}}$$

Figure 5.34B diagramatically shows that the series capacitors maintain the same plate area but increase the spacing between plates (by a factor of three in this example). [See Heathkit Learning Programs (5) for further discussion of capacitors in series.]

TIME CONSTANT

When, as in Fig. 5.35A, a battery is connected across a capacitor through a resistor and the switch is closed at position 2, it takes time for the capacitor to become fully charged. This is due to the resistance in the circuit. For a fixed value of C, the larger the resistance, the longer the

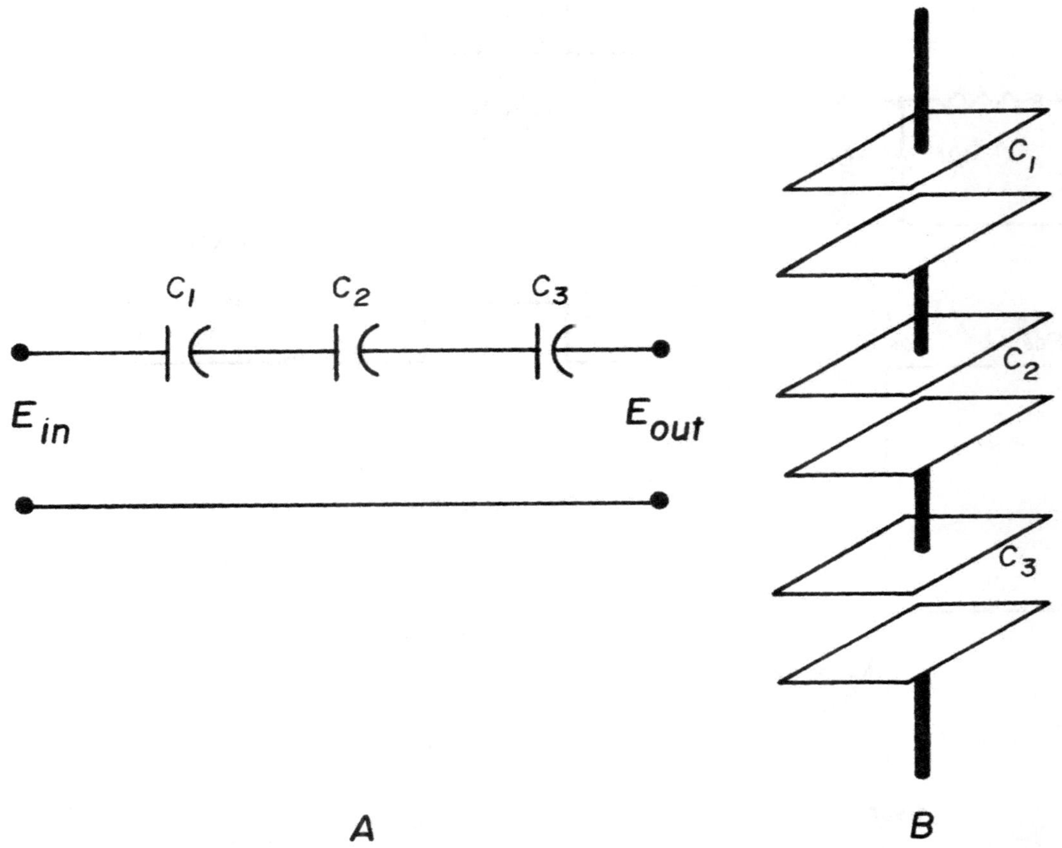

FIG. 5.34. A: Schematic diagram of capacitors in series. **B:** Pictorial diagram of **A** illustrating increase in spacing of plates.

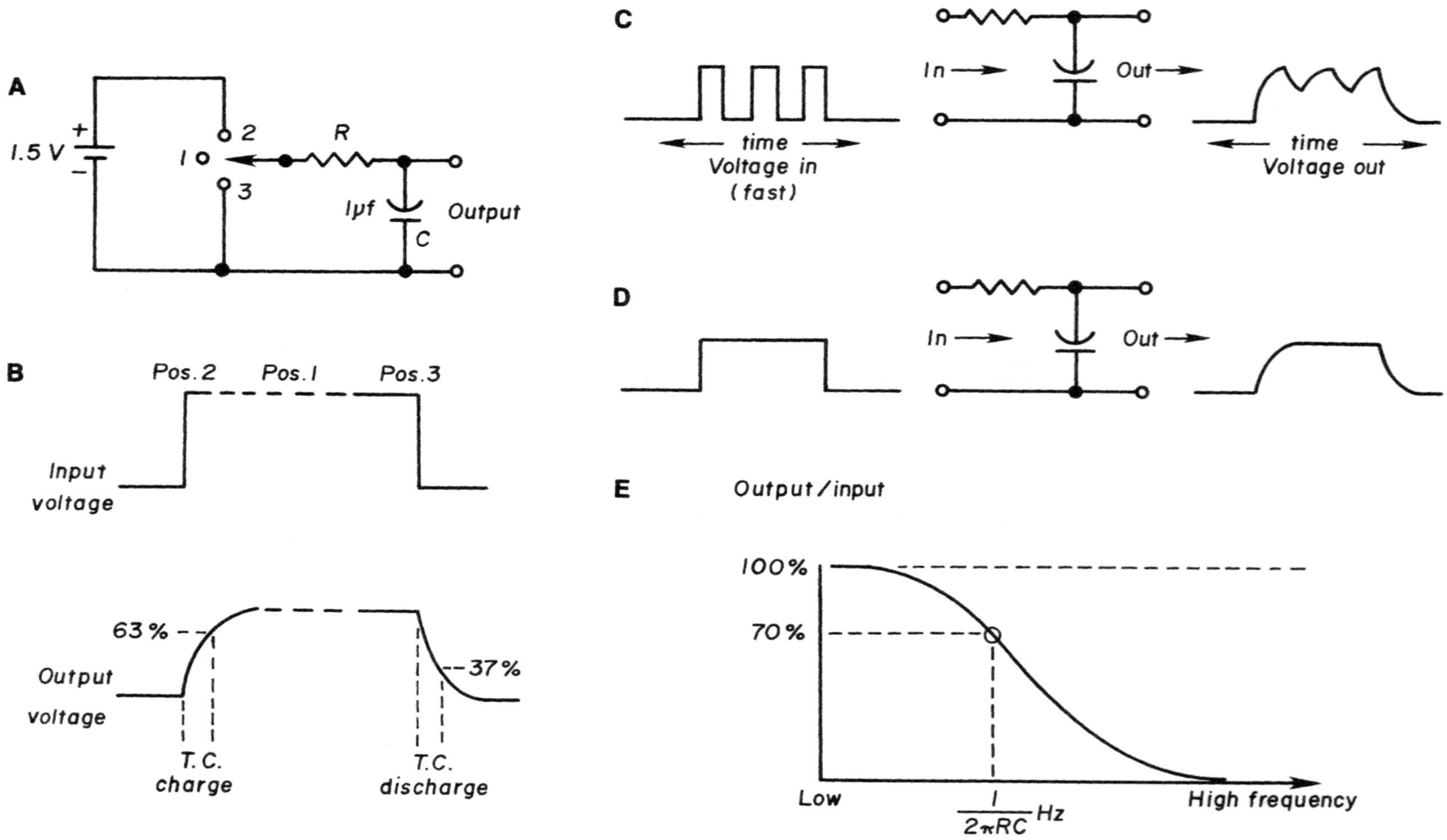

FIG. 5.35 A: Charging a capacitor through a resistor when switch is at position 2. B: Input voltage at switch positions 2, 1, and 3, and corresponding output voltage at each switch position. C: Basic configuration of a high frequency filter with output across a capacitor. Change in output voltage when switch in A alternates rapidly between positions 2 and 3. D: Change in output voltage when switch in A cycles slowly between positions 2 and 3. E: Cut-off frequency defined for high frequency filter. (See text for further discussion.)

time required for the capacitor to become fully charged. If the switch is moved to "1," the charge remains on the capacitor, as previously discussed. If the capacitor now is discharged through the resistor by moving the switch to position 3, it will take a finite period of time for the discharge to be completed.

If a voltmeter is placed across a charged 1-μF capacitor which has been charged from a 1.5 V DC source, the measured voltage will initially be 1.5 V. As measurement continues, the voltage will slowly decrease, eventually reaching zero. The time required to return to zero will depend on the internal resistance of the meter, which acts as R in Fig. 5.35A. In the same way that the charging time was determined by the value of the resistance in the circuit, so was the discharge time determined. These times are a function of the capacitance and the resistance.

Refer to Fig. 5.35B in conjunction with Fig. 5.35A. The time required for the 1-μF capacitor to charge to 63% of its full charge when the switch is closed (i.e., moved from position 1 to position 2) is the *time constant* (TC) of the capacitor-resistor circuit. This is often called the rise time constant since it is measured on the rise of the output. After the capacitor is charged, when the switch is again moved to position 1, the charge is stored. If moved to position 3, C will discharge. The time required for this discharge to decay to 37% of the full charge (or to reach 63% of complete discharge) also equals the time constant of the circuit. The time constant can be computed by the formula:

$$\text{TC} = \text{C (farads)} \times \text{R (ohms)}.$$

In practical units, this is:

$$\text{TC} = \text{C } (\mu\text{F}) \times \text{R (megohms)}.$$

If C is 1 μF and R is 1 MΩ, it will take 1 sec for the capacitor to charge to 63%, or to discharge to 37% of the full charge value. [See Cooper et al. (2), Geddes and Baker (3), and Heathkit Learning Programs (5) for further discussion of the time constant.]

HIGH FREQUENCY FILTER

As we have seen, the step response of the circuit in Fig. 5.35B is a "slowly" rising voltage that eventually equals the input voltage. If the switch is moved rapidly between positions 2 and 3, the total input simulates a high frequency input. The output will just start to rise when the input drops back to zero (Fig. 5.35C). If the switch is slowly cycled between positions 2 and 3, the output will have time to follow the input (Fig. 5.35D). The circuit passes low frequencies but attenuates high frequencies. It acts as a *high frequency filter,* reducing the amplitude of high frequencies.

The circuit responds to sine waves by allowing low frequency sine waves to pass without attenuation, whereas high frequency sine waves are attenuated. It also is called a *low-pass filter* because it does not attenuate low frequencies. The dividing point between low and high frequency is $1/2\pi$ RC Hz, where $\pi = 3.1416$. This is called the cut-off frequency (Fig. 5.35E). At the cut-off frequency, the output voltage will be 70% (actually, $\sqrt{2}/2$) of the input. This is a 30% decrease in the amplitude of the output. Signals with higher frequency components above the cut-off will be increasingly attenuated as their frequencies increase.

The high frequency filter setting $1/2\pi$ RC Hz is inversely proportional to the time constant, RC. Thus the longer the rise time constant, the lower the high frequency filter setting. In order to vary the high frequency filter setting, R is usually fixed and various capacitors are selected by the high frequency filter switch.

Phase Shift in High Frequency Filter

The high frequency filter not only attenuates the output, but it may, when the output is compared to the input, shift its apparent occurrence in time (Fig. 5.36A). This is called *phase shift.*

Channel 1 of Fig. 5.36A is a circuit without filters. Its input and the inputs of channels 2, 3 and 4 are the same. The HF filters on these channels are set at 70 Hz, 35 Hz, and 15 Hz, respectively. The peaks of the waves have been shifted at the outputs of the channels with filters, indicated by the dotted line. The outputs of channels 3 and 4 are attenuated.

An intuitive approach to phase shift is to imagine half of a sine wave input to a circuit with a rise time constant (Fig. 5.36B). Multiply the wave by the rising curve and the result is an attenuated wave shifted to the right or delayed in time. If the frequency of the input is low, the output will not be attenuated and the phase difference will be zero (positive and negative peaks of the input and output occur simultaneously). As the input frequency approaches $1/2\pi$ RC, the output is attenuated and shifted to the right (appears at a later time) compared to the input. At the cut-off frequency,

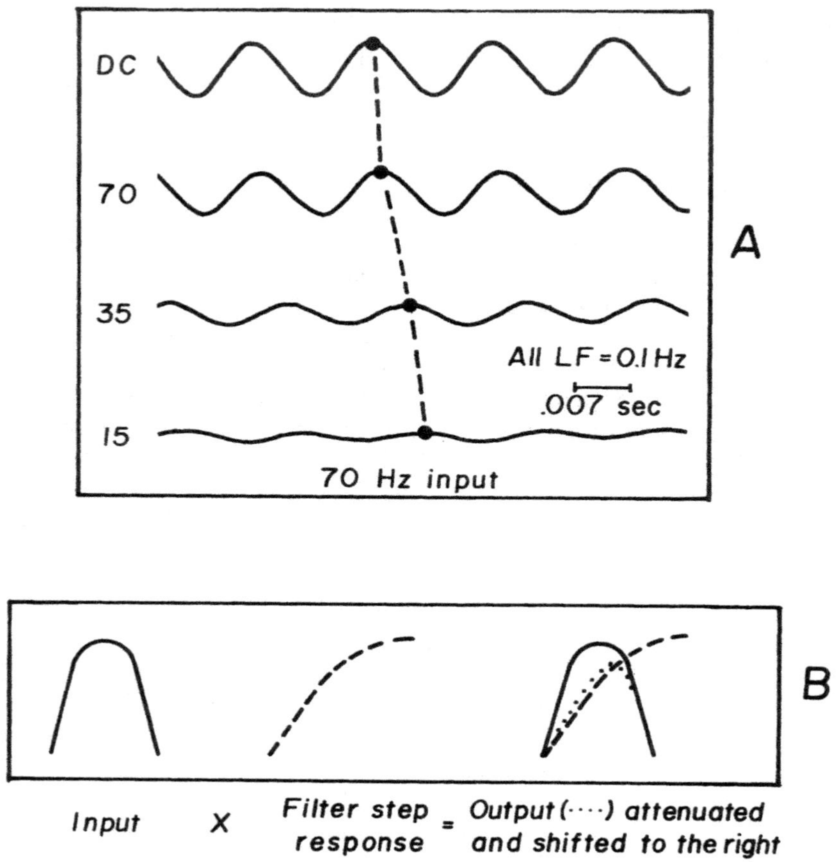

FIG. 5.36. Phase shift: high frequency filter (A). Diagrammatic explanation of phase shift and attenuation (B).

1/2π RC, the output is 70% of the input and is delayed by 45° or one-eighth of the full cycle of 360°. The phase shift introduced by high frequency filters usually is disregarded in clinical EEG. At 15 Hz, the duration of one cycle is 1/15th sec, or 0.067 sec. Thus 45° of this would be only 0.0083 sec. At a chart speed of 30 mm/sec, this would be 30 × 0.0083, or approximately 0.25 mm. Even at "the worst case" (LF 15-Hz filter), the measured delay would be less than the width of the line made by the recording pen. [See Heathkit Learning Programs (6) for further discussion of phase shift and high frequency filters.]

LOW FREQUENCY FILTERS

If the positions of the resistor and the capacitor in Fig. 5.35A are reversed, the filter is changed from a high frequency filter to a *low frequency filter*. This configuration is shown in Fig. 5.37A. This is also called a *high-pass filter*. [See Heathkit Learning Programs (6) for further discussion of phase shift and low frequency filters.]

The step or calibration response of the low frequency filter can be deduced because we know the waveforms of the input voltage and the voltage across the capacitor (the high frequency filter response, rise time constant) (C). When a DC calibration voltage is applied to a resistor and capacitor in series, the voltage across the capacitor plus the voltage across the resistor must equal the input voltage. The output of the low frequency filter is the voltage across the resistor (Fig. 5.37A). Thus, this voltage can be obtained by subtracting the voltage across the capacitor (response of the high frequency filter to calibration) from the input voltage. This is done graphically in Fig. 5.37B.

The input (a) immediately rises to 100%, while the voltage across the capacitor (b) starts rising from 0. The voltage across the resistor (c) must start at 100% of the initial value. Although the rise time constant of the high frequency filter (the voltage across the capacitor) is measured at 63%, the decay time constant of the low frequency filter (the voltage across the resistor) is measured at 37%.

When the calibration button is released, the input voltage immediately drops to 0. The voltage across the capacitor is 100% at this point (and decays to 0). The voltage across the resistor must start at 0% minus 100%, or −100%. The output of the low frequency filter now goes in a direction opposite to that when the voltage was first applied. The pen responds by dropping below baseline when the calibration button is released.

The low frequency filter passes high frequencies and attenuates low frequencies. The dividing point between low and high frequencies (the cut-off frequency) is 1/2π RC Hz. (Fig. 5.36C). At this frequency, the output signal is 70% of the amplitude of the output signal. The same inverse relationship exists between the decay time constant and the filter setting. Thus the longer the decay time constant, the lower the low frequency filter setting.

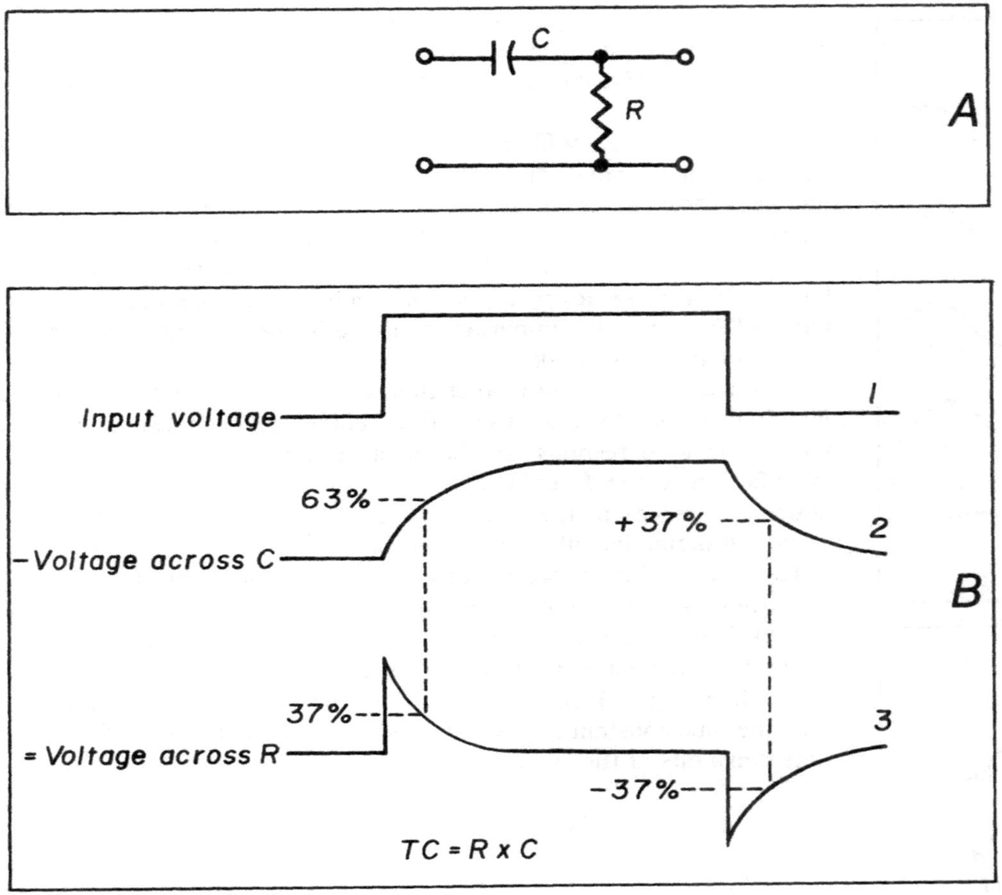

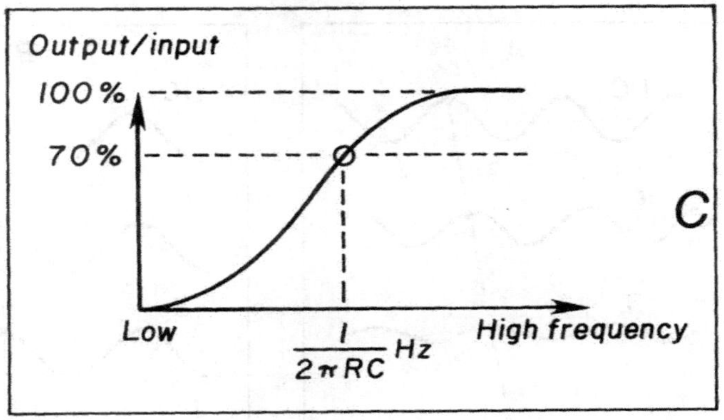

FIG. 5.37. A: Basic configuration of a low frequency filter with output across a resistor. **B:** DC voltage applied to input and voltage across C and R. **C:** Cut-off frequency defined for low frequency filter. (See text for discussion.)

Phase Shift in Low Frequency Filters

The output not only is attenuated, but it also is shifted in time. Figure 5.38A, B compare input and output with four low frequency filters (0.1, 0.3, 1, and 5 Hz) at two low input frequencies. These are typical EEG low frequency filter settings. The phase shift and the attenuation are seen clearly. The low frequency filter shifts the output to the left, or earlier in time. Again, an intuitive explanation may be seen in Fig. 5.38C where half a sine wave is multiplied by the decay time constant. The time constant falls before the input reaches its peak and thus the output appears shifted ahead in time. If the input frequencies to the low frequency filter are high enough, the output is not attenuated or shifted. If the input frequency equals $1/2\pi$ RC Hz, the output is attenuated by 30% and shifted 45° to the left.

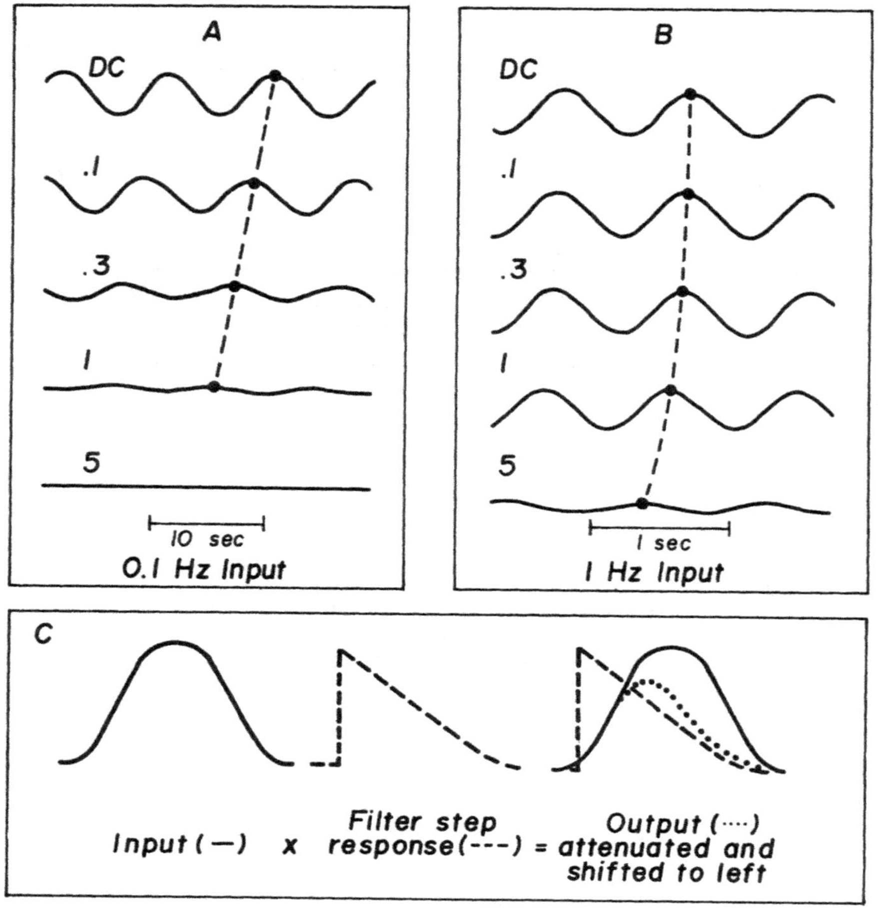

FIG. 5.38. Phase shift in low frequency filters. A: Effect of 0.1-, 0.3-, 1-, and 5-Hz filters on 0.1-Hz sine wave input. DC channel has no filter. *Dotted line* shows shift in phase. B: Effect of same filters on 1-Hz sine wave input. C: Diagrammatic explanation of phase shift and attenuation (see text).

If the low frequency filter is set at 1 Hz ($1/2\pi$ RC = 1), a 1-Hz wave is shifted 45° or 1/8 wave. This is 1/8 sec, or 125 msec. At a chart speed of 30 mm sec, the apparent peak of the 1 Hz is displaced by nearly 4 mm. Consequently the phase shift of low frequency filters is important in clinical EEG. It should be noted, however, that the phase shift caused by both high and low frequency filters can be much more critical in evoked potential studies, where the important measure is latency and amplitude measures usually are secondary.

In actual practice, a few other things affect the above theory. First, at high frequencies, the response of the oscillograph becomes important and affects the total response of the electroencephalograph. Second, some manufacturers label filters to define cut-off as 20% instead of 30% attenuation. References to the frequency response for each particular instrument will define its cut-off frequencies.

The relationship between decay time constant of the low frequency filter and its component values holds only for single stage filters (Fig. 5.39A). If there are two or more stages of filtering in series the decay no longer is a simple exponential curve and there will be overshoot on return to baseline (Fig. 5.39B). The time constant of filters in series will be less than the time constant for any single section. It can be estimated from the time constants of the single stages:

$$TC \cong \frac{1}{\frac{1}{TC_1} + \frac{1}{TC_2} + \frac{1}{TC_3} + \cdots}$$

INDUCTANCE

Inductance is the property a circuit possesses that causes a voltage to be induced in the circuit when there is a variation in current flow. As shown in Fig. 5.40A, there will be a change in voltage in the circuit when

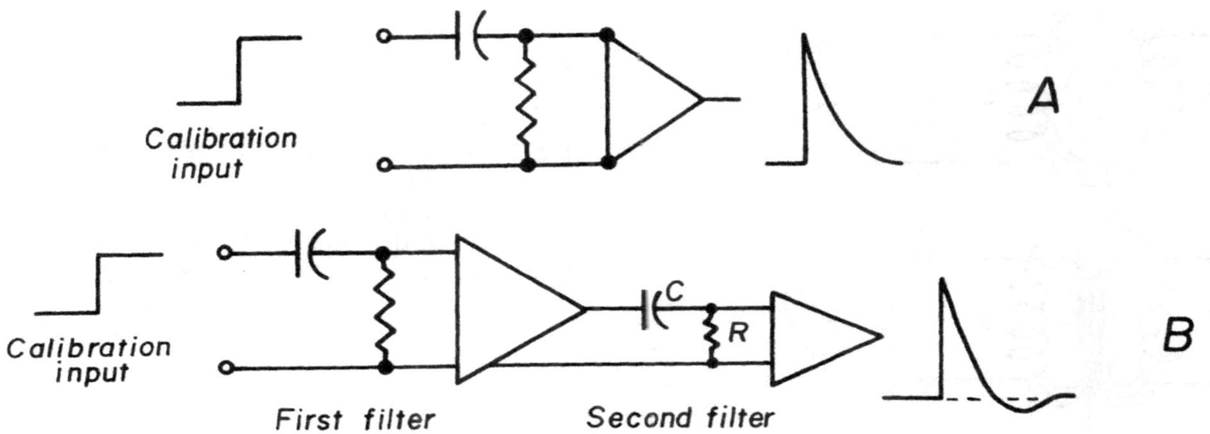

FIG. 5.39. A: Single-stage RC filter output. B: Two-stage RC filter and output.

the switch is closed (A). Current starts to flow in the circuit and a magnetic field is built up rapidly around the wires connecting the battery, switch, and inductance (B). The buildup of the magnetic field "cuts" the wires and induces an opposing voltage *in the same circuit*. This is a "counter EMF." The induced current opposes the original current; however, the induced voltage will be short-lived and will not continue. When the switch is opened (C) current stops flowing and the magnetic field collapses. The collapse of the field again induces voltage in the circuit. The direction of current flow induced by the voltage will be in the same direction of the original current. The effect is analogous to inertia; inductance opposes any change in current.

The unit of inductance is the *henry*, and the symbol for inductance is L. Straight wires have some inductance, but more practical inductors are formed by coils (refer to Fig. 5.15). The more turns in the coil, the larger the inductance. By placing the coil over an iron core, a further increase in inductance occurs. [See Heathkit Learning Programs (5,6) and Rusgrove and Woodward (11) for further discussion of inductance.]

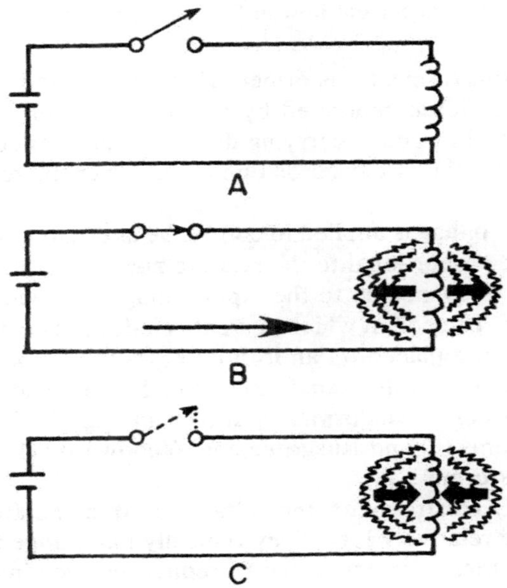

FIG. 5.40. A: Current will flow when switch is closed. B: Current flows when switch is closed and magnetic field builds up in circuit represented by R. C: Current stops flowing when switch is opened; magnetic field reverses.

TRANSFORMERS

When two coils are placed adjacent to each other, the flow of current in one coil generates a magnetic field that induces current flow in the sec-

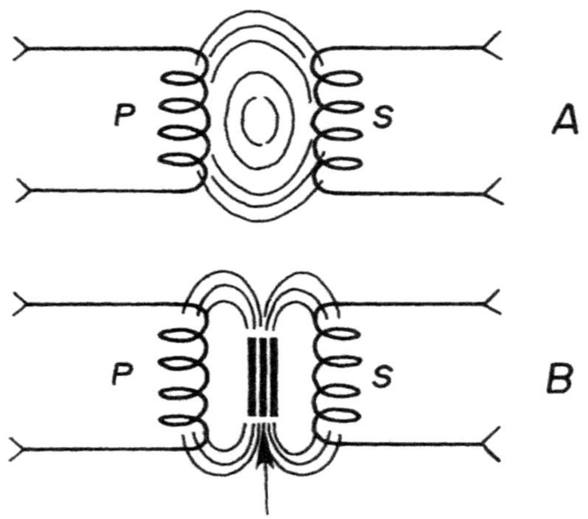

FIG. 5.41. A: Air core transformer. Current flow in second coil induced by magnetic field resulting from current flow in first coil. **B:** Iron core transformer.

ond. The two coils form a transformer. This is illustrated in Fig. 5.41. The magnetic lines of force generated by coil P "cut" coil S, and induce a voltage in coil S. In circuits carrying direct current, induction will occur only when the switch is closed or opened or when there is a change in voltage.

When an AC voltage is applied to coil P, the alternating voltage induced in coil S will be proportional to the relative number of turns in each coil. The coil which is connected to the input voltage is called the *primary* of the transformer. The coil in which current is induced is called the *secondary*. If the coils are placed on an iron core, there will be a considerable increase in efficiency of the transformer (Fig. 5.41B). The schematic symbol for an iron core transformer is shown in Fig. 5.15. [See Heathkit Learning Programs (6) and Rusgrove and Woodward (11) for further discussion of transformers.]

In modern EEG instruments, the voltages used to operate the electronic components are relatively low. They typically may range from 1.35 to 12 and 24 V. It is therefore necessary to reduce the nominal 117 V of the mains to the required operating voltages. This is done by the use of transformers, having a smaller number of turns in the secondary coil than in the primary.

REACTANCE AND IMPEDANCE

Capacitive Reactance

The capacitor opposes changes in voltage. When alternating current is placed across a capacitor, it is alternately charging and discharging. The time required for the charge and discharge causes opposition to the changes in applied voltage, and this in turn causes opposition to the flow of current in the circuit. This opposition is called capacitive reactance. Capacitive reactance is a resistance and it impedes current flow. It has a special symbol: X_C. It is measured in ohms. Its value is determined by the frequency of the AC voltage and by the size of the capacitor:

$$X_C = \frac{1}{2\pi\ fc}$$

where $\pi = 3.1416$, f = frequency in hertz, and c = capacitance in farads. This can be simplified as:

$$X_C = \frac{0.1592}{fc}.$$

A 10-Hz EEG signal is applied in series with a 2 μF capacitor. What is the reactance of the capacitor at this frequency?

$$X_C = \frac{1}{2\pi\ (10 \times 2 \times 10^{-6})}$$

$$= \frac{1}{0.000126}$$

$$= 7{,}937\ \Omega.$$

Inductive Reactance

When current begins to flow in an inductor, there is counter EMF which opposes the applied voltage. The opposition (impedance) to current flow has the same effect as a resistor and lowers the total voltage. This is inductive reactance, X_L. It is measured in ohms and is expressed:

$$X_L = 2\pi\ fL$$

where $\pi = 3.1416$, f = frequency in hertz, and L = inductance in henrys.

For practical purposes, X_L is negligible in EEG amplifiers compared to X_C and R. Inductance, however, is a factor in power supplies.

Impedance

The combined effect of resistance and reactance is called impedance (Z). Sometimes the term impedance is used in a general sense, even though a circuit has only resistance. In such a case, the proper term is "resistive impedance." Although a capacitive (or an inductive) impedance is expressed in ohms, it is not correct simply to add a resistive impedance and a capacitive impedance. The proper formula for adding series resistance and capacitive (or inductive) reactance is:

$$Z = \sqrt{R^2 + X^2}.$$

In the circuit shown in Fig. 5.42, if R = 3 kΩ and X_C = 4 kΩ, the total impedance is 5 kΩ.

If there are resistive, capacitive, and inductive impedances (in series) to be added, then:

$$Z = \sqrt{R^2 + (X_C - X_L)^2}.$$

[See Heathkit Learning Program (6) and Rusgrove and Woodward (11) for further discussion of impedance.]

GROUND

In electronic instruments, there are three grounds: (a) earth (the building or power outlet) ground, (b) the chassis, or case ground, and (c) the common connection of the electronic circuitry. The symbol for each is shown in Fig. 5.43. The similarity between earth and building ground is seen in Fig. 5.44, and the relationships between patient ground, circuit ground, and earth ground are diagrammed in Fig. 5.45. [See Heathkit Learning Programs (5) for further discussion of ground.]

The National Electrical Code (10) requires that the chassis of instruments such as the electroencephalograph (which is used in critical care areas) be connected to earth or power ground. Any current leaking to the chassis (for example, from a power supply circuit) then may flow harmlessly to earth ground (see Chapter 6). In the United States, earth

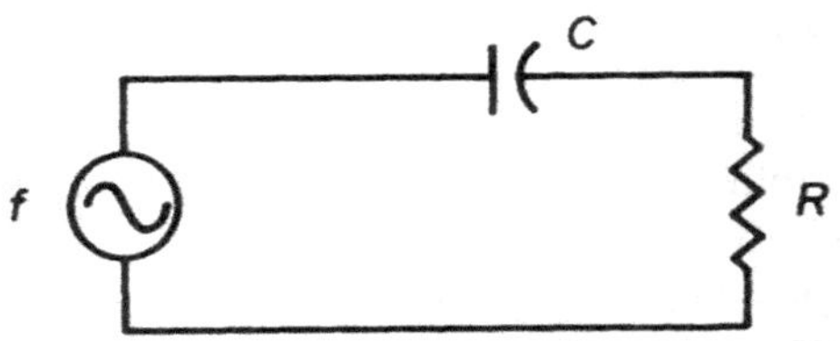

FIG. 5.42. Impedance (Z) is determined by frequency (f), C, and R.

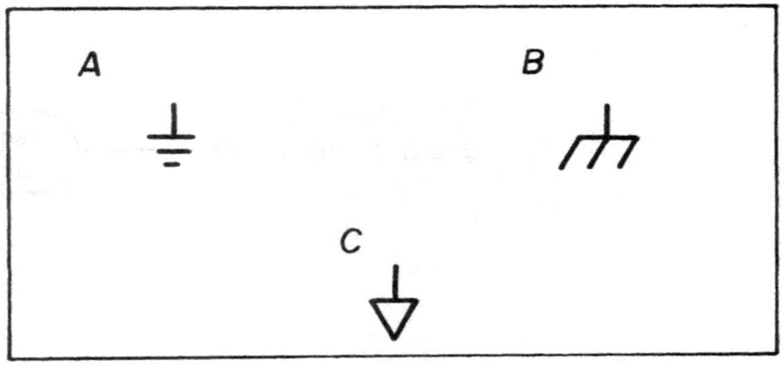

FIG. 5.43. Symbols for ground. A: Earth ground. B: Chassis (case) ground. C: Common connections of circuit.

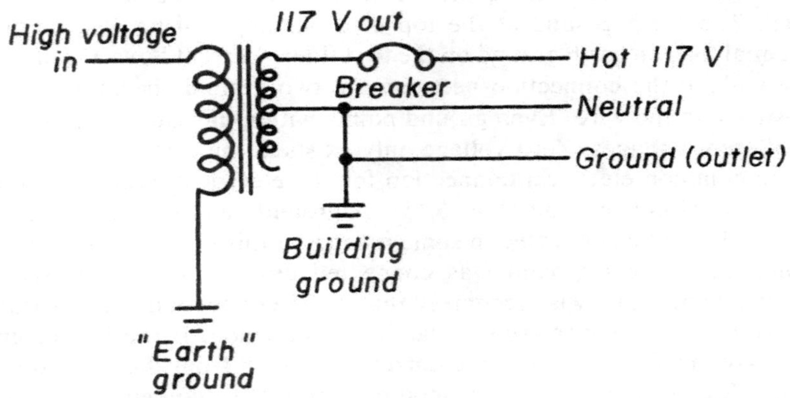

FIG. 5.44. Schematic representation of high voltage line supplying a building, and relationships of grounds—earth, building, and receptacle.

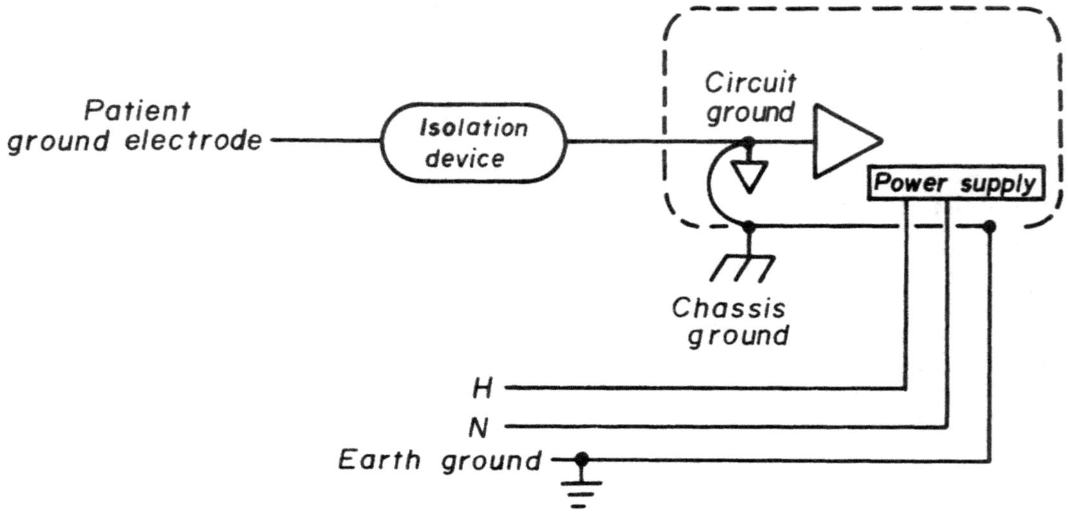

FIG. 5.45. Diagrammatic relationships between grounds in an EEG laboratory: earth, chassis, circuit, and patient.

and chassis ground must be connected, and they are often considered the same.

It should be noted, however, that not all earth grounds are exactly equal. The earth ground at the top of a building will be at a different potential than an earth ground on the first floor. Current flows through the wire making the connection between the two grounds because there is resistance in the wire. Even ground points within the same room may be at different voltages. Zero voltage only exists at the earth.

The common electrical connection for the electrical circuitry is often called the circuit ground (Fig. 5.45). A ground electrode attached to a patient should be connected in some manner at this point. In older instruments, the patient ground was connected directly to the chassis and power ground. It now is recognized that direct connection of the patient's electrode to the power ground should not be made. If the instrument's earth ground fails, any leakage current will flow from the ground electrode, through the patient, to another ground. If another device is attached to the patient, its leakage current could find a direct path to ground through the patient to the EEG ground electrode. Therefore, it is present-day practice to place some type of isolation device in the patient ground circuit (Fig. 5.45).

Currents also can flow into or from other patient connections (amplifier inputs) although the path is not direct. These inputs have high impedance only as long as the input voltages are in the microvolt or millivolt range. At higher voltages, these inputs have a much lower impedance. This is due to circuit elements such as protective diodes that start conducting at approximately 0.7 V, or reverse biasing field effect transistors, in which case, they exhibit low resistances.

AMPLIFICATION

The most important application of electronics to EEG deals with amplification. Amplification involves the electronic processing of very small voltages so that they control much larger voltages or currents, which can be more easily measured. [See Cannon and Luecke (1), Heathkit Learning Programs (8), and Rusgrove and Woodward (11) for further discussion of amplification.]

To facilitate thinking about amplifiers, a schematic symbol may be used in place of a full circuit diagram (see Fig. 5.15). Figure 5.46 shows a single-ended amplifier that accepts a voltage at "IN" and delivers a voltage at "OUT." The voltage at each location is with reference to ground. The output voltage is larger than the input voltage, i.e. it is amplified. The ratio of the output voltage to the input voltage is the amplification factor of the amplifier (also called the "gain"). If 0.01 V IN produces 10 V OUT, the amplification factor is 10/0.01 or 1,000.

The amplifier does not increase the original 0.01-V input signal. A voltage source (provided by the power supply) is connected to the amplifier (E_{E+} + E^-; Fig. 5.46). The original input voltage controls the resistance from E^+ to output and E^- to output. When the input is 0.0 V, there is no output. At input levels between 0 and 0.01 V, the output is proportional: 0.001 IN, 1.0 OUT; 0.002 IN, 2 OUT; 0.005 IN, 5 OUT, for example. By analogy, the amplifier functions as if the input voltage controlled the potentiometer, shown in Fig. 5.46. Variation in the position of the arm of the potentiometer changes the output voltage, E_{out}. It should be emphasized that the source of the output voltage, E_{E+} and E^-, the power supply of the power amplifier, is entirely independent of the input voltage.

A single-ended amplifier is not readily adaptable to EEG instrumentation. If pairs of scalp electrodes are connected to such amplifiers, one electrode of every pair will be grounded. As shown in Fig. 5.47, electrodes 2, 3, and 4 are connected to ground. They are short circuited, and Input 2 of each amplifier is at ground potential. There can be no voltage difference between electrodes 2 and 3 (channel 2) and 3 and 4 (channel 3).

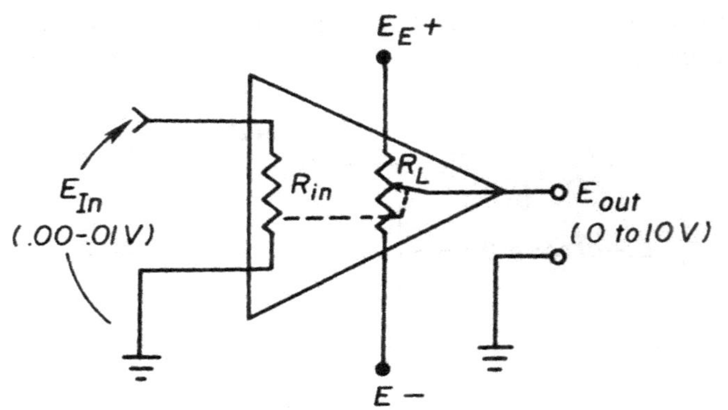

FIG. 5.46. Single-ended input amplifier (model). *Dotted line* indicates that the current flowing in R_{in} by analogy controls the arm of potentiometer, R_L, which varies E_{out}. (See text.)

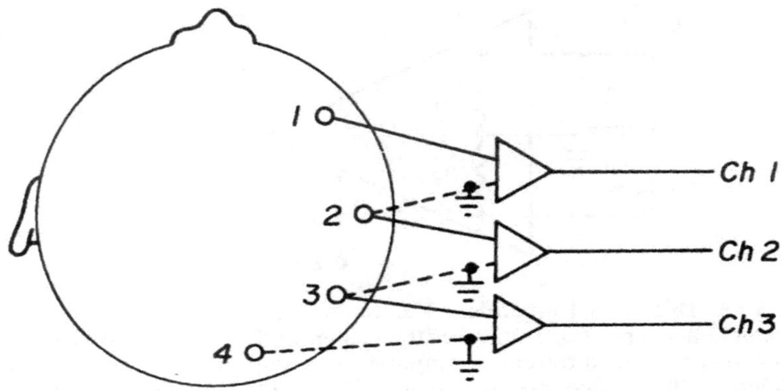

FIG. 5.47. Problem with single-ended amplifiers (see text).

Differential Amplifier

A differential amplifier is used in electroencephalography. It amplifies only the difference in voltage between the two inputs, neither of which is at ground potential. It does not amplify equal (common) voltages at the two inputs. [See Heathkit Learning Programs (8) for further discussion of differential amplifiers.]

A differential amplifier is shown schematically in Fig. 5.48. Inputs 1 and 2 are separated from ground by a very high impedance (Ri_1 and Ri_2) and from each other by an impedance of twice that value. The output may be single-ended (E_C), although it may be differential ($E_{C1}-E_{C2}$), as shown in Fig. 5.49. Differential amplifiers allow the use of multiple electrode derivations, using electrodes in common, but with minimal interaction (Fig. 5.50).

In Fig. 5.50, the same electrode (electrode 2) may be connected to two amplifiers and not be grounded directly. Some impedance imbalance develops when two inputs are connected to one electrode, however, since R_{A2} and R_{B1} are connected in parallel (Fig. 5.51) between electrode 2 and ground. If R = 10 megohms (M), the imbalance is:

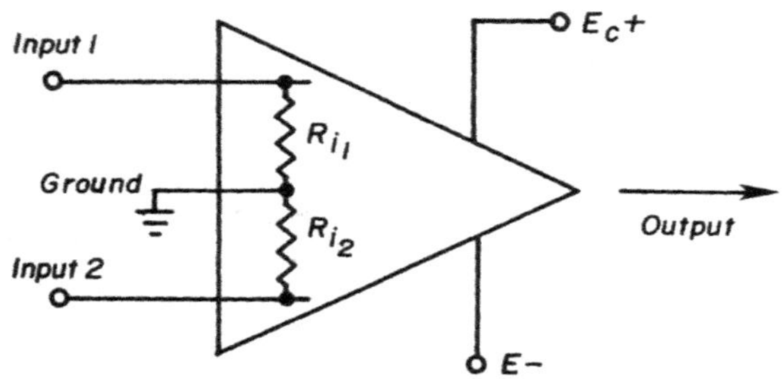

FIG. 5.48. Differential amplifier. Values of Ri_1 and Ri_2 are typically 5–10 megohms. Each input stage amplifies the voltage *at that* input, relative to ground. In this regard, the differential amplifier is composed of two single-ended amplifiers. If the voltages are equal (e.g., 100 μV), then there is no difference and the output, relative to ground, will be zero.

$$10\text{ M}: X$$

$$\text{where } X = \frac{R_{A2} \times R_{B2}}{R_{A2} + R_{B2}} = \frac{10\text{ M} \times 10\text{ M}}{20\text{ M}} = \frac{100\text{ M}^2}{20\text{ M}} = 5\text{ M}.$$

The imbalance is 10M to 5M (or 2:1).

When referential montages (see Chapter 13) are used, the imbalance becomes much greater, since 8 or 16 (or more) inputs, all from the reference electrode, are connected in parallel. External interference is much more evident when using referential montages, because the imbalance causes interference to be amplified unequally. This effect may be avoided through the use of special preamplifiers.

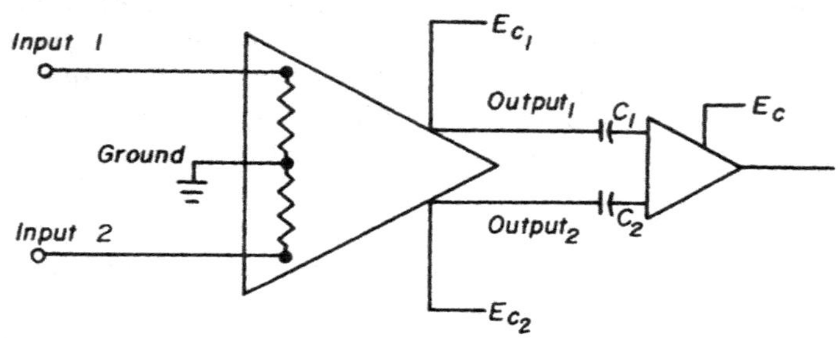

FIG. 5.49. Two stages of differential amplification with single-ended output of second stage.

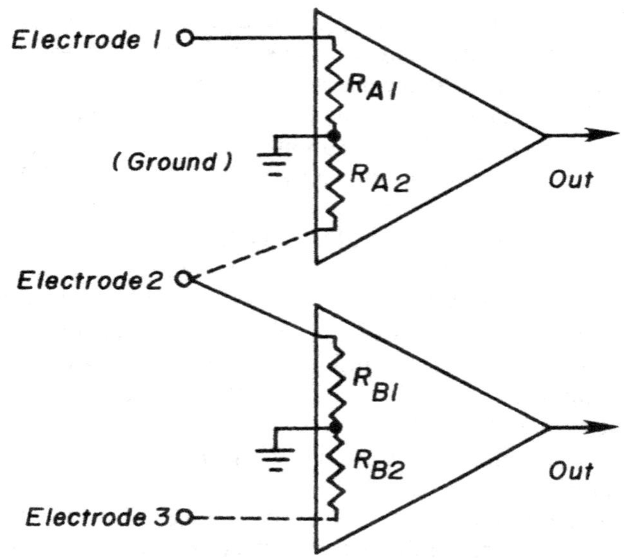

FIG. 5.50. Use of differential amplifiers to record from a common electrode (electrode 2) with maximal isolation from ground and with minimal inter-channel interaction. Compare with Fig. 5.47.

One advantage of the balanced differential amplifier lies in its ability to reject external interference. A radiating electrical field such as can originate in the 60-Hz AC mains is diagrammed in Fig. 5.52. It equally affects Inputs 1 and 2 of a differential amplifier. This is called a *common mode*

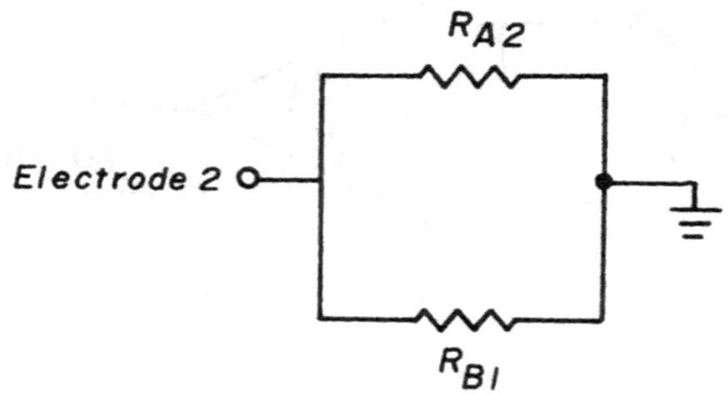

FIG. 5.51. Equivalent circuit of electrode 2 in Fig. 5.50. R_{A2} is resistor in first channel and R_{B1} is resistor in second channel (see text).

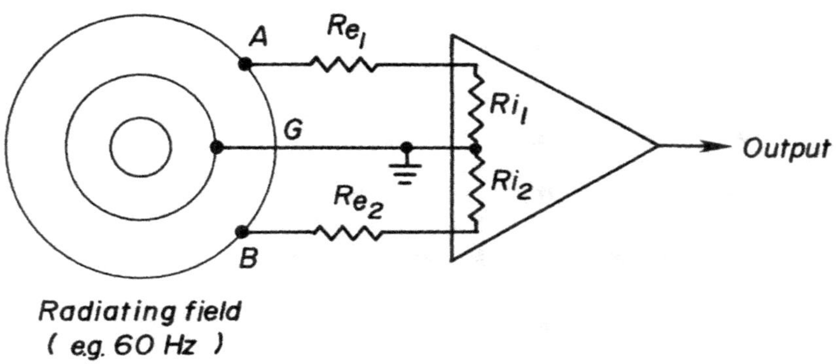

FIG. 5.52. A and B are electrodes in EEG derivation; G is ground electrode on patient. Re_1 and Re_2 are electrode resistances. Ri_1 and Ri_2 are amplifier input impedances.

signal. Current will flow from each input to ground through R_1 and R_2. If the resistances are absolutely equal, the currents will be equal, and there will be no voltage appearing at the output. If there is a difference in the current flow in the input resistors, then the amplifier will have an output proportional to its amplification factor. As discussed above, if the amplification factor is 1,000 and if the voltage difference between the inputs is 0.001 V, the output will be 1.0 V.

The degree to which an amplifier will reject a common mode signal is expressed as a figure of merit, called the *common mode rejection ratio* (*CMRR*). The CMRR is determined by the method shown in Fig. 5.53A, B. A voltage is applied simultaneously to the two inputs of a differential amplifier and ground (Fig. 5.53A). This is a common mode signal. The input voltage that is required to produce a 10-mm deflection of the recording pen is determined. The input voltage now is connected between the inputs (Fig. 5.53B). This is the differential signal. The voltage necessary to produce an equal output, 10-mm deflection, is determined. The ratio of the voltage of the common mode signal to the voltage of the differential signal is then computed (E_{CM}:E_{Diff}). This is the common mode rejection ratio.

If the voltage required to produce a 10-mm deflection in the common mode input configuration is 500 mV and the voltage required to produce a 10-mm deflection in the differential configuration is 50 μV, the CMMR is 10,000 to 1, a typical value for an EEG amplifier. [See Cooper et al. (2), Grass Instrument Company (4), and Heathkit Learning Programs (8) for further discussion of the common mode rejection ratio.]

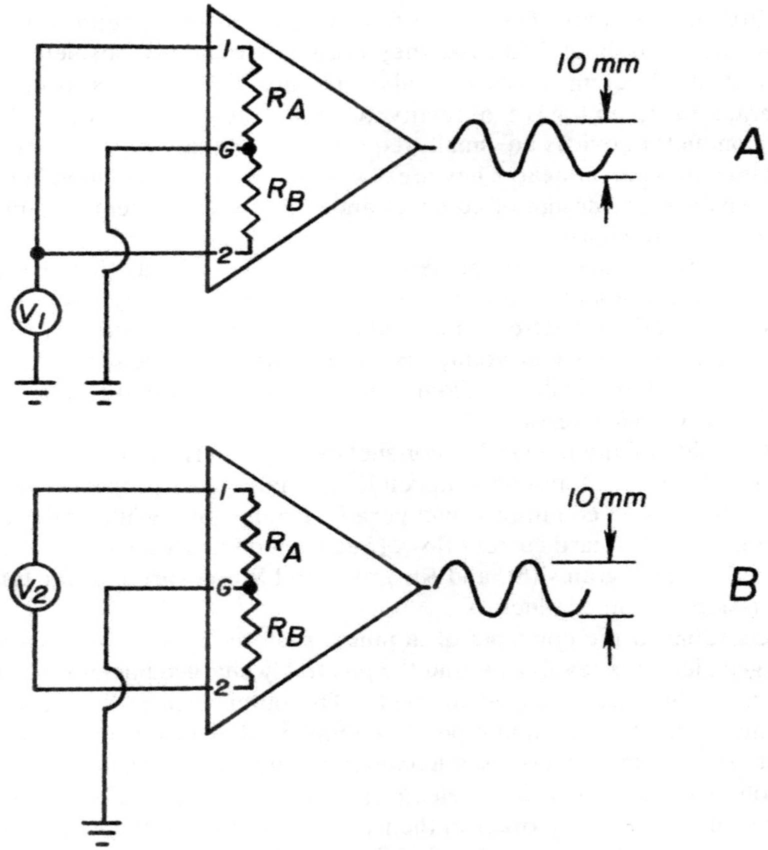

FIG. 5.53. Determining common mode rejection ratio (CMRR). CMRR = common mode input voltage to produce 10-mm deflection (A) ÷ differential mode input voltage to produce 10-mm deflection (B).

SEMICONDUCTORS

Today, amplification is achieved almost universally through the use of semiconductor devices. Only a few years ago, vacuum tubes were used to amplify small signals. They were first introduced in neurophysiological applications in about 1920, but they became essentially obsolete in the early 1970s. Vacuum tubes are bulky, require high voltages to operate, generate heat, and have a relatively short life. On the other hand, semiconductor devices are small, require low voltages, and do not generate large amounts of heat. They are stable, have a relatively long life, and have enabled the design of compact and efficient equipment for amplification of small signals.

From a technical standpoint, semiconductors are exactly that. They are neither good conductors nor good insulators, although they have characteristics of both conductors and insulators, as well as another important characteristic: If a small voltage is suitably applied to a semiconductor device, it can be switched from acting as an insulator to acting as a conductor (or vice versa).

The ability of any material to conduct electrons is related to the number of free electrons. A usable semiconductor must have properties which, under the desired conditions, will permit current flow, while under other conditions, will retard current flow. [See Cannon and Luecke (1), Heathkit Learning Programs (6), and Rusgrove and Woodward (11) for further discussion of semiconductors.]

According to the concepts of atomic structure (p. 31), the negatively charged electrons revolve around the positively charged nucleus in orbits, and the orbits are arranged in shells. The outer shell is known as the valence shell. The maximum possible number of electrons in this shell is eight. Two commonly used semiconductor materials, germanium (Ge) and silicon (Si) have four valence electrons in their valence shells. Ge (or Si) atoms adjacent to each other in their crystal form share the valence electrons of single atoms with those of four neighboring atoms, as shown in Fig. 5.54. [See Heathkit Learning Programs (7) for further discussion of silicon and germanium semiconductor crystal structure.] It is as if each atom has a stable configuration of eight electrons in its outer shell. This causes bonding, which keeps the atoms together. A shared electron forms a covalent bond.

If an electron escapes from the lattice position in the covalent bond, a vacant space or "hole" occurs. [See Heathkit Learning Programs (7) for further discussion of "hole-electron pair."] An absence of negativity in this instance is the equivalent of a positively charged particle. This empty space becomes a relatively positive hole. Schematically, what has occurred is the creation of a hole-electron pair (also shown in Fig. 5.54). An electron has been knocked out of orbit and is now free to move. In its absence, there is a relatively positive hole that can attract any free electrons that are in the vicinity.

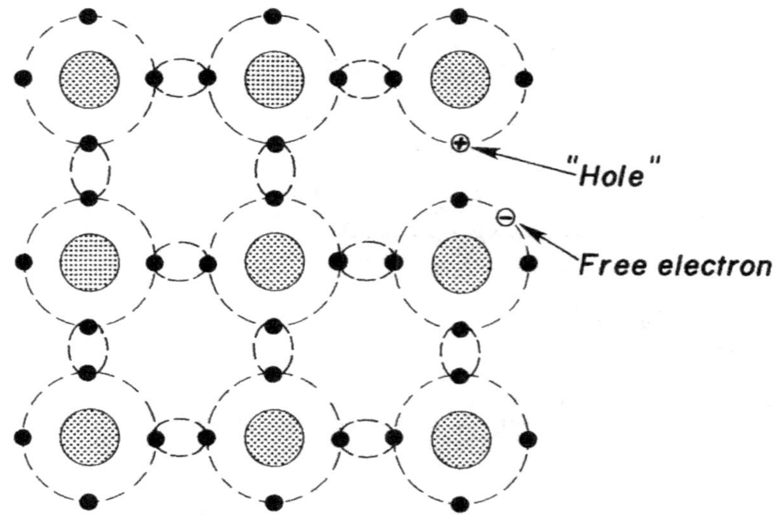

FIG. 5.54. Crystal structure of silicon semiconductor. ● = Shared electrons in outer shells; ⊖ = free electron; ⊕ = "hole" left by free electron.

Because of random drift, electrons occasionally escape from the covalent bond and create a paired hole, and other free electrons are drawn from their covalent bond to fill the first hole. When an electron moves to fill one hole, it then creates another hole. The hole will appear to move in a direction opposite to the movement of the electron. If this process can be controlled, the electron movement will cause current flow.

When a source of EMF is placed across a semiconductor (Fig. 5.55), any free electrons will be forced to move to the positive pole. The holes created by the free electron will move toward the negative pole. The number of holes that move will be equal to the number of electrons that move.

This is to be contrasted with current flow in a pure conductor. Current flow in such a conductor involves only electrons. In a semiconductor, current flow involves the movement of both electrons and holes.

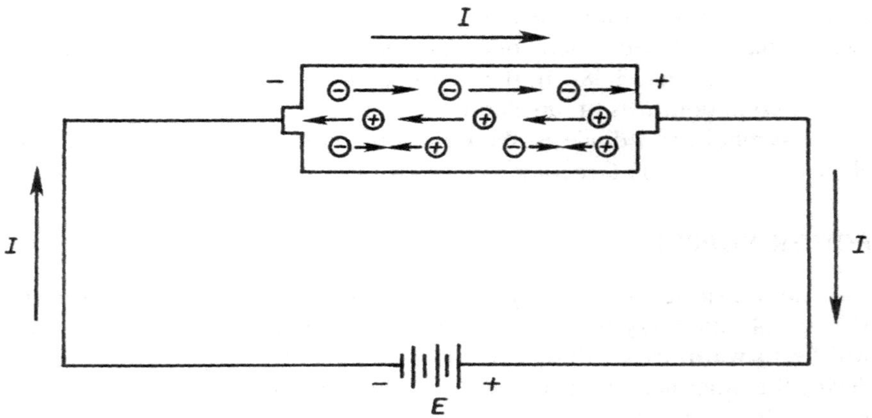

FIG. 5.55. Conduction in semiconductor.

Doping

Under normal conditions, pure semiconductors have available only a small number of free electrons and holes, so they do not conduct readily. It is technically possible to create special semiconductor materials by adding controlled impurities to make them more conductive. This process is called doping. [See Cannon and Luecke (1) for further discussion of doping.] One element commonly used for doping is arsenic (As), which has five electrons in its valence ring; thus As is pentavalent. An arsenic atom has one more valence electron than Ge and Si (which are tetravalent). If As and Ge are crystallized together, arsenic atoms can replace some of the germanium atoms in the crystal lattice. In so doing, the fifth electron, an extra electron which is not bonded, is easily set free. With the proper mixture of As and Ge, a large number of free electrons becomes available. This material is called an N-type, or negative type, semiconductor because the surplus electrons make it negative. If an EMF is placed across an N-type semiconductor, the electrons donated by the As will move to the positive pole. A few free electrons from the Ge also will move to the positive pole. The holes they leave move toward the negative pole.

If silicon is doped with an element such as gallium (Ga) or boron (B), which is close to its atomic structure but has only three electrons in its valence ring, a crystal lattice is formed that has an excess of holes. There will be seven electrons available which is one too few to establish a covalent bond with eight electrons. The surplus holes act like positively charged particles. Therefore, this material is known as a P-type, or positive-type, semiconductor. When an EMF is placed across this material, holes move toward the negative pole and any free electrons move to the positive pole.

Diodes

An elementary but important semiconductor device can be constructed by placing a piece of N material in contact with a piece of P material. This device is a *junction diode*. Its intrinsic behavior is shown in Fig. 5.56.

Holes migrate from the P-type material to the N-type material, and electrons from the N-type material migrate to the P-type material. This continues until the imbalance in charge is great enough to prevent the migration from continuing. This imbalance in charge is called the *barrier voltage* and is approximately 0.3 V for Ge diodes and 0.7 V for Si diodes. Holes and electrons in the junction area combine and form a depletion region, depleted of holes or electrons.

If a voltage is impressed across the diode with negative connected to the N-type material and positive to the P-type material (Fig. 5.57), current will not flow until the voltage exceeds the barrier voltage. As the applied

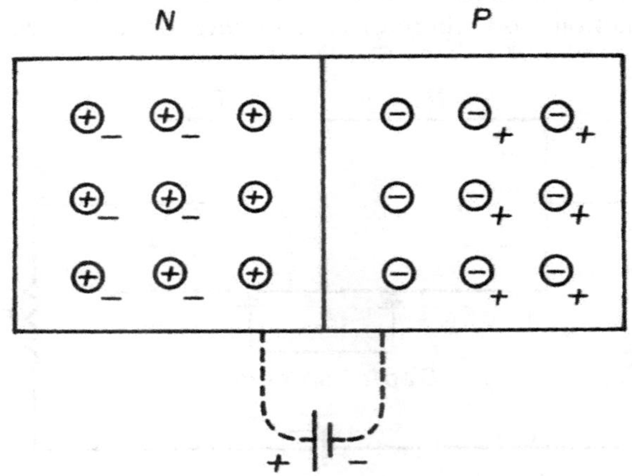

FIG. 5.56. Barrier voltage in junction diode (*dotted lines*).

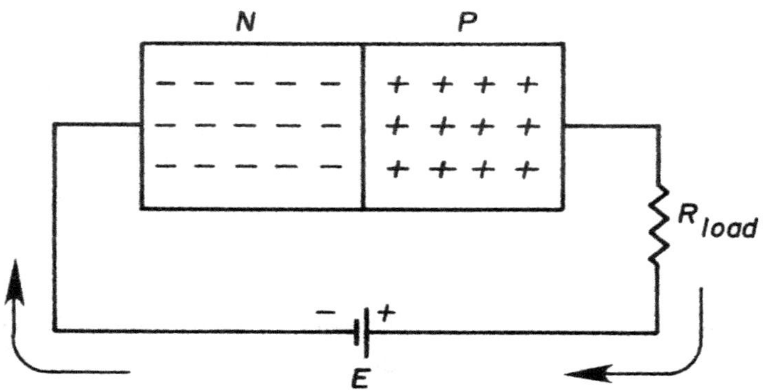

FIG. 5.57. Forward-biased PN junction diode. When E, the external EMF, exceeds the barrier voltage, current will flow through the diode.

negative voltage reaches and exceeds the barrier voltage, holes are forced from the P-type material to the junction and electrons are forced from the N-type material to the junction. The diode is said to be "forward-biased," conducting current.

When the external EMF is reversed (Fig. 5.58), no current flows through the diode. The diode now is "reverse-biased." The positive voltage applied to the N-type material attracts the free electrons, while the negative voltage applied to the P-type material attracts the holes. The result is a large, insulating depletion area and little current can flow.

The PN junction diode therefore is a unidirectional device, conducting

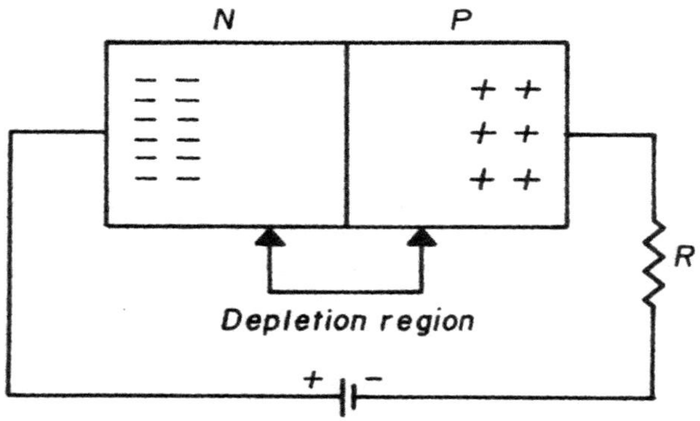

FIG. 5.58. Reverse-biased PN junction diode (see text).

current in one direction and not in the other. It can be described as a switch that is closed when forward-biased (Fig. 5.57) and open when reverse-biased (Fig. 5.58). In the first condition, it is a conductor. In the second condition, it is an insulator.

The symbol for a diode is shown in Fig. 5.59. In normal conduction, electrons flow in the direction opposite to the arrow in the symbol.

POWER SUPPLIES

A diode can be used readily to convert alternating current, which reverses polarity every half cycle, to direct current (AC to DC). The diode will be forward-biased during one half cycle and will be reverse-biased during the other half cycle. Current will flow through the diode during the positive half cycle, but not the negative half cycle. The diode rectifies the AC (Fig. 5.60 A, B, C).

If a capacitor is placed across the output of the rectifier, the DC envelopes will be smoothed (Fig. 5.61). Energy is stored in the capacitor when the voltage rises and is supplied to the load when the input voltage drops. In this circuit there is output voltage only during alternate half cycles. This type of power supply is called a *half-wave rectifier*.

A *full-wave rectifier* provides smoother output characteristics and better voltage regulation. The basic circuit of such a power supply is shown in Fig. 5.62. The voltage will depend on the transformer characteristics.

In most power supplies, it is important to maintain constant voltage at the output. This is achieved by a variety of circuits, all employing solid state devices. A commonly used device is the Zener diode, which can maintain constant voltage over a required range of current flow.

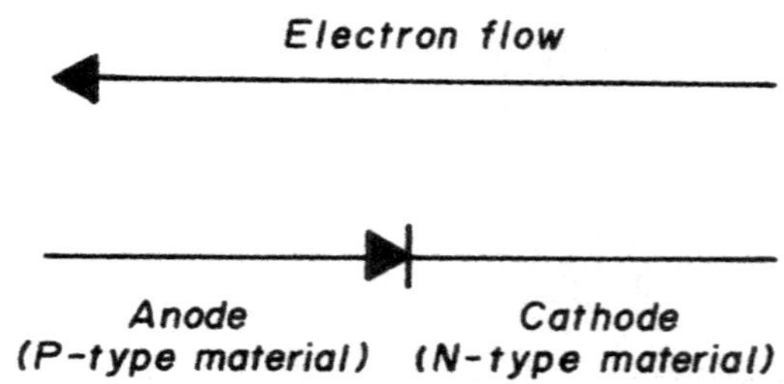

FIG. 5.59. Direction of electron flow (**upper**) through PN diode (**lower**) (see text).

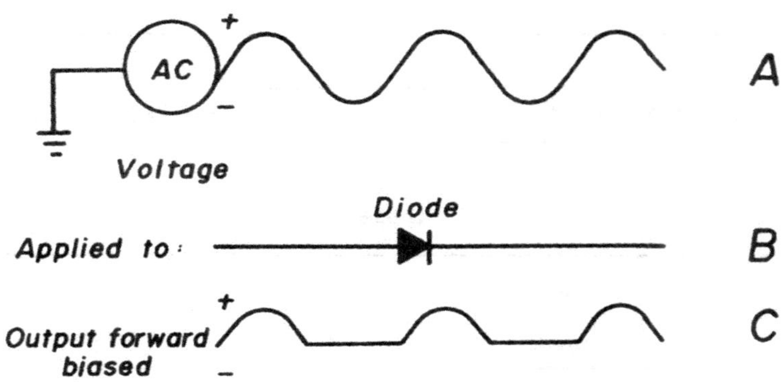

FIG. 5.60. Current flows only on positive half cycles (see text).

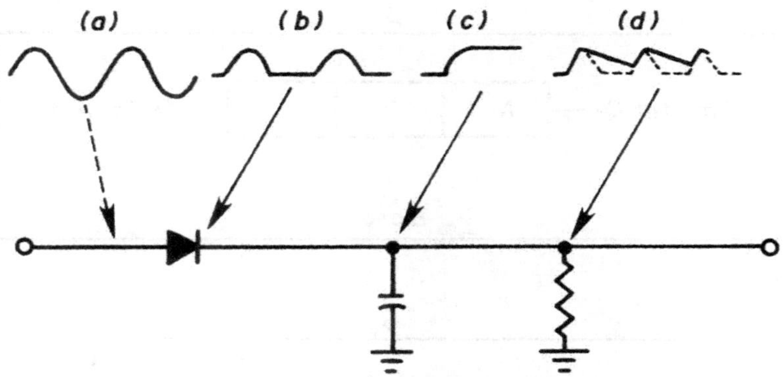

FIG. 5.61. AC (a) converted to half-wave rectified DC (b), then smoothed by capacitor (c). Ripple occurs (d) when the load (R) draws current from the capacitor (C) between peaks. The decay between peaks is the familiar RC decay, with TC = R × C.

A more complete and better regulated power supply is shown in Fig. 5.63. The output voltage will depend on the design characteristics of the transformer and on the Zener values. Complex voltage regulators are now fabricated as integrated circuits (see below). These include circuitry that compensates for temperature changes and limits current to a maximum value. [See Heathkit Learning Programs (8) and Rusgrove and Woodward (11) for further discussion of power supply regulation.]

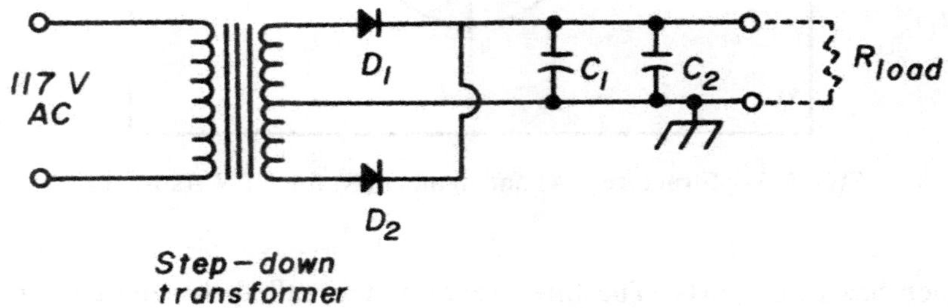

FIG. 5.62. Full-wave rectifier.

TRANSISTORS

A semiconductor device capable of more complex functions than a diode, including amplification, is made by nesting a slice of P material between two slices of N material (Fig. 5.64A). This is an *NPN transistor*,

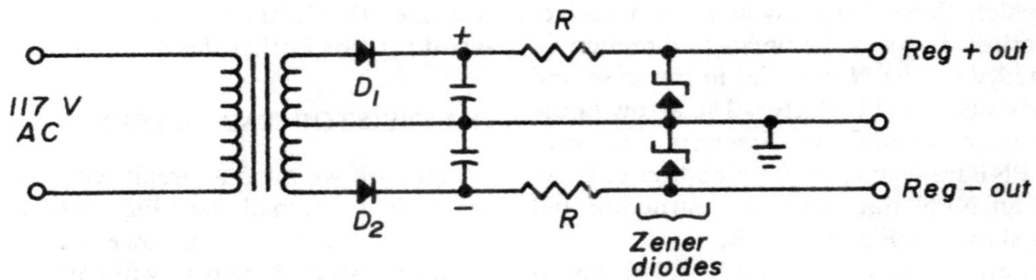

FIG. 5.63. Circuit diagram of power supply with full-wave rectifier and voltage-regulated output. D_1, D_2 = diodes.

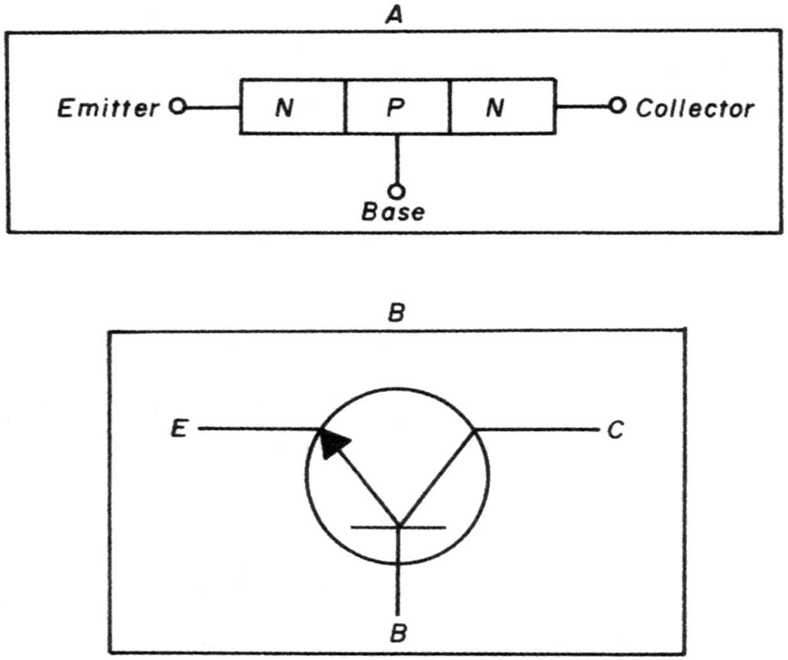

FIG. 5.64. Structures (A) and symbol (B) for NPN transistor.

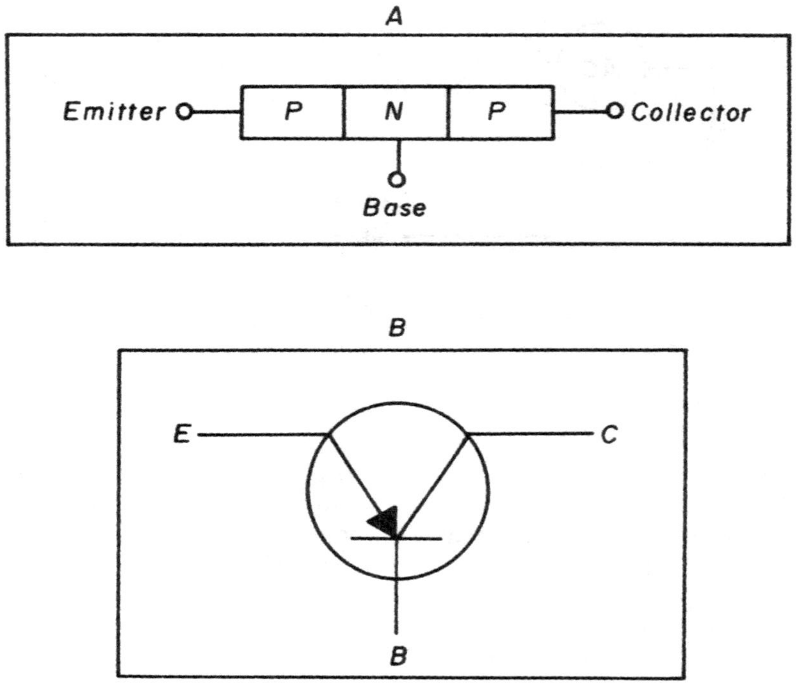

FIG. 5.65. Structure (A) and symbol (B) for PNP transistor.

which has three parts. The three sections are called the emitter (an N-section), the base (the P-section), and the collector (the other N-section).

The symbol for an NPN transistor is shown in Fig. 5.64B. The arrow indicates that the direction of current flow is from the base to the emitter. This is conventional current, which flows from positive to negative. Electron current, as discussed earlier, flows in the opposite direction.

A *PNP transistor* is constructed with the N material in the base and with the P material serving in the emitter and collector. The arrow in the schematic symbol of the emitter again indicates the direction of conventional current flow, which in the PNP transmitter is from emitter to base. This is opposite in direction to an NPN transistor. The structure and symbol for the PNP transistor is shown in Fig. 5.65A, B.

The transistor must be biased (i.e., voltages of the proper polarity must be applied to insure normal operation). In effect, the NPN transistor operates so that a small amount of current flowing from the P-type base allows a much larger amount of current to flow from emitter to collector. The PNP transistor functions so that electrons flow into the N-type base and control current flow from collector to emitter. [See Cannon and Luecke (1), Heathkit Learning Programs (7), and Rusgrove and Woodward (11) for further discussion of NPN and PNP transistors.]

TRANSISTOR AMPLIFIERS

Suppose we have a circuit with a variable resistance (R_v) that can be controlled externally (see Fig. 5.66). If R_v is in series with a fixed resistor (R_f) and placed across a power supply, the output at the junction of the series resistors R_v and R_f will vary as R_v varies.

A transistor is a device that performs this type of function. A small

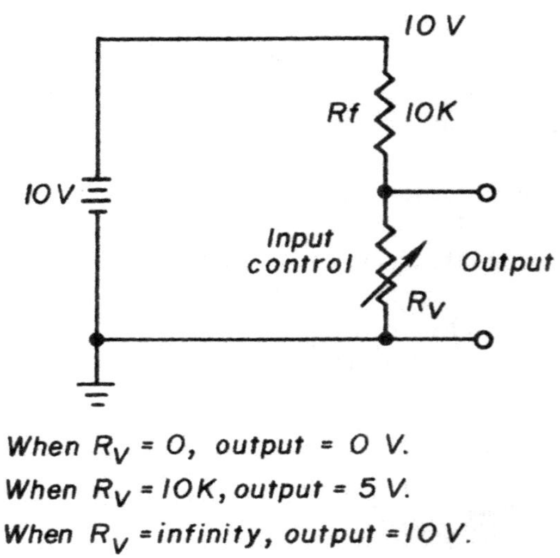

FIG. 5.66. Hypothetical model of device for controlling output voltage.

current flowing through the base can control the flow of 100 to 1,000 times as much current through the collector and its load resistor (Fig. 5.67). The analogy with Fig. 5.66 is obvious. [See Heathkit Learning Programs (7,8) and Rusgrove and Woodward (11) for further discussion of transistor amplifiers.]

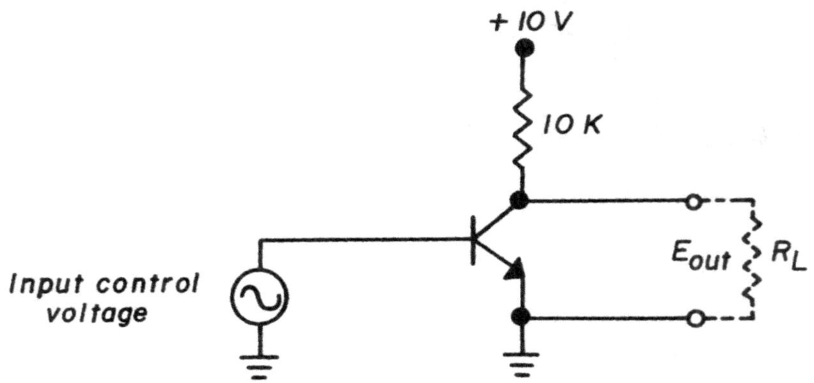

FIG. 5.67. The transistor as amplifier. (See also Figs. 5.46, 5.66, and text.)

Further advances in transistor technology were made with the development of the *junction field effect transistor* (*JFET*). The JFET has a high input impedance and is suitable for use in the input circuits of EEG amplifiers. It may be of N or P type. An *N channel* type is shown in Fig. 5.68A, B. When negative voltage is applied to the *gate*, an electrostatic charge is created and a *field* develops. Because of the high impedance, it is a reversed biased PN junction. Current flow between the *source* and the *drain* is controlled by the width of the conducting N channel which, in turn, depends on the charge of the field. An even higher input impedance

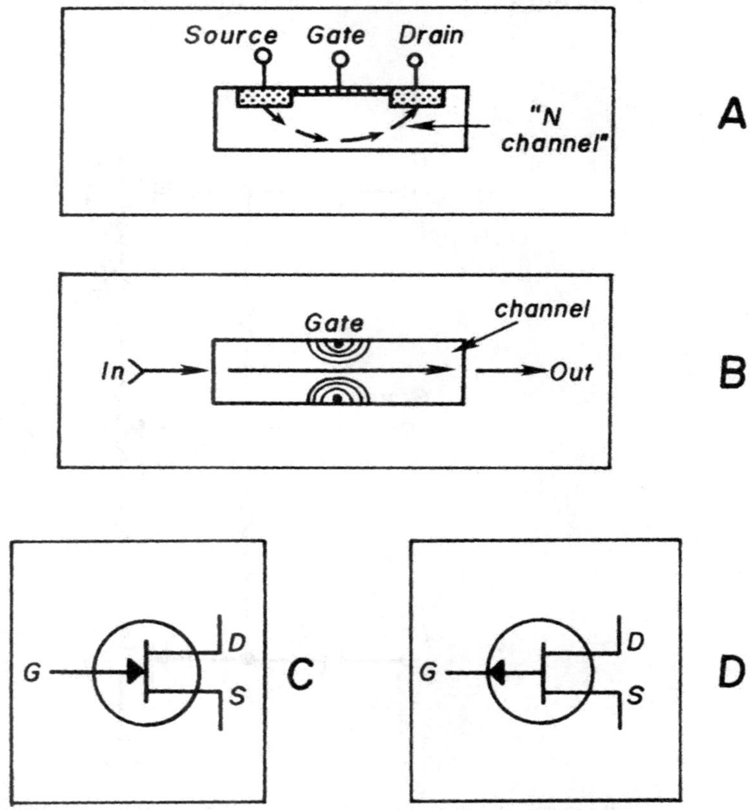

FIG. 5.68. Junction field effect transistor. **A:** Side view. **B:** Top view. **C:** N-channel. **D:** P-channel.

is achieved in the *insulated gate FET* (*IGFET*). The channel acts as a variable resistor. A very small voltage applied to the gate allows a larger voltage to develop across the source to drain. This type of transistor can serve as a voltage amplifier and is used in the input circuits of EEG amplifiers. It also may be used as a remote switching device to control amplifier functions such as sensitivity, low frequency, and high frequency settings. The symbols for N and P channel JFETs are shown in Fig. 5.68C, D. [See Heathkit Learning Programs (7) and Rusgrove and Woodward (11) for further discussion of field effect transistors.]

Other broad advances in solid state electronics have made possible new devices called *integrated circuits* (ICs). The active area of a transistor is small. In an integrated circuit, several transistors, diodes, capacitors, and resistors are packed into one small structural unit, which may be only a few millimeters square. These often are called *chips*. Several ICs may be combined to make up an amplifier for use in other services. A configuration of integrated circuits used in the input of a typical EEG amplifier (with the necessary additional capacitors and resistors, and supply voltages) is shown in Fig. 5.69. The functions are described in the legend. [See Cannon and Luecke (1), Heathkit Learning Programs (7), and Rusgrove and Woodward (11) for further discussion of integrated circuits.]

Thus, the single transistor already has gone the way of the vacuum tube. Even the early form of the integrated circuit has been replaced by

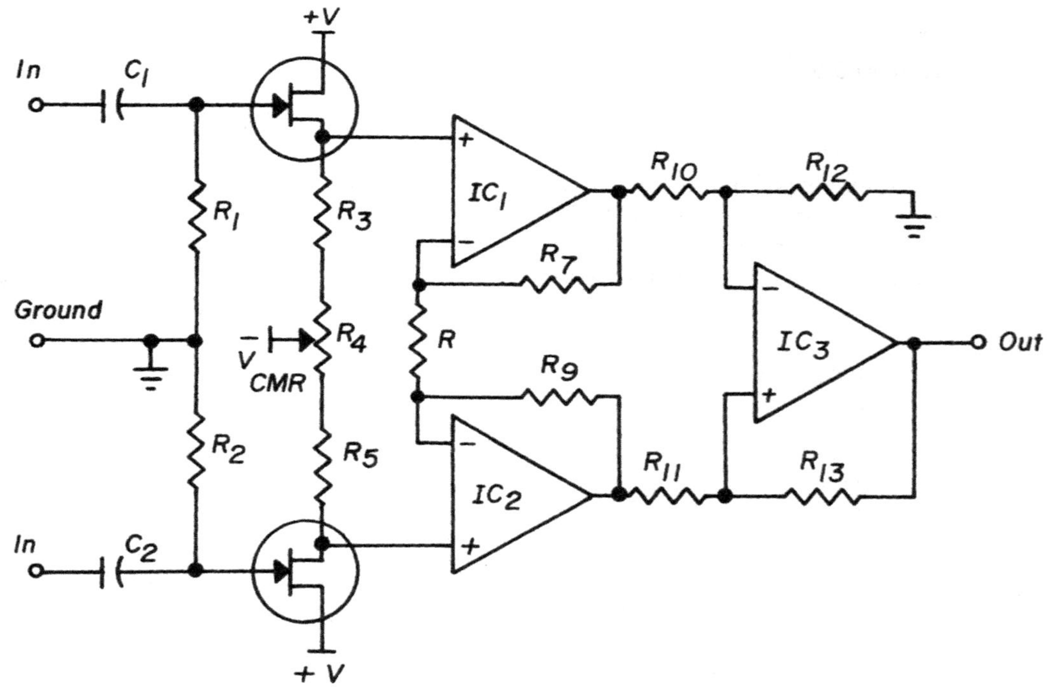

FIG. 5.69. Typical input circuit for an EEG amplifier, using FET transistors at the input. C_1 and C_2 are input capacitors. R_1 and R_2 are the input resistors, typically 10 MΩ. IC_1 and IC_2 are integrated circuits forming a differential amplifier. Potentiometer R_4 adjusts the common mode rejection ratio. IC_3 converts the differential output to a single-ended output.

medium and large scale integration (LSI) components, which combine a multitude of unit devices into a single relatively small package. We are now in the generation of very large scale integration (VLSI).

INK-WRITING RECORDERS

The output voltage of the EEG amplifier is applied to an *oscillograph* or *galvanometer* which carries an ink-writing pen or stylus. [See Cooper et al. (2) and Geddes and Baker (3) for further discussion of ink-writing recorders.] This is an electromechanical transducer, converting electrical energy to mechanical movement. Movement of the pen from the baseline must be proportional to the input voltage (Fig. 5.70). A nonlinear output would make it impossible to determine input voltage.

A typical ink-writing recorder may be made up of a precisely designed and mounted coil of wire, located between the poles of a powerful magnet (Fig. 5.71A, B). When current flows in the coil, an electromagnetic field is created. This interacts with the stationary field between the north and south poles of the magnet, causing the coil to turn. In effect, the ink-writing galvanometer is a recording meter. Zero is in the center position, rather than at one end of the scale. In the oscillograph, the direction of movement of the pen up or down depends on direction of current flow.

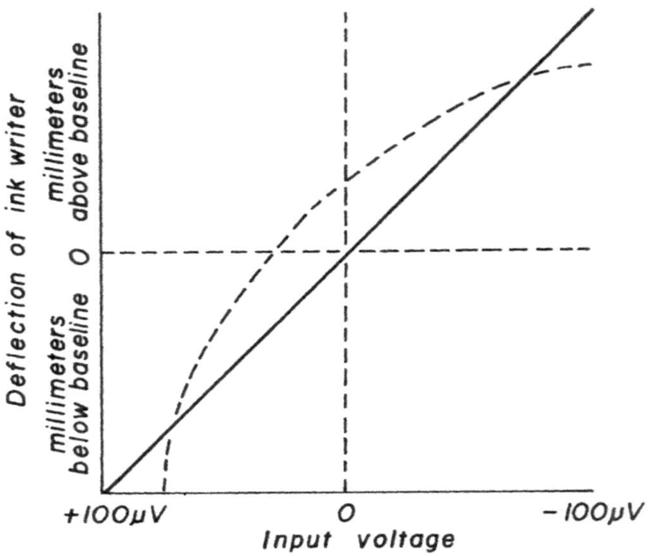

FIG. 5.70. Hypothetical input-output relationship of ink-writing oscillographs. *Solid line:* Linear relationship. *Dashed line:* Nonlinear relationship.

The position of the coil changes, as the input voltage to the amplifier changes, moving the pen. The result, as the recording paper moves beneath the pen, is a graphic display of the variations in voltage between a pair of EEG electrodes.

THE EEG INSTRUMENT

There are many similarities and many differences between modern EEG instruments and early ones. Figure 5.72 combines the analysis of the typical EEG instrument given in Chapter 2 and the electronic principles discussed in this chapter into a hypothetical schema of an equally hypothetical EEG instrument. The functions, and for the most part the names, of the operating controls of a contemporary electroencephalograph are unchanged from those of an instrument designed in the 1940s. However, the components and circuits employed to provide the functions are quite different. D (Fig. 5.72) is the differential amplifier (input) stage. The input impedance, the CMRR, and the stability are greater than that of the 1940 or 1950 instrument, and the instrument noise is less. Amplifier modules $A_{1,2,3}$ and A_4 are integrated circuits. A_5 is a power amplifier furnishing the high currents (at low voltage) needed to drive the oscillograph. Older power amplifiers required much higher voltage, although they used less current. The sensitivity and filter controls function in the same manner as those found in older instruments. However, some switching in today's instrument is performed by field effect transistors instead of mechanical switches. The total package is smaller, weighs less, and generates less heat.

Future instruments also may be expected to retain the basic functions of electrode selection, control of sensitivity (amplification), and choice of pass band (LF and HF cut-off points). However, the manner in which these functions are carried out will change with advances in the state of the electronic art. For example, electronic switching will probably replace mechanical switching, and some manual functions may be taken over by technologist-controlled electronic devices. These changes should free the technologist to make more intelligent use of the instrumentation available, to the advantage of the patient.

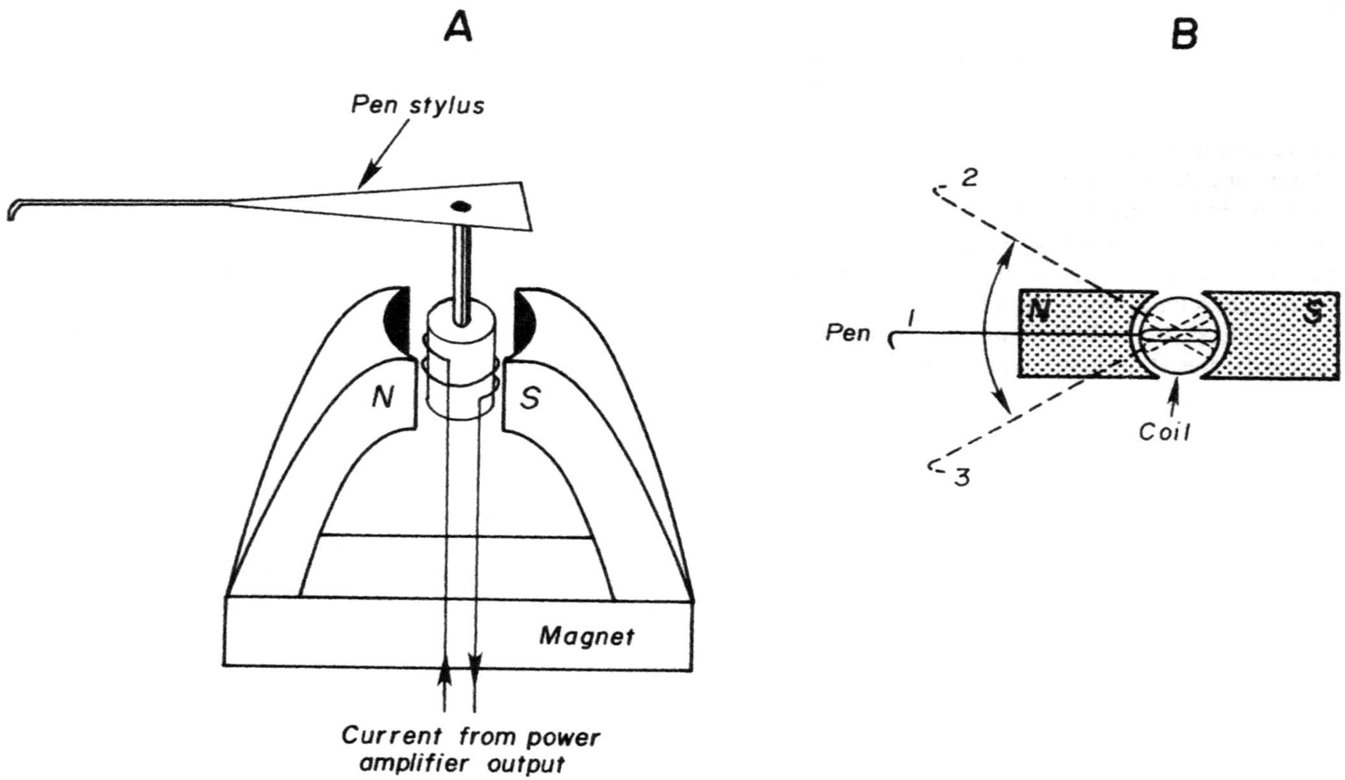

FIG. 5.71. Schema of hypothetical ink-writing galvanometer. A: Side view. B: Top view: (1) center position, (2) maximum upward deflection, (3) maximum downward deflection.

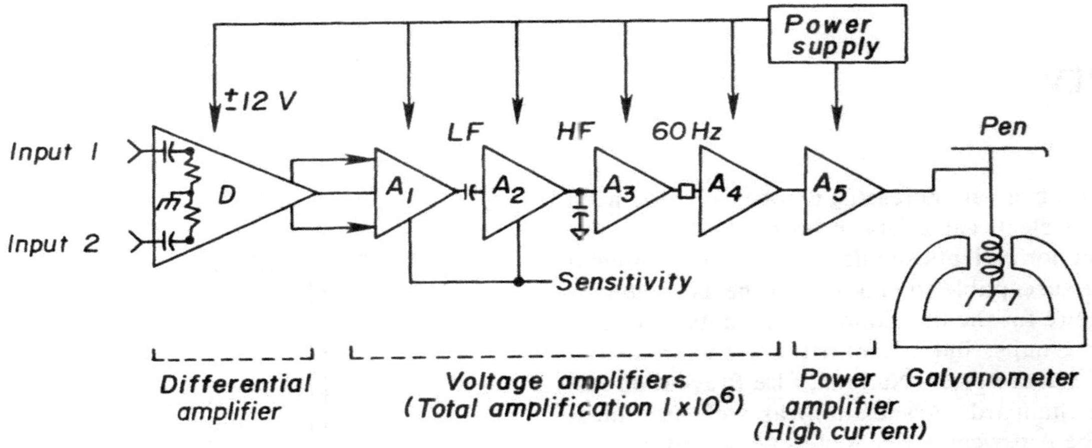

FIG. 5.72. Typical amplifier stages and controls of an EEG instrument.

The purpose of the EEG instrument is to reproduce faithfully at its output the voltages generated in the brain. Continuing expansion in applications of the field of electronics will enhance this purpose, and the field of electroencephalography will gain. One should, however, maintain caution in adopting new techniques simply because they are new to avoid degrading the practice of EEG technology through compromise with acceptable standards of excellence in performance. EEG instruments do not run themselves. Indeed, the effective use of modern instruments requires a technologist with the appropriate technical and operational sophistication.

REFERENCES AND SUGGESTED READINGS

1. Cannon, D. L., and Luecke, G., editors (1978): *Understanding Solid State Electronics*, (3rd ed.) Texas Instruments Learning Center, Dallas, Texas.
2. Cooper, R., Osselton, J. W., and Shaw, J. C. (1980): *EEG Technology*, 3rd ed. Butterworths, London.
3. Geddes, L. A., and Baker, L. E. (1975): *Principles of Applied Biomedical Instrumentation*. John Wiley, New York. Ch. 13, p. 584–605.
4. Grass Instrument Company (1973): *Grass Model 8 Instruction Manual, Part II: Theory and Application*. Quincy, Massachusetts.
5. Heathkit Continuing Education—Individual Learning Program (1975): *DC Electronics*. Benton Harbor, Michigan.
6. Heathkit Continuing Education—Individual Learning Program (1975): *AC Electronics*. Benton Harbor, Michigan.
7. Heathkit Continuing Education—Individual Learning Program (1975): *Semiconductor Devices*. Benton Harbor, Michigan.
8. Heathkit Continuing Education—Individual Learning Program (1977): *Electronic Circuits*. Benton Harbor, Michigan.
10. McPartland, J. F., editor (1981): *National Electrical Code Handbook*, 17th ed. McGraw-Hill, New York.
11. Rusgrove, J., and Woodward, G., editors (1981): *The Radio Amateur's Handbook, 58th ed*. American Radio Relay League, Newington, Connecticut.
12. *Webster's Third New International Dictionary* (1971): G. & C. Merriam Co., Springfield, Massachusetts.

Chapter 6

Electrical Safety

Since the late 1960s there has been an increasing emphasis on the need to establish basic principles of electrical safety in hospitals. Obviously, neither professional personnel nor patients should receive any accidental shock. Patients may be more susceptible to shock than the average person. Much of the initial pressure for the development of safety rules and codes came from consumer groups, but manufacturers and industrial safety groups (Underwriters' Laboratories, National Fire Prevention Association, and the Canadian Standards Association) as well as professional EEG groups (such as the American EEG Society) have led the way toward improved safety practices. The United States Food and Drug Administration is currently establishing instrument standards that include electroencephalographic apparatus (7).

A potentially hazardous situation would arise if a patient could come in contact with a water pipe (a ground) and, at the same time, with a metal lamp with an internal short circuit, putting its frame 117 V above ground. If such double contact occurred, serious injury or death could result. (Fig. 6.1). In all likelihood, such situations have occurred in one form or another, involving electrically operated beds, steam vaporizers, or other electrical apparatus. This situation also occurs in homes, in kitchens, and in bathrooms. It is conceivable that it could occur in the EEG laboratory.

Not all safety problems are as obvious as the one just described, and it should be realized that there are hundreds of medical devices that involve the use of electricity in their operation. These range from hearing aids to devices placed within the heart. In modern intensive care units, and sometimes in the patient's own room, there may be several electrical devices simultaneously recording from and perhaps stimulating the patient. In such situations, it is important that care be taken to avoid creating any current-carrying circuit that includes the patient as a part of the pathway.

A restatement of this point can be made for (and continually should be made by) the EEG technologist: *The technologist must be certain that no unsafe currents from any source can pass through the patient because of the EEG electrodes attached to the patient.*

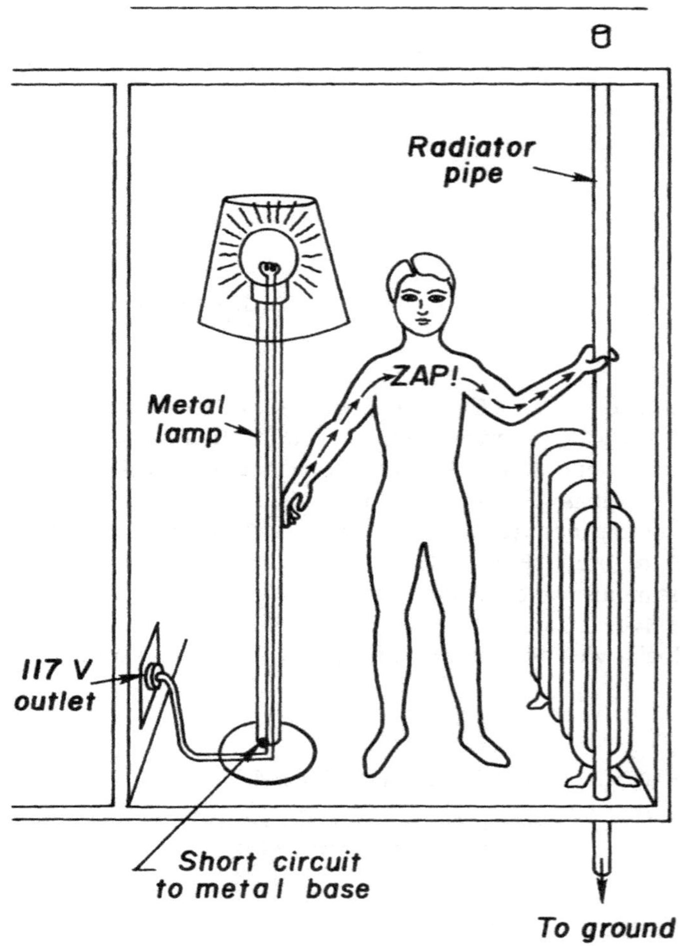

FIG. 6.1. Hazard created by short circuit in lamp base and nearby grounded conductor; if patient makes simultaneous contact, death may result (see text).

THE POWER SOURCE

The normal source of all externally powered equipment in a hospital comes from the AC power mains. This system is schematized in Fig. 6.2. The high voltage of the transmission line from the power plant is reduced to the 117 V domestic operating voltage by means of a transformer. One side of the service line is 117 V above ground. (This is a nominal value; it may range from 105–130 V.) The 117 V, or hot side, of the line is carried by a wire which is color-coded *black* (for death). The return wire to the transformer is called neutral, and it is color-coded *white*. A third wire carries the return to building (earth) ground and is color-coded *green*.

In older installations there may be only two contacts in the wall receptacle, one hot at 117 V, and the other neutral. Without testing the receptacle, it is not possible to tell one from the other. Although neutral is equivalent to ground in a two-wire system, there may be a small voltage at the neutral wire relative to building ground. This wire will have some (though minimal) resistance. The conductor used in house wiring is usually 14-gauge copper wire that has a resistance of 0.02 Ω per 100 feet. A 100-foot return to the building ground with a 5-A current will cause 0.1 V of EMF to appear at the neutral contact of the wall outlet relative to true ground. The typical 18-gauge wire used for extension cords has a resistance of 0.06 Ω per 100 feet. If a 25-foot extension cord is used, a 5-A current would create 0.075 V of EMF in the neutral wire. This would increase the voltage of neutral by 57% beyond the original 0.1 V.

The greatest danger of a two-wire system (Fig. 6.3A) lies in the accidental short circuiting of the device to its own case or chassis, which is usually metal, as in the example of the lamp. If a person contacts both the case and a ground of any kind, severe shock, burn, or death may occur (see Fig. 6.1).

The modern three-wire system helps to prevent this because the metal case or chassis of the device is returned directly to ground through the third (green) wire in the power cord. If a short circuit develops in the device (for example, in the power supply of an EEG instrument), current will reach the chassis. This current then can flow through the green wire attached to the instrument frame directly to ground. When this occurs, the current rapidly exceeds a critical value (10–15 A, typical) and the fuse will blow or the circuit breaker will open and current no longer can flow (Fig. 6.3B). Because it takes time for a fuse to blow, the protection is not instantaneous. [See Seaba (4) for further discussion of these various points.]

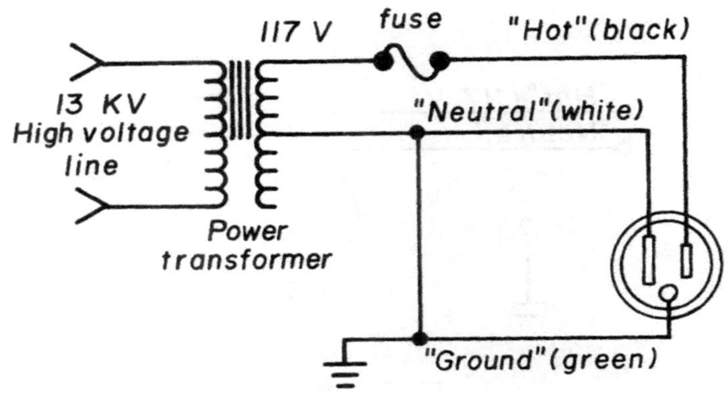

FIG. 6.2. Schematic of high voltage input to hospital and 117-V distribution to EEG laboratory. Ground return of service line is to building ground.

The EEG technologist must be certain that the ground wire of the power cord of the EEG instrument is indeed intact so that any current accidentally reaching the instrument case will flow safely to ground. The green ground wire of the cord can break or it can become disconnected at the instrument or inside the plug. Checks on continuity of the ground should be a part of every laboratory's maintenance schedule. These checks are easily carried out with an ohmmeter (Fig. 6.4). The meter is placed on the 1× Ω scale. One probe from the meter is placed in contact with the ground contact of the plug (the long, round, or semicircular pin or blade). The other probe from the meter is placed in contact with a metal surface of the EEG instrument. If there is a designated ground on the instrument, this would be the best point of contact.

If the ohmmeter shows a very low resistance (less than 0.1 Ω), there is obviously continuity (Fig. 6.4A) and the circuit's integrity has been demonstrated. However, even if the meter reads 5 Ω, there is danger, as a 30-A fuse or circuit breaker would still conduct up to 23 A (I = 117/5 = 23.4 A). *In no case should the instrument be used until the absolute integrity of the ground circuit is restored.* If resistance is infinite, there is a serious defect, and the cord must be repaired or replaced (Fig. 6.4B).

LEAKAGE CURRENTS

Not all voltages that may reach the frame or chassis of an electrical instrument are caused by short circuits or faults in the equipment. Every

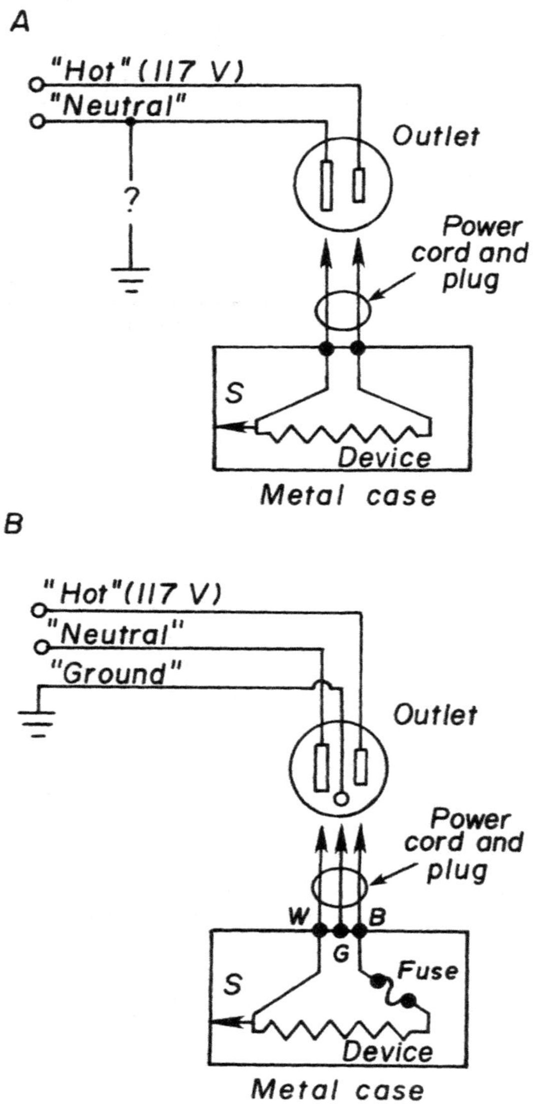

FIG. 6.3. Effects of short circuit to metal case, with two-wire system **(A)**and with three-wire system **(B)**. ? = uncertain ground; S = short circuit.

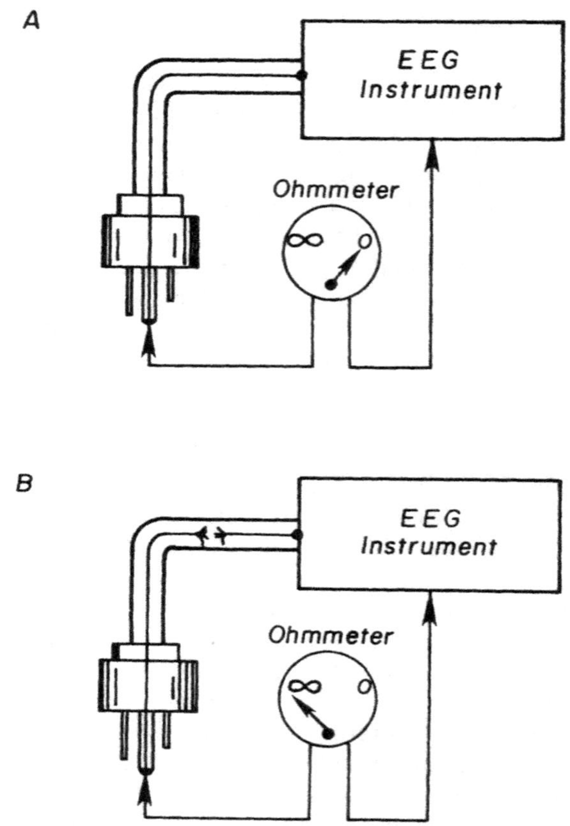

FIG. 6.4. A: Continuity of ground circuit. Resistance below 0.1 Ω when meter leads are placed on ground blade of three-wire plug and on instrument frame. **B:** Discontinuity of ground circuit. Infinite resistance (open circuit) when meter leads are placed on three-wire plug and on instrument frame.

instrument has what are called leakage currents. The instrument is designed to keep these at a very low level. Such leakage currents concern EEG and other electromedical technologists. If excessive leakage current develops, the integrity of the ground wire can prevent a fatal accident.

Stray Capacitance

The most common source of leakage current is stray capacitance in the instrument's power cord and power supply. Wires running parallel to each other and separated by insulating material, in addition to being conductors, act as plates of a capacitor. Figure 6.5A shows the typical construction of a three-wire cable. Fig. 6.5B illustrates the equivalent circuit, which has a 117-V AC source and three capacitors.

The conductors (wires) are acting as the plates of capacitors (C_1, C_2, and C_3). The insulation around the wires is the dielectric. Since the voltage is AC, the capacitors alternately charge and discharge. Current flows between the hot and the ground wires (C_3), and between the hot and the neutral wires (C_1). The neutral and ground wires form capacitor C_2. The amount of current (i.e., the leakage current) flowing in the neutral and ground wires will be determined by the length and diameter of the wires (total surface area of the plates), by the dielectric constant of the insulating material and by the distance between the wires in the power cord. The physical construction of the power cord, including its length, is critical.

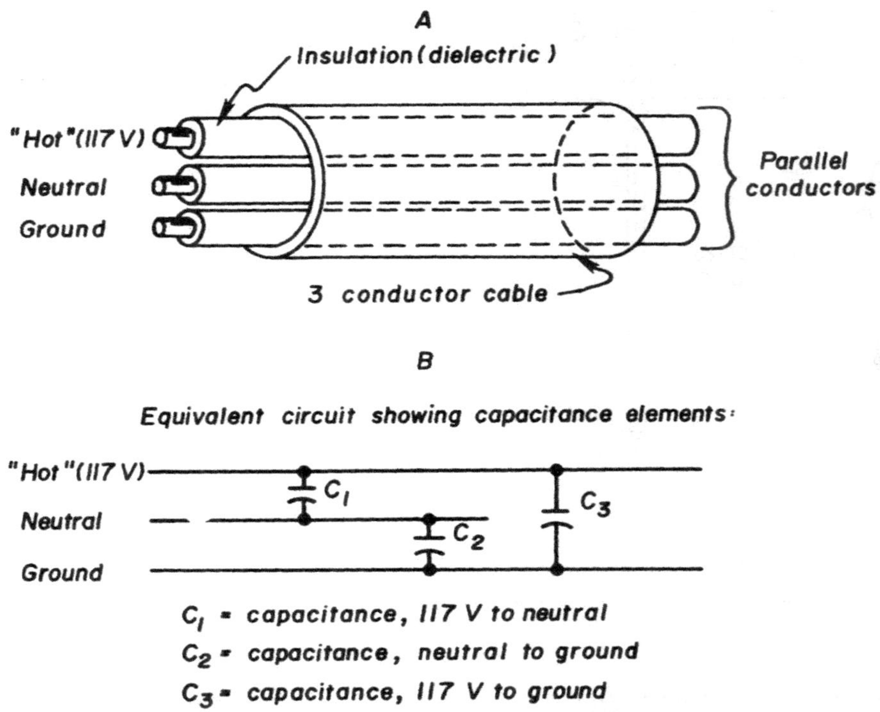

FIG. 6.5. A: Pictorial diagram of a three-conductor cable. B: Equivalent circuit of A, illustrating the capacitive elements.

Manufacturers select power cords on the basis of their capacitance per foot (or meter). A 6-foot power cord is reported to contribute a leakage current of 7 μA, although in some cords, it may run as high as 40 to 60 μA. For this reason, *extension cords should never be used between an AC outlet and the three-prong plug of the EEG instrument's cord. The use of an extension cord will increase the leakage current by an unknown and potentially dangerous amount.*

Further sources of stray capacitance are found in the wiring inside the instrument, particularly in components such as transformers, within the power supply. Instrument manufacturers consider all these factors in designing equipment, including the quality of the components and their orientation inside the instrument.

Stray Inductance

Another source of leakage current is stray inductance. AC passing through an inductor—and any wire which carries current acts as an inductor—creates an electromagnetic field that alternately expands and collapses. All wires within that field will have current generated coincident with each cycle in the circuits of which they are a part. Leakage current from this source is much less than that caused by stray capacitance. Designers allow for such currents, however, in computing the total leakage current in an electromedical device.

So far we have said that (a) current can kill, (b) there are inherent sources of leakage current that are subject to partial control through design features, and (c) the undesired voltage on exposed surfaces of equipment can be reduced to zero by proper grounding procedures. Since some patients are much more susceptible to shock than healthy people, it takes less current to kill them and, therefore, extreme caution should be taken when using electrical equipment attached to them.

FAULT CURRENTS AND GROUND LOOPS

As we have seen, any instrument has some current leaking to ground. Even if there is a fault in an instrument, causing excessive leakage current, an intact ground circuit will allow the current to pass harmlessly to ground. However, voltage between two "grounds" may not be zero. If a patient is connected to two instruments, each using a different ground, a voltage difference will cause current to flow through the patient. There are two main causes of such a voltage difference.

Consider the following situation, illustrated in Fig. 6.6. Two instruments are attached to the patient, each connected to a different AC outlet. The ground returns of the outlets are of different lengths. The resistances of the paths to ground will be low, but not zero (here represented as R_1 and R_2). Since the leakage currents from the two instruments will be different, and R_1 and R_2 also are different, the voltage at the ground terminals of outlet 1 and outlet 2 will be different. The presence of two ground electrodes on the patient will permit current to flow from one instrument to the other through the patient. If instrument 2 developed a fault current (i.e., a high leakage current) the voltage at outlet 2 would increase appreciably. This would then increase current flow through the patient to the EEG ground. If a defect occurred in the ground of outlet 2, all of the fault current could flow through the patient to the EEG ground.

In addition to fault currents producing voltage differences between outlet grounds, magnetic fields in the area will induce currents in the ground wiring. In Fig. 6.6 the patient completes a loop. This ground loop acts as the secondary of a transformer in which a small voltage but a large current may be developed (5).

In either case, the solutions are the same: (a) use outlets in the same cluster; (b) use only one ground electrode on the patient; (c) be certain that the patient ground has a current-limiting device in it.

A ground loop need not involve a patient. If two instruments already are interconnected by a common ground, making another connection between them (Fig. 6.7) may cause 60-Hz interference. The "loop" acts like a secondary of a transformer by picking up all magnetic radiation in its vicinity. There is no need for the extra wire, as the two instruments

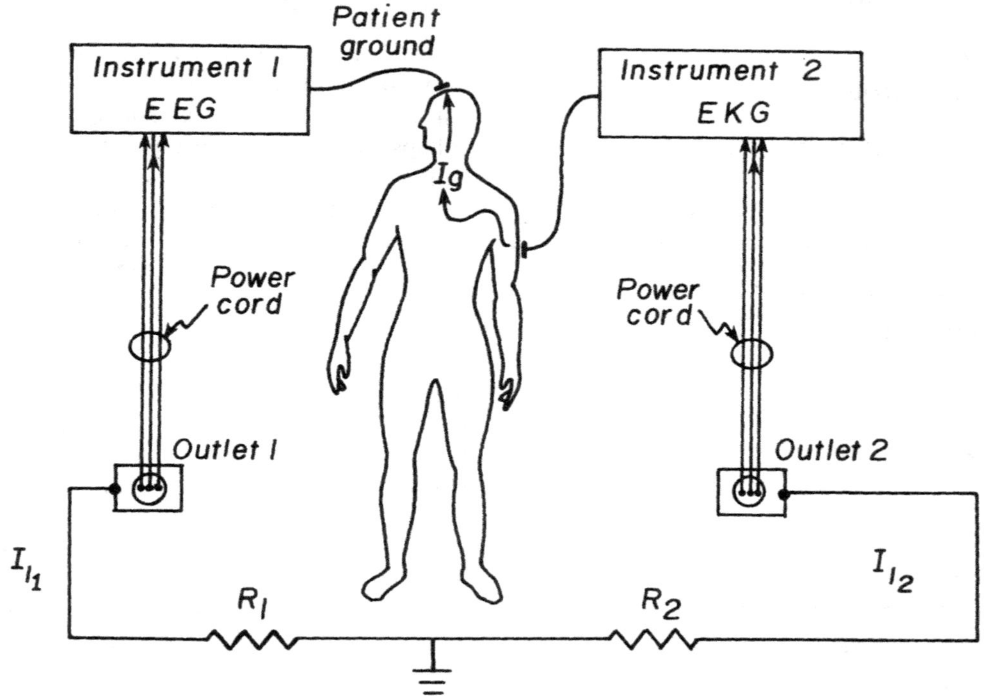

FIG. 6.6. Effect of having two grounds on a patient. The EEG ground is on the patient's head; the EKG ground is on the leg or arm. This creates a ground loop. If the EKG power cord has a defective ground wire, current will flow from EKG ground on patient to EEG ground. (See text for discussion.)

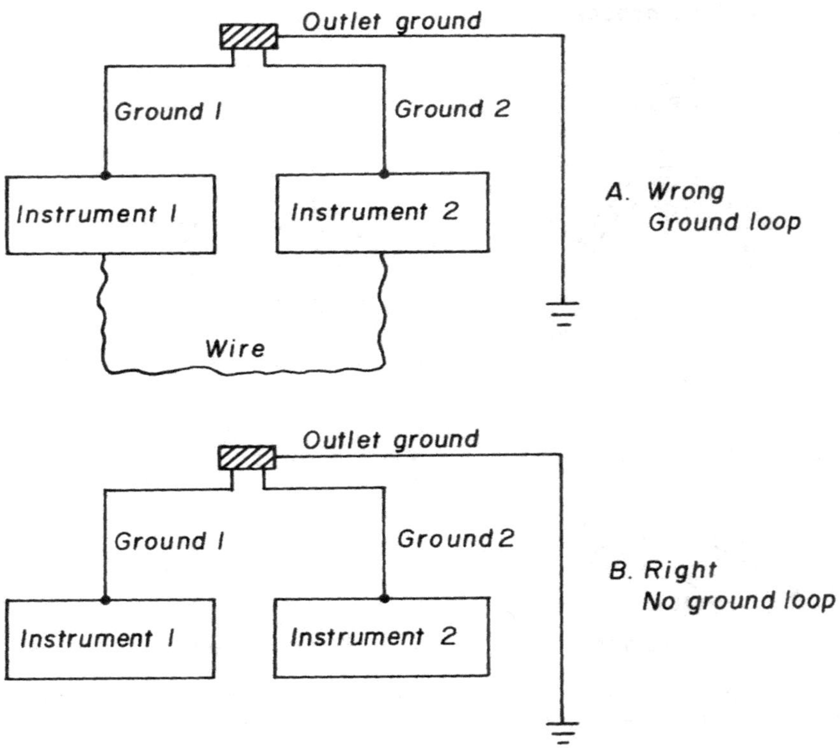

FIG. 6.7. A: Ground loop caused by redundant interconnection of two instruments. **B:** Proper connection is via a single ground.

share a common ground at the outlet. An example in ordinary EEG practice could involve an EEG instrument and a photic stimulator. They should have a common 117-V receptacle to provide them with a common ground point, and no other interconnection should be made.

Sometimes it may be necessary to place a "redundant" ground on an EEG instrument. This is a separate, heavy-gauge wire attached to the metal of the console. The other end of this wire often is connected to a cold water pipe, since such a pipe is usually regarded as a good ground. However, the potential of the pipe and of the AC receptacle ground may not be equal. The EEG instrument completes the loop, and current flows through the instrument from one ground to the other. The redundant ground should reach the ground point of the AC outlet (Fig. 6.8). Such a connection can be established by using a receptacle ground outlet that permits the attachment of other instrument grounds to the same wall receptacle ground (a typical unit is Ohmic model RGO). The allowable potential difference between conductive surfaces (which presumably are grounded) is 40 mV (3).

Technologists sometimes find it necessary to ground the patient's bed to avoid 60-Hz interference. If a water pipe or radiator is used to ground the bed, a ground loop will be created. The rule to be followed is that *all devices should go to one* (*common*) *ground*. In an EEG laboratory, if there are four devices such as (a) the EEG instrument, (b) a photic stimulator, (c) a lamp, and (d) a portable air compressor for drying collodion when applying electrodes, the grounds should all return to one point. If a bed requires a ground, it also should go to the same point. In critical care areas, there should be six outlets per bed to provide ground returns for six instruments. In addition, there should be jacks for grounding nonelectrical metal surfaces such as beds. All conductive surfaces within seven feet of a patient's bed should be grounded to this common ground (3).

SHOCK

It is true that current kills, but not *all* current kills. Very small currents may be perceived as a mild shock (those near 1 mA, or sometimes much

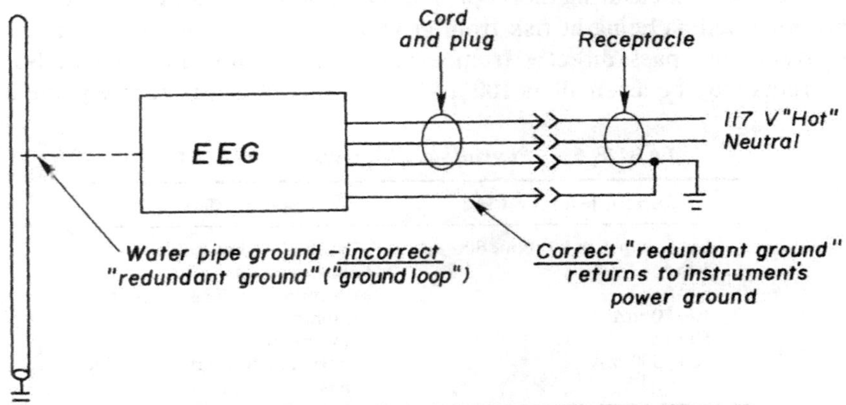

FIG. 6.8. Incorrect versus correct "redundant ground" connection, avoiding ground loop (see text).

less). Some direct currents can be perceived, may not be lethal, but may cause burns to the skin. Alternating currents may be more easily perceived (300 μA) and are more likely to be lethal at some frequencies than others (e.g., 60-Hz AC has lower thresholds for perception, pain, and death than currents of other frequencies). Table 6.1 presents typical ranges of current, from perceptible to lethal. The effects will depend in part on the actual pathway through the body.

Macroshock

The type of shock referred to in Table 6.1 is called macroshock. Macroshock involves large and quite perceptible currents passing from one external surface area to another (Fig. 6.9A). The body is partly protected from current by its high skin resistance. When a person's skin is wet, less voltage is required to produce a lethal current. Ohm's law (I = E/R) (see Chapter 5) can help predict these dangers. If a person completes a circuit between a 117-V source and earth and his or her resistance is 10 kΩ, only 11 mA will flow. If the skin resistance is 250 Ω, 468 mA will flow. This could be lethal. [See Strong (5).]

Microshock

Microshock is a term used to describe very low currents that nevertheless may be lethal. Patients with indwelling electrodes in the heart (catheters for measuring blood pressure and other implanted transducers) are regarded as being at risk from ground loop and other stray currents. Current may pass directly from exterior to interior (Fig. 6.9B). Such currents may be as small as 100 μA. Although 100 μA is barely perceptible when applied between the arms, or from arm to leg, it may be lethal when introduced directly to the heart. [See Strong (5).] The pathways of macro- and microshock are compared in Fig. 6.9.

TABLE 6.1. *Physiological effects of 60-Hz AC*[a]

Current level for 1 sec	Bodily effect
Less than 1 mA (about 300 μA)	"Can feel" (threshold)
1 mA	Pain threshold
5 mA	Maximum harmless current
10–20 mA	"Cannot let go"
50 mA	Pain, injury
100–300 mA	Ventricular fibrillation; possible death

[a] See Olson (3) and Strong (5).

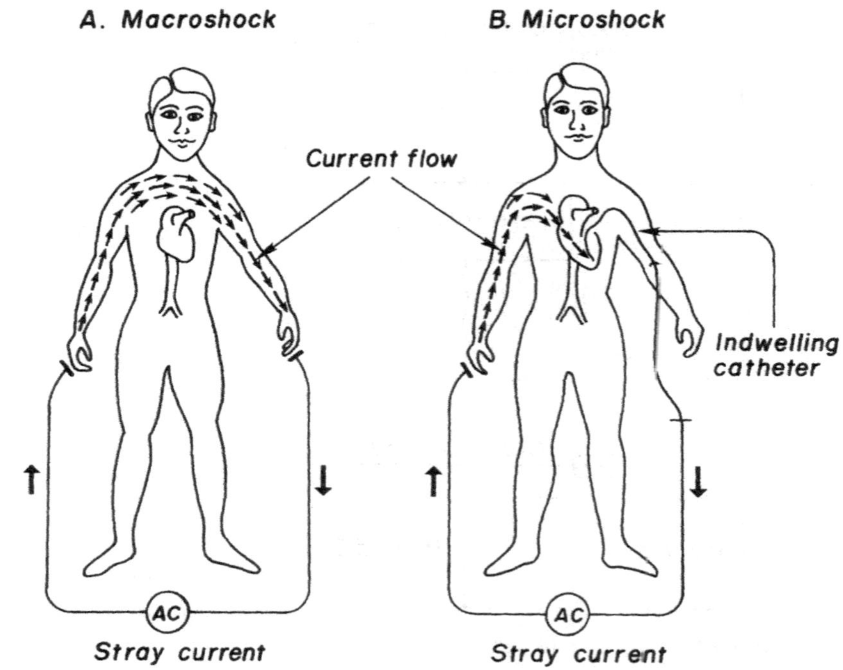

FIG. 6.9. A: Macroshock: current directly passes through arm-to-arm pathway. B: Microshock: current concentrates in heart-to-arm pathway.

ELECTRICAL INSTRUMENTATION AND PATIENT RISK

There are three general situations in which electrical instrumentation is used in hospitals. One involves the connection of an instrument to electrically susceptible patients. These patients, at high risk for stray or accidental sources of current, include neonates and patients who have an external source of voltage that connects with indwelling electrodes making contact with the heart. Such patients often have several instruments attached to them.

A second, less potentially dangerous situation involves a single electrical instrument attached to a patient. A properly designed, approved, and tested instrument should have no chassis leakage currents over 100 μA when the chassis is ungrounded, and no patient lead current greater than 50 μA. A third situation involves the use of electrical equipment that makes no contact with the patient, such as a stroboscopic light used to test photic sensitivity. Its exposed metal surfaces and its metal chassis must have an acceptable return to ground.

It is the responsibility of the technologist to be absolutely certain that no electrical contact between devices can occur other than through a common three-wire power receptacle or a ground bus, as described earlier in this chapter.

Use of EEG with Other Electrical Equipment

When a patient has an EEG instrument and another AC-powered device attached to him, such as an EKG monitor or an electrically powered blood pressure monitor, *no EEG ground electrode should be attached to the patient,*[1] unless you are certain the instrument has a current-limiting device in the ground lead and that it is functioning properly.

The ground system of the other device, connected through the green wire in its power cord, will provide a patient ground and there should be no 60-Hz interference in the EEG. Should the ground wire in the other device be defective and if leakage currents develop in that instrument, an EEG ground electrode on the patient's head would permit the leakage current to flow to ground through the EEG ground lead. If this current passed through the heart, death or cardiac damage conceivably could occur.

A hypothetical situation in which an EEG instrument and an EKG instrument are attached to the same patient is shown in Fig. 6.10; a ground loop also occurs. Both instruments should have the same ground point, and *there should be only one ground electrode attached to the patient.* If the EKG ground develops a fault, leakage current from the EKG instrument will flow to ground through the patient. If the EEG instrument's ground is defective, any leakage current from the instrument will reach ground through the EKG ground.

[1] When the EEG is used in the operating room, another ground will already be on the patient. *Do not apply an EEG ground.* It is unnecessary and could be hazardous to the patient.

LEAKAGE CURRENT LIMITS

To insure the safety of patients, strict leakage current limits have been specified for instrumentation. These are continuously under scrutiny and revision. The maximum allowable chassis leakage current (mostly affecting the operator) when the green/ground wire of the power cord is disabled is 100 μA.

There are additional paths through which current may flow and put the patient at risk. Every functioning EEG electrode provides a potential pathway for current flow. In the event that the chassis ground of the EEG instrument is interrupted, stray currents could flow back through the input leads (i.e., the recording electrodes). In ordinary EEG recording, leakage currents up to 50 μA per electrode may be tolerated (1,4).

It always is necessary to specify conditions for the "worst case." Such would occur if, when all or some electrodes were secured to the scalp, one EEG electrode made contact with a 117-V line. Provisions must be made to limit the current flow to 20 μA, which defines an isolated input (1,4,6). It would seem that an input resistor with a nominal value of 10 MΩ would limit current to 12 μA ("worst case," 117 V, 10 MΩ; see Fig. 6.11). Some EEG amplifiers will have diode protection for the field-effect transistors in the differential input stage, which will trip at 0.7 V and the input resistance will sharply drop. This can increase current flow in nonisolated inputs.

The technologist should be informed about the characteristics of the equipment being used so that proper precautions can be taken to meet the needs for safety in each application.

When recording an EEG in an intensive care unit or a cardiac care unit, an "isolation jack box" or "biopotential isolator" electrode board provides necessary protection. Units are commercially available that will limit any accidental current flow from electrode to scalp typically at 1 μA or less. One device uses a solid state component that acts like a resistor (the nominal value, typical, 6 kΩ) at low current flow. If the current exceeds a specified value, the resistance increases infinitely, thus preventing dangerous levels of current from being reached. Another form of this system utilizes a current-limiting device in the patient ground lead only. This provides a measure of safety to the ground line only. Optical isolation also is used in some systems.

Measurements of leakage current of electromedical equipment should be carried out in hospitals at regular intervals by qualified biomedical

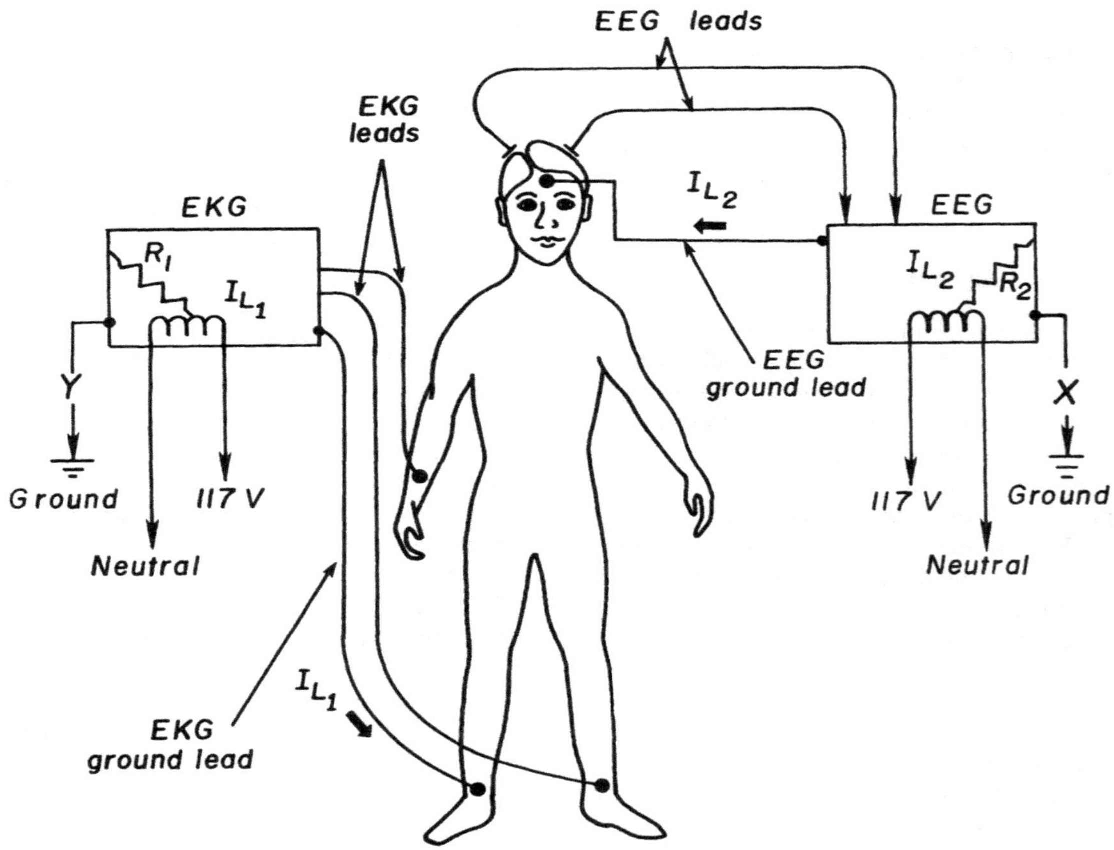

FIG. 6.10. If EEG ground (X) is not continuous, then leakage current in the EEG instrument will flow through the patient to the EKG instrument ground. Conversely, if the EKG ground is interrupted (Y), current will flow to EEG ground. $R_{1,2}$ = resistance in instrument carrying leakage current. $I_{1,2}$ = leakage current in EKG and EEG.

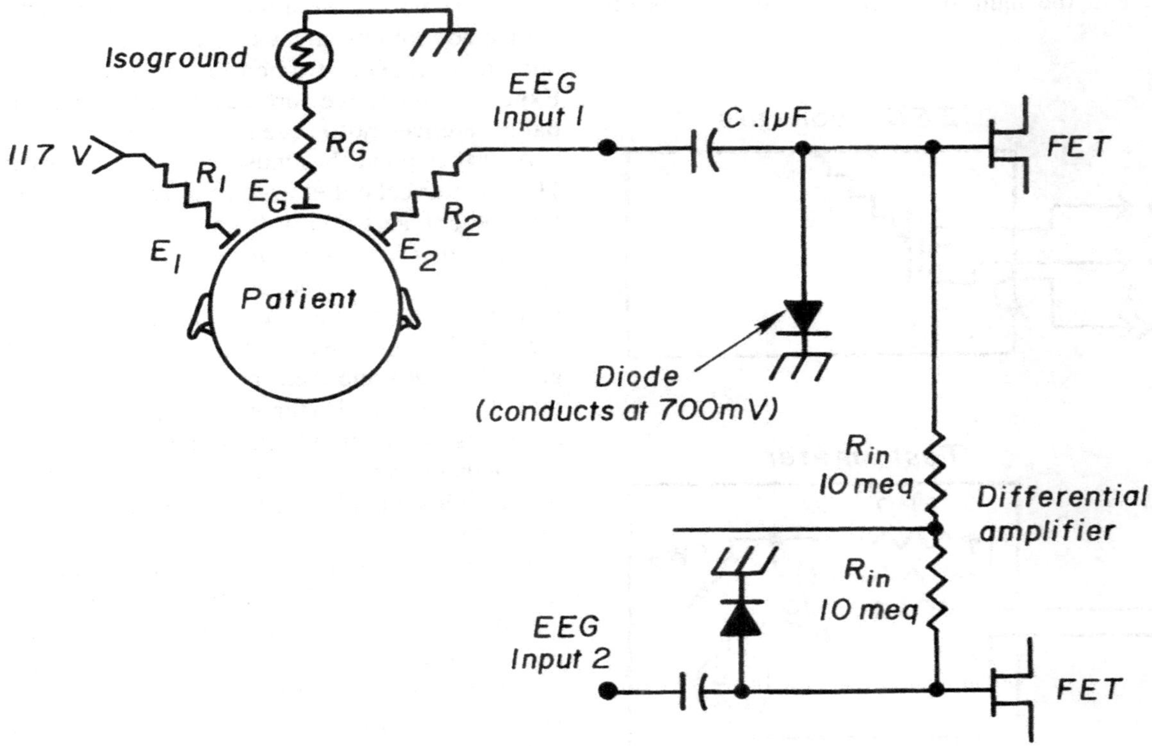

FIG. 6.11. Inherent protective circuitry with C–R input (and protective diode) of typical EEG amplifier. E_1 and E_2 = EEG electrodes. E_G = EEG ground electrode. R_1, R_G, R_3 = resistance of EEG electrodes E_1, E_G, and E_2. Isoground (protective diodes).

engineers. The procedures used are shown in Fig. 6.12. The ground return in the three-wire power cable is purposely broken at A and B, and any leakage current (I_L) will then be measured when SW_2 is closed. A polarity reversing switch (SW_1) is used to reverse the 117-V input so that the normal neutral wire of the instrument is connected to the 117 V hot line and the hot side connects to the neutral side of the power source. Leakage current again is measured, and the highest reading (worst case) is recorded. Maximum level of chassis leakage is 100 μA. Current from patient input to ground (instrument ungrounded) should be limited to 50 μA.

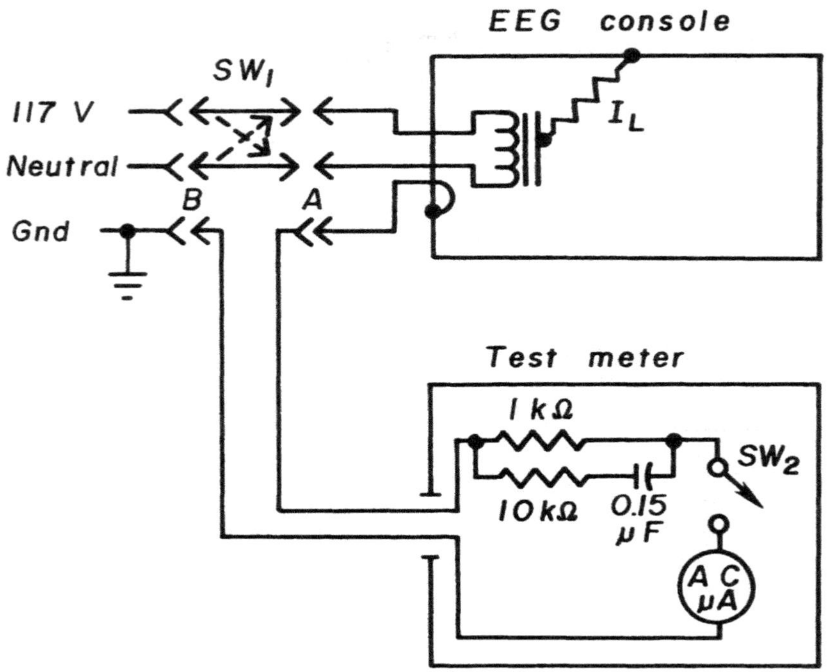

FIG. 6.12. Measurement of leakage current from EEG chassis to ground. The normal ground wire is disabled at A and B. A safety test instrument is inserted at A and B and any AC (flowing as leakage current, I_L) in μA is measured as it flows through a 1-kΩ load, in parallel with a low-pass filter (the 10-Ω and 0.15-μF branches). SW_1 is a reversing switch that can shift the normal neutral of the power plug to 117 V (hot) and the 117 V to the instrument's neutral conductor. SW_2 is the test switch.

PREVENTIVE MAINTENANCE AND SAFETY PRECAUTIONS

EEG technologists in office practice rarely deal with high-risk patients but they must still be aware of the dangers involved when ground circuits are interrupted through faults in the equipment or in the building wiring. Under no circumstances is it acceptable to use two-wire AC circuits to operate an EEG instrument or any other device within the patient area. Exposed conductive surfaces must be adequately grounded, their potential differences not exceeding 40 mV.

A further point that must always be considered is the adequacy of the 117-V electrical outlet used to operate the EEG instrument. One assumes that the contacts in a wall outlet are correctly wired, but *sometimes the contacts in a wall outlet are not correctly wired.* A relatively inexpensive device called a *receptacle inspector* (or analyzer) will indicate the correctness of the wiring by the appearance of a pattern of lights. (One type is the Ohmic model RIN.) This indicates the status of hot, neutral, and ground circuits and their interrelation. If the receptacle analyzer indicates that there is a fault (for instance, if hot and neutral are reversed, or if ground is nonfunctioning), do not use that outlet. Report it to the electrical engineer, who can carry out a more sophisticated test. The correction of the fault should be verified by a qualified electrician before the outlet is used again.

The spring pressure of the contacts in a wall outlet must provide a firm, tight contact, especially the ground contact. A simple spring-scale tester, called a *receptacle contact tension tester,* also can be used to measure the contact tension of a wall receptacle (Ohmic model RC-2). A defective wall receptacle should be reported to the hospital or building electrician. It should not be used for EEG recording until it has been replaced. Both of these test devices should be part of the equipment carried to the bedside when portable EEG recording is done. Their use will reduce the possibility of placing a patient at risk because of defective electrical equipment such as AC receptacles.

If the plug of the EEG power cord is loose and not fully inserted into an outlet, it leaves an exposed area on any or all of the three contacts: hot, neutral, and ground. If a metal object falls into the exposed area, there may be a short circuit and damage may occur to the equipment. If one end of an electrode slipped against the hot contact, either the patient or the technologist (or both) could receive a lethal electrical shock.

To illustrate the potential hazard: in a laboratory formerly directed by one of the authors, a technologist was recording an EEG at bedside. A loose AC plug for a lamp was near the bed and one end of the metal tape the technologist used for measuring electrode positions fell into the exposed region of the plug. Results: (a) Short circuit between hot and ground pins of the plug. (b) Destroyed tape measure, now in two pieces. (c) One startled but fortunately unharmed technologist. These dangers really exist and such accidents can occur.

All hospital and EEG laboratory electrical receptacles and plugs should be hospital grade. These must be mated so that no conductor is visible. Hospital grade outlets and instrument plugs are identified by a green dot signifying that the highest standards of construction and dependability of operation are met.

It was emphasized at the beginning of this chapter that the technologist should be on guard against any faults in the EEG instrument that could create electrical hazards. In addition, the technologist always must be on the alert for faults in other electrical equipment within the EEG environment. The example of the tape measure provides warning of how the unexpected can happen. All electrical connections of other equipment must be safe and all wiring must be safe.

Scientists and engineers often refer to a well-known set of humorous principles known as Murphy's laws. The basic "law" states that "Whenever anything can go wrong, it will." The EEG technologist must make it impossible for this rule to operate.

In the United States, all EEG instruments should be approved as medical instruments (UL544) by the Underwriters' Laboratoris, Inc. (6). In Canada, the Canadian Standards Association also has minimal specifications for approval. An instrument that is type-approved by both organizations has passed the most stringent and exacting set of tests.

Not all hazards in the practice of EEG are caused by stray currents, ground loops, or loose plugs. Whenever switches are turned on or off there is a spark. Sparks can ignite explosive vapors. EEG instruments are frequently used in operating rooms. The ordinary clinical instrument is not fitted with an explosion-proof switch for turning on the power supply, the individual amplifiers, or the chart drive motor. Therefore, it is important that the EEG not be used in the operating room if a flammable anesthetic agent is being used. Preoperative consultation with the surgeon and anesthesiologist is necessary. The technologist should ask, "Are any explosive anesthetics being used today?" If the answer is "Yes," the technologist should explain the danger. By the use of a long electrode cable (*not an extension power cord*), the instrument usually can be placed out of the danger area.

It is the EEG technologist's responsibility to be certain that proper care is taken in all recording situations to insure the safety of the patient and all personnel.

SUMMARY

Hundreds of electrical devices are used in medicine. Some are potentially hazardous. Any domestic AC-operated 117-V line and equipment operating from it poses dangers to the operator or to patients. Battery-operated equipment also can pose problems. Direct short circuits in a device present the greatest danger. The maintenance of a safe and certain ground is the only protection against hazard.

Leakage currents are present in any AC-operated equipment. They arise from stray capacitance and stray inductance. An intact ground system removes these and prevents dangers to the operator or patient.

Ground loops and ground faults can cause current to flow between two instruments. A common ground point for all instruments is essential.

When multiple ground electrodes are attached to a patient, current from ground loops and ground faults can flow through the patient. There should be only one ground electrode on a patient.

There are different levels of shock and risk. Macroshock is measured in milliamperes and applies to patients and instrument operators. Microshock is measured in microamperes. Patients with indwelling cardiac monitors and other cardiac electrodes (pacemakers) and neonates are regarded as at risk from microshock. Limitations should be placed on possible current flow into their bodies from other devices such as EEG or EKG instruments.

Leakage current from chassis to ground should not be more than 100 μA. Leakage current (non-isolated inputs) from any EEG amplifier input to ground should not be more than 50 μA. For isolated inputs, if 120-V AC should be applied accidentally to a susceptible patient, no current in excess of 20 μA should flow into the EEG inputs. These stringent limits may require the use of isolated inputs in (electrode) circuits.

When using EEG equipment in the operating room, another hazard exists: ignition of explosive anesthetics. This hazard must always be considered and prevented.

The technologist must carry out preventive maintenance and routine instrument checks to be certain that the patient is never at risk.

REFERENCES

1. Grass Instrument Company (1976): *An Introduction to Electrical Safety* (Bulletin X705476). Grass Instrument Co., Quincy, Massachusetts.
2. McPartland, J. F., editor (1981): *National Electrical Code Handbook,* 17th ed. McGraw-Hill, New York.
3. Olson, W. H. (1978): Electrical safety. In: *Medical Instrumentation: Application and Design,* edited by J. G. Webster. Houghton-Mifflin, Boston.
4. Seaba, P. J. (1980): Electrical safety. *Am. J. EEG Technol.,* **20**:1–13.
5. Strong, P. (1973): *Biophysical Measurements,* pp. 249–267. Tektronix, Beaverton, Oregon.
6. Underwriters' Laboratories, Inc. (1976): *Standards for Medical and Dental Equipment, UL 544,* 2nd ed. Underwriters' Laboratories, Inc., Northbrook, Illinois.
7. United States Regulatory Council (1978): Classification of neurological devices, part III. *Federal Register,* 43:54640–55732, November 28, 1978.

Chapter 7

Measurement of Frequency and Voltage

EEGs are described in terms of the frequency of the activity present and its voltage. These are primary dimensions that can be described in quantitative terms. The technologist should be able to determine the frequencies present in an EEG and the voltage of each frequency.

FREQUENCY

Frequency is defined in hertz (cycles, or waves, per sec). If activity is rhythmic, all that is necessary is to mark off 1 sec on the record and count the number of waves. Since the standard paper speed used to record EEGs is 30 mm/sec, 1-sec intervals can be designated easily. If the chart speed is 15 mm/sec or 60 mm/sec, a suitable change in scale is made. However, if a single wave is isolated and does not form part of a rhythmic sequence, it can be assigned a frequency by determining its duration in seconds and converting this into its equivalent hertz.

Figure 7.1 is a sample of EEG. The paper speed is 30 mm/sec. In channel 3, T_3-A_1 shows several large waves appearing in the center of the sample. A 1-sec interval is marked off between A and B. Starting to count waves at A and stopping at B, the number of waves is observed to be two. Therefore this activity has a frequency of 2 Hz.

The frequency of each individual wave also may be determined. The distance from A to a is 15 mm. The paper speed is 30 mm/sec, so 15 mm represents 0.5 sec. The duration of the wave marked off as A–a is therefore 0.5 sec.

These measurements were made from the top of one wave to the top of another. The same result is obtained by measuring from the bottom of the waves, A′ to B′, and A′ to a′, a′ to B′.

The equivalent frequency of each wave can be computed by taking the reciprocal of 0.5 sec: 1/0.5. The equivalent frequency is 2 Hz.

A slightly more complex example of frequency measurements is also found in Fig. 7.1. The distance C to D in channel 4 (T_4-A_2) represents 1 sec. There are seven waves in this 1-sec period of time. The peak directly beneath C is at zero time and, counting to the right (the end of the 1-sec interval), the seventh peak is directly below D. However, a close examination of the individual waves in this segment leads to the conclusion that they are not all of the same duration. Measurement of the distance between individual peaks, made with a ruler marked in millimeters, demonstrates the variation.

The measurements estimated to the nearest 0.5 mm are given in column 2 of Table 7.1. The interpeak distances range from 4 to 5 mm with several measured at 4.5 mm. When the individual distances in the 30-mm sample were summed, it was found that the total, 30.5 mm, was in error by 0.5 mm. This is an error of only 1.7% and is permissable when using such a crude instrument as a ruler marked to the nearest millimeter.

Column 3 of Table 7.1 gives the duration of each wave. This is computed by dividing the distances, or wave length (in millimeters), by the number of millimeters in 1 sec. Thus, 4/30 = 0.13 sec. To check for error in the measurement and computations, the individual wave durations are added together. They should equal 1 sec. The actual sum is 1.01 sec. The error is 1%.

When the duration (in sec) is known, the frequency can be computed. The frequency is the reciprocal of the duration (1/duration). Column 4 gives the equivalent frequency for each of the seven waves measured in Fig. 7.1. The range of frequencies, wave by wave, is from 5.9 to 7.7 Hz. The average of the individual equivalent frequencies is 7 Hz. This was the original frequency value obtained by counting the total number of peaks in the designated 1-sec interval. When the equivalent frequency is computed from the average of the individual durations, it is (1/0.144) 6.9 Hz. The error (compared to the original count, or to the average equivalent frequency) is 1%, which is not serious.

The equivalent frequency of any isolated wave also can be determined. The wave lettered E in channel 3 of Fig. 7.1 has a duration of 0.3 sec (9 mm length, e to e′, divided by 30). The equivalent frequency is 3.3 Hz. In channel 2 of Fig. 7.1, there is a single slow wave, lettered F. Its duration is

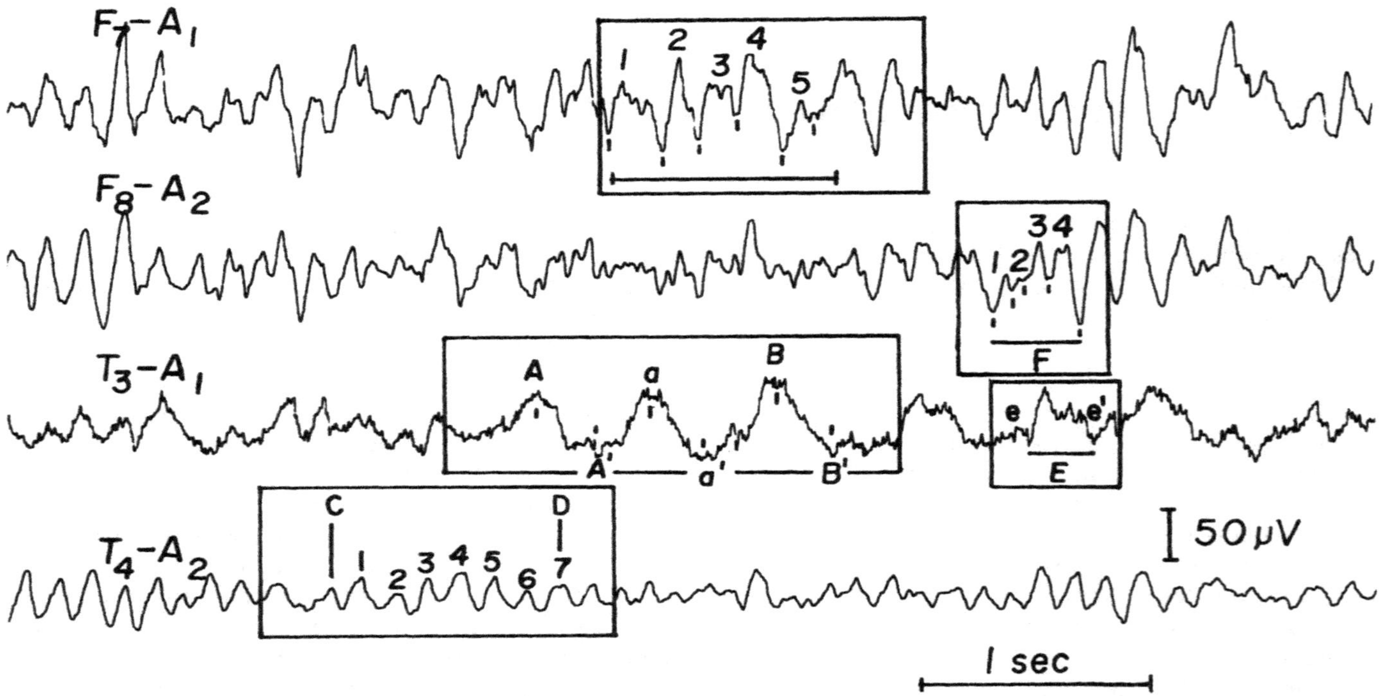

FIG. 7.1. Measurement of EEG frequencies (see text for details).

0.38 sec (11.5 mm/30 mm) and its equivalent frequency is 2.6 Hz. Superimposed on this wave are several smaller waves, numbered 1, 2, 3, and 4. The durations of these are:

wave 1: 0.12 sec (8.3 Hz)
wave 2: 0.05 sec (20 Hz)
wave 3: 0.12 sec (8.3 Hz)
wave 4: 0.13 sec (7.5 Hz)

The section of record marked F, therefore, has various frequencies present within it. Superimposed on the 2.6-Hz wave are smaller waves, two of them with a frequency of 8.3 Hz, one with a frequency of 20 Hz and one with a frequency of 7.5 Hz.

In channel 1, the 1-sec interval that has been marked encompasses about 5½ "waves." Their equivalent frequencies are:

wave 1: 4.0 Hz
wave 2: 6.0 Hz
wave 3: 6.0 Hz
wave 4: 5.0 Hz
wave 5: 8.5 Hz

The average of these equivalent frequencies is 5.9 Hz. This is approximately the number of waves counted within the 1-sec segment. However, this value is not a frequency in the sense of a rhythmic, repetitive process. It is the average equivalent frequency.

TABLE 7.1. *Conversion of distance to duration to frequency of individual EEG waves*[a]

Interval	Distance (mm)	Duration (sec)	Frequency (Hz)
C–1	4	0.13	7.7
1–2	5	0.17	5.9
2–3	4	0.13	7.7
3–4	4.5	0.15	6.7
4–5	4.5	0.15	6.7
5–6	4.5	0.15	6.7
6–D	4	0.13	7.7
Total	30.5	1.01	49.1
Average	4.4	0.14	7.0

[a] See Fig. 7.1, T_4–A_2, channel 4.

Estimates of equivalent frequency are obtained easily by using a cursor, a special ruler made of clear plastic with windows of various widths that represent different equivalent frequencies. When a single wave fits into a window, the equivalent frequency is read off directly.

Most manufacturers provide EEG paper with lines drawn vertically every 30 mm and with slightly lighter lines dividing the larger sections into 6-mm segments. When the recording speed is 30 mm/sec, each large division represents 1 sec and the smaller segments represent 0.2 sec. With the aid of the 0.2-sec lines, the frequency of most activity can be estimated visually with a fair degree of accuracy. If there are three waves in a 0.2-sec interval, the frequency is 15 Hz. If there are 1.5 waves in 0.2 sec, the frequency is 7.5 Hz, and so on.

VOLTAGE

Voltage is expressed in microvolts, although exceptionally large voltages may be expressed in millivolts. The voltage of any EEG wave can be computed by multiplying its amplitude (in mm) by the sensitivity (in μV/mm): ($V = A \times S$). The amplitude is determined by measuring the height of the wave from the point where it begins to rise to the point where it reaches its maximum height. The measurement, in ordinary language, is from the trough to the peak but in EEG terms this is called peak-to-peak amplitude (1,2).

Figure 7.2 is a detail of Fig. 7.1; the slow waves of channel 3 have been isolated for closer examination. An upward arrow defines the point at which each wave was judged to start its rise. A dotted line has been drawn, parallel to baseline, at the point of maximum rise. A vertical line then has been drawn from the arrow to the dotted line. This defines the amplitude of each wave. The measured values are shown in Table 7.2.

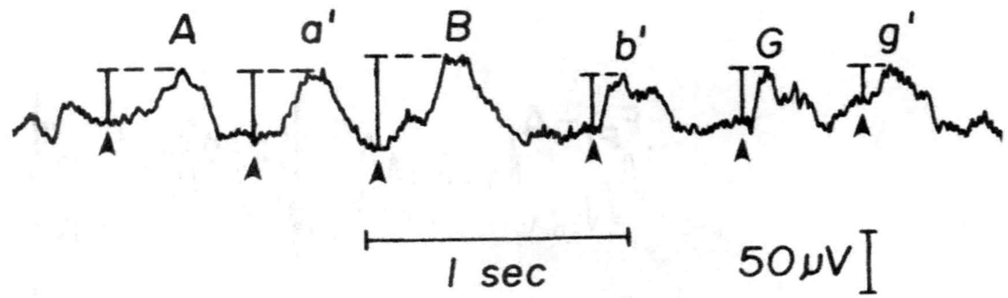

FIG. 7.2. Measurement of EEG amplitudes (see text for details).

The sensitivity used to record this EEG was 7 μV/mm. From the formula just given, the voltages were computed. The third column of Table 7.2 gives the voltage of each of the slow waves. The average voltage of the six waves was 49.6 μV. Figure 7.2 and Table 7.2 thus illustrate the basic principle of determining voltage in the EEG.

Figure 7.3 provides additional examples of practical voltage measurements. There is dominant rhythmic activity in the first two channels at a frequency of approximately 11.5 Hz. The distance from line A to line B is 30 mm, indicating a 1-sec duration. The peak amplitude of each wave

TABLE 7.2. *Voltages of slow waves*[a]

Wave	Amplitude (mm)	Voltage (μV)
A	6.5	45.5
a'	8	56
B	10.5	73.5
b'	5.5	38.5
G	6	42
g'	6	42
Totals	42.5	297.5
Averages	7.1	49.6

[a] See Fig. 7.2 (S = 7 μV/mm).

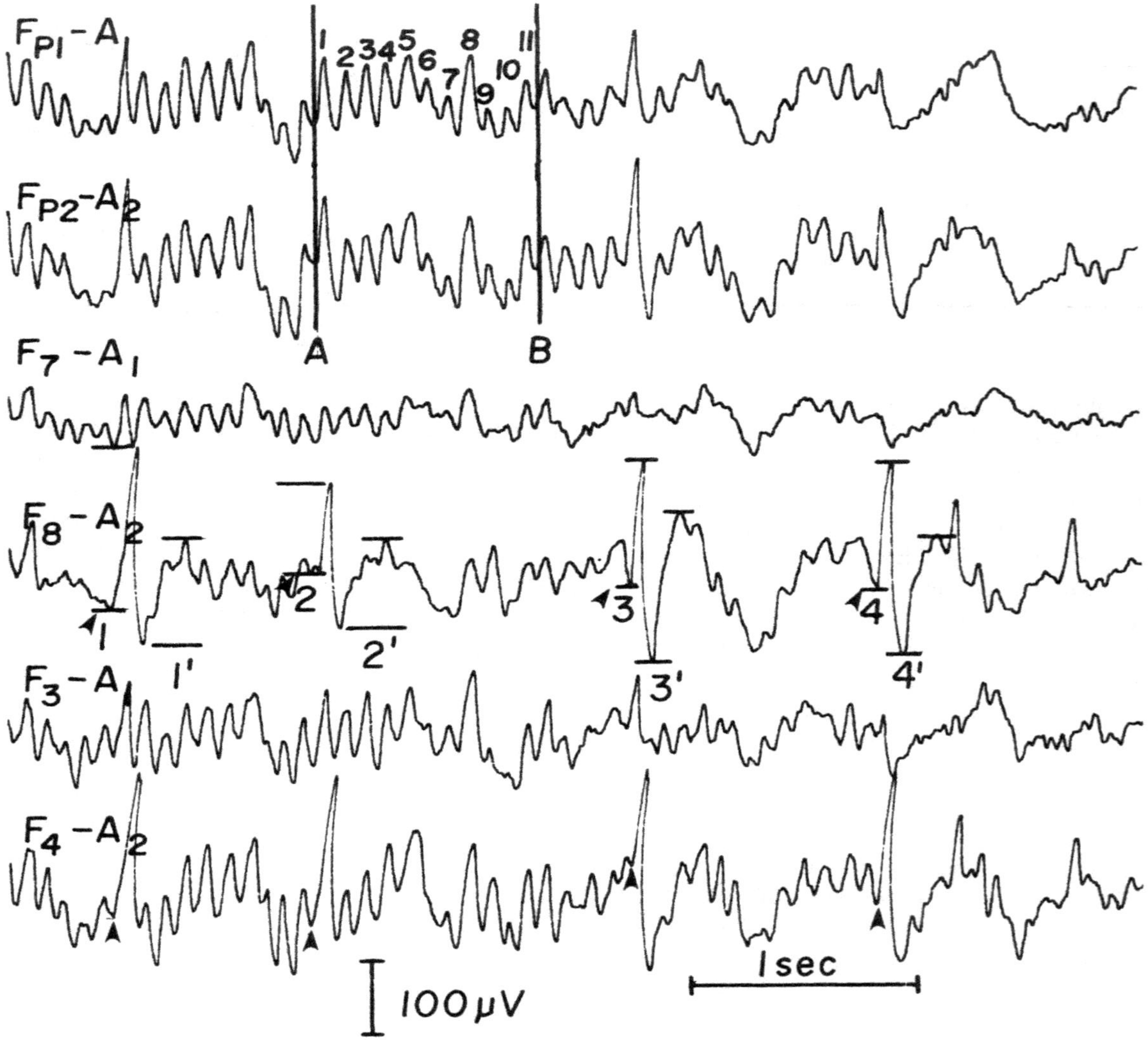

FIG. 7.3. Measurement of EEG frequencies and amplitudes (see text for details).

of the eleven rising waves in the designated 1 sec was measured to the nearest 0.5 mm in both channels 1 and 2; the results are given in columns 2 and 4 of Table 7.3. The sensitivity was 10 μV/mm, and the voltages for each wave are given in columns 3 and 5.

There was considerable wave-to-wave variability in voltage. In channel 1, the range was from 30 to 110 μV. In channel 2 it was 20 to 120 μV. Although waves appearing simultaneously in channels 1 and 2 did not always have identical voltage, they tended to get larger or smaller at the same time. The average voltage of the 11-Hz rhythm in this sample was about 64 μV in both channels.

In Fig. 7.3, another interesting EEG characteristic is the presence of high voltage sharp transients. These are particularly obvious in channels 2, 4, and 6. Following each sharp transient, there is a somewhat lower amplitude slow wave. The voltage of the sharp transients in channel 4 are shown in Table 7.4. First, the start of the rise was defined by an arrow. The distance (in mm) of the maximum rise was measured in the same way as the slow waves in Fig. 7.2 were measured. The four sharp waves varied in voltage from 120 to 220 μV (Table 7.4, column 3). The average voltage was 168.8 μV (or 169 μV).

The slow waves that followed the sharp waves in channel 4 were also measured (Fig. 7.3). Table 7.4 shows the amplitudes (column 5) and the voltages (column 6); the average slow wave voltage was 157.5 μV.

Two arbitrary decisions must be made in measuring voltage. First, Where does the wave start? Second, Where does it reach its peak? There is no particular difficulty in answering these questions in the case of the sharp waves. Their "take-off" points and their peaks are quite clear. In the case of the slow waves, the start of the rise is clear. The point of the peak becomes slightly subjective because of the superimposed 11.5-Hz activity. This may have added 2 mm to the amplitude measurement of waves 1′ and 2′. In the case of wave 4′, the decision was made to take the earliest peak as the slow wave peak, and the 11-Hz wave at the peak was disregarded in determining the amplitude.

The working examples above demonstrate the procedures to be followed in computing voltage of EEG activity. First, the amplitude of a wave is measured in millimeters. This is then converted to voltage by multiplying the amplitude by the sensitivity. Generally speaking, one should refer to an EEG as showing "low voltage activity," not "low amplitude activity." A record could be of low amplitude (for example, 5 mm on the average). If the sensitivity was 20 μV/mm, this would be fairly high voltage: 100 μV. However, if the sensitivity was 3 μV/mm, the voltage would be low: 15 μV.

TABLE 7.3. *Voltage of L and R F_p 11-Hz activity*[a]

Wave	Channel 1 Peak amplitude (mm)	Channel 1 Voltage (μV)	Channel 2 Peak amplitude (mm)	Channel 2 Voltage (μV)
1	9	90	9	90
2	8	80	8	80
3	7	70	6	60
4	8.5	85	8	80
5	7	70	6.5	65
6	3	30	2	20
7	3	30	2.5	25
8	11	110	12	120
9	3	30	4	40
10	4	40	4	40
11	7	70	9	90
Totals	70.5	705	71.0	710
Averages	64.1	64.1	6.45	64.5

[a] See Fig. 7.3, channels 1 and 2 (S = 10 μV/mm).

SUMMARY

Frequency is defined in hertz (Hz). If the activity is apparently rhythmic, its frequency can be determined by counting the number of

TABLE 7.4. *Voltage of sharp transients*[a]

Wave	Channel 4, sharp waves Amplitude (mm)	Channel 4, sharp waves Voltage (μV)	Wave	Channel 4, slow waves Amplitude (mm)	Channel 4, slow waves Voltage (μV)
1	22	220	1′	14	140
2	12	120	2′	12.5	125
3	16.5	165	3′	20	200
4	17	170	4′	16.5	165
Totals		675			630
Averages		168.75			157.5

[a] See Fig. 7.3, channels 2,4,6 (S = 10 μV/mm).

waves appearing in 1-sec. Usually, waves are not exactly the same and vary in duration. The duration of the wave can be determined by measuring its length (in mm) and converting this measurement to time. When the duration (in sec) is known, the equivalent frequency is the reciprocal (1 divided by the wave duration). Random, nonrhythmic waves can be referred to by their equivalent frequency.

Voltage is computed by measuring the amplitude of a wave from its lower-most point to the following peak. The vertical distance of rise (in mm) is multiplied by the sensitivity of the amplifier (in μV/mm). This gives the voltage. The computations of voltage are carried out in the same manner for waves of all frequencies.

REFERENCES

1. Chatrian, G. E., Bergamini, L., Dondey, M., Klass, D. W., Lennox-Buchthal, M., and Petersén, I. (1974): A glossary of terms most commonly used by clinical electroencephalographers. *Electroencephalogr. Clin. Neurophysiol.*, 37:538–548.
2. Cooper, R., Osselton, J. W., and Shaw, J. C. (1980): *EEG Technology*, 3rd ed. Butterworths, London, pp. 123–147.

Chapter 8

The EEG Amplifier and Its Controls

The EEG amplifier is a device that magnifies the input signals from the brain so that they can be easily observed and measured at the output. The input voltages and the input frequencies must be reproduced accurately. An ideal amplifier would give a faithful reproduction of all electrical signals generated in the brain, ranging from slow DC shifts to fast activity in the vicinity of 3 kHz. In conventional EEG applications, only a relatively small portion of this range, from approximately 0.5 Hz to 60 or 70 Hz, is of clinical relevance. An amplifier whose output reproduces the input over most of this frequency range would meet the necessary requirements (2).

The ink-writing recorder (the pen galvanometer or oscillograph) has electrical and mechanical limitations. The pen can be moved only within a fixed distance above and below the baseline (zero or center position). In addition, there are limitations on the rapidity with which it can be moved (4,13). An amplifier that is linear from 0.1 Hz to 1 kHz, for example, cannot drive a galvanometer beyond its high frequency limit, which may be 70 to 100 Hz. The practical frequency range of linearity then would be from 0.1 Hz (the amplifier's lower limit) to 70 Hz (the galvanometer's upper limit). Therefore, the characteristics of the galvanometer must be considered along with those of the amplifier when discussing the accuracy of reproduction of EEG signals (11,12,14). In practical terms, the amplifier and the galvanometer must be considered as a system for the display of the EEG.

The four main controls on the amplifier (Fig. 8.1) are (a) Sensitivity; (b) Low Frequency Filter, (c) High Frequency Filter, and (d) 60-Hz Rejection Filter. All of these controls have one thing in common: they act as *attenuators*. The sensitivity control acts to decrease equally the output amplitude of the system at all input frequencies when the sensitivity is decreased. When the sensitivity is increased, there is less attenuation and output amplitude is increased equally at all input frequencies.

The low frequency (LF) filter decreases the output amplitudes over selected ranges of low frequencies and leaves higher frequencies unattenuated. The high frequency (HF) filter decreases the ouput amplitudes over selected ranges of high frequencies, but it does not change the amplitudes of lower frequencies. The 60-Hz rejection filter sharply reduces the amplitude of 60-Hz activity, with diminishing effects on frequencies just above and below 60 Hz.

SENSITIVITY CONTROLS

The sensitivity control, as it appears to the EEG technologist, is simply a dial on the panel of the instrument. Behind the dial is a voltage divider composed of a number of resistors placed across the output of an amplifier stage (Fig. 8.2). By selection of the output at particular points in this string of resistors, more or less voltage can be passed on to the next amplifier stage. When the sensitivity control is at maximum (typically, 1 μV/mm), all of the output voltage is available. When a lower sensitivity is used, the sensitivity switch selects a different point on the voltage divider and only a part of the total signal voltage is passed on to the next amplifier stage. More technical details are discussed in Chapter 5.

Assuming that the amplifying system is linear from 0.1 Hz to 100 Hz

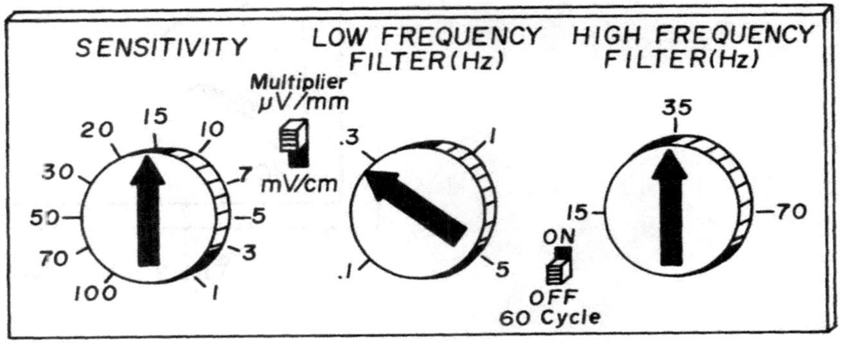

FIG. 8.1. Principal controls of an EEG amplifier.

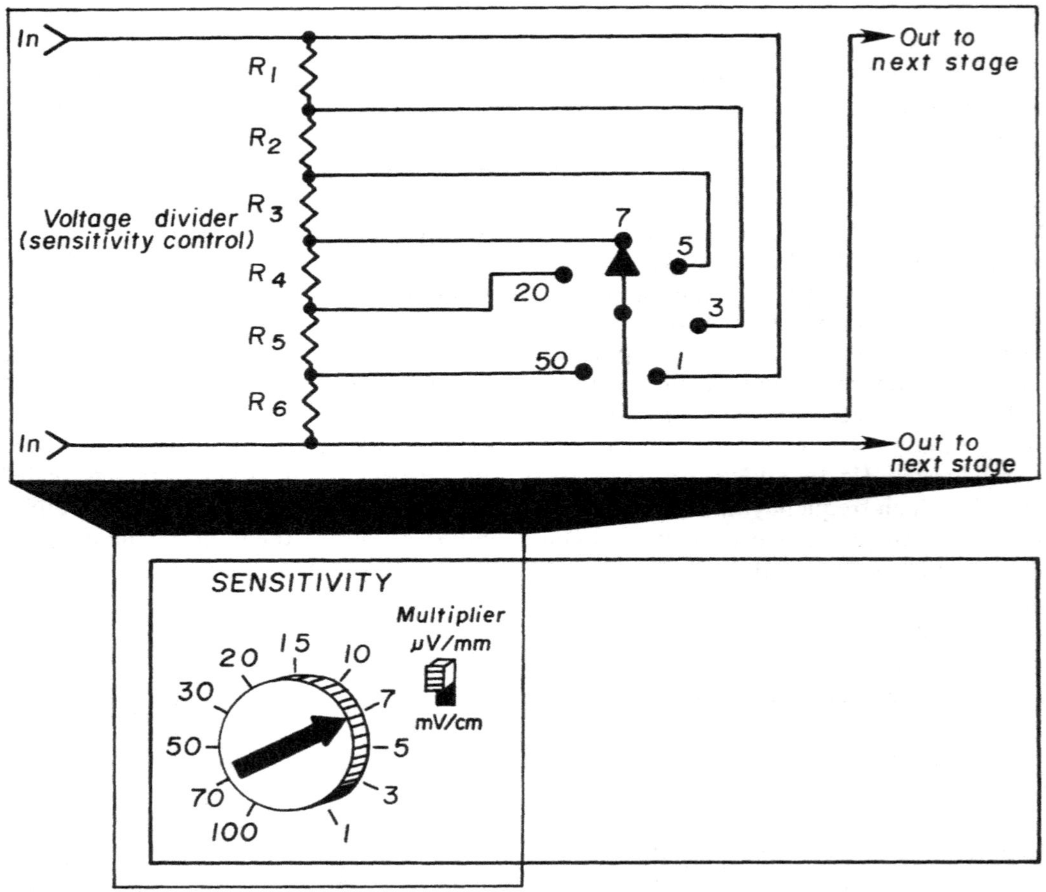

FIG. 8.2. Sensitivity dial and circuit it controls.

when the sensitivity control is set at 10 μV/mm, a 100-μV input signal with a frequency of 0.1 Hz, 1 Hz, 10 Hz, 50 Hz, or 100 Hz will produce a galvanometer pen deflection of 10 mm. Any increase or decrease of 10 μV input voltage over this range of frequencies will increase or decrease the amplitude of the pen's deflection by 1 mm.

These statements are based on the definition of sensitivity as the ratio between input voltage (in μV) and output amplitude (pen deflection in mm) (3). The basic formula is, then:

$$S = \frac{V}{A}$$

where S = sensitivity, V = μV input signal voltage, and A = amplitude (pen deflection).

This also can be expressed as:

$$V = S \times A, \text{ or}$$

$$A = \frac{V}{S}.$$

The basic linear relationship that is assumed is shown as a graph in Fig. 8.3. However, this relationship can hold only within the limits of the pen's deflection.

Figure 8.4 reproduces one channel of EEG recorded at S = 10 μV/mm. As indicated by the arrows, the record is "squared off" because the pen could move no further up or down. The total range of this deflection was 37 mm. We know that the voltage represented by the distance from A to B was at least 370 μV (V = S × A), but we cannot know how much more it might have been. To know the actual peak voltage, it would have been necessary to record at a lower sensitivity, for example, 20 μV/mm.

Typically, the maximum peak-to-peak pen deflection of an EEG system will be about 35 mm. The International EEG Federation (3) recommends a range of "at least" 20 mm.

Dynamic Range

The range of input voltages between the least voltage that can be measured and the maximum voltage that can be measured may be considered the dynamic range of the system. The maximum voltage that can be

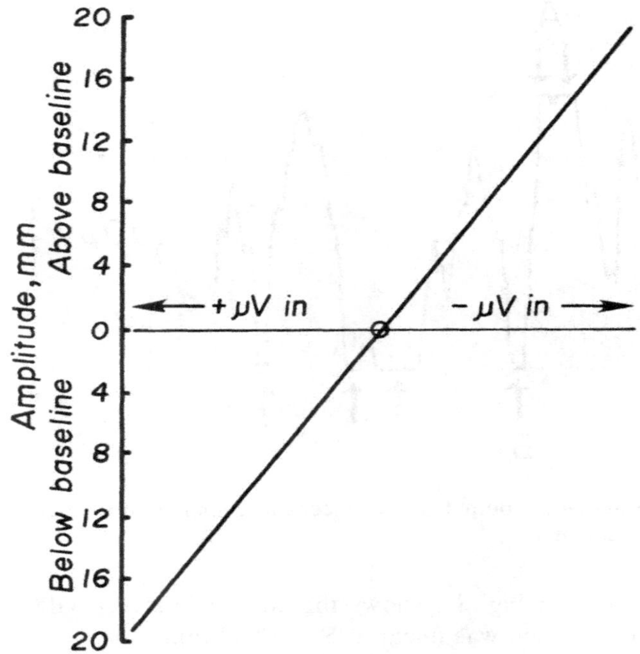

FIG. 8.3. Linear relationship between amplitude and voltage.

measured will depend on the mechanical limitations of the pen and galvanometer and on the sensitivity setting used. Fig. 8.5 is based on an instrument with a typical maximum pen deflection of 35 mm. When S = 7 μV/mm, the upper limit of measurable voltage is 245 μV. However, if the input voltage suddenly increased to 275 μV, the amplitude that would be necessary to maintain a linear input-output would be 39 mm. In order for the system to accommodate this larger voltage at the output, the sensitivity would have to be reduced to 10 μV/mm. This would produce a 28-mm deflection of the pen, which is well within the upper limits of the dynamic range (350 μV) of the new setting. If the input voltage reached 400 μV, it would be necessary to reduce the sensitivity to 15 μV/mm to keep within the upper limit of the dynamic range (525 μV).

Figure 8.6 shows an EEG that reached, at A, a peak voltage of 2,200 μV. It was necessary to use S = 100 μV/mm to keep within the dynamic range.

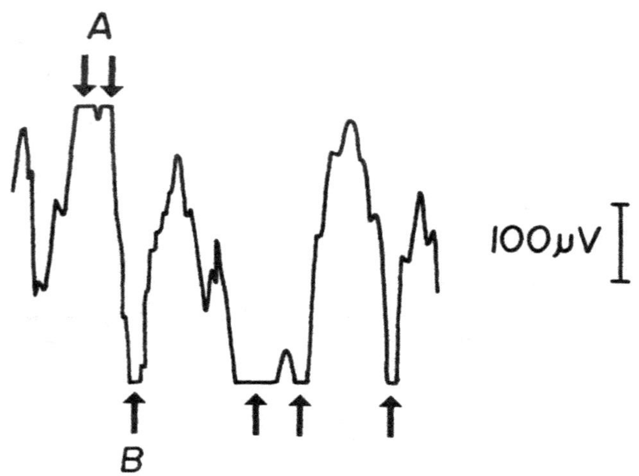

FIG. 8.4. Squared-off output due to mechanical limitation of oscillograph (see text). S = 10 μV/mm.

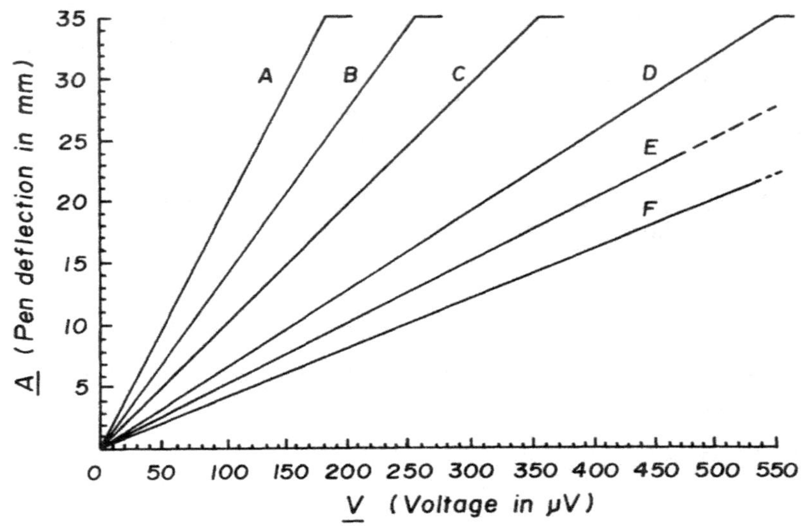

FIG. 8.5. Dynamic range as a function of sensitivity of the recording system (square wave unit). The maximum pen excursion of this instrument was 35 mm peak to peak. Sensitivity of 5 μV/mm (*A*) is higher than the "conventional" sensitivity setting of 7 μV/mm (*B*), but the dynamic range of 175 μV at higher sensitivity is less than dynamic range of 245 μV at conventional setting. A wider dynamic range, 350 μV, occurs at a sensitivity setting of 10 μV/mm (C). *A:* 5 μV/mm, *B:* 7 μV/mm, *C:* 10 μV/mm, *D:* 15 μV/mm, *E:* 20 μV/mm, *F:* 25 μV/mm. (See text for discussion.) Modified from Snodgrass and Knott (14).

The dashed line in Fig. 8.6 shows the amplitude that would have been reached if the system was linear at S = 10 μV/mm.

Dynamic range is set by (a) the limits of pen deflection and (b) the sensitivity. The lower the sensitivity, the greater the dynamic range.

The upper limit of dynamic range at any sensitivity setting can be determined by multiplying the peak-to-peak limits of pen deflection by sensitivity. Assuming the galvanometer provides a 35-mm peak-to-peak deflection, dynamic ranges will be established at the sensitivity settings shown in Table 8.1.

On the other hand, input voltages can be so small that they are difficult to perceive and measure unless sensitivity is increased. A 3-μV signal recorded at S = 7 μV/mm produces a deflection with an amplitude of 0.5 mm, which is only slightly greater than the width of the tracing. The *least voltage change* that can be measured at any given sensitivity setting establishes the *resolution* of the system (8). Figure 8.7 illustrates the effect of changing sensitivity on resolving the voltages present in a sample of EEG. It is obvious that at S = 50 and 30 μV/mm, accurate measurement of less than 20 μV is virtually impossible. Little activity can be perceived until sensitivity is increased to 15 or 10 μV/mm. Measurement becomes more precise as the amplitude of the output becomes larger. A resolution of at least 2 μV is required in some clinical applications (1).

Dynamic range and resolution are inversely related, and the technologist must use a sensitivity for a particular recording that keeps the EEG signals at useful output amplitudes.

Sensitivity Multiplier

The sensitivity multiplier changes the dynamic range in large steps. One type of multiplier shifts the sensitivity scale from μV/mm to mV/cm. Since there are 1,000 μV in a millivolt and 10 mm in a centimeter, when measured in μV/mm, sensitivity is increased by a factor of 100 as opposed

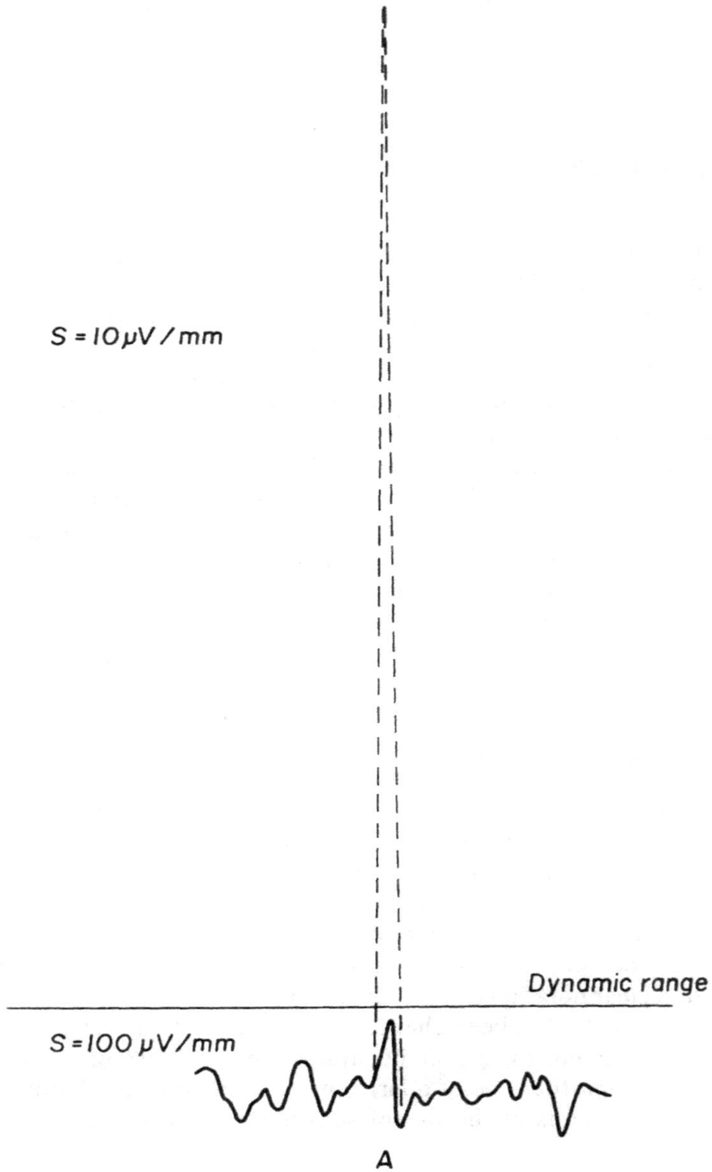

FIG. 8.6. Peak voltage of 2,200 μV within dynamic range, and (*dashed line*) as it would have appeared if system was linear at S = 10 μV/mm. LF = 0.3 Hz; HF = 70 Hz.

TABLE 8.1. *Dynamic range at nine sensitivity settings (peak-to-peak limits of pen deflection × sensitivity)*

Sensitivity (μV/mm)	Dynamic range (μV)
1	35
2	70
5	175
7	245
10	350
15	525
20	700
50	1,750 (1.75 mV)
70	2,450 (2.45 mV)

to the mV/cm scale. A sensitivity of 1 mV/cm is the same as a sensitivity of 100 μV/mm. When monitoring the electrocardiogram, for example, a lower sensitivity may be needed. Special monitoring devices, such as those used to measure tremor or respiration, also may require very low sensitivity. The multipliers are installed in the individual amplifiers and do not have a master control.

At least one EEG instrument uses multipliers of another type. Basic sensitivity is set by a single sensitivity control that serves all amplifiers. The individual amplifiers have no standard sensitivity control, but only multiplier switches with typical values of 20, 4, 2, 1, 0.5, and 0.25; these normally are set with the multiplier on "1." If the basic sensitivity control is set at 7 μV/mm, a change of the multiplier to 0.5 on a single channel will increase its sensitivity from 7 μV/mm to 3.5 μV/mm. A change of the multiplier to 0.25 will shift sensitivity to 1.75 μV/mm.

Decreases in sensitivity can be set at three levels: 2×, 4×, and 20×. Starting at 7 μV/mm, these would be 14 μV/mm, 28 μV/mm, and 140 μV/mm, respectively. The technologist must compute these values, and the individual channel sensitivity values will depend on the basic setting of the basic control, multiplied by the multiplier factor of each individual

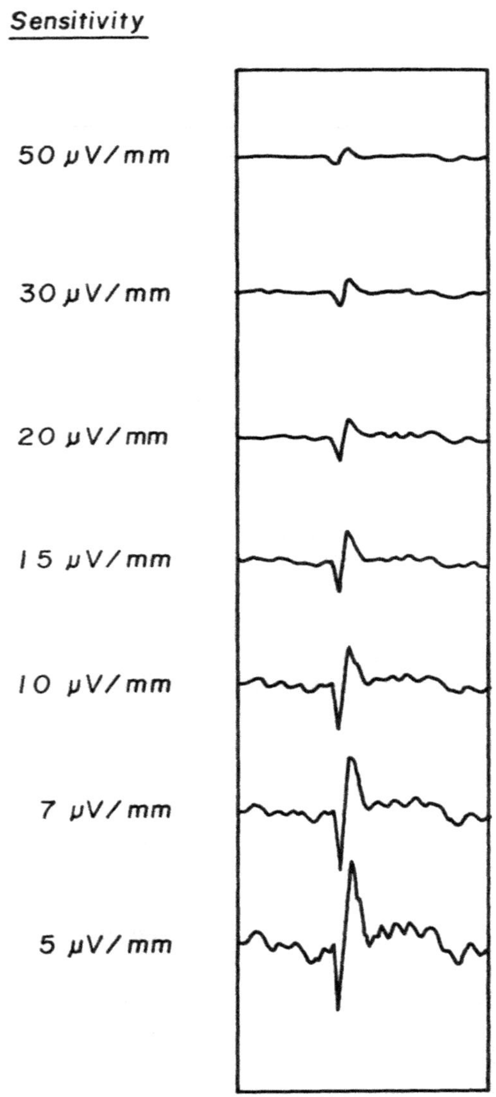

FIG. 8.7. Effect of changing sensitivity on resolving the voltages present in a 1-sec sample of EEG. HF = 70 Hz; LF = 1 Hz.

channel. One must remember that 20× does not make the channel 20 times more sensitive, but 1/20 as sensitive. The necessity of including terminal calibrations at all deviations from the basic setting of the multiplier control should be obvious.

Master Sensitivity Control

Clinical EEG instruments are equipped with a master sensitivity control that simultaneously sets the sensitivity for each channel. (Some instruments have an individual channel "override" provision that allows the channel to operate on its own individual, calibrated sensitivity control.) The master control is calibrated in μV/mm.

Some older instruments have "all-channel" controls that are not calibrated in μV/mm, although the individual channels are so calibrated. The all-channel control can be set at "+1," "0," "−1," "−2," and "−3." If an increase in sensitivity in all channels is desired, the control is moved to "+1." Decreases in sensitivity can be accomplished typically at three levels. The actual sensitivities for these levels must be computed from calibrations. They often will prove to be near the appropriate step changes of the individual channel μV/mm scale. If individual channels are set at 7 μV/mm, the all-channel "+1" may become approximately 5 μV/mm; changes of "−1", "−2," and "−3" may be approximately 10 μV/mm, 15 μV/mm, and 20 μV/mm.

Using the Sensitivity Controls

The settings on the sensitivity controls should be changed during the course of the recording whenever it is necessary to keep activity within the system's dynamic range. The sensitivity chosen should be such that resolution of small voltage differences can be preserved to the best possible degree. This is usually accomplished by changing the master sensitivity control; no recording time is lost. Whenever a sensitivity setting is changed, a clear notation of the fact should be made on the recording, and the value of what it has been changed *from* and what it is being changed *to* should be indicated. Figure 8.8 illustrates the adroit use of a master sensitivity control at the time of a large increase in voltage. (Further examples and discussions of the use of sensitivity controls may be found in ref. 10.)

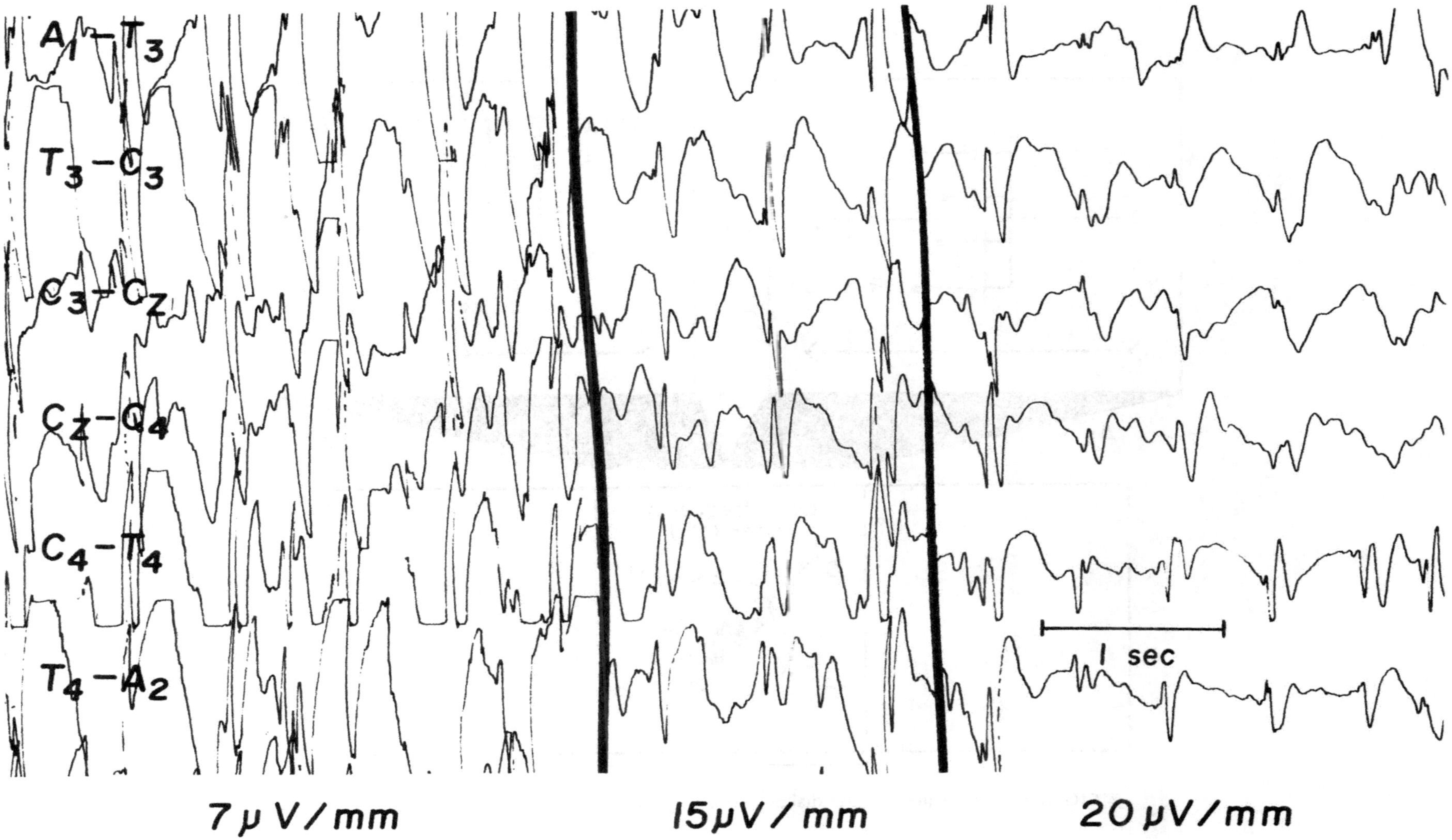

FIG. 8.8. Effects of changes in sensitivity settings during recorded seizure.

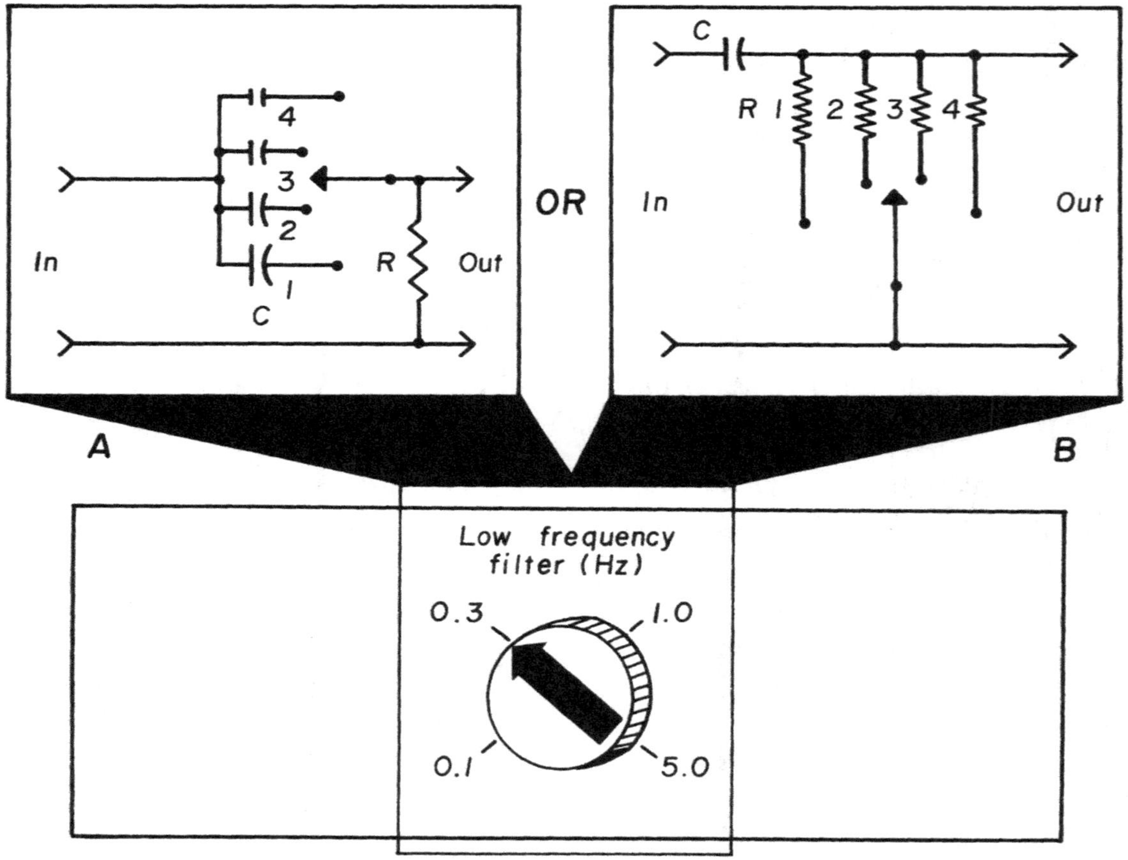

FIG. 8.9. Low frequency filter dial and circuit it controls. (See text for discussion.)

Most EEG recordings begin with a sensitivity level of 7 μV/mm, since most activity falls inside the dynamic range of this setting. Variations in sensitivity then may be made as needed, depending on the voltages encountered. At the end of the record, calibrations must be made for each sensitivity setting used.

LOW FREQUENCY FILTER

The low frequency (LF) filter control appears as another dial, with another set of numbers, on the panel of the EEG instrument. Behind the panel, there are four possible capacitive–resistive configurations, any one of which can be selected and placed in series between amplifier stages to determine the low frequency response of the system. Figure 8.9A shows the classical system, which uses four capacitors and a fixed resistor to establish the low frequency response. Figure 8.9B shows an alternative system, which utilizes one capacitor and four selectable values of resistance.

This capacitive–resistive configuration (as discussed in Chapter 5) has the ability to attenuate low frequencies. This is determined by the size of the capacitors (C_1, C_2, C_3, and C_4) in microfarads and the value of the resistor (R_1) in megohms. C_1 is the largest capacitor, and attenuates very low frequencies the least. C_4 is the smallest capacitor, and attenuates very low frequencies the most. By choosing the value of the capacitor in conjunction with the value of the resistor, it is possible to define the lowest frequency in the EEG that will be recorded without significant attenuation. (The term "significant attenuation" will be discussed shortly.) The numbers on the LF dial represent the frequencies above which attenuation is disregarded and below which there is significant attenuation. For example, if the LF filter is set at 1 Hz, there will be acceptable linearity at all frequencies above 1 Hz. Frequencies below 1 Hz will not be linearly amplified.

Some LF controls have a second set of numbers on the dial. These are the time constants of the capacitive-resistive circuits switched in by the LF control (Chapter 5). The value of the time constant, in seconds, has less direct meaning to the technologist, in on-line applications, than does the value of the cut-off frequency, in Hz. The latter indicates the specific frequency above which the amplifier is linear and below which activity in the EEG becomes distorted. The practical usefulness of the time constants is limited to calibration procedures, and quick visual assessment of the integrity of the LF filters. This is discussed later in this chapter, and in Chapter 9.

The practical effects of LF filters on EEG activity are shown in Fig. 8.10. The same activity (Fp_1-O_2) goes to the input of each of four amplifiers. The sensitivity control is set at 7 μV/mm and the HF is set at 70 Hz in each channel. The LF filters are different in each: channel 1 = 0.1 Hz, channel 2 = 0.3 Hz, channel 3 = 1 Hz, and channel 4 = 5 Hz.

It is obvious that there are differences between the outputs of the four amplifiers, although their inputs are identical. The most obvious differences are between Channel 4 and the others. However, careful observation shows many differences between channels 1, 2 and 3, seen as variations in amplitude and morphology (shape) of the waves. Wave A in Fig. 8.10 has an approximate equivalent frequency of 1 Hz. In channel 3 (LF = 1 Hz), its amplitude is lower than in channels 1 and 2. In addition, owing to phase shift, the peak of wave A occurs earlier when LF = 1 Hz is used (see Chapter 5). Wave A has become so attenuated and distorted in channel 4, in which LF is set at 5 Hz, that it cannot be identified.

Similar effects appear in wave B. This wave has an approximate equivalent frequency of 0.67 Hz. Comparison of channel 2 (LF = 0.3 Hz) with channel 1 (LF = 0.1 Hz) shows that the amplitude of the wave is attenuated 6%. In channel 3 (LF = 1 Hz), it is attenuated 41%. Further, the character of the 0.66 Hz wave is destroyed and only the three waves superimposed upon it (Channels 1 and 2) appear. In Channel 4, the 0.66 Hz is attenuated 100% and the superimposed waves also are attenuated. There also is phase shift, as seen by comparing the times of the peak voltage in the various channels.

Although the effects that LF filters have on the display of EEG activity can be demonstrated roughly by examples of the type used in Fig. 8.10, it is more difficult to grasp the principles of filter functions when the input frequencies are not under the control of the observer, as is the case when essentially random EEG activity is recorded. By inputting sine waves whose frequencies can be controlled by the observer, the amplitudes and phase shifts at the outputs can be measured, tabulated, and graphically displayed. A technologist can, by examining the results of these observations, learn what LF filters actually do to modify the appearance of the EEG, which is made up of many frequencies. This will provide the necessary foundation for the optimal use of LF filters in clinical recording situations.

Figure 8.11 schematically shows the influence of LF filters on low

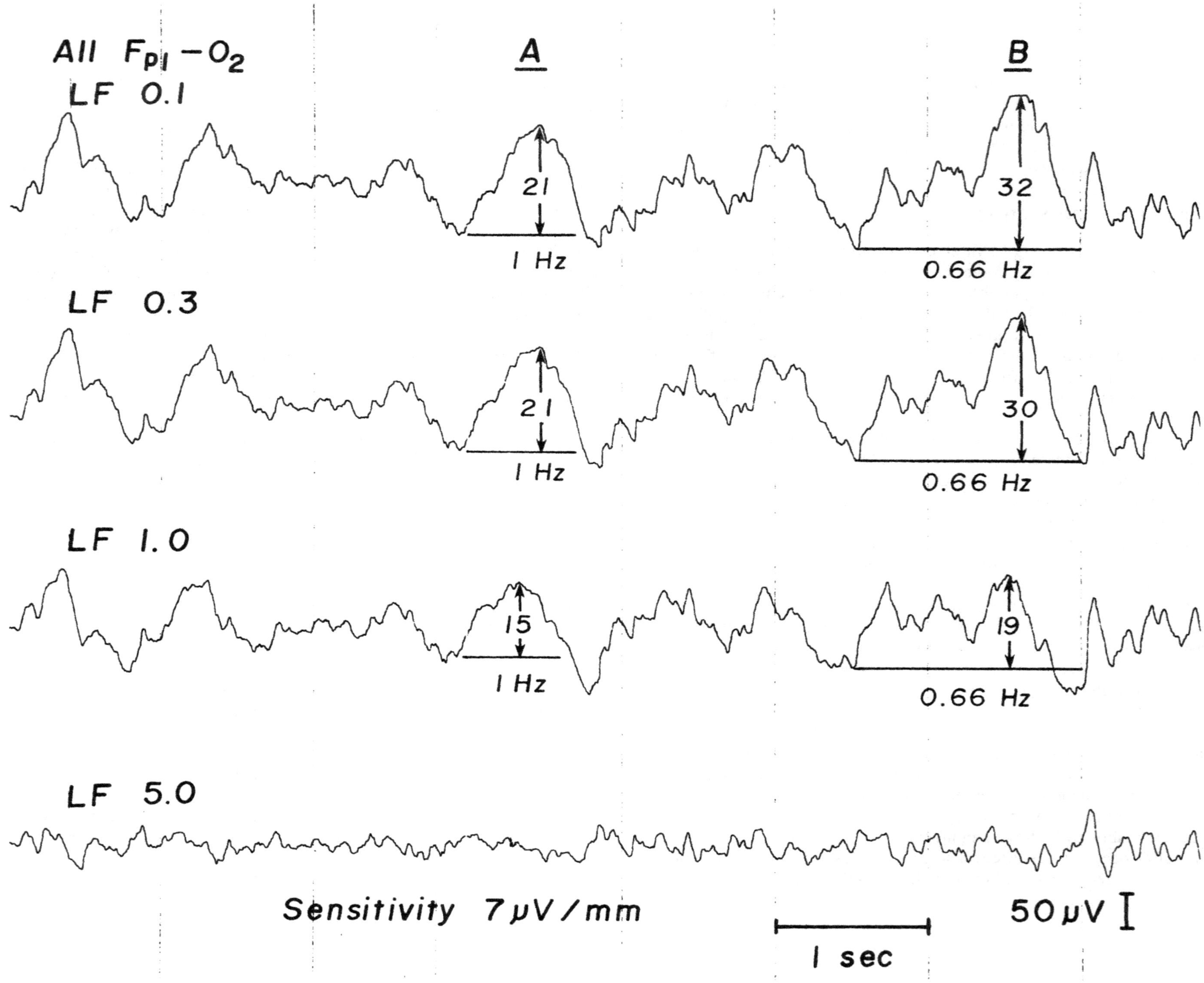

All $F_{p1} - O_2$
A
B
LF 0.1
21
1 Hz
32
0.66 Hz
LF 0.3
21
1 Hz
30
0.66 Hz
LF 1.0
15
1 Hz
19
0.66 Hz
LF 5.0
Sensitivity 7 μV/mm
1 sec
50 μV

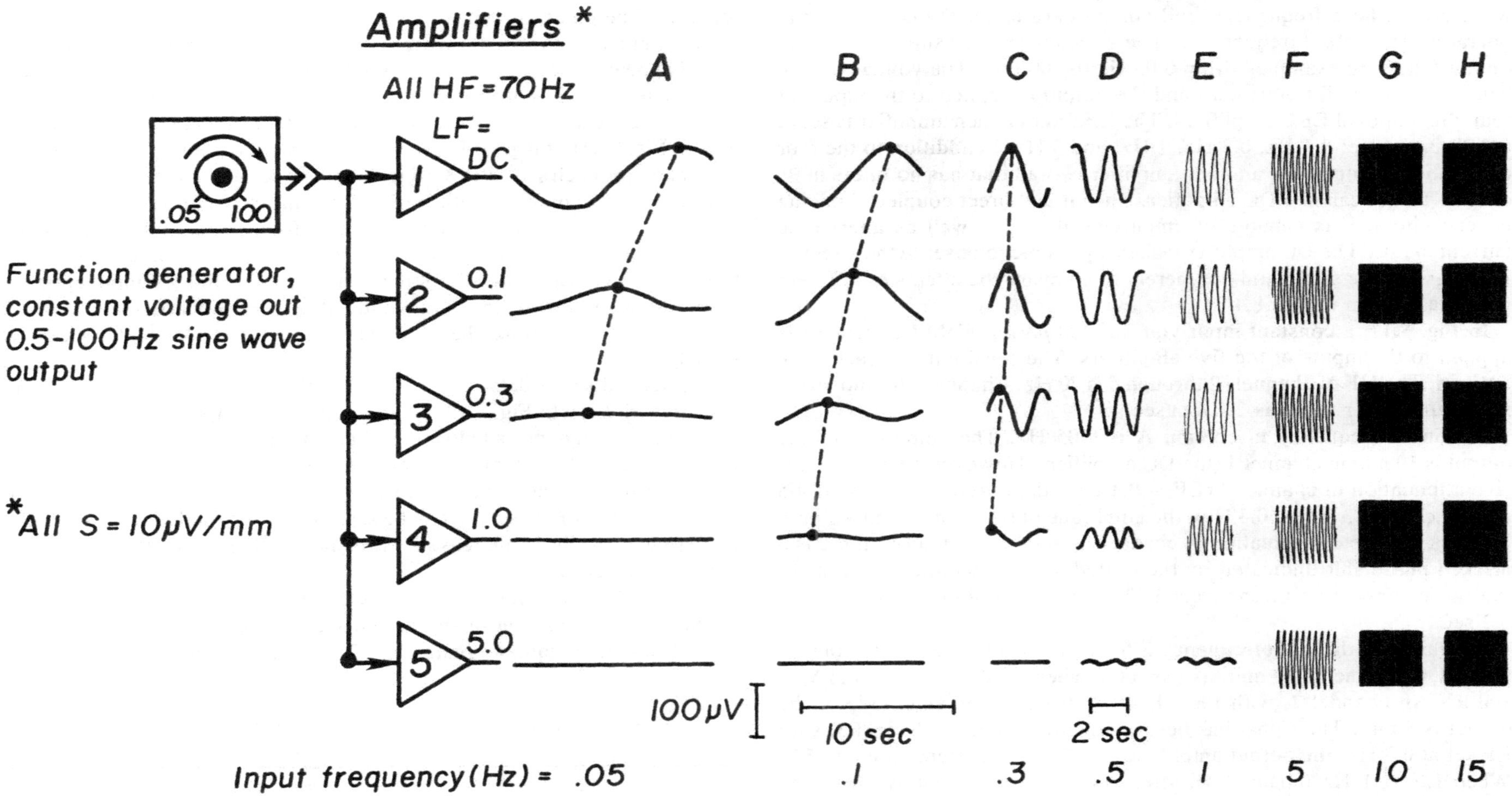

FIG. 8.11. Frequency response characteristics of LF filters 0.1 Hz, 0.3 Hz, 1 Hz, and 5 Hz compared with unfiltered channel (DC). S = 10 μV/mm; HF (channels 2–5) = 70 Hz.

FIG. 8.10. Effect of LF filters on delta activity. S = 7 μV/mm; HF = 70 Hz.

frequency sine waves. The sine waves are produced by a function generator, which is an electronic device capable of producing a variety of waveforms whose frequencies and voltages are under the control of the operator. The output frequency can be varied from very slow to very fast (in the following examples, from 0.05 Hz to 100 Hz). The voltage can be held constant at all frequencies and the output is applied to the inputs of four conventional EEG amplifiers. The LF filter of each amplifier is set at a different value: 0.1 Hz, 0.3 Hz, 1 Hz, and 5 Hz. In addition to the four conventional amplifiers, another amplifier is used that has no filters in its circuit. This is called a DC amplifier, since it is "direct coupled," having no capacitors; it is capable of amplifying direct as well as alternating current inputs. The DC amplifier makes it possible to observe the effect of LF filters on the signal and not merely to compare the effects of different filters, as shown in Fig. 8.10.

In Fig. 8.11, a constant input voltage, 100 μV, at eight frequencies is applied to the inputs of the five amplifiers. The sensitivity of each is 10 μV/mm. The HF of channels 2 through 5 is 70 Hz. Channel 1 has no HF in its circuit. Paper speed is 2.5 mm/sec.

The input frequency in column A is 0.05 Hz. The amplitude of the output is 10 mm in channel 1 (the DC amplifier). However, there is extensive attenuation in channel 2 (LF = 0.1 Hz); the output amplitude is 4.5 mm. In channel 3 (LF = 0.3 Hz), the amplitude of the output is only 1 mm. There is complete attenuation in channels 4 and 5. In addition, there is a marked phase shift indicated by the dotted line connecting the peaks of the waves appearing in channels 1, 2, and 3. The shift in channel 2 is 5.2 sec.

In column B, the input frequency is 0.1 Hz. The amplitude of the output of the DC channel is 10 mm, as expected when S = 10 μV/mm and V = 100 μV. In channel 2, with the LF set at 0.1 Hz, the amplitude of the output is 8 mm. The signal has been attenuated 20%. In channel 3, with LF set at 0.3 Hz, the output amplitude is 3.5 mm, an attenuation of 65%. When LF = 1 Hz (channel 4), attenuation is approximately 90%, and when LF = 5 Hz (channel 5), it is 100%.

Although the amount of phase shift (in time) is less at this frequency than it was when the input frequency was 0.05 Hz, it still is large in channel 2 (LF = 0.1 Hz); the phase shift is 2 sec. In channel 3, the phase shift is nearly 3.5 sec, and in channel 4, it is almost 4.5 sec.

When the input frequency is again increased, to 0.3 Hz, a different set of output data appear (column C, Fig. 8.11). The amplitudes may be measured as before, and the phase shift noted.

The output amplitudes at each input frequency of each channel are presented in Table 8.2. Figure 8.11 and Table 8.2 should be examined together. The point to understand is that if, at these frequencies, 100 μV signals were simultaneously present in an actual EEG, the voltage of each would appear to be different and the time relationships between the three frequencies would appear to be changed at each LF setting (5,12).

By using the amplitude data from Table 8.2 (based on measurements of data in Fig. 8.11), it is possible to draw a graph of the output at each input frequency for each LF filter setting. The first set of data, from channel 1, is based on an amplifier with no LF filter in its circuit (Fig. 8.12). The amplitude of the output is 10 mm at all input frequencies. When plotted on a graph, the values of the Y-axis, on the left, appear as percent attenuation and, on the right, as dB attenuation. Since the 100-μV input appears as a 10-mm output (S = 10 μV/mm) at all frequencies, there is zero attenuation. Connecting the dots that represent these points yields a straight line.

The second set of data, based on LF = 0.1 Hz, is plotted in Fig. 8.13. By comparison with Fig. 8.12, it can be seen that amplitude progressively decreases at frequencies below the filter setting. Full output, however, is not reached until the input frequency is above the filter setting.

The third set of data, based on LF = 0.3 Hz, is shown in Fig. 8.14. By comparison with Fig. 8.13, it can be seen that when the LF filter setting is increased, there is an increase in attenuation of the lowest frequencies, particularly below 0.2 Hz.

Figure 8.15 plots attenuation versus frequency when LF = 1 Hz. There is extensive attenuation of the lowest frequencies below 0.3 Hz, and a good deal of attenuation (greater than 20%) at all frequencies below 1 Hz.

TABLE 8.2. *Output amplitude (mm) at eight input frequencies at five LF filter settings*[a]

LF filter (Hz)	Input frequency (Hz)							
	0.05	0.1	0.3	0.5	1	5	10	15
None[b]	10	10	10	10	10	10	10	10
0.1	4.5	8	10	10	10	10	10	10
0.3	1	3.5	8	9	10	10	10	10
1	—	0.5	3	4	8	10	10	10
5	—	—	—	0.5	1.5	8	9.5	10

[a] HF = 70 Hz; S = 10 μV/mm; input = 100 μV.
[b] No HF in this channel.

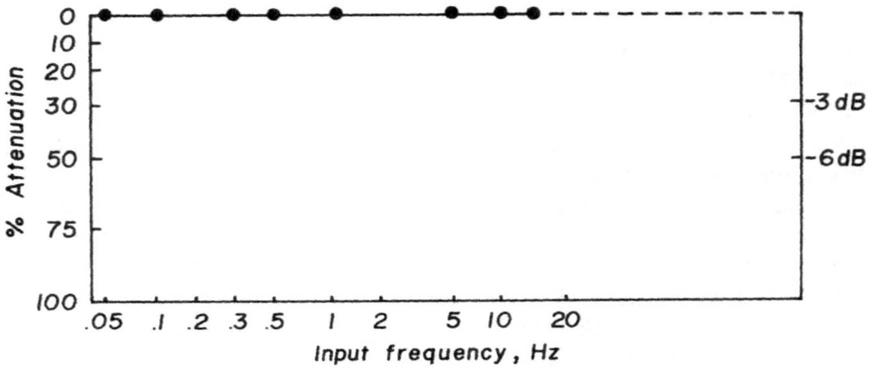

FIG. 8.12. Frequency versus attenuation for DC amplifier, no LF filter.

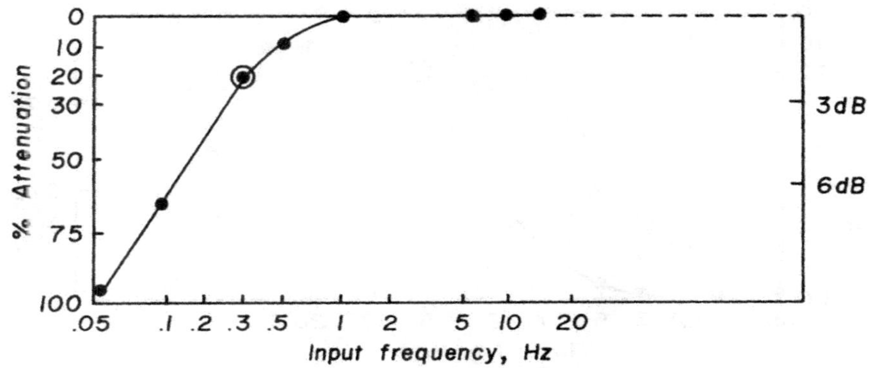

FIG. 8.14. Frequency versus attenuation, LF filter 0.3 Hz. Based on frequency response curve published by Grass Instrument Company (1973), with permission.

When LF = 5 Hz, there is more than 50% attenuation at all frequencies below 3 Hz, as shown in Fig. 8.16.

Each of the five graphs (Figs. 8.12 to 8.16) is a *frequency response curve,* which describes the low frequency characteristics of the filter in use. As can be seen by using the DC channel as a standard for comparison, LF filters attenuate output, both above and below the setting of the filter. As the input frequency is decreased below the filter setting, the attenuation increases. As the input frequency is increased above the filter setting, the attenuation decreases. Note, however, that the decrease in attenuation is gradual and that full output (zero attenuation) does not occur immediately as the frequency increases above the filter setting.

From Table 8.2 and from this series of frequency response curves, a common feature appears: The input frequency that is attenuated 20% is the same frequency as that of the filter setting. This point on the frequency response curve arbitrarily is called the *cut-off frequency*. This point is circled in Figs. 8.13 to 8.16. Attenuation greater than 20% is

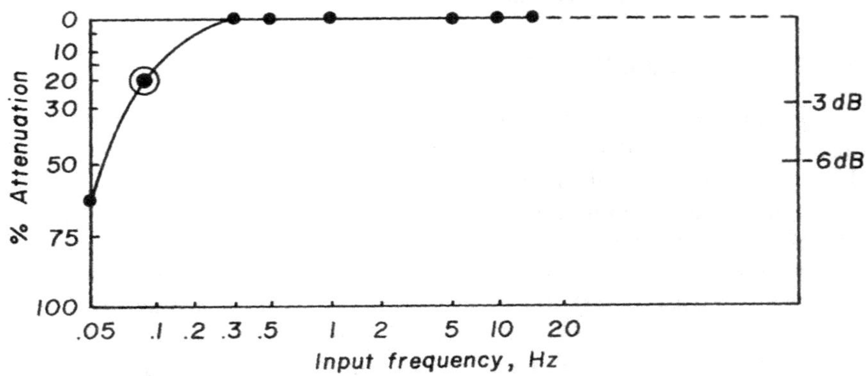

FIG. 8.13. Frequency versus attenuation, LF filter 0.1 Hz. Based on frequency response curve published by Grass Instrument Company (1973), with permission.

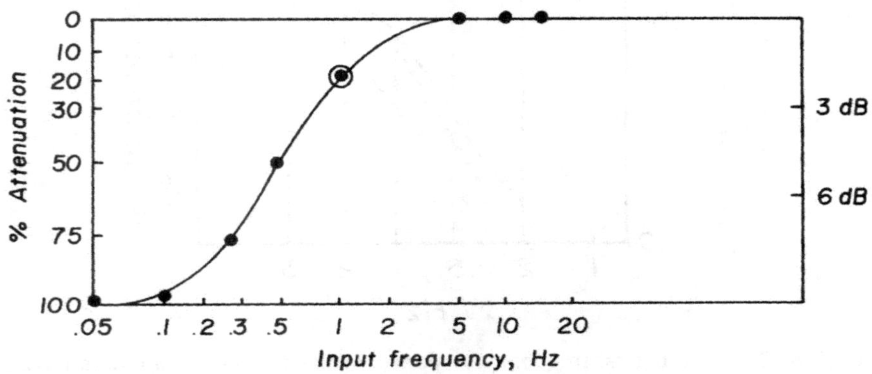

FIG. 8.15. Frequency versus attenuation, LF filter 1 Hz. Based on frequency response curve published by Grass Instrument Company (1973), with permission.

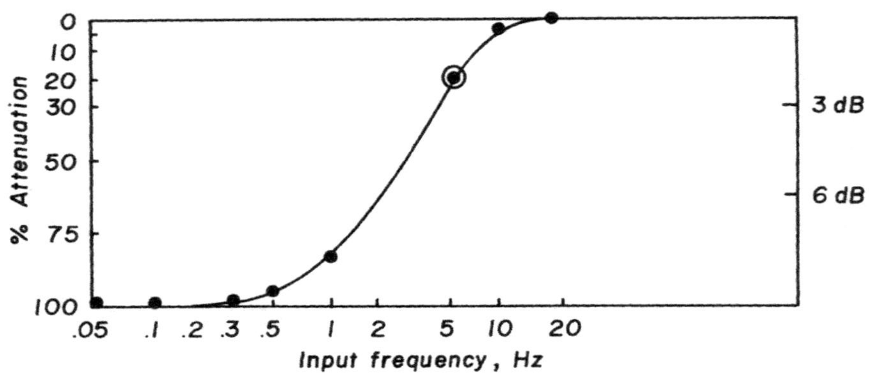

FIG. 8.16. Frequency versus attenuation, LF filter 5 Hz. Based on frequency response curve published by Grass Instrument Company (1973), with permission.

"significant attenuation." The relationship between input and output voltage at frequencies above the LF cut-off is regarded as being "linear."

If the frequency is reduced by 50% (e.g., from 1 Hz to 0.5 Hz), it is said to have been changed by one *octave*. A change from 0.5 to 0.25 Hz is also

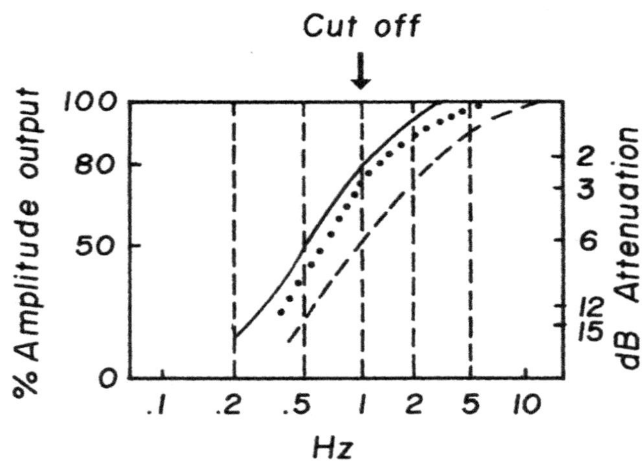

FIG. 8.17. Hypothetical frequency response curves for three amplifiers having different definitions of 1-Hz cut-off. *Solid line:* 20% attenuation. *Dotted line:* 3 dB attenuation. *Dashed line:* half-amplitude.

a change of one octave. With each reduction of the input frequency by one octave, the output amplitude typically will be reduced by 50%. This is called the *roll-off*. The slope of the roll-off is usually designed to be 6 dB per octave, or a 50% change of amplitude as the frequency is halved or doubled. Another slope could be established (such as 12 dB per octave, using series filters) and sometimes is.

Although cut-off frequency has been defined in this instance as the frequency at which output is reduced 20%, the International EEG Federation (2) follows common engineering practice and defines cut-off frequency as a reduction of 3 dB, or the preservation of 0.707 of the original signal. The value −3 dB thus becomes, in practical terms, 30% attenuation. The dB attenuation has been indicated in all relevant figures.

If one instrument defines cut-off as the frequency at which attenuation is 20% and another instrument defines it as −3 dB, when the cut-off frequency is the same for the two instruments, the first will have less attenuation at that particular frequency. Furthermore, the first instrument will reach zero attenuation (100% output) at a lower frequency than the second instrument if the roll-off is the same. In addition, the second instrument (−3 dB) will attenuate each frequency below cut-off to a greater extent than the first one (20%).

One type of amplifier used for special EEG recording has been designed with the cut-off frequency specified as "half-amplitude" (which is −6 dB). This amplifier will have a different frequency response curve than an amplifier having a cut-off defined as 20% attenuation or an amplifier with a −3 dB cut-off definition. Hypothetical curves for these three amplifiers, each with a cut-off of 1 Hz, are shown in Fig. 8.17.

HIGH FREQUENCY FILTER

The high frequency (HF) filter control is the third control to be considered on the panel of the EEG instrument. Behind the panel (Fig. 8.18) there are three possible resistive-capacitive configurations, any one of which may be selected and placed in parallel with the output of an amplifier stage to determine the high frequency response of the system. Fig. 8.18A shows a classical HF filter, which selects one of three capacitors. Figure 8.18B shows an alternative method, which employs a single capacitor in parallel and three selectable series resistors. This resistive–capacitive configuration, which was discussed in Chapter 5, has the ability to attenuate high frequencies, depending (Fig. 8.18A) on the

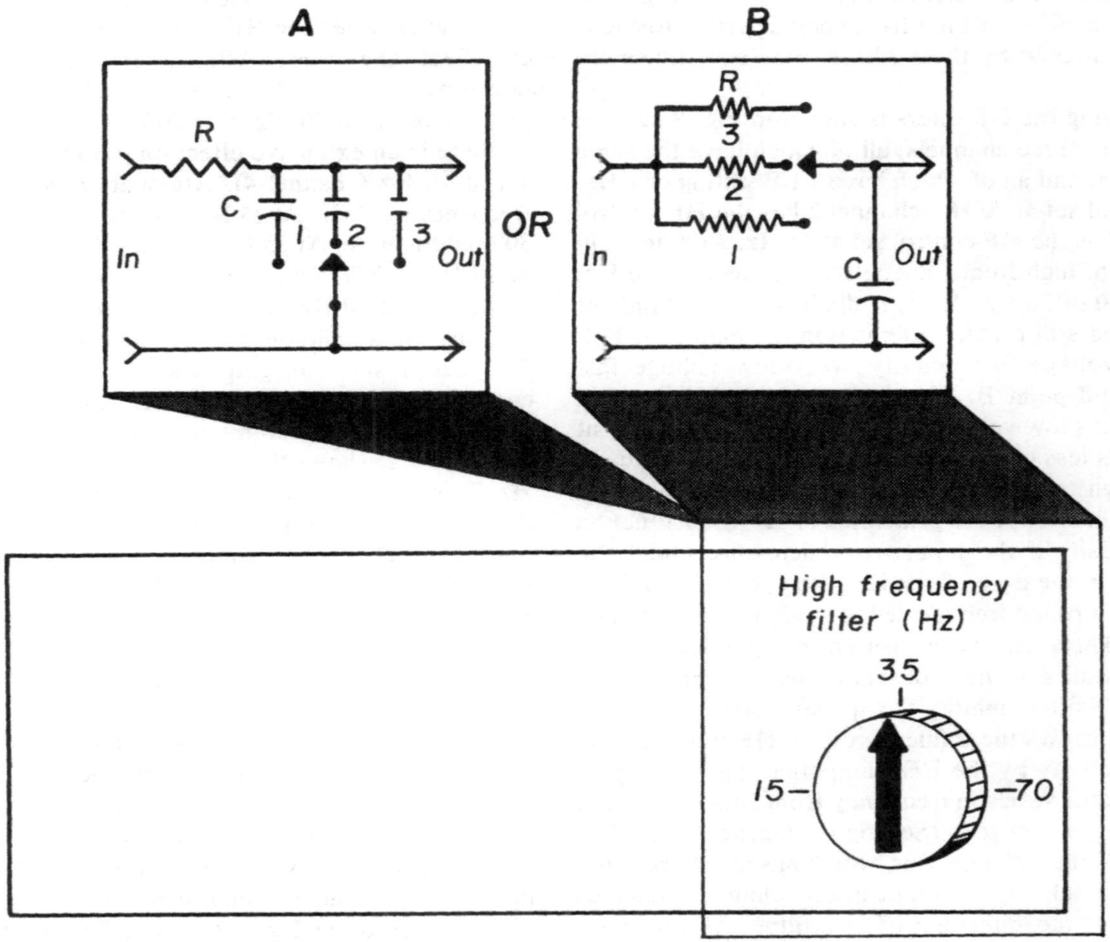

FIG. 8.18. HF filter dial and circuit it controls (see text for discussion).

size of the capacitors: C_1, C_2, and C_3. The larger the capacitor, the greater the degree of attenuation of high frequency activity. C_1 is the largest capacitor, and attenuates activity that approaches the higher limits of the alpha frequency band. If resistors are switched (Fig. 8.18B), the larger the resistor, the greater the attenuation of high frequency activity. Because low frequencies are not attenuated by these filters, they sometimes are called low-pass filters (9).

The practical effects of using the HF filters is shown in Fig. 8.19. The same activity is being fed into three channels, all of which have the same sensitivity setting (7 μV/mm) and all of which have a LF setting of 1 Hz. Channel 1 has the HF control set at 70 Hz; channel 2 has the HF control set at 35 Hz, and channel 3 has the HF control set at 15 Hz. At point A in the record, there is a burst of high frequency activity, exceeding 40 Hz, and probably approaching 60 or 70 Hz. There is diminished amplitude of this activity in channel 2 and still greater attenuation in channel 3. Following the burst of high voltage fast activity, very low voltage fast activity occurs at and around point B. This includes beta activity at a frequency of about 30 Hz. This low voltage, fast activity is seen clearly at point B in channel 1, but it is less obvious in channel 2, and it is virtually absent in channel 3. Although some of the effects of the HF filters can be demonstrated by using EEG activity, the principles of HF filter function can be understood more easily if the input frequencies are under the control of the observer. As in the case of the LF filters, it is possible to use pure sine waves with controlled frequencies to study attenuation and phase shift at the output. These can be measured and graphically displayed. By examining the results of these observations, it is possible to understand precisely how HF filters modify the appearance of the EEG.

Figure 8.20 schematically shows the influence of the HF filters on the display of high frequency activity by the EEG amplifier. The input produced by the function generator varies in frequency from 5 to 100 Hz and the voltage is held constant at 100 μV. (See figure legend for further details.) Channel 1 again uses the DC amplifier, which has no filters in the circuit. The amplitude of the ink-writer output in this channel indicates the system response without the influence of any filter. As the input frequency is raised from 5 to 100 Hz, there is attenuation of the signal beginning at about 60 Hz. At 70 Hz, the attenuation is 20%, and at 100 Hz, the attenuation is 65%. This is due to inherent electromechanical characteristics of the oscillograph.

When the HF is set at 70 Hz (channel 2), the same degree of attenuation occurs as appeared in the DC channel. This indicates that, in this instrument, the response of the ink-writing oscillograph was the limiting factor at high frequencies, not the high frequency filters. (See also Seaba, ref 13.)

However, when the HF is changed to 35 Hz (channel 3), a rather different effect takes place. Attenuation starts at 20 Hz, the output being reduced by 5%. At 25 Hz, it is reduced by 10% and attenuation continues progressively; at 70 Hz, it is 70%.

There is an extensive effect on output amplitude when the HF filter is set at 15 Hz (channel 4). Attenuation is first observed when the input frequency is 10 Hz. At 15 Hz, the attenuation is 20%, and at 20 Hz, there is 30% attenuation. At 35 Hz, the signal is reduced by 55%. The attenuation at 40 Hz is 70%, and from that point onward, little activity is left to be measured; at 70 Hz there is 90% attenuation.

Using the amplitude data in Table 8.3 based on the data presented in Fig. 8.20, a series of graphs was drawn to plot the output amplitude at each input frequency for each HF filter setting. This is the same procedure that was followed for the low frequency data.

Figure 8.21 shows the frequency response curve for an HF setting of 70 Hz. This curve drops rather sharply, faster than the usual 6 dB per octave described in the LF filters. This sharp drop is due not to the filter alone, but to the electromechanical characteristics of the ink-writing oscillograph in conjunction with the filter (13). Figure 8.22 shows the frequency response curve for an HF setting of 35 Hz. It is obvious that much high frequency activity passed by HF-70 Hz is attenuated by HF-35 Hz.

Figure 8.23 shows the frequency response curve for an HF setting of 15 Hz. Again, the loss of amplitude of high frequency components, particularly those beyond 35 Hz, is apparent.

As in the case of the LF filters, the cut-off frequency is defined arbitrarily as that frequency at which amplitude is attenuated 20% (or, if the International recommendations are used, −3 dB). In Figs. 8.21 to 8.23, the cut-off frequency is indicated by a circle. Roll-off is (typically) 6 dB per octave, although some instruments provide a fast roll-off of 12 dB per octave at 30 or 35 Hz to attenuate more effectively frequencies arising from the activity of muscles.

Phase shift is much less significant with HF filters than with LF filters because a time shift of one cycle is exceedingly short, as discussed in Chapter 5. (Reference to Fig. 5.36 will show the amount of phase shift

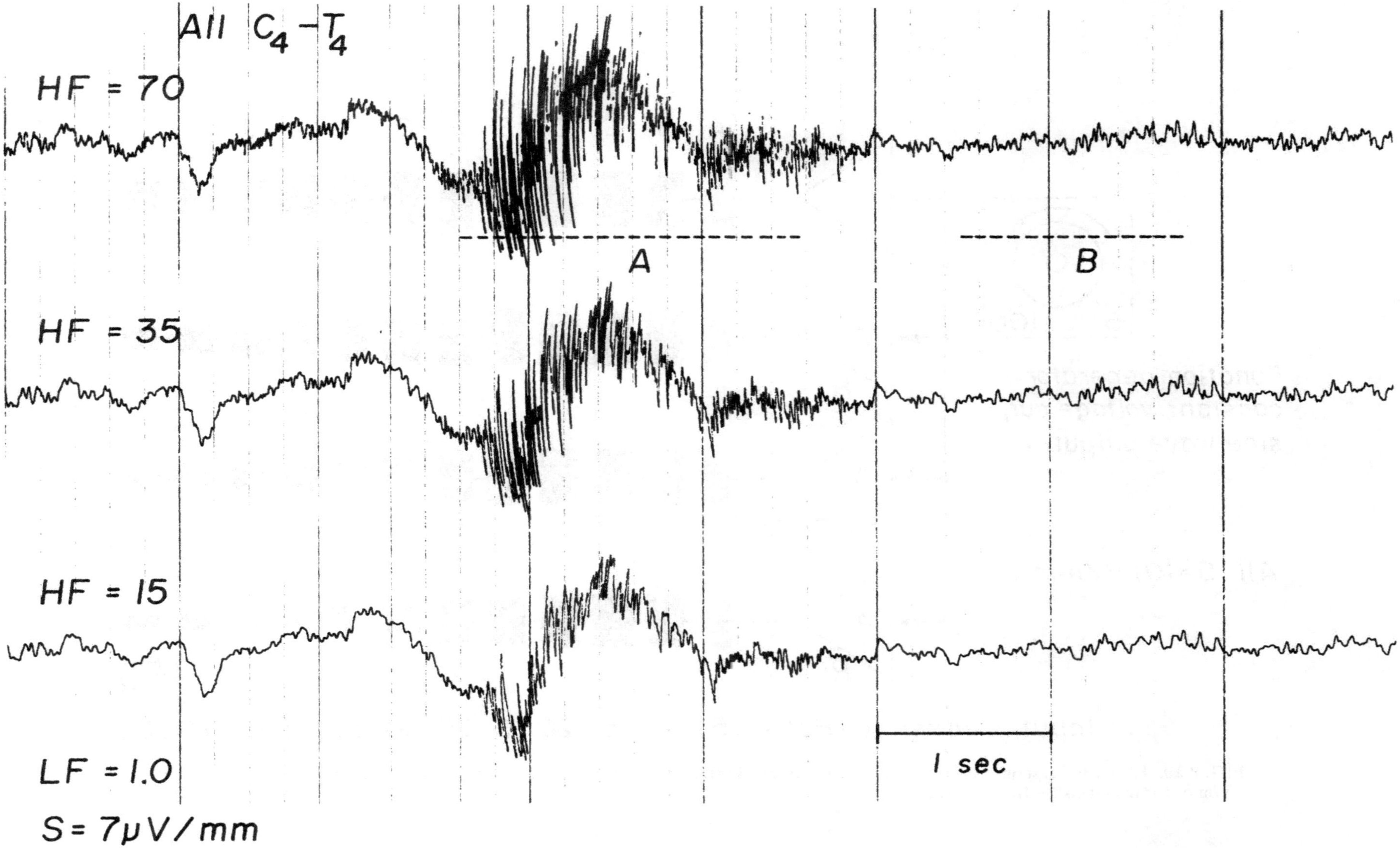

FIG. 8.19. Effects of HF filters on high voltage, fast activity. LF = 1 Hz; S = 7 μV/mm.

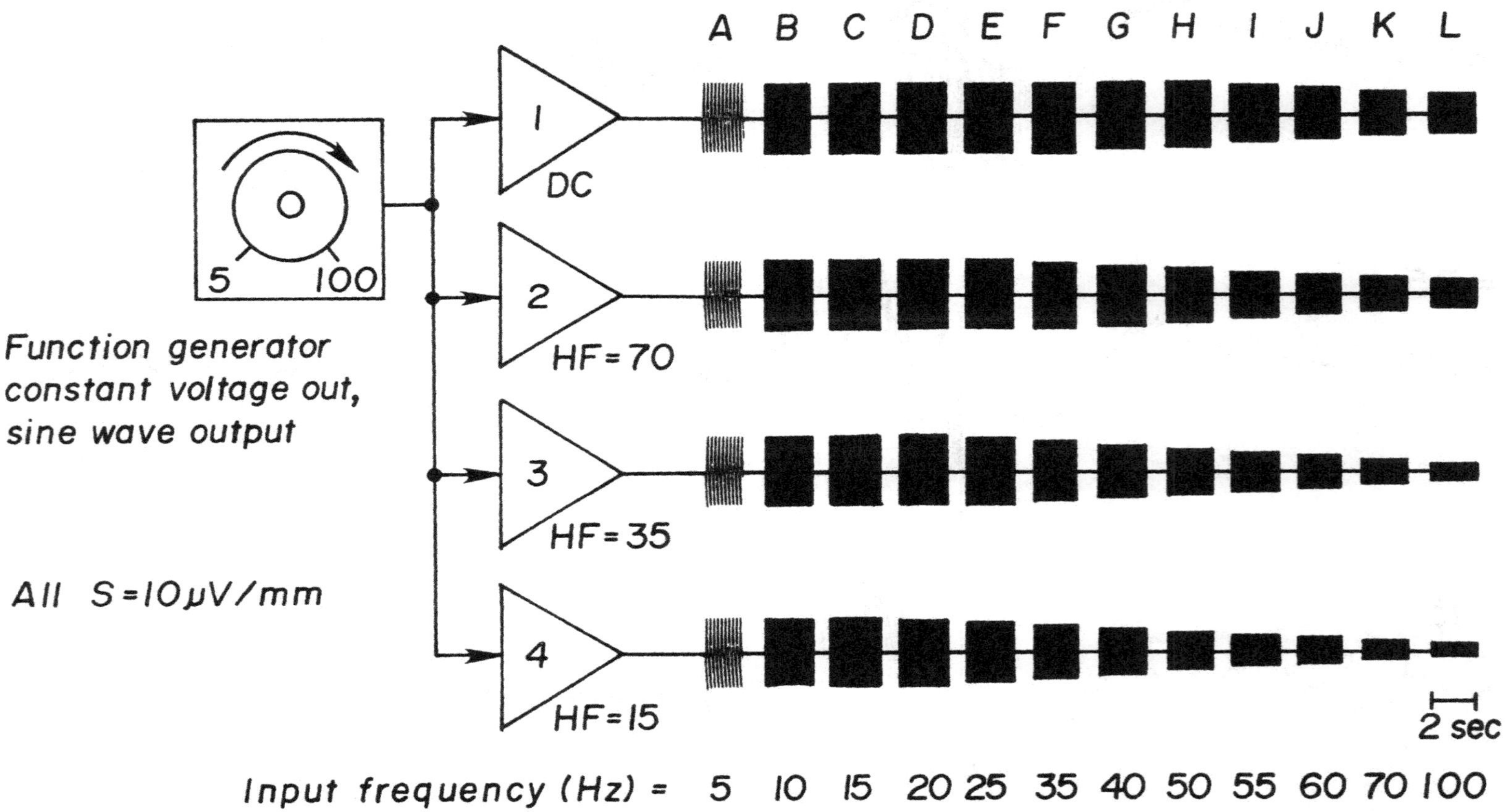

FIG. 8.20. Frequency response characteristics of HF filters 70 Hz, 35 Hz, and 15 Hz compared with unfiltered channel (DC). S = 10 μV/mm; LF (channels 2–4) = 0.1 Hz.

TABLE 8.3. *Output amplitude (mm) at twelve input frequencies at three HF filter settings*[a]

HF filter (Hz)	Input frequency (Hz)											
	5	10	15	20	25	35	40	50	55	60	70	100
None[b]	10	10	10	10	10	10	10	10	10	9.5	8	3.5
70	10	10	10	10	10	10	10	10	10	9.5	8	3.5
35	10	10	10	9.5	9	8	7.5	7	6	5	3	2
15	10	9	8	7	6	4.5	3	2.5	2	1.5	1	1

[a] LF = 0.1 Hz; S = 10 μV/mm; input = 100 μV.
[b] No LF in this channel.

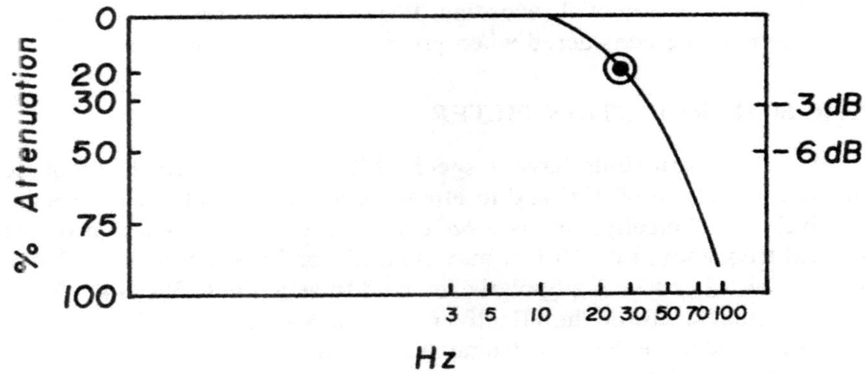

FIG. 8.22. Frequency versus attenuation, HF filter 35 Hz. Based on frequency response curve published by Grass Instrument Company (1973), with permission.

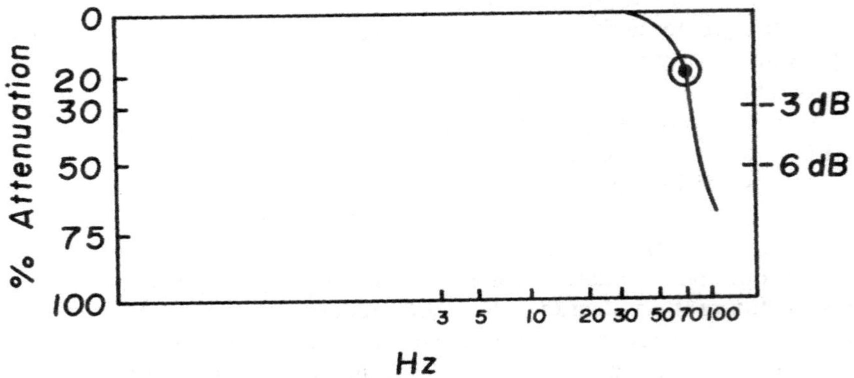

FIG. 8.21. Frequency versus attenuation, HF filter 70 Hz. Based on frequency response curve published by Grass Instrument Company (1973), with permission.

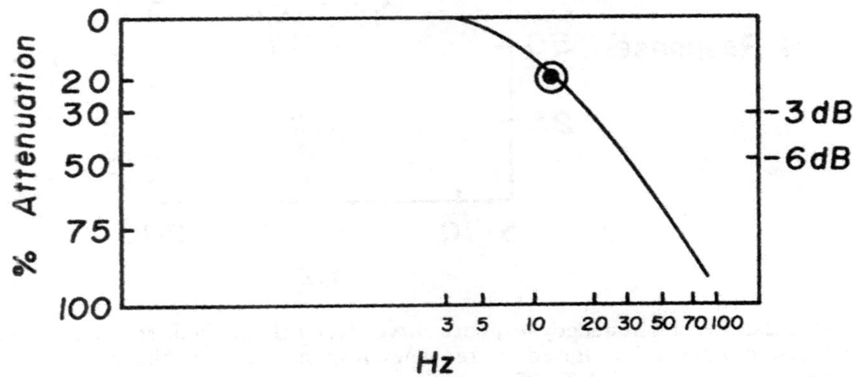

FIG. 8.23. Frequency versus attenuation, HF filter 15 Hz. Based on frequency response curve published by Grass Instrument Company (1973), with permission.

resulting from the use of HF-70 Hz, HF-35 Hz, and HF-15 Hz when compared to the DC amplifier.) Because this is a negligible shift, it is ignored in clinical electroencephalography. However, it cannot be ignored in evoked potential recording. Phase shift changes apparent latencies and must be considered when procedures are established.

THE 60-Hz REJECTION FILTER

All EEG instruments have a special filter that is tuned to attenuate activity sharply at 60 Hz[1] and to attenuate adjacent frequencies less extensively. Technically, this is a *band-stop* filter (9). Attenuation of the critical frequency, i.e., 60 Hz, may typically be by a factor of 1000:1 or more. This filter also is popularly referred to as a *notch filter* (4,9).

The actual width of the effectiveness of a 60-Hz filter will vary with different models of EEG instruments, and there is no universal design curve. A typical frequency response curve is shown in Fig. 8.24. The response of this filter is broad, with cut-off frequencies (−3 dB) at approximately 40 Hz and 80 Hz. In practice, the upper cut-off frequency is never seen because of the limitation of the galvanometer.

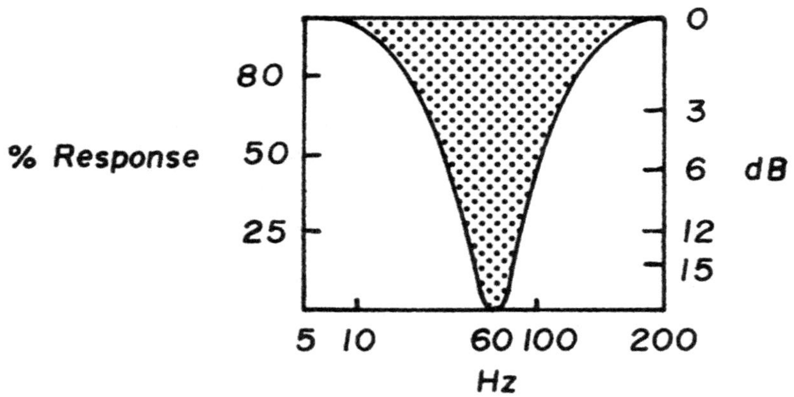

FIG. 8.24. Typical frequency response curve of a 60-Hz notch filter. Shaded area is region of attenuation. Based on frequency response curve published by Grass Instrument Company (1973), with permission.

[1] This is the standard AC mains frequency in the United States. Some countries have 50-Hz AC mains frequency. The filter used in those areas is a 50-Hz filter. The same rules apply.

The effect of the 60-Hz filter on a sine wave input that rapidly increases from 10 Hz to 100 Hz is shown in Fig. 8.25. This shows the interaction of the 60-Hz filter with each HF filter: 70, 35, and 15 Hz.

The interaction should be contrasted with the response of each HF filter without the 60-Hz filter. The effect of inserting the 60-Hz filter on the performance of the 35 and 15 Hz HF filters is clear: The roll-off is steeper when the notch filter is inserted.

An example of the practical use of this filter is shown in Fig. 8.26. The EEG is totally masked by high amplitude 60-Hz interference caused by an external electrical appliance near the patient. Turning the 60-Hz filter to the ON position attenuates the interference and the EEG now can be seen.

It is important always to remember that *when the 60-Hz interference is attenuated, all EEG activity within the range of the filter is also attenuated*. An epileptiform spike may have its apparent amplitude affected because some components of the spike have frequency characteristics above 30 or 40 Hz.

There are other undesirable features of 60-Hz filters. The first is their tendency to "ring" when set into activity by a fast transient. The ringing is a damped oscillation of 60 Hz. In general, the narrower the notch of the filter, the greater is the ringing effect. Fig. 8.27 shows the ringing caused by a square wave calibration pulse in an amplifier with a narrow filter. The second undesirable feature is the introduction of phase shift at frequencies above and below 60 Hz. This phase shift can be disregarded in clinical EEG, but it can have serious effects on evoked potential latencies.

Because of its extensive effect on the performance of HF filters, the 60-Hz filter should be used only in emergency situations. If a laboratory has serious 60-Hz interference, the source of the interference should be sought out and eliminated rather than taking refuge in permanently used 60-Hz filters that degrade the EEG record. Portable, bedside, and operating room recording may sometimes require the use of the 60-Hz filter, but it never should be used in the main laboratory. Need to do so may indicate an electrical safety problem.

If 60-Hz interference appears only in one or two channels, in all probability the problem lies in the electrodes inputting the involved channel(s). The 60-Hz filter should not be used. The resistance of the electrode(s) should be reduced, or they should be reattached, as necessary.

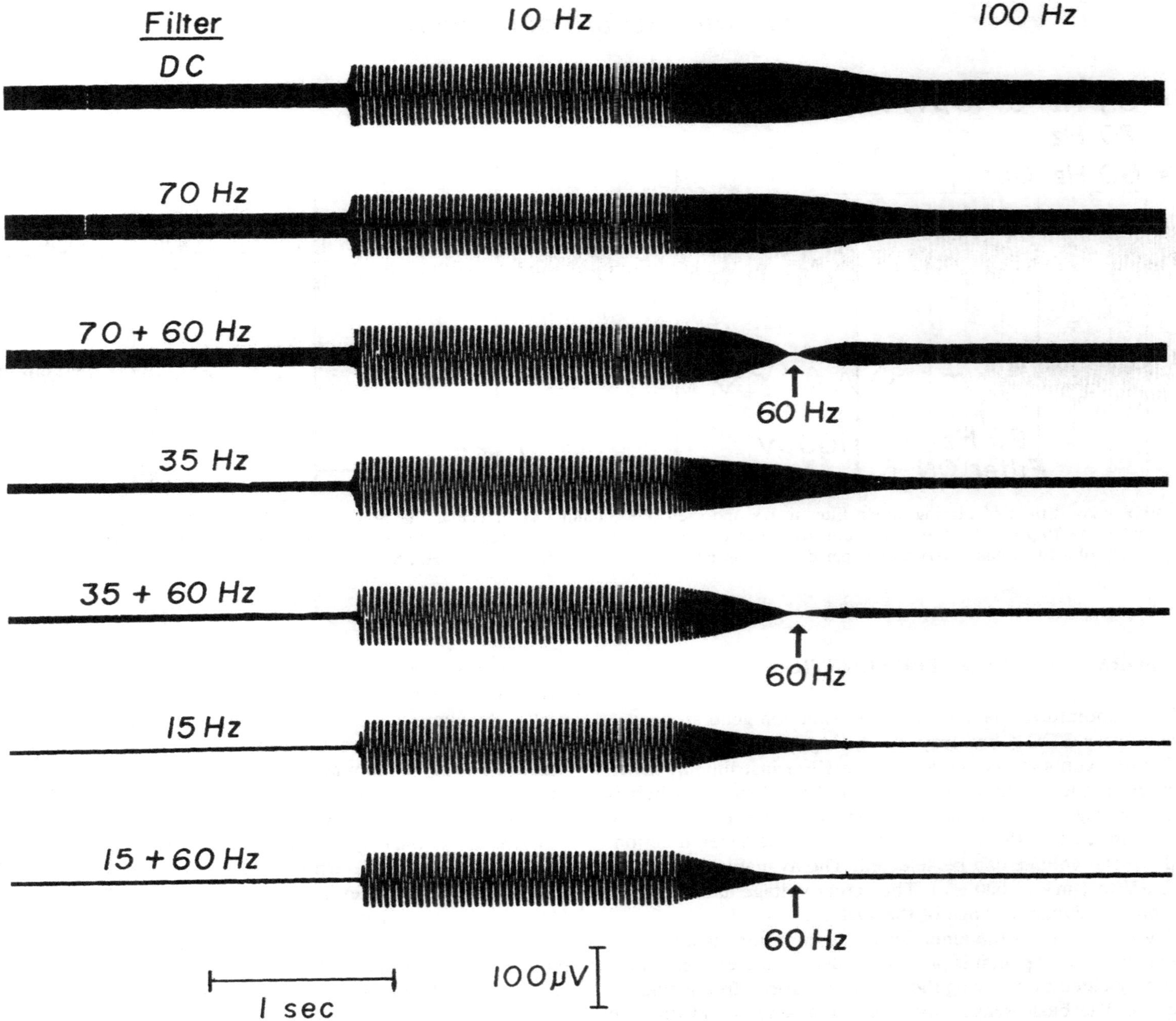

FIG. 8.25. Effect of 60-Hz filter on sweep of input frequency from 10 to 100 Hz. All LF filters are 0.1 Hz. HF filters and position of 60-Hz filter are indicated. *Arrows* show the maximum attenuation of output in channels with 60-Hz filter when sweep passes through 60 Hz. (See text for details on interaction of filters.)

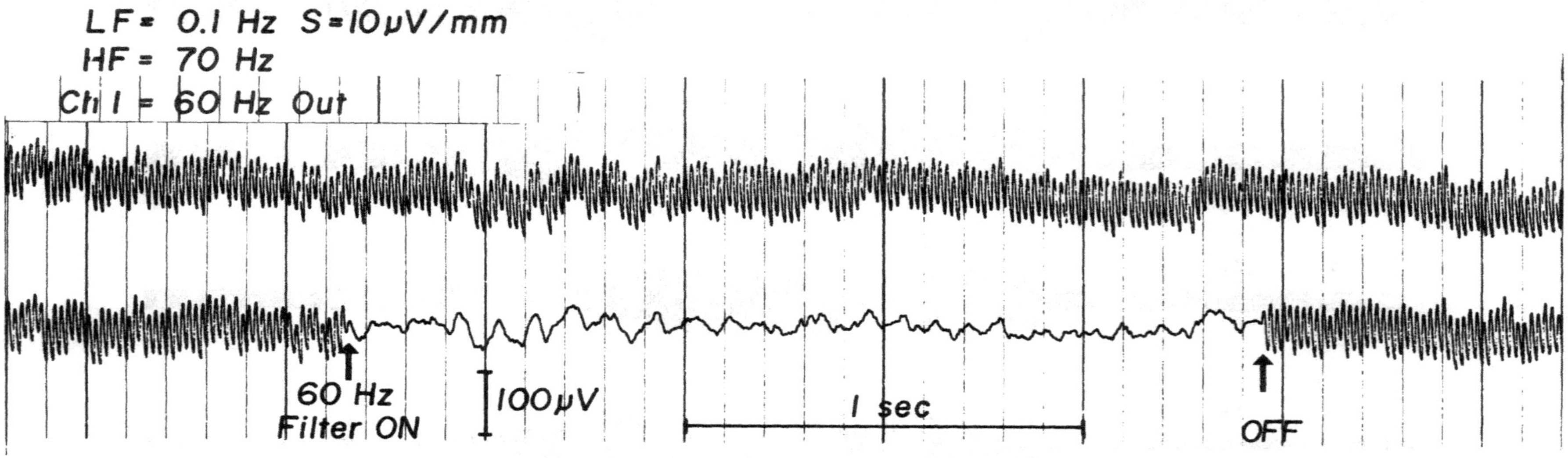

FIG. 8.26. Effect of turning 60-Hz filter to ON and then OFF (channel 2). Irregular, medium voltage (20–40 μV), 11-Hz activity is masked by 70-μV, 60-Hz artifact from nearby electrical appliance. Paper speed is 60 mm/sec to make positive identification of frequency of artifact easier (six waves per division on paper). LF = 0.1 Hz; HF = 70 Hz; S = 10 μV/mm.

FILTER PERFORMANCE AND STEP FUNCTION

Very few EEG laboratories have a sine wave function generator available. However, every EEG laboratory has a simple step function generator. This is the CALIBRATION section of the EEG instrument. When the instrument is in the CALIBRATION mode and the "CAL" switch is closed, a precise voltage is instantaneously impressed on the inputs of all channels and continues until the switch is opened. This is a step function. The magnitude of the voltage can be selected. The available range typically is from 1 μV to 1 mV (1,000 μV). The actual voltage used must, of course, be within the dynamic range of the system.

By examining the output of the amplifier to a calibration signal as displayed by the galvanometer pen, it is possible to deduce a great deal of the same information yielded by studying the effects of various frequencies of sine wave inputs. The basic reason for this is that any waveform that is not a sine wave can be mathematically analyzed into its sine wave components. Conversely, the waveform can be synthesized from the sine wave components if voltage and phase relationships are maintained correctly. A square wave can be synthesized from its equivalent sine wave components. A 1-sec square wave has a fundamental sine wave equivalent to 1 Hz. By combining the fundamental and odd numbered harmonics (e.g., 3, 5, 7, 9 Hz) and subharmonics (e.g., 1/3, 1/5, 1/7, and 1/9 Hz), it is possible to construct a square wave with a duration of 1 sec (6).

The shape of the response of the EEG instrument to the step function or square wave input is determined by the filter settings, both LF and HF. In Fig. 8.28 A, the LF filter in channels 2, 3, 4, and 5 is set at 0.1, 0.3, 1 and 5 Hz, respectively. Channel 1 is the DC system. The step input in channel 1 causes an instantaneous rise at the output, which stays at constant amplitude until the signal is terminated. In channel 2, however, the output response slowly drops back toward baseline. In channel 3, it returns more rapidly. Channels 4 and 5 have progressively more rapid returns.

If we define a point of return at 37% of the peak amplitude, the time

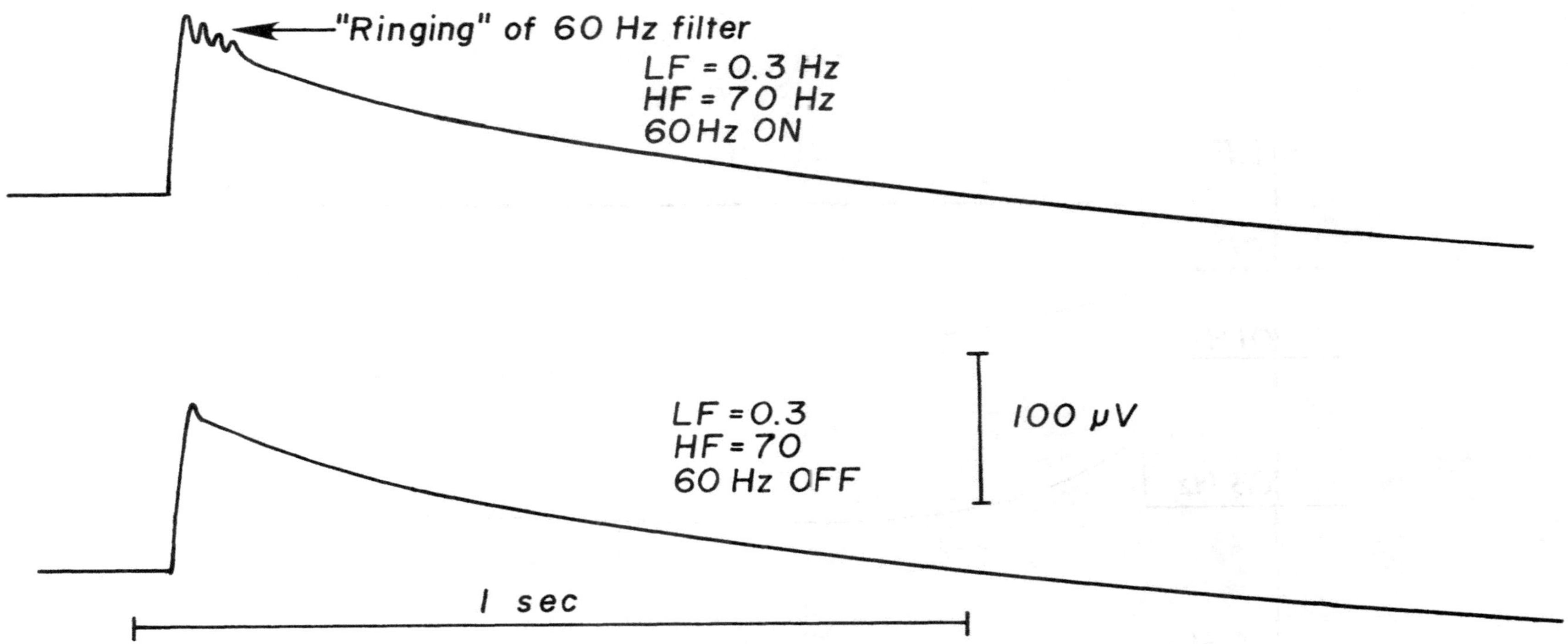

FIG. 8.27. Example of ringing of 60-Hz filter. (Effect enhanced during tracing of original.)

from the maximum rise to 63% return will be the decay time constant (TC), as discussed in Chapter 5. The time constant also can be computed by multiplying the size of the capacitor (in farads) by the resistance (in ohms): TC = C (in farads) × R (in ohms) or in practical units, TC = C (μF) × R (MΩ).

Figure 8.28B demonstrates the measurement of the time constant. Table 8.4 lists the values obtained from these data. [Slight variations occur between individual instruments; these are close to the published data for these amplifiers (7).]

The general rule: the lower the low frequency cut-off, the longer the decay TC. The longer the TC, the more accurately will low frequency activity be reproduced at the output. That is, there will be less attenuation and less phase shift.

The setting of the LF filter can be deduced easily by looking at square wave calibrations. This also makes it possible to discover whether there are faults in an amplifier and its capacitive–resistive circuit that require repair. Generally speaking, as discussed earlier in this chapter, the technologist is concerned primarily with cut-off frequency and only secondarily with the time constant *per se*.

The amplitudes of the square waves in channels 2 through 5 of Fig. 8.28A decrease slightly but progressively as the time constant decreases because the sine wave equivalent low frequencies are being attenuated by the filters. The square wave will be reproduced more faithfully with an LF setting of 0.1 Hz. It will be least accurately reproduced when the LF is set on 5 Hz. Recall the frequency response curve with the sharp attenuation of all low frequencies below 5 Hz, and this will be easier to understand.

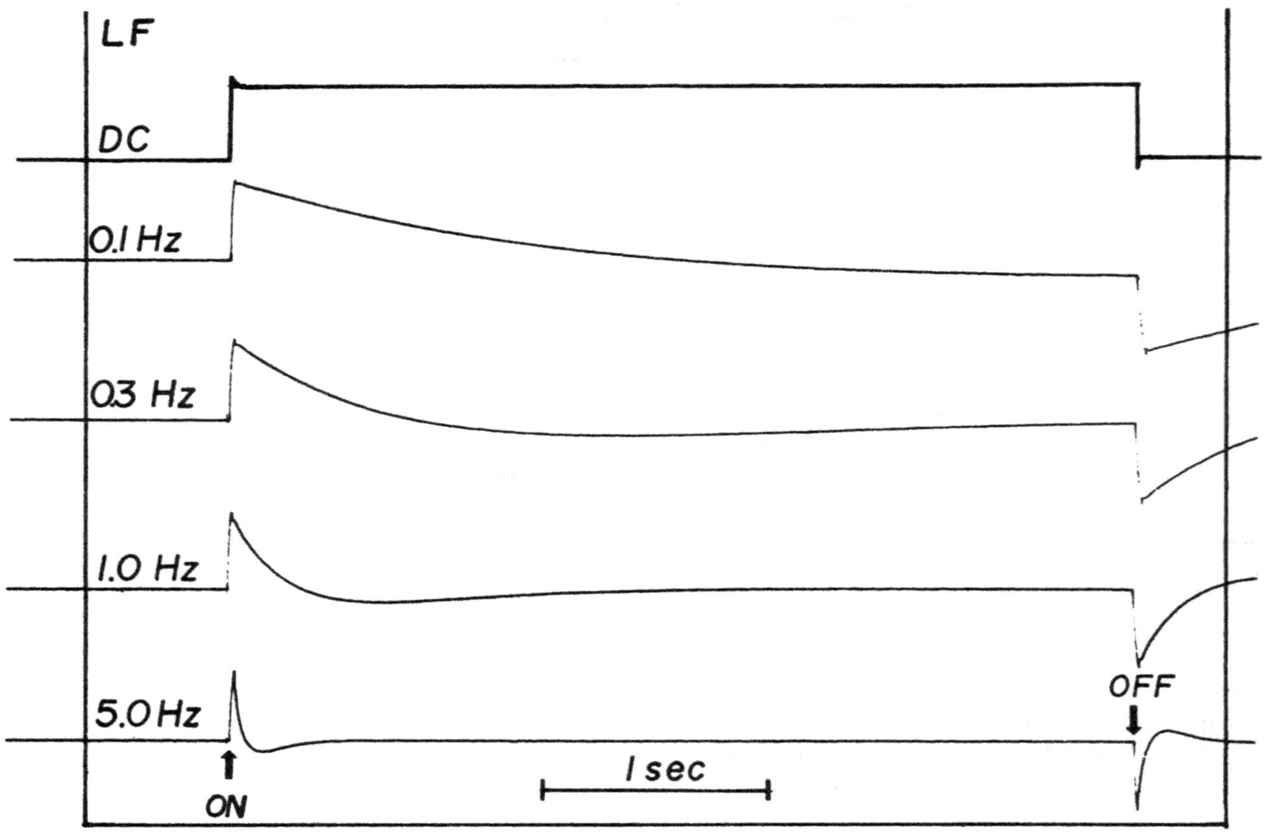

FIG. 8.28. A: Step response of DC and four capacity-coupled amplifiers. Note that the response in the DC channel is maintained throughout the duration of the calibration voltage (ON to OFF). The channels with filters decay to baseline; the rapidity of the decay is directly proportional to the cut-off frequency of the filter: LF = 0.1 Hz has the longest decay time and LF = 5 Hz has the shortest.

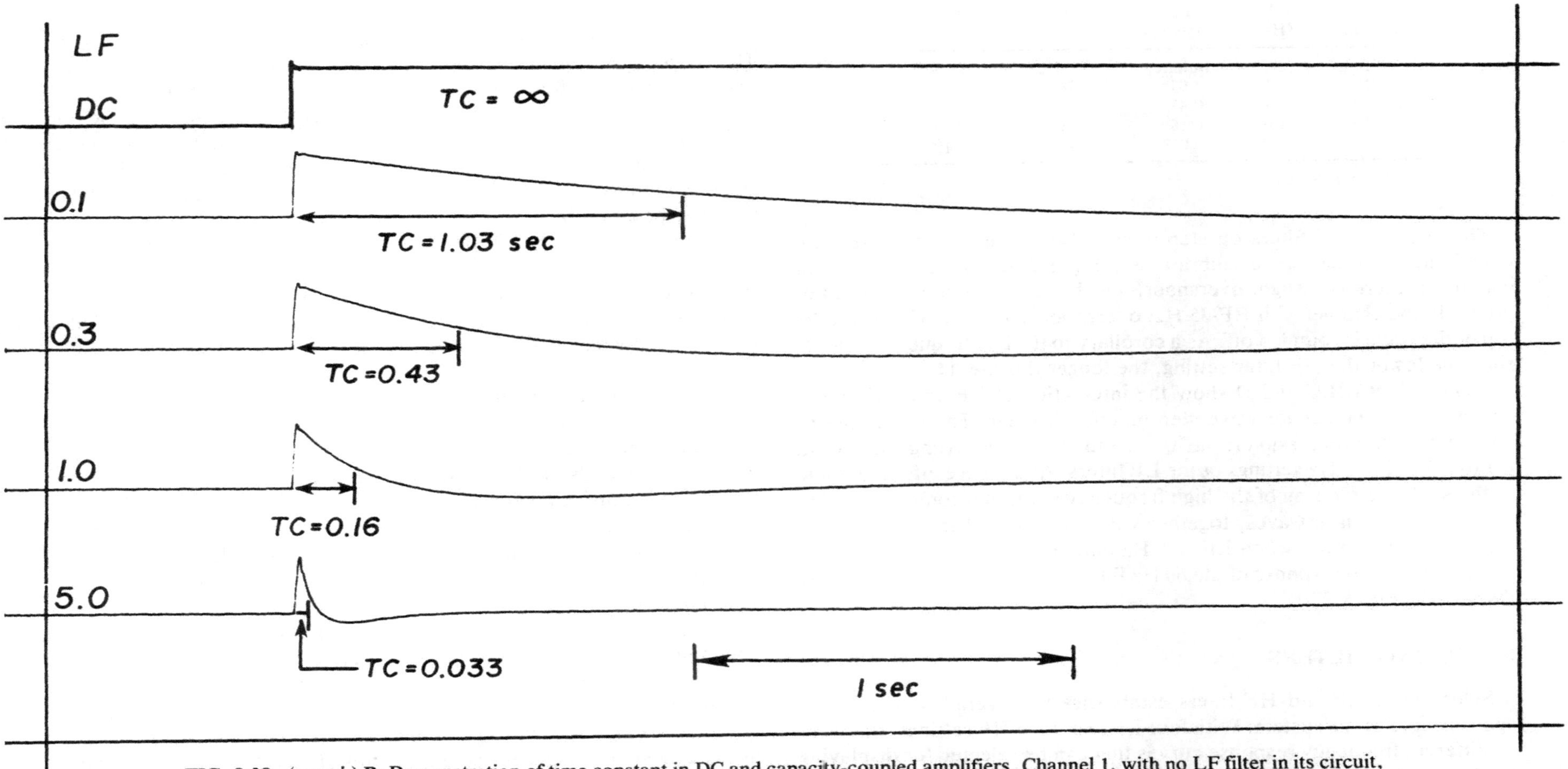

FIG. 8.28. (*contd.*) **B:** Demonstration of time constant in DC and capacity-coupled amplifiers. Channel 1, with no LF filter in its circuit, has an infinite time constant (TC = ∞). Channel 2, LF = 0.1 Hz, has a measured TC = 1.03 sec; channel 2, TC = 0.43 sec; channel 3, TC = 0.16 sec; channel 4, TC = 0.033 sec.

TABLE 8.4. *Typical values obtained from measurement of TC*[a]

Channel	LF (Hz)	TC (sec)	Relative amplitude (%)	Attenuation (%)
1	DC	Infinite	100	0
2	0.1	1.03	100	0
3	0.3	0.43	100	0
4	1.0	0.16	100	0
5	5.0	0.033	85	15

[a] See Fig. 8.28B.

The effect of HF filters on step inputs also is fairly easy to see. By examining the square wave calibrations in Fig. 8.29A, it is apparent that in channel 1, there is a slight overshoot, which is a function of the oscillograph. In the channel with HF-35 Hz, overshoot is lost. At HF-15 Hz, the top of the wave is rounded off. As a corollary to the low frequency general rule, the lower the HF filter setting, the longer the rise TC.

Figures 8.29A,B,C and D show the interaction of LF and HF filters. The effect on the square wave step function is clear. There is a loss of amplitude with progression from 70 to 35 to 15 Hz HF settings, and from 0.1 to 0.3 to 1 to 5 Hz settings of the LF filters. All of these effects are due to the selective filtering of the high frequency harmonic components that compose the square waves, together with LF filters. The 100 μV input looks like only 65 μV when LF = 5 Hz and HF = 15 Hz.

The calibration response of the 60 Hz filter shows ringing, as previously discussed. (Fig. 8.27.)

SELECTING FILTERS

Selection of LF and HF filters establishes the overall frequency response curve of the system. With four LF and three HF settings, there are 12 different frequency response curves that can be selected for displaying the EEG. The 60-Hz filter also must be considered: There are 24 possible frequency response curves that can be selected by the technologist at the time of recording. Seven of these will be reviewed and compared with the ideal frequency response curve of the DC amplifier.

Figure 8.30 shows the frequency response curve of the system based on the DC amplifier with no filters in its circuit. The shaded area at the high frequency end may be considered as a curtain in a window. The curtain is the relative attenuation introduced by the electromechanical properties of the ink-writing oscillograph, which significantly obscures our view of activity beyond 70 to 80 Hz.

Figure 8.31 shows the effects of using LF = 0.1 Hz and HF = 70 Hz. The shaded areas again represent curtains at the sides of a window. Very low and very high frequencies are obscured. The loss of information is proportional to the degree to which the window is occluded by the curtain. All activity in the EEG from approximately 0.5 Hz to 45 Hz is seen with no attenuation. Activity between 0.1 Hz and 0.5 Hz, and 45 Hz and 70 Hz is seen with up to 20% attenuation. Below 0.5 Hz and above 70 Hz, the view becomes increasingly obscured.

Figure 8.32 shows the effects of closing the curtain somewhat further at the low frequency end. This is the frequency response curve resulting from the use of LF = 0.3 Hz and HF = 70 Hz. Compared with Fig. 8.31, it is apparent that below 0.3 Hz much information is lost. A typical LF filter setting used by most EEG technologists is 1 Hz together with HF = 70 Hz (Fig. 8.33).

By comparing the LF curtains at 1 Hz and 0.3 Hz, it is clear that very slow activity from 0.4 Hz down is occluded when LF = 1 is used. One must also remember that LF = 1 causes not only attenuation of slow frequencies, but also different amounts of phase shift at the various slow frequencies, causing an alteration of the characteristics of the EEG. Figures 8.10 and 8.11 should be reviewed together with Figs. 8.31 and 8.32.

Figure 8.34 illustrates the curtain effect produced by LF = 5 Hz and HF = 70 Hz. This is a low frequency filter for use only on limited conditions. The most appropriate condition involves recording electromyographic activity, as is routinely required in certain types of sleep recording. Sometimes it may be defensible to attenuate very high voltage, slower activity (below 2 Hz) to maintain adequate sensitivity to perceive faster frequencies (20–40 Hz), as for example to clarify the spike component in spike-wave discharges where the spike may be very low voltage, relative to associated slow activity. However, this should be used only for brief periods. It must be remembered that those low frequencies that still appear in the record will have been subjected to extensive phase shift (5,12). If this LF setting is used without proper identification, the EEG will be misrepresented grossly and could be misinterpreted.

Figure 8.35 illustrates a combination of HF and LF settings that may be more commonly used than many would care to admit: LF = 1 Hz and HF

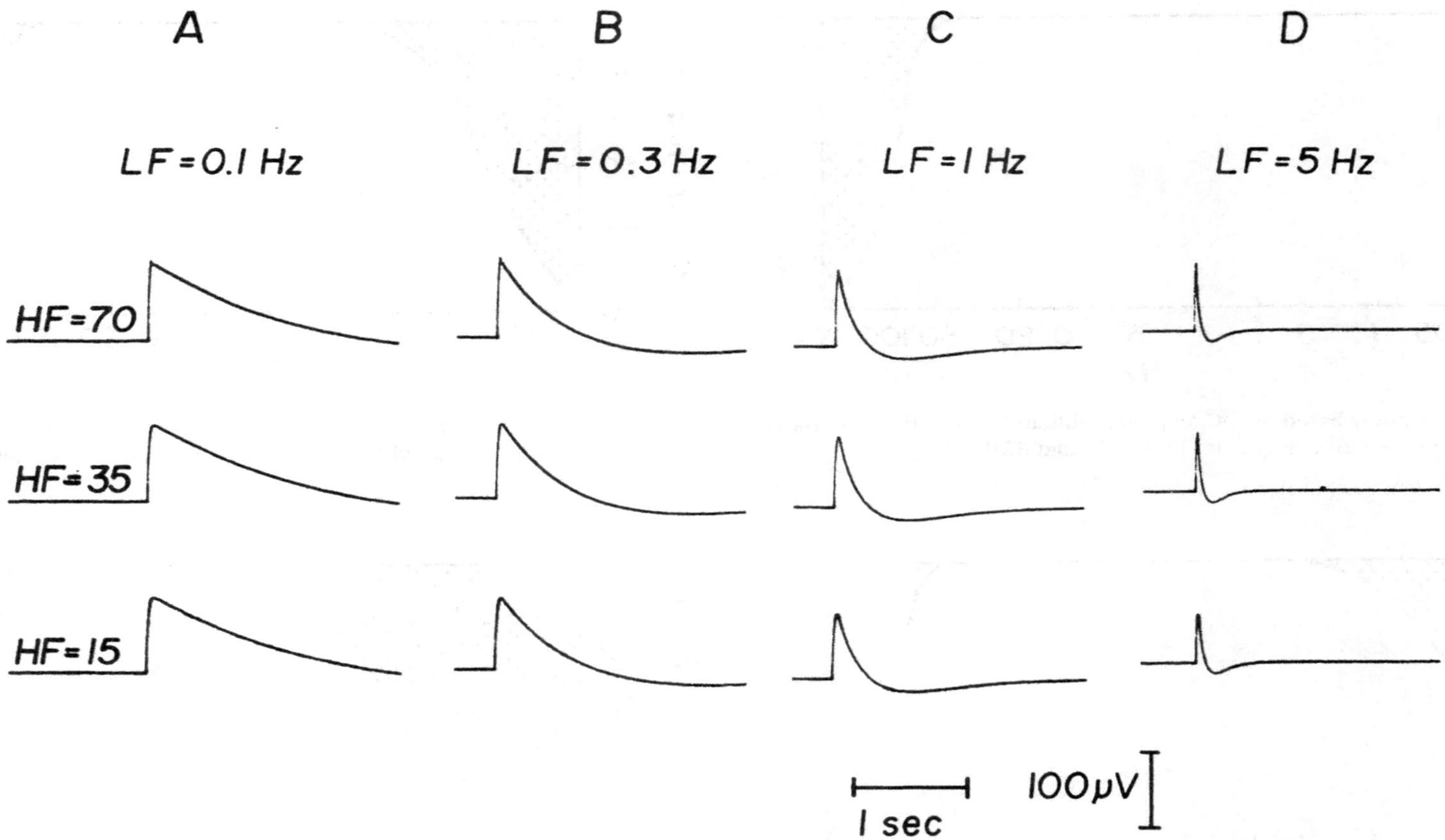

FIG. 8.29. Interactive effects of LF and HF filters on step function. (Note decreased amplitude as HF cut-off is lowered and LF cut-off is increased.) Paper speed = 15 mm/sec. S = 10 μV/mm. Input = 100 μV.

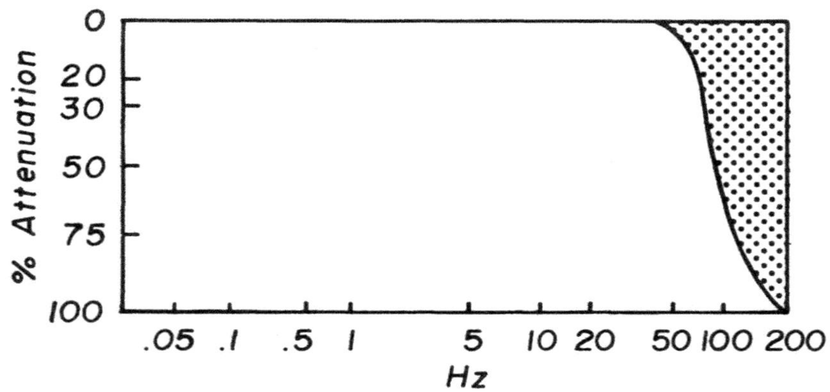

FIG. 8.30. Ideal window based on DC amplifier without LF or HF filters. Based on frequency response curve data from Figs. 8.11 and 8.20.

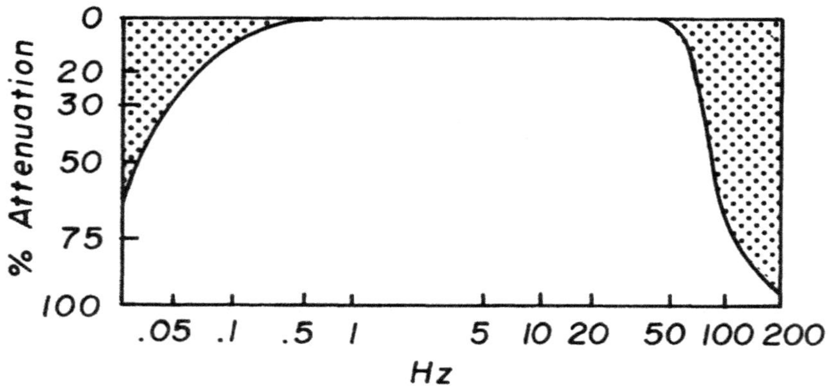

FIG. 8.31. Window based on LF filter 0.1 Hz and HF filter 70 Hz. *Shaded area* indicates frequencies in which information is lost. The distance the curtain extends downward indicates the degree of loss. Based on frequency response curve published by Grass Instrument Company (1973), with permission.

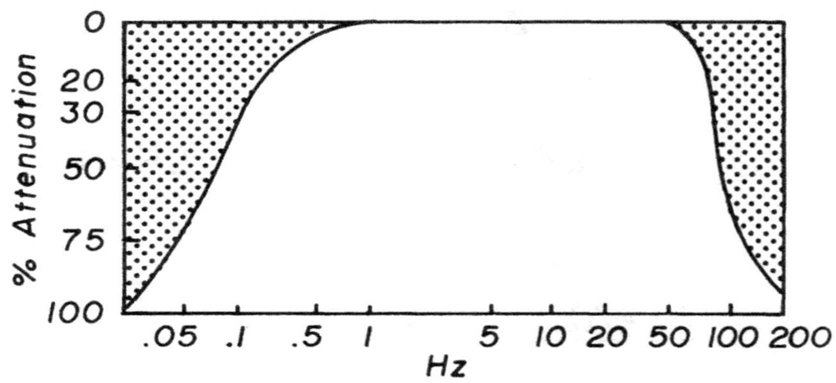

FIG. 8.32. Window based on LF filter 0.3 Hz and HF filter 70 Hz. Based on frequency response curve published by Grass Instrument Company (1973), with permission.

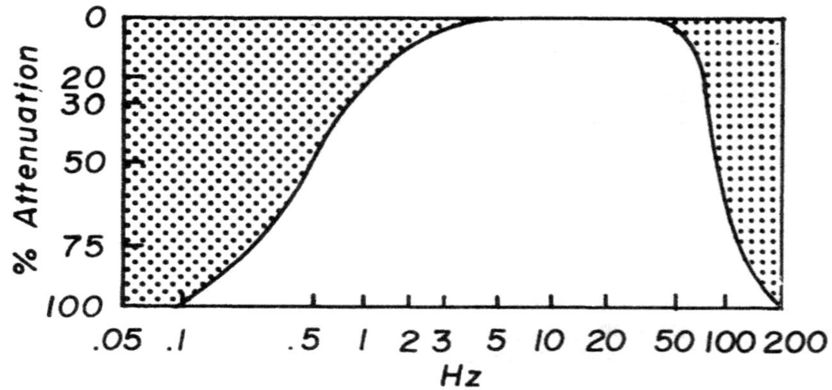

FIG. 8.33. Window based on LF filter 1 Hz and HF filter 70 Hz. Based on frequency response curve published by Grass Instrument Company (1973), with permission.

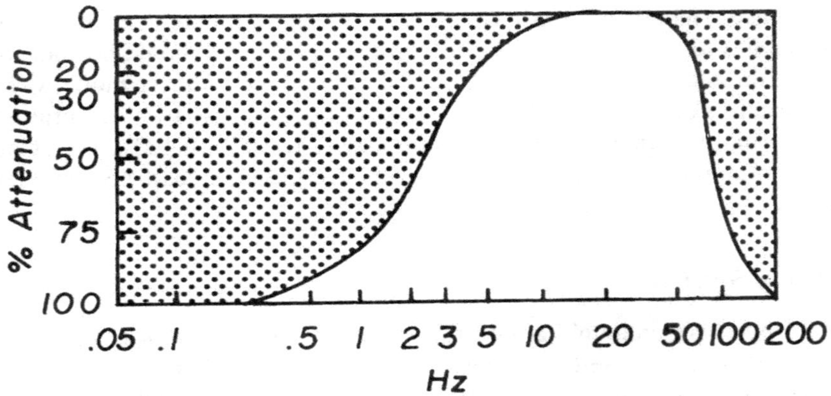

FIG. 8.34. Window based on LF filter 5 Hz and HF filter 70 Hz. Based on frequency response curve published by Grass Instrument Company (1973), with permission.

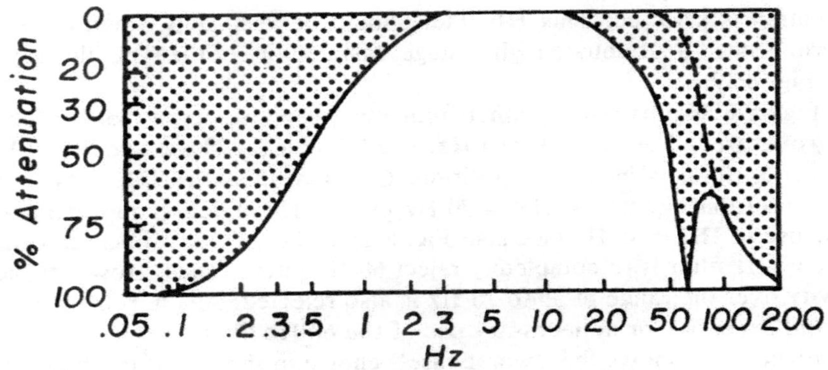

FIG. 8.36. Window based on LF filter 1 Hz, HF filter 70 Hz, and 60-Hz filter ON. *Dotted line* shows curtain with 70-Hz filter (see text). Based on frequency response curve published by Grass Instrument Company (1973), with permission.

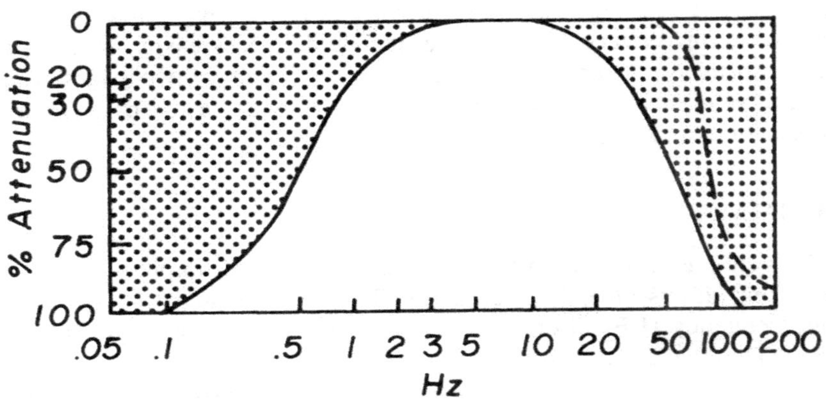

FIG. 8.35. Window based on LF filter 1 Hz and HF filter 35 Hz. *Dotted line* indicates the position of curtain when HF = 70 Hz (see text). Based on frequency response curve published by Grass Instrument Company (1973), with permission.

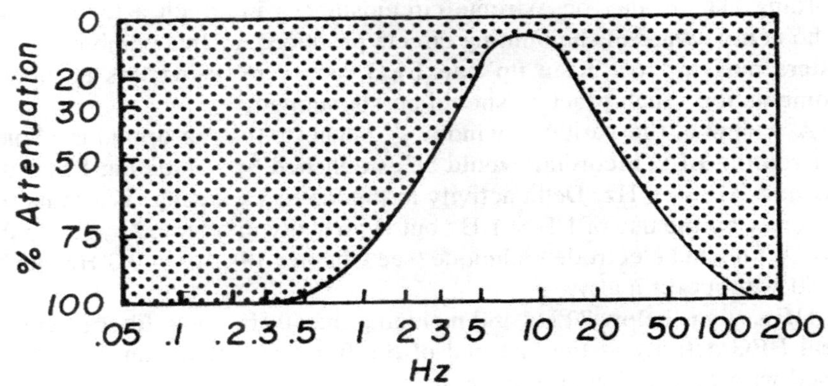

FIG. 8.37. Window based on LF filter 5 Hz and HF filter 15 Hz, showing band pass filter effect (see text). Based on frequency response curve published by Grass Instrument Company (1973), with permission.

= 35 Hz. The dotted line in this figure shows the position of the curtain when the HF is at 70 Hz. It is quite clear that considerable information about high frequency activity is lost (15 Hz and above) when this combination is selected. This HF filter should be used only when there is serious need to attenuate high voltage, fast activity of the type illustrated in Fig. 8.19.

Figure 8.36 illustrates another frequency response curve that is probably overused. The LF is set at 1 Hz. The HF is set at 70 Hz, and the 60-Hz rejection filter is in the ON position. Compare this with Fig. 8.34. It is apparent that the use of HF = 70 Hz plus 60-Hz rejection approximates the use of HF = 35 Hz (see also Fig. 8.25). The only advantage to using the 60-Hz filter is to completely reject 60-Hz interference. However, activity over the range of 35 to 70 Hz is also rejected. Again, remember to avoid excessive or unnecessary use of the 60-Hz filter.

Figure 8.37 shows the "worst case" choice in the use of the filters on the EEG instrument. The LF is set at 5 Hz and HF is set at 15 Hz. The curtains have been drawn on most of the activity present in any EEG, normal or abnormal. Although the peak of visibility is at 10 Hz, there is some loss of information at this basic alpha frequency. The choice of these filters creates a band-pass filter (9) at 10 Hz. Obviously, this is a choice of filter positions that never should be used in clinical EEG recording. There may be extreme circumstances in which a technologist who is not aware of the limiting effects produced by this combination of filters may try to "clean up" an EEG record by using this particular combination. Such practice should be abandoned.

A review of the various "windows" suggests that an optimum choice for routine EEG recording would be established by combining LF = 0.3 Hz and HF = 70 Hz. Delta activity in the 0.5 to 1 Hz range is attenuated severely by the use of LF = 1 Hz but is virtually unaffected by LF = 0.3 Hz. With good electrode technique (see Chapter 10), LF = 0.3 Hz can be used without difficulty.

HF settings below 70 Hz and including the 60 Hz notch filter attenuate real EEG activity at the fast end of the frequency range and should be used with care and good judgment.

The use of LF = 0.1 Hz may be reserved for recording in special situations. Monitoring respiration requires use of a very low frequency filter for adequate display of slowly changing activity, for example. The display of slow eye movements also demands an adequate low frequency response. (See Chapters 14 and 16.)

MASTER FILTER CONTROLS

Modern EEG instruments provide master LF and HF controls, as well as a master 60-Hz filter control. These provide a convenient means of changing settings when necessary. However, provision should be made to permit individual channels to be switched out of the master mode when necessary. For example, if two channels are to be used for respiratory monitoring, they may be changed individually to LF = 0.1 Hz. If a channel is required simultaneously for EMG recording, it can be switched individually to LF = 5 Hz.

PAPER SPEED

Although not an amplifier control, the chart speed selector is an important control that is used to enhance the display of the EEG. The standard 30 mm/sec paper speed gives an adequate degree of resolution of the frequency of most EEG activity. However, if there is very fast activity present, it can be more easily measured at fast paper speeds, which will increase the distance between successive peaks. Slower paper speeds may be used to compress periodic discharges in the EEG, as well as to group low voltage discharges of slow activity, so that they can be more easily perceived. For example, if there is a low amplitude discharge appearing once every 15 to 20 sec, it would be less easily noticed at a paper speed of 30 mm/sec because one and a half to two pages would separate the discharges. At 15 mm/sec, two or more discharges would appear on every page.

SUMMARY

This chapter has reviewed the functions of the EEG amplifier's controls and their effects on EEG recordings. The controls are 1) sensitivity, 2) low frequency (LF) filter, 3) high frequency (HF) filter, and 4) 60-Hz filter. They have a common function: They attenuate activity.

The sensitivity control equally attenuates EEG activity at all frequencies. Sensitivity is the ratio between input voltage and output amplitude, and is commonly expressed in μV/mm. At any given sensitivity setting, the output amplitude will be limited by the mechanical capabilities of the ink-writing oscillograph, beyond which the response becomes nonlinear. The range from the least voltage that can be measured to the maximum voltage that can be linearily recorded is the dynamic range of the amplifier-inkwriter system. High sensitivity reduces the dynamic range; low sensitivity increases it. The least change in voltage that can be measured establishes the resolution of the sensitivity setting in use. Optimally, the EEG sensitivity should be chosen to provide an effective dynamic range and an acceptable degree of resolution. Not all EEGs can be recorded at the same sensitivity setting.

The LF filters attenuate low frequencies. Each LF filter is defined by its cut-off frequency, which is that frequency at which the output is reduced by a given amount. In EEG practice, the cut-off frequency is defined either as an attenuation of 20%, or of 30%, depending upon the manufacturer. The attenuation of the input increases at frequencies below cut-off, and decreases to zero at some frequency above cut-off. The higher the LF cut-off frequency, the greater the attenuation of low frequencies.

The HF filters attenuate high frequencies. The cut-off frequency of an HF filter is defined in the same way as LF filters. The higher the input frequency is above cut-off, the greater the attenuation. The lower the cut-off frequency of the filter, the greater the attenuation of high frequencies.

The 60-Hz rejection, or notch, filter sharply attenuates 60-Hz activity. It also attenuates adjacent frequencies and should be used only when necessary.

Filters, in addition to attenuating activity in certain frequency ranges, cause phase shift (a displacement, in time, of output relative to input). LF filters are particularly likely to cause phase shift that can change waveform and the relative appearance of peak voltages at different frequencies.

Frequency response curves are graphs which show amplifier output amplitude, in response to a constant voltage input, over a wide range of frequencies. Different LF and HF filters combine to give different frequency response curves. The curves define the frequency range over which the amplifier responds linearly.

The filters of choice for least distortion of significant EEG signals are LF = 0.3 Hz and HF = 70 Hz. The use of the 60-Hz filter at these settings is equivalent to changing the HF to 35 Hz.

Careful selection of filter and sensitivity settings by the technologist will provide a recording most closely conforming to the input characteristics of the EEG actually generated in the brain.

REFERENCES

1. American EEG Society (1980): 4. Minimum technical standards for EEG recording in suspected cerebral death. In: *Guidelines in EEG—1980*. American EEG Society, Tucker, Georgia.
2. Barlow, J. S., Kamp, A., Morton, H. B., Ripoche, A., Shipton, H., and Tchavdarov, D. B. (1978): EEG instrumentation standards (revised 1977): Report of the Committee on EEG Instrumentation Standards of the International Federation of Societies for Electroencephalography and Clinical Neurophysiology. *Electroencephalogr. Clin. Neurophysiol.*, 45:144–147.
3. Chatrian, G. E., Bergamini, L., Dondey, M., Klass, D. W., Lennox-Buchthal, M., and Petersén, I. (1974): A glossary of terms most commonly used by clinical electroencephalographers. *Electroencephalogr. Clin. Neurophysiol.*, 37:538–548.
4. Cooper, R., Osselton, J. W., and Shaw, J. C. (1980): *EEG Technology*, 3rd ed. Butterworths, London, pp. 55–89.
5. Geddes, L. A. (1951): A note on phase distortion. *Electroencephalogr. Clin. Neurophysiol.*, 3:517–518.
6. Geddes, L. A., and Baker, L. E. (1975): *Principles of Applied Biomedical Instrumentation*, pp. 584–595. John Wiley, New York.
7. Grass Instrument Company (1973): *Grass Model 8 Instruction Manual Part II: Theory and Application*. Grass Instrument Co., Quincy, Massachusetts.
8. Grass Instrument Company (1981): *Glossary of Terms Used in Electroencephalography, Including Evoked Potentials and Computer Terminology*. Grass Instrument Co., Quincy, Massachusetts.
9. Heathkit Learning Publications (1975): *AC Electronics*. Heath Co., Benton Harbor, Michigan.
10. Henry, C. E. (1979): Optimal display of EEG activity. In: *Current Practice of Clinical Electroencephalography*, edited by D. W. Klass and D. D. Daly, pp. 179–220. Raven Press, New York.
11. McGee, F. E., Jr., and White, R. J. (1981): EEG Instrumentation. In: *Current Clinical Neurophysiology—Update on EEG and Evoked Potentials*, edited by C. E. Henry, pp. 1–49. Elsevier-North Holland, Amsterdam.
12. Saunders, M. G., and Jell, R. M. (1959): Time distortion in electroencephalograph amplifiers. *Electroencephalogr. Clin. Neurophysiol.*, 11:814–816.
13. Seaba, P. J. (1975): Understanding frequency response, *Am. J. EEG Technol.*, 15:20–41.
14. Snodgrass, L., and Knott, J. R. (1962): Some effects produced by three sets of EEG controls: Amplification, low frequency filters and high frequency filters. *Am. J. EEG Technol.*, 2:65–81.

Chapter 9

Adjustments to the EEG Instrument

Before recording an EEG, the technologist must carry out a series of checks to detect any faults in the instrument or any errors in the setting of the controls. The procedure is known as calibrating the instrument.

CALIBRATION PROCEDURES

A known DC voltage is applied simultaneously to the input of each amplifier. The generally accepted settings are S = 7 μv/mm; LF = 1 Hz; HF = 70 Hz. The deflections of the ink-writing oscillographs are then examined. The amplitude of the deflections should be equal in all channels and the calibration waveforms should match the standard for the instrument settings selected. Figure 9.1 is a sample of the expected output if the applied calibration voltage is 50 μV, the amplifier's sensitivity is 7 μV/mm, the LF is set at 1 Hz, the HF is set at 70 Hz, and the paper speed is 30 mm/sec. Figure 9.2 shows the output of an EEG instrument, using a 50-μV input signal. It is obvious that the 8 channels are not yielding equal outputs to the same input. By examining the calibration in each channel, the technologist can identify the causes of the differences.

CALIBRATION ADJUSTMENTS

With a basic knowledge of sensitivity and filters and a good mental image of the standard calibration signal, the technologist can solve the problems presented by the calibrations shown in Fig. 9.2.

Channel 1. The calibration signal matches the standard of S = 7, LF = 1, HF = 70.

Channel 2. The sensitivity is too low, as is obvious from the 5-mm deflection. LF = 1 and HF = 70. Return S to 7.

Channel 3. S = 10, and LF = 1. HF = 35, as can be deduced from the slightly rounded peak of the 5 mm calibration pulse. Return S to 7, and HF to 70.

Channel 4. The sensitivity is too high. The pen deflects 17 mm, so S = 3. The decay time constant (return to baseline) is longer than in channel 1. LF = 0.3. The peak is not rounded, so HF = 70. Return S to 7 and LF to 1.

Channel 5. The sensitivity is higher than 7 μV/mm. The deflection of the calibration signal is 11 mm, so S = 4.5, which is within 10% of the 5-μV/mm setting. LF = 0.1, as deduced by noting the long time required to return to baseline. The peak of the calibration is slightly rounded, so HF = 35. To restore to the standard settings, return S to 7, LF to 1, and HF to 70.

Channel 6. The deflection is nearly 7 mm. The peak shows no rounding. However, the time constant is very short. LF = 5. Set LF at 1 to return this channel to its usual condition.

Channel 7. The amplitude of the calibration is lower than expected. It is 4.5 mm, which is within 10% of the 5-μV/mm setting. The peak of the pulse is rounded off excessively. HF = 15. To return to standard, set S at 7 and return HF to 70.

Channel 8. The amplitude of the signal is 3.5 mm, which is 5% higher than expected of S = 15, but this is acceptable. The LF setting is lower than usual, being 0.3 Hz. To return to standard settings, set S at 7 and LF at 1.

The calibrations should be accurate to 10% or 0.5 mm. This is attained by adjusting the amplifiers' sensitivity equalizers (Figs. 2.8 and 2.14).

To carry out the usual calibrating procedure, the calibrator input is fed into all amplifiers by placing the master selector in the calibration mode and activating the calibration switch. When the calibration button is depressed, Input 1 becomes negative with respect to Input 2 and the pens deflect upward (see Chapter 12). Releasing the calibration button allows the capacitors of the amplifiers to discharge and the pens deflect downward. This downward deflection should be equal in distance to the first upward deflection. At least 1.5 or 2 sec should elapse between depressing and releasing the calibration button when using a low frequency setting of 1 Hz (time constant 0.12 sec). It is necessary to allow time for the pens to

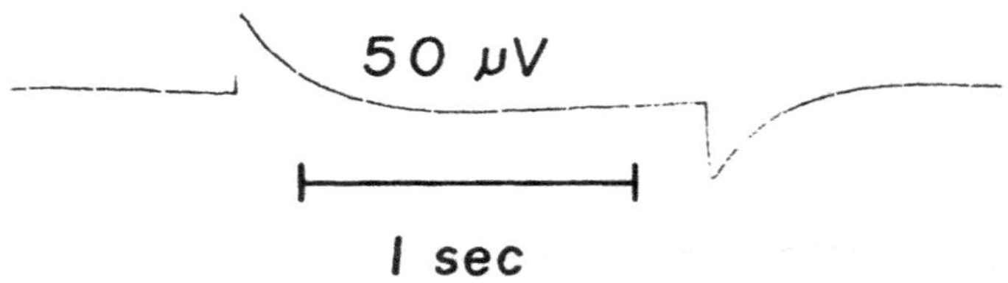

FIG. 9.1. Example of a standard calibration. A 50-μV square wave was applied to the amplifier input. The sensitivity was 7 μV/mm; LF was set at 1 HZ; HF was set at 70 HZ. The paper speed was 30 mm/sec.

return fully to baseline between successive deflections so that all characteristics of the amplifier response can be observed. In general, the interval between deflections should be about five times the duration of the time constant used.

A minimum of three ON-OFF, 50-uV calibration signals should be recorded at the beginning of each EEG record. These should be compared within each channel to be certain that transient influences induced by turning on the amplifiers and the chart drive have not affected, for the first deflections, the amplitudes or the apparent time constants characteristic for the filter setting. It also is useful to calibrate with several input voltages, for example, 50 μV, 20 μV, and 10 μV. A 5-μV calibration also may be advantageously included. There are two reasons for inputting several different calibration voltages. First, it makes certain that each channel is responding properly over the dynamic range of the sensitivity setting in use. Sometimes there may be an instrument fault in a single channel that appears only with a low voltage input. An increase in inertia or "drag" that occurs when an oscillograph and its pen develop excessive tension, for example, can cause a low voltage deflection to be seriously attenuated. This will be apparent with a low voltage square wave calibration that will be rounded off. Second, instrument faults can develop within the circuit of a calibrator. By comparing the relative deflections of several input voltages, such a fault can be more easily detected. If the calibration voltage is faulty, the EEG record may be inaccurately described and interpreted. Further, if three calibration signals are recorded at each of three input voltages in a continuous strip, an estimate can be made of stability of the baseline and excessive amplifier noise.

Measurements of both upward and downward deflections should be made in each channel. This may be done with preset calipers or with a millimeter ruler (Fig. 9.3). The height of the pen excursion should be measured from the baseline to maximum for both the upward and the downward excursions. These should be equal. Do not include the slight overshoot often seen when the HF setting is on 70 Hz. If the calibration signal is 50 μV and the sensitivity setting is 7 μV/mm, all deflections should be 7.1 mm. (This value is determined by dividing 7 into 50 μV.) If S = 10 and the calibration signal is 100 μV, the deflection should be 10 mm. If S = 2 and the calibration signal is 20 μV, the deflection should be 10 mm.

Notations of the paper speed, filter settings (including 60-Hz filter), calibration voltage, and sensitivity settings should be made on the recorded calibrations. If there is any doubt about the performance of an amplifier at any point during the recording, the calibration procedures should be repeated at that time.

Biological calibration, sometimes referred to as "bio-cal" or as an "equalizing run," usually is done after the initial calibration. The bio-cal compares all channels, using as their input the EEG activity from one pair of scalp electrodes connected to every channel. Each channel should be set at the same HF, LF, 60-Hz, and sensitivity settings. The bio-cal affords a check of the electrode cable, the two electrodes being used, the amplifiers, the galvanometers, and the pens. A visual comparison will indicate whether there are differences in performance on the different channels that may not appear on square wave calibration. The use of Fp_1 on Input 1 and O_2 on Input 2 will give the widest frequency and voltage ranges for this comparison. (See Figs. 1.3 and 11.1 for locations.)

At the end of every recording, another set of square wave calibrations must be obtained, using all the filter and sensitivity settings that were employed during the course of the recording. These calibrations will detect amplifier faults that might occur at settings other than those used on the initial calibration or those that develop during recording. The settings and calibration voltages should be noted directly on these final calibrations.

MECHANICAL BASELINE

Unequal spacing between the lines of the various channels with the amplifiers in the OFF or STANDBY position indicates that the mechanical baseline of the pens needs adjustment. Misalignment can affect the limit

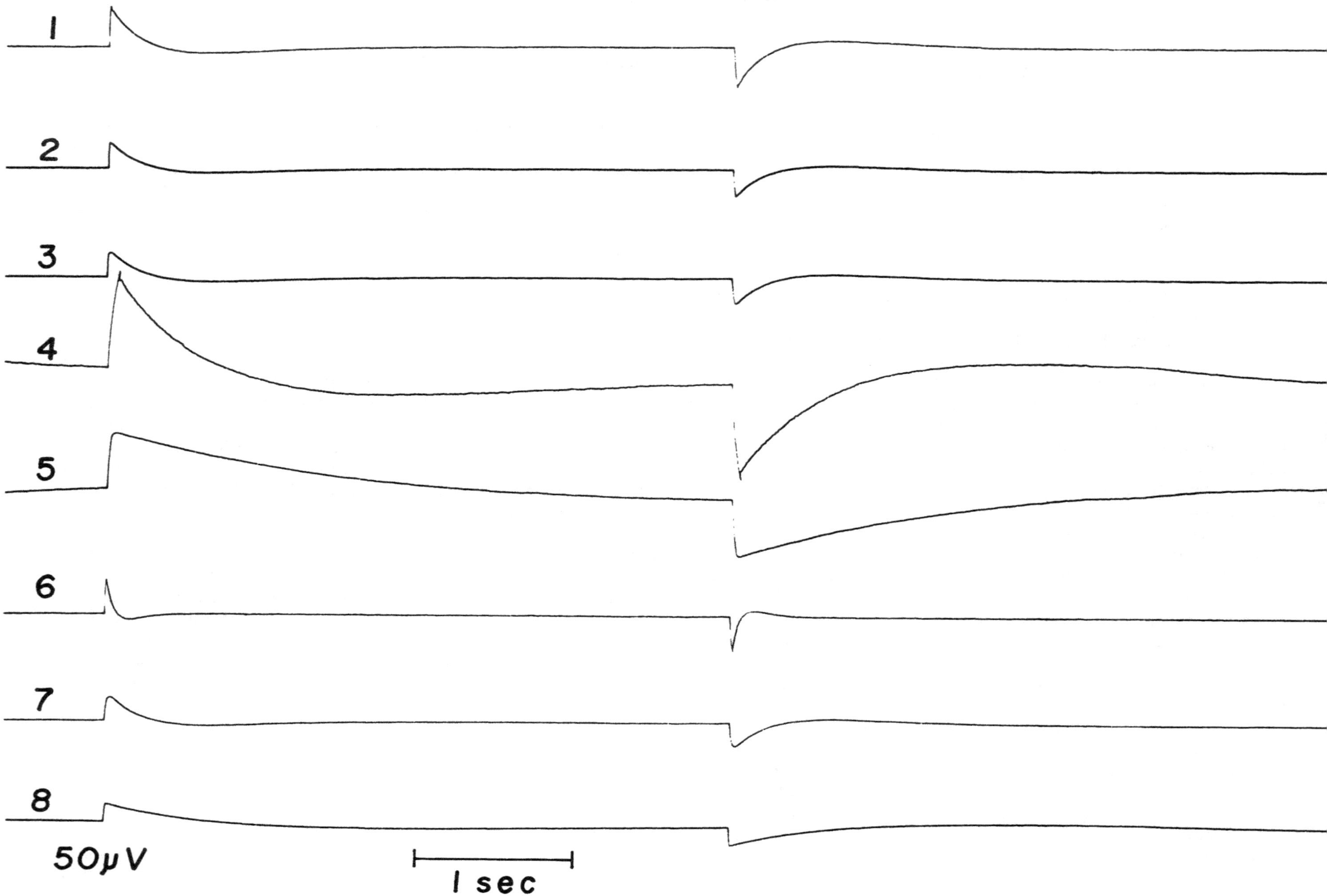

FIG. 9.2. Sample calibrations revealing different instrument settings (see text for details).

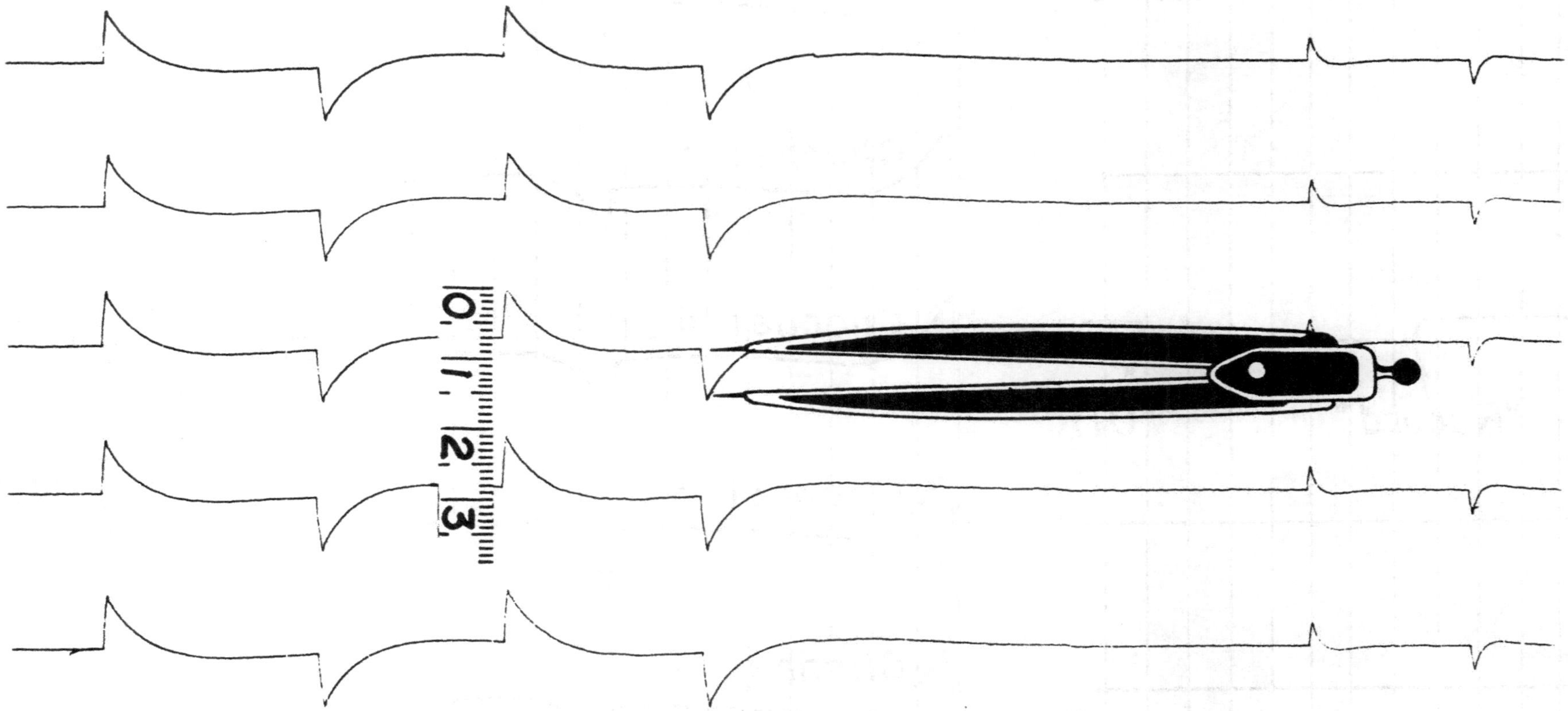

FIG. 9.3. Measuring a calibration pulse with calipers and with a millimeter ruler. Use of calipers permits rapid and precise interchannel comparison.

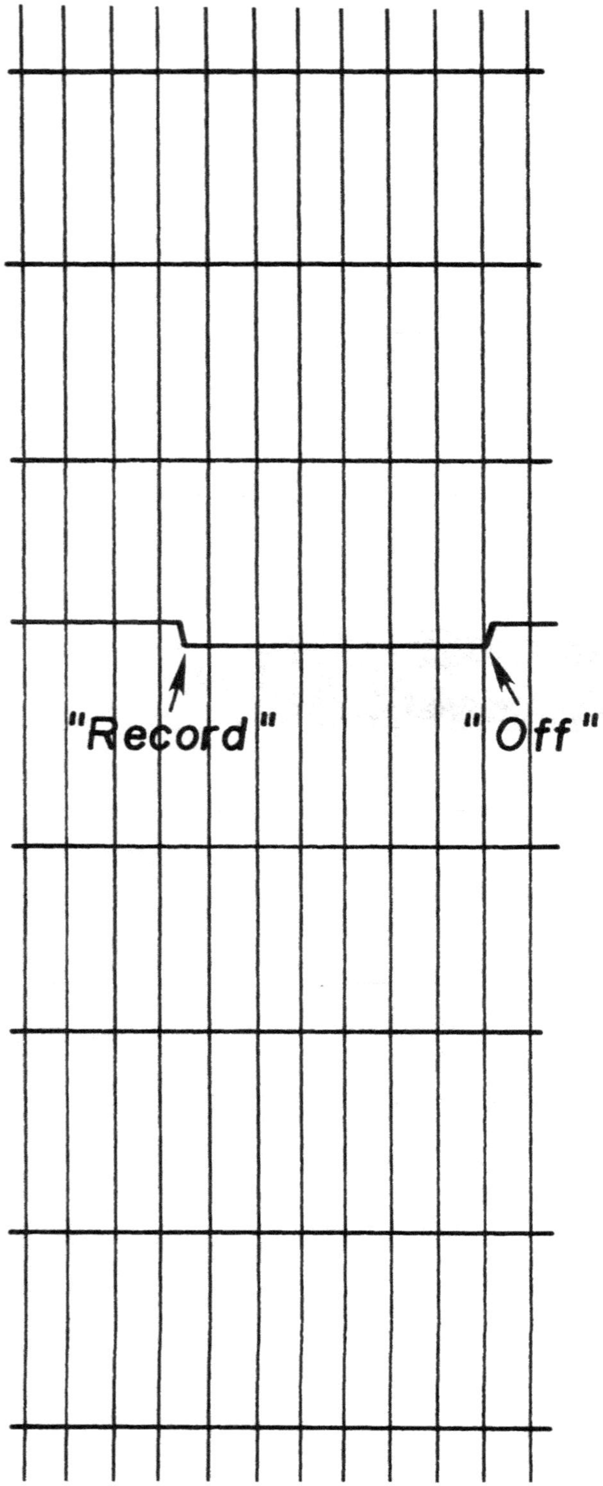

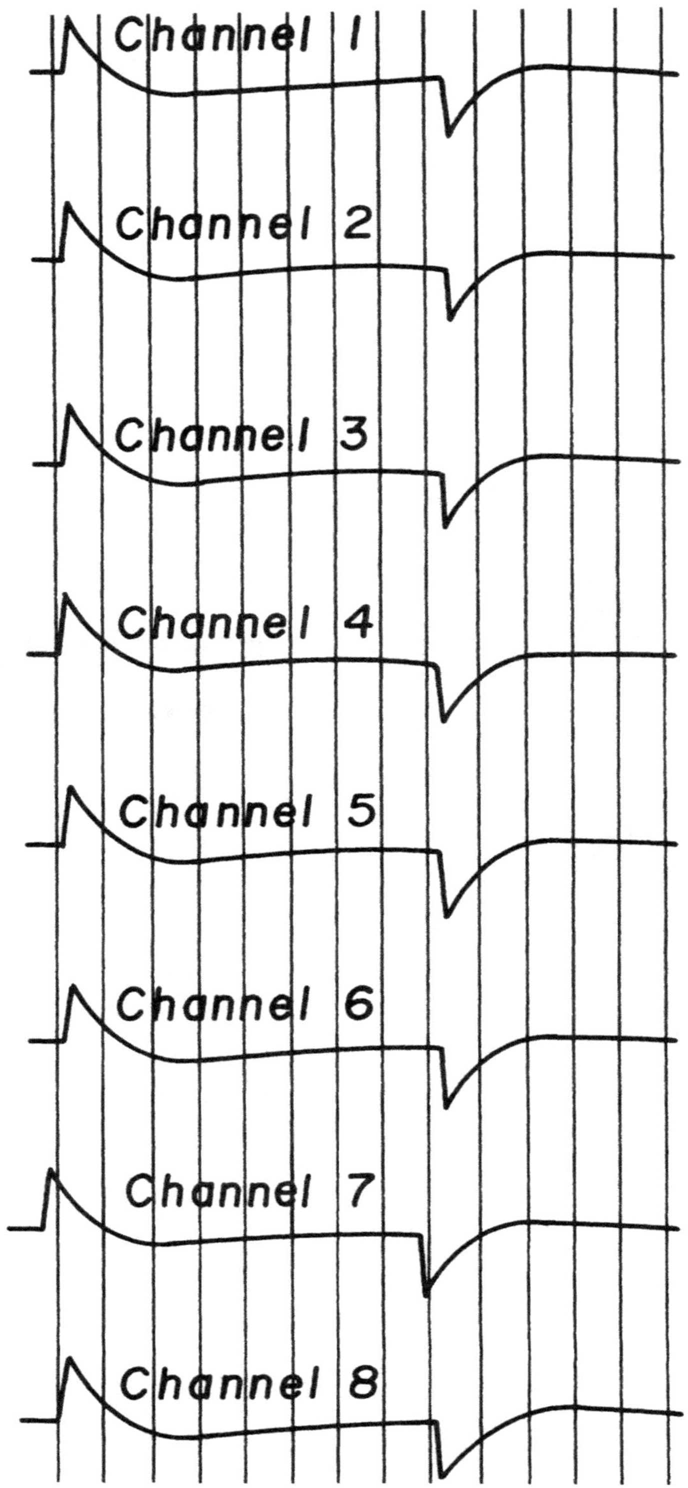

FIG. 9.4. (*left*) Electrical baseline. Pen moves up or down from its mechanical baseline when the writer switch is turned to record and input is in CAL mode (see text).

FIG. 9.5. (*right*) Time axis alignment. There is misalignment in 6 of 8 channels. Channel 1 lags behind channels 4 and 8 by 2 mm. Channels 2, 3, 5, and 6 lag by 1 mm. Channel 7 leads by 2 mm (see text for discussion).

of a pen's deflection. Correction is accomplished by following the manufacturer's instructions for mechanical centering of the pens.

ELECTRICAL BASELINE

If, in the calibration mode, a pen moves up or down from its mechanical baseline when the writer switch is turned to RECORD, and returns to baseline when turned to OFF, an adjustment of the electrical baseline control is indicated (Fig. 9.4). On some instruments this is a simple operation; a control on the front panel of each amplifier can be adjusted as necessary. Reference should be made to the service manual of the instrument regarding correction of a faulty electrical baseline.

TIME–AXIS ALIGNMENT

If any pen leads or lags behind the others when a calibration signal is applied (Fig. 9.5), the time axis alignment of that channel requires adjustment. A slight variation may be difficult to observe unless the calibration deflection occurs over a time line on the paper. Errors in alignment are seen more easily at a paper speed of 60 mm/sec. "Hitting" a time line can be accomplished by applying the calibration signal frequently. Measurements also can be made by using a drafting triangle aligned with the top or bottom of the paper, drawing a line through the signal from one channel, and comparing the position of other channels to it. It also is possible to use a caliper or ruler to measure from a common vertical axis to the deflection of the calibration signals. Follow the directions given by the manufacturer for correcting misalignment of the time axis.

The sample shown in Fig. 9.5 has 6 channels that do not begin their deflections at the first vertical time line on the recording paper. Five channels lag and one channel leads. Only channels 4 and 8 are on the vertical line. The maximum misalignment, channel 7 contrasted with channel 1, is 4 mm. At a paper speed of 30 mm/sec this represents 0.13 sec. It is obvious that this particular EEG instrument is in need of adjustment. If a clinical recording had spike activity in all channels, the apparently earlier event in channel 7 could easily lead to misinterpretation, the first spike being presumed to represent a primary focus of discharge and the later spikes representing areas of secondary discharge.

SUMMARY

The technologist should check the instrument before recording each EEG and make any adjustments necessary to correct errors in instrument settings and to detect instrument faults. It is necessary for all test procedures to be made again at the end of each recording. The terminal calibrations should include all instrument settings actually used. If the initial and final calibrations are identical, it shows the integrity of the instrument during the recording.

Chapter 10

Electrodes

EEG electrodes are the first instrumental link between the electrical generators in the brain and the EEG record itself. In an overly elementary sense, EEG electrodes are pieces of metal held against the scalp with a conductive jelly beneath them and with wires connecting them to the inputs of the EEG amplifiers. The events that occur at the interface of the electrode and the conductive jelly (called an electrolyte) are of great importance, for it is at this interface that current flow within the body becomes electron flow in the electrode and all following sections of the EEG instrument. The degree to which the output of the EEG instrument can be modified by the characteristics of the electrodes used for recording has been known for many years (15).

When any metal is placed in contact with an *electrolyte* (the body fluids in the scalp and the conductive jelly both contain free chloride ions and collectively are the electrolyte), a voltage develops between the metal and the electrolyte, due to the formation of a layer of electrical charges on the surface of the electrode and another layer of opposite charges in the electrolyte. Figure 10.1 schematically represents the formation of the charged layers of the electrode–electrolyte interface. In an ideal electrode, there will be an equilibrium in the migration of positive and negative charges at the interface, and the voltage difference between metal and electrolyte will be constant. In practice, electrodes have some drift and noise because of continuous variability in the electrode potential (7,11,12).

The formation of two closely spaced and opposing charges is equivalent to the plates of a charged capacitor (see Chapter 5). Consequently, an EEG electrode placed against the scalp has the property of a capacitor.

Different metals develop different voltages when immersed in the same electrolyte. By using one electrode material as a standard, the voltage between it and other materials can be determined. Every metal, whether it is an element (e.g., silver), a compound (e.g., silver chloride), or a metal alloy (e.g., stainless steel), has its own electrode potential relative to the standard electrode. This electrode potential is called a half-cell potential because the single electrode is acting as half of a battery. Typical half-cell potentials for several materials used in the construction of electrodes are given in Table 10.1. Electrodes also have the property of a battery. They also have resistance.

The equivalent circuit of the electrode–electrolyte interface is shown in Fig. 10.2. The voltage source (E) is in series with the capacitive (C) and resistive (R and r) elements of the electrode (13). Since a practical EEG record requires two electrodes connected to the inputs of each amplifier, further information about the effects of electrode properties can be derived from a review of the equivalent circuit of a pair of electrodes and the input to the first stage of the EEG amplifier, shown in Fig. 10.3 (13,14).

This schema is less complex than it first looks. Consider G, the generator of EEG activity, to be the source of activity with a frequency of 2 Hz. This activity is conducted to the surface of the head through resistive pathways that include the internal resistances of the generator (Rg) and other tissues (Rt), including brain coverings, skull, and scalp (Rs). Contact is made at the surface of the head with the electrodes. Together, the electrodes form a source of DC potential and their capacitive and resistive elements form an impedance (Z_1 and Z_2) that is in series with the amplifier input impedances $R_{in\ 1}$ and $R_{in\ 2}$. Alternating current with a frequency of 2 Hz flows through each input circuit through the resistive and capacitive elements of the electrodes and through R_{in}. Ideally, the resistances and capacitances in each of these circuits will be equal, and any DC voltage appearing at the two inputs also will be equal. Otherwise, DC current will flow in the circuit formed by the electrodes on the scalp and the input resistors in the amplifiers. This will be small if the input impedance of the amplifier is large. The flow of DC current will cause baseline drift of the amplifiers, particularly when long time constants are used. Extreme polarization can convert an electrode into a diode so that current will flow only in one direction; this would distort an AC signal.

If the impedances of the electrodes are unequal, there will be imbalance of input to the amplifiers. This can have an adverse effect on the amplifier's common mode rejection capabilities.

Because an electrode has a capacitance in series with a resistance, it

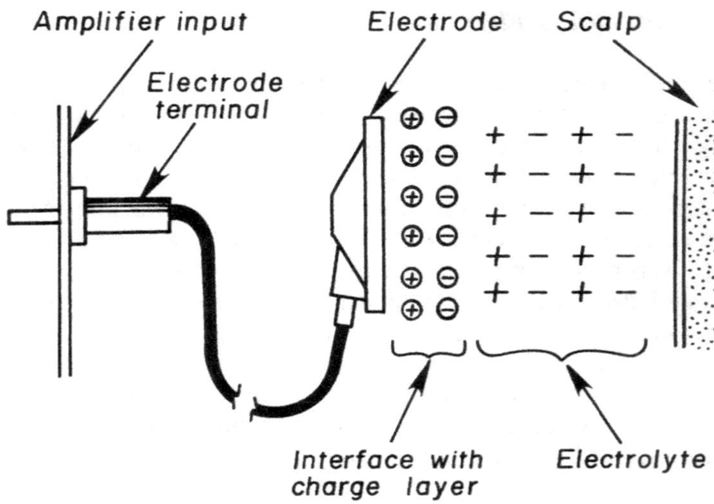

FIG. 10.1. Charge layer at electrode–electrolyte interface. Modified from Geddes (13).

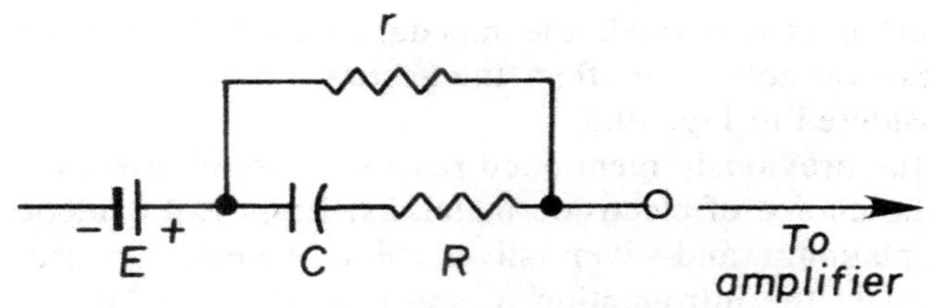

FIG. 10.2. Series equivalent circuit of a single electrode in contact with an electrolyte. Redrawn from Geddes (14).

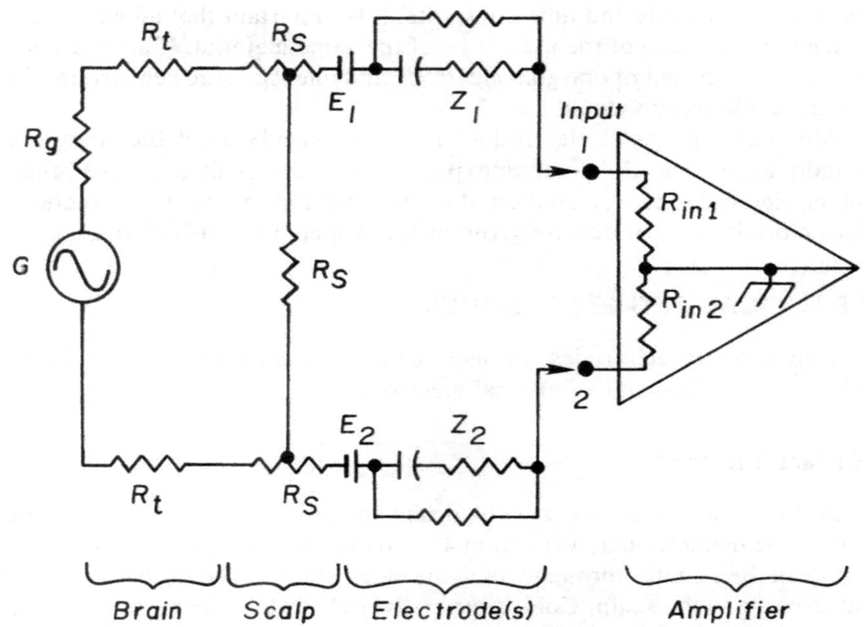

FIG. 10.3. Equivalent circuit of electrode pair with input to an EEG amplifier. G = Cerebral generator; Rg = internal resistance of generator; Rt = tissue resistance; Rs = scalp resistance; $E_{1,2}$ = electrode potential; $Z_{1,2}$ = capacitive and resistive properties of electrodes; $R_{in,1}$ and $R_{in,2}$ = input resistance (impedance) of amplifier. Redrawn from Geddes (14).

has properties of a low frequency (high-pass) filter and has a time constant. It has been shown (6,15) that different electrode materials have different effects on low frequency input signals. Not only may the time constants differ with the material used for constructing an electrode, but so may the effects of frequency on electrode impedance differ. In general, electrodes present high impedances to very low frequency signals and low impedances to higher frequency signals. Also, when the electrode–elec-

TABLE 10.1. *Typical half-cell potential values*

Electrode material	Electrode potential (V)
Lead (Pb)	−0.13
Tin (Sn)	+0.14
Silver chloride (AgCl)	+0.22
Copper (Cu)	+0.52
Silver (Ag)	+0.80
Platinum (Pt)	+0.86
Gold (Au)	+1.50

trolyte interface is very small, the impedance will be higher than when it is large. These variables can affect the accurate reproduction of the 2-Hz signal considered in Fig. 10.3.

For all the previously mentioned reasons, careful attention should be given to the choice of electrode materials. Empirical evidence suggests that gold, platinum, and silver–silver chloride electrodes are among the best. To avoid the introduction of spurious signals to the input of the amplifiers, it is important to choose a material that has minimum drift of electrode potential and a very long time constant. Chlorided silver disc (Ag–AgCl) electrodes have the best properties of all materials. Gold also is a useful electrode material, having little drift and a long time constant. Stainless steel has drift and a short time constant and, depending on the type of stainless steel, extraneous DC potentials may be introduced (6).

Because of the differences between electrode materials with respect to electrode potentials and time constants, it is important that all electrodes placed on the scalp of the patient be of the same material. If an electrode pair was composed of one gold electrode and one Ag–AgCl electrode, the potential difference would be 1.28 V.

Although Ag–AgCl electrodes are commercially available, they are usually expensive. Relatively inexpensive, commercially available bright silver electrodes can be converted to Ag–AgCl at low cost. Instructions for chloriding electrodes are given in the Appendix to this chapter.

PRACTICAL EEG ELECTRODES

Two types of electrodes are used commonly for recording the EEG. These are surface and subdermal electrodes.

Surface Electrodes

Surface electrodes, as usually designed, are metal discs or shallow cups. The diameter may vary from 4 to 10 mm. Some cup electrodes have a hole in their center through which the electrolyte can be introduced after attachment to the scalp. Gold, silver–silver chloride, bright silver, and tin are typical materials used in the construction of surface electrodes. Gold electrodes, however, are not pure gold. They are gold plated over pure silver, the thickness being sufficient to insure against bimetallic action of the electrolyte, which would introduce DC signals. Theoretically, a potential of 0.7 V could develop across such an interface.

Application of Surface Electrodes

Before surface electrodes are applied, the scalp must be prepared properly. This requires topical cleaning at the measured locations. Local scrubbing with a gauze pad or a cotton swab, using alcohol, acetone, or a mild detergent, will remove local oils and reduce scalp resistance. Proprietary materials that contain a mild abrasive also are available. After the local area is cleaned, an electrolyte, usually an ECG paste containing free chloride ions, is rubbed into it. This expedites ion movement from scalp to electrode and also lowers scalp impedance. It is important to restrict the area of application of the electrolyte to avoid creation of a short circuit between electrodes via a "salt bridge" on the scalp. A small amount of electrolyte is then spread on the surface of the electrode to be placed against the scalp. A cup electrode is filled with the electrolyte. The electrode then is placed on the prepared surface and secured by appropriate means.

The most effective method of securing an EEG electrode to the scalp is to use collodion. The electrode is held in position, and collodion may be placed directly around its edges and over it. Alternatively, a 2 × 2 cm square of collodion-impregnated gauze is placed over the electrode. The collodion is dried quickly with a stream of compressed air. Compressed air may be installed permanently in the laboratory, or a small, relatively quiet and portable air compressor may be used. Electrodes that are attached properly with collodion will withstand several pounds of direct pull and will not be inadvertently pulled away from the scalp during movement, which may occur in a restless child or convulsing patient. Electrodes attached with collodion may be left in place for many hours (up to several days). Additional electrolyte may be introduced through a small hole in the center, if necessary, to maintain a satisfactory impedance. Adequate ventilation is required when applying collodion.

An alternative method of applying a surface electrode is to use a conductive electrode cream or paste that has adhesive properties sufficient to hold an electrode at the desired scalp location. The electrode site must be cleaned, as described above. The hair is then separated at the electrode site and the electrode cup, filled with the paste, is pressed against the scalp; a small amount of paste will overflow the rim of the cup. A square of gauze or absorbent paper is placed over the electrode–paste assembly. This helps hold the electrode in place, and retards drying of the paste during the examination period.

Some technologists apply the paste directly to the scalp in a small mound, insert the disc in the paste, and cover the combination with cotton or paper. This is a less satisfactory procedure because the "electrode" now has become the entire area of the paste in contact with the scalp. Not only may asymmetries of placement inadvertently develop, but interelectrode spacing will vary, and effective short circuiting of a pair of electrodes can occur.

The use of adhesive paste has an advantage in speed and perhaps ease of application, but it has the disadvantage of mechanical instability. If a patient has a convulsion, electrodes easily become detached from the scalp, and valuable information is lost. If the patient is restless, individual electrodes may slide, and their locations no longer are precisely defined; interelectrode distances will be changed and asymmetries will occur. The sliding effect is enhanced by perspiration.

When selecting an electrode cream or paste, the technologist should be aware that materials in some may be irritative to the skin and that some patients may be specifically sensitive to particular chemical agents. There have been several reports of serious skin sensitivity to bentonite, particularly in the presence of calcium chloride (5,23). Some proprietary adhesive–conductive pastes have warning statements printed on their containers indicating discretion in use when recording infants and persons with sensitive skin. The technologist always should read all literature concerning any proprietary electrolyte or material used for skin preparation.

Subdermal Electrodes

Subdermal electrodes are usually made of platinum alloy or stainless steel. Platinum alloy has a relatively long time constant; stainless steel does not. The diameter is approximately 0.5 mm and typical length is approximately 12 mm.

Application of Subdermal Electrodes

Subdermal, or needle, electrodes are inserted just beneath the skin, parallel to the surface of the scalp. They should be embedded the full length of the needle. Scalp preparation involves thorough cleaning so that the small puncture wounds remain clean.

Subdermal electrodes must be inserted symmetrically over homologous brain areas to avoid artificial (artifactual) amplitude asymmetries (24). Figure 10.4 shows an experimental example of this effect. Two pairs of subdermal electrodes are arranged to record from a common generator. The electrodes are symmetrical, relative to the source, but one pair has the needle tips facing away from, the other pair facing toward, each other (Fig. 10.4A). Those facing toward each other yield less amplitude (Fig. 10.4B). Figure 10.5 shows the effects of electrode orientation on an actual EEG. Fig. 10.5A shows the positions of the electrodes, and Fig. 10.5B illustrates the effects on the EEG. When the tips of subdermal electrodes

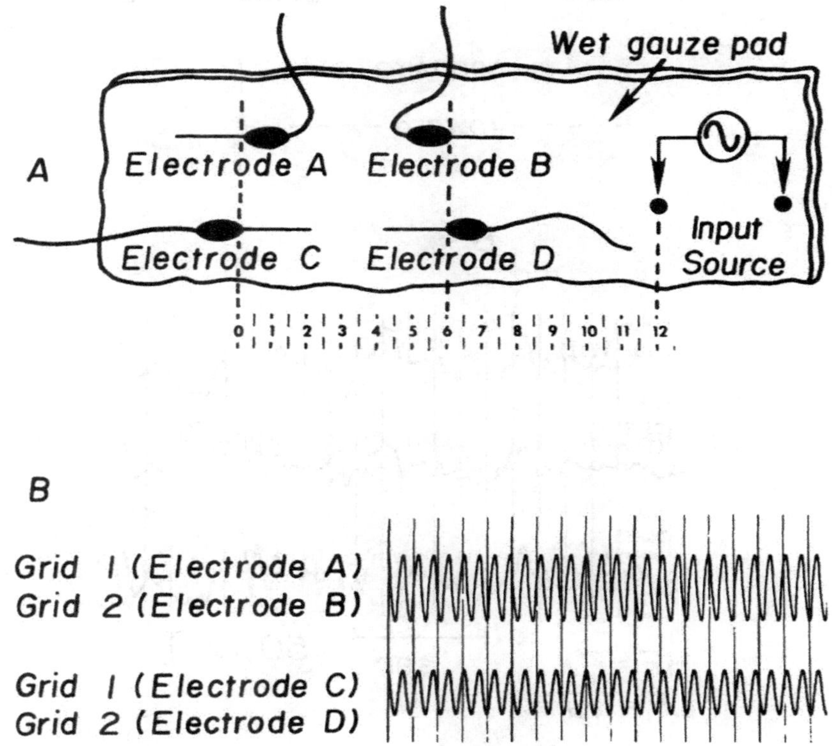

FIG. 10.4. A: Orientation of recording electrodes. B: Amplitude asymmetry of function generator signal induced by orientation of recording electrodes. From Tyner and Knott (24).

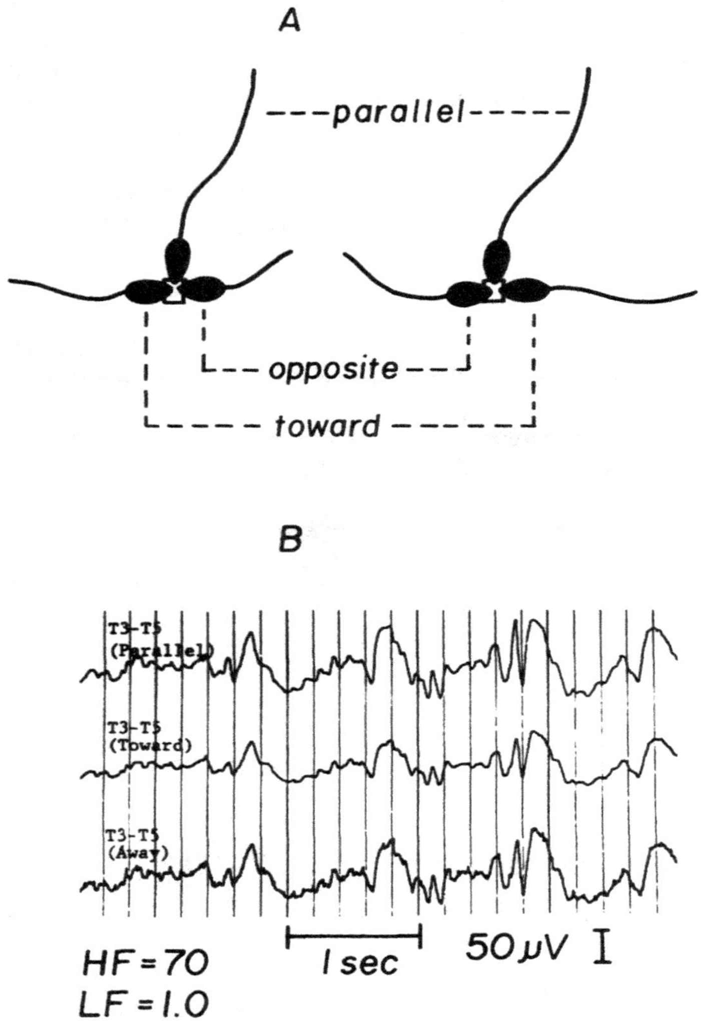

FIG. 10.5. A: Direction of subdermal insertions using human subjects. B: Amplitude variability due to directional orientation of subdermal electrodes. From Tyner and Knott (24).

face each other, the amplitude is lower. These effects are due to differences in the potential fields recorded by the different electrode orientations (see Chapter 12).

Subdermal electrodes must be sterilized after each use, and require careful handling at the time of application to preserve sterility. (Electrode sterilization is discussed below.)

Because of the many problems presented by the use of needle electrodes, including the need for sterilization, the American EEG Society states that they "are not recommended for use under ordinary laboratory conditions" (2), and "Needle electrodes should never be used" when recording newborn infants and "They are not needed and are not advised" for recording in infants and young children (3). Needle electrodes should not be used to record from any patient suspected of having viral hepatitis or Creutzfeldt-Jakob disease (see Sterilization of Electrodes, below).

MEASUREMENT OF ELECTRODE IMPEDANCE

Regardless of the method of application and the type of electrode used, the impedance (Z) of every electrode should be measured before recording begins. Measurement of electrode impedance is carried out using an AC impedance meter.

The impedance of subdermal electrodes is typically higher than the impedance of surface electrodes, being limited in part by surface area. A subdermal electrode with a diameter of 0.5 mm and an effective length of 12 mm has a surface area of 20 mm^2. This may be compared with the surface area of a 10-mm disc electrode, which is 78.5 mm^2, and of a 7-mm disc electrode, which is 38.5 mm^2. Only a 4-mm disc would present a smaller area, 12.6 mm. The impedance of a needle electrode cannot be lowered by topical treatment with an electrolyte, as is possible with surface electrodes.

The impedance of most electrodes varies with the frequency of the signal being recorded, particularly below 10 Hz. Platinum alloy needles have been depicted as having an impedance of 21 kΩ at 10 Hz and 105 kΩ at 1 Hz, whereas the impedance of Ag–AgCl surface electrodes remains constantly low, from 10 Hz to less than 1 Hz (7). Others (26) confirm the poor impedance of subdermal electrodes at low frequencies, especially below 0.5 Hz.

The use of a DC ohmmeter to determine resistance (only) involves the measurement of DC current from a standard voltage source which is converted into resistance (R = E/I) (see Chapter 5). It does not include any capacitive component. Further, when using a DC ohmmeter, direct current flows through the electrodes under test, causing them to become polarized in the process of measuring their resistance. This in turn may cause them to become electrically unstable. Depending on the amount of current flowing in the circuit, the patient may experience an unpleasant sensation (22). This type of meter should not be used to measure the resistance of EEG electrodes.

In recent years, the use of AC impedance meters has become almost universal. The measurement is made by using a 10 to 30 Hz alternating current, which is within the range of EEG frequencies. The current level is very low (a few microamperes). Electrode polarization is minimized, and it is rare that this current is perceived by a patient.

Electrode impedance meters may be connected directly to the electrode board of the EEG, which expedites measurement. All electrodes except the one being tested are interconnected within the device, and the impedance of the electrode selected for test is measured against the impedance of the others in parallel. A switch consecutively selects electrodes for test. One should be certain that the impedance of the ground electrode applied to the patient also is checked.

Acceptable impedances of surface electrodes should be below 5 kΩ (2). After a recording has started, it may be necessary from time to time to recheck the impedances, particularly if there are unusual asymmetries or if there is 60-Hz artifact in only one or a few derivations. Many modern EEG instruments have a built-in impedance checking system that permits rapid in-line evaluation. If an electrode's impedance rises above 5 kΩ, it should be reduced by adding electrolyte, or the electrode should be replaced as necessary.

ELECTRODE REMOVAL

Electrodes applied with collodion are removed by using alcohol and acetone applied to a ball of cotton in small amounts. Initial moistening of the electrode area with water is helpful. A metal or plastic comb, pulled gently through the area, breaks up the collodion and brings it free of the hair. Alternating acetone application with a few drops of water facilitates the break-up of the collodion. Topical application of baby oil will assist in soothing the scalp. Dry the scalp and hair with a dry towel. This method is especially recommended for infants (17).

Acetone is flammable and also somewhat toxic. It must be used with care. There should be no open flame or sparking in the environment. It must not be used in an isolette or any small closed space. The patient's eyes should be protected. When removing electrodes, rubbing with acetone should not be so vigorous that it is painful.

Electrodes applied with an adhesive paste electrolyte are removed with water (a wet cloth or ball of cotton). In general, adhesive creams harden rather quickly after application, and removal may be time consuming. A comb helps to break up the residual paste and pull it free of the hair.

Some pastes (especially bentonite) are radio-opaque. If radiological examination of the head follows the EEG examination, residual paste will show up as a shadow in the X-ray or CT scan. The technologist must remove *all* electrode paste.

Needle electrodes usually are removed by deftly pulling them out. An alcohol swab should be applied to the area of puncture. If the wound bleeds, it should be wiped with sterile gauze and pressure applied until bleeding stops.

The principle should be followed that the patient shall leave the laboratory with a thoroughly clean head, and no patient shall show evidence of just having had an EEG examination.

STERILIZATION OF ELECTRODES

When surface electrodes have been used to record the EEG of patients with infectious disease, they require sterilization. Subdermal electrodes always require sterilization after each use because they can transmit viral diseases. The two diseases that are especially dangerous in this regard are viral hepatits, which is not uncommon, and Creutzfeldt-Jakob disease, which is uncommon but lethal.

Needle electrodes must always be sterilized by steam autoclaving. Routine sterilization requires 15 min at 121 to 127° at 15 psi (16), but to achieve adequate sterilization after contamination by Creutzfeldt-Jakob virus, autoclaving for 1 hr at 121°C and 20 psi is recommended. A suggested alternative is to soak contaminated electrodes in 5% sodium hypochlorite solution (household bleach). For complete safety, the electrodes may be incinerated (10).

Gas sterilization of electrodes is not recommended. A comparative study of steam autoclaving versus gas sterilization showed only steam sterilization to be 100% effective (16).

The same rules apply to sterilization of surface electrodes used to record from patients with infectious disease.

CARE OF ELECTRODES

Surface electrodes, which use an electrolyte in contact with them, must be cleaned thoroughly after each use. Electrolytic paste never should be allowed to dry on electrodes between applications, as this will affect impedance, reduce effective surface area, and create an unstable battery effect, thus increasing noise at the amplifier input. After use, the electrodes should be washed in warm water, and residual electrolyte or adhesive should be removed with a small, soft brush. Care should be taken not to damage the surface of Ag–AgCl electrodes, as this could create a local battery at an interface between the silver electrode material and the AgCl coating. Scratching gold-plated electrodes must be avoided for the same reasons.

Platinum alloy needles are easily bent, and they also can acquire small burrs or barbs at their tips that create discomfort on insertion and withdrawal. The needles should be checked frequently for such defects by pulling the needle through a piece of cotton; any defects should be eliminated by sharpening. The needles also may be examined with an 8× magnifying glass to insure a sharp and barbless point.

Subdermal electrodes require careful cleaning after each use because blood and plasma, when dried, reduce effective surface area, increase impedance, and lead to instability. Subdermal electrodes, like surface electrodes, should be cleaned immediately after use and then sterilized. If not cleaned before steam sterilization, the heat will harden residual contaminants and render the electrodes useless. Ultrasound may be utilized to remove dried substances from electrodes. (Small ultrasound units are commercially available at reasonable prices.) When cleaning gold-plated electrodes by this method, care must be taken not to expose them too long to the ultrasound as it is possible to remove the plating by an overly robust treatment. The technologist should be exceedingly careful when handling unsterilized needle electrodes because viral and blood-borne infections could be transmitted through a scratch or skin puncture. Should the technologist receive a skin puncture from an unsterilized needle electrode, it should be reported immediately to the medical director of the laboratory.

All electrodes have a point of basic weakness, which is the junction between the wire (the conducting pathway from the electrode to the electrode board) and the electrode material. This region is particularly vulnerable to penetration by water and electrolyte materials. If this area is penetrated, an active battery is created. Wire strands may become weakened through corrosion and may be fractured by mechanical stresses. The result will be massive noise artifact at the input to the amplifier. Well-made commercial electrodes use special seals at the wire–electrode junction to minimize the penetration of moisture and strengthen the mechanical junction. Nevertheless, the technologist should keep this region clear of electrolyte, dry or wet, and should not bend or pull excessively at the junction.

The electrical integrity of electrodes should be checked frequently. A DC ohmmeter can be used to determine continuity between the electrode surface and the terminal tip that inserts into the jack of the electrode box. The resistance should be less than 0.1 ohm. An electrode that is intermittently "open" (that is, whose continuity is variable) should be discarded.

SPECIAL ELECTRODES

There are a variety of special electrodes that sometimes are used in EEG practice.

Nasopharyngeal Electrodes

Nasopharyngeal electrodes are the most commonly used special electrodes. They are usually made of silver wire, appropriately insulated, approximately 12.5 cm long, with a silver ball exposed at the tip. The nasopharyngeal electrode is classified as a basal electrode, in contrast to a surface electrode. It is inserted via the nostril, and the ball tip makes contact with the roof of the nasopharynx (20). It has been estimated that the tip lies about 2 cm from the anterior mesial surface of the temporal lobe (20). It is presumed to record from that area. Some laboratories use these electrodes relatively routinely, whereas others use them sparingly or perhaps not at all. Nasopharyngeal electrodes may be utilized when a patient is suspected of having seizures of temporal lobe origin. There are documented instances in which nasopharyngeal electrodes have yielded significant localizing data (8). There are also instances in which nasopharyngeal electrodes may provide data that are easily overinterpreted (25) (see Chapter 14—small, sharp spikes).

In many laboratories, nasopharyngeal electrodes are inserted by a technologist (21). We believe, however, that a technologist should insert nasopharyngeal leads only when a physician is available, in case of emergency. There have been instances in which rapid edema of nasal passages occurred after insertion, so that removal became difficult and painful. It also is possible for internal trauma and bleeding to occur during insertion or removal, during struggling, or during a seizure. Nasopharyngeal electrodes should be sterilized after each use.

Tympanic Electrodes

Tympanic electrodes are less frequently used as a basal lead than are nasopharyngeal electrodes. They were developed for use in conjunction with nasopharyngeal electrodes to form bipolar derivations from mesial to lateral aspects of the temporal lobe (4,5). Tympanic electrodes are short wires (6 cm long) with a ball tip, and are inserted in the external auditory meatus. The tip originally was covered with moistened felt and placed next to the tympanic membrane. It has been estimated that the tip of the electrode lies 0.5 to 0.75 cm from the inferior temporal lobe. Tympanic electrodes should be sterilized after each use.

Sphenoidal Electrodes

Sphenoidal electrodes are another type of basal lead (19). It is assumed that they record the electrical activity of the inferior lateral surface of the temporal lobes. The electrode is placed by insertion through the zygomatic arch, which is at the mandibular notch. The tip of the electrode should be in contact with the trigone, in the region of the foramen ovale. If all goes well, this will be near the tip of the temporal lobe. The electrode is a platinum wire inserted through a cannula, which is removed after the electrode is in place (18,19). Insertion of these electrodes may be painful, and local anesthesia in the area of the insertion may be necessary. Sphenoidal electrodes must always be inserted by a physician. Recording may be carried out for a relatively long period of time. Sterilization of these electrodes is necessary.

Indwelling Electrodes

Indwelling electrodes are sometimes placed directly into the substance of the brain for the purpose of evaluating patients for the surgical treatment of epilepsy. These implanted electrodes usually are constructed so that several recording points are situated on a long, narrow-diameter shaft. After surgical placement under sterile conditions, they may be left in place for several days or weeks to evaluate the EEG over long periods of time. The electrode materials must be chosen carefully to minimize pathological reactions in cerebral tissue. Silver and silver chloride cause severe cellular damage; gold and stainless steel cause relatively little (7,9). Once the electrodes have been implanted under sterile conditions, recording can be carried out at the bedside or in the EEG laboratory. Thoroughly clean, although not necessarily surgically sterile, conditions should prevail at the time of such recording and care must be taken to preserve any sterile zones on the head.

Indwelling electrodes must be sterilized after each use. If implanted in a patient with Creutzfeldt-Jakob disease, they should be destroyed (10).

Electrocorticographic Electrodes

Recording from the cortical surface may be carried out in the operating room to localize focal epileptogenic areas. The use of this method of recording is limited to centers that are concerned with the surgical treatment of seizure disorders. The electrodes, usually 12 to 16, are arranged in a holder that is clamped to the skull after a bone flap has been turned. Each electrode, which may be a small silver ball or a wet cotton wick attached to a silver wire, is moveable in three dimensions via a ball joint. These electrodes are placed on the cortical surface and manipulated by the surgeon, not by the technologist. Due to pulsation of the brain, frequent artifacts may occur and be difficult to reduce. Sterilization of the electrodes is necessary before and after each use.

An alternative method of recording directly from the surface of the brain uses electrodes embedded in a square or strip of plastic (Ag–AgCl may be used, since the time in place is relatively brief). The assembly can be inserted between the cortex and the dura (7). Artifact caused by pulsation of the brain is less likely to occur because the electrodes "float" on the cortical surface. This electrode assembly must be sterile, and location and manipulation must be carried out by the surgeon.

SUMMARY

In this chapter we have learned that:

1. EEG electrodes are not simply passive conductors of electrical current.
2. An electrode is, in effect, one-half of a battery, and two electrodes form a small source of potential, the voltage depending on the metals used to make the electrodes.
3. Electrodes have resistance and capacitance, and different metals have different time constants; their impedance varies with frequency.
4. Electrical and mechanical stability of electrodes is essential to good EEG recording. Electrode impedances should be less than 5 kΩ.
5. Electrodes must be capable of being sterilized; needle electrodes must be sterilized after every use; in some types of infectious diseases (specifically, Creutzfeldt-Jakob disease), electrodes, once used, should be destroyed.
6. Special electrodes include those that record indirectly from the brain: nasopharyngeal, tympanic, sphenoidal. These require special placement procedures and are used to supplement information from scalp electrodes. In addition, there are special electrodes for recording from within or from the surface of the brain: intracerebral (implanted) and electrocorticographic. These must be placed under sterile procedures, and their use usually is limited to centers for surgical treatment of seizures.

APPENDIX

How to Make Silver–Silver Chloride Electrodes

Silver–silver chloride (Ag–AgCl) electrodes can be prepared by using commercially available bright silver electrodes. The silver electrodes should be cleaned thoroughly and then placed in a sodium chloride (NaCl) solution in a nonmetallic container and attached to the positive pole of a battery or other source of direct current. The concentration of the solution can vary from 0.9% to 5%. A second silver electrode is then placed in the middle of the container and attached to the negative pole of the voltage source. Assuming this to be 1.5 or 3 V, a 1,500- to 3,000-Ω resistor should be placed in series with the electrode to be chlorided to limit current to 1 mA. As the process proceeds, the chlorided electrode (anode) will darken slowly, to a uniformly gray color. There will be bubbles given off from the negative electrode (cathode).

As many as 21 or more electrodes can be chlorided simultaneously by adapting an electrode jack box as shown in Fig. 10.6, with an inexpensive AC to DC converter used as a power source. Alternatively, a battery may be used. The rate of chloriding is dependent upon the current flow through each electrode. Current-limiting resistors should be put in series with each electrode to limit current to approximately 1 mA. Chlorided electrodes should be maintained with care. If it is necessary to rechloride them, they first may be dechlorided by reversing the current in the above circuit.

Gold electrodes should never be chlorided because the electrolytic process involved will destroy the gold plating.

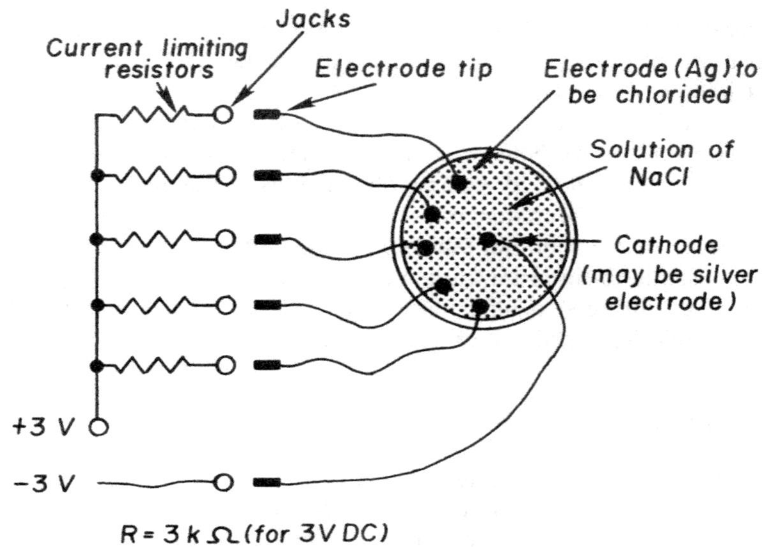

FIG. 10.6. Chloriding via use of an electrode jack box. Voltage source may be an AC/DC adapter for radio or calculator. If a 6-V adapter is used, change R to 6 kΩ.

REFERENCES

1. Allen, A., McKillop, J. A., Sorensen, G. M., West, W. L., Wilbert, L., and Royce, M. W. (1979): Skin injury from electrode paste used in electroencephalography. *Am. J. EEG Technol.*, 19:97–101.
2. American EEG Society (1980): 3. Minimum technical requirements for performing clinical electroencephalography. In: *Guidelines in EEG—1980*. American EEG Society, Tucker, Georgia.
3. American EEG Society (1980): 6. Minimal technical standards for pediatric electroencephalography. In: *Guidelines in EEG—1980*. American EEG Society, Tucker, Georgia.

4. Arrelano, A. P. (1949): A tympanic lead. *Electroencephalogr. Clin. Neurophysiol.*, 1:112–113.
5. Arrelano, A. P., and Schwab, R. S. (1949): Tympanic leads and their application to the Maclean nasopharyngeal leads for basal recording of the EEG. *Electroencephalogr. Clin. Neurophysiol.*, 1:524.
6. Cooper, R. (1963): Electrodes. *Am. J. EEG Technol.*, 3:91–107.
7. Cooper, R., Osselton, J. W., and Shaw, J. C. (1980): *EEG Technology*, 3rd Ed., pp. 15–31. Butterworths, London.
8. deJesus, P. V., and Masland, W. S. (1970): The role of nasopharyngeal electrodes in clinical electroencephalography. *Neurology*, 20:869–878.
9. Fischer, G., Sayre, G. P., and Bickford, R. G. (1961): Histological changes in the cat's brain after introduction of metallic and plastic-coated wire. In: *Electrical Stimulation of the Brain*, edited by D. E. Sheer, pp. 55–59. University of Texas Press, Austin.
10. Gajdusek, D. C., Gibbs, C. J., Asher, D. M., Brown, P., Diwan, A., Hoffman, P., Nemo, G., Rowher, R., and White, L. (1977): Precautions in medical care of, and in handling materials from, patients with transmissable virus dementia (Creutzfeldt-Jakob disease). *N. Engl. J. Med.*, 297:1253–1258.
11. Geddes, L. A. (1972): *Electrodes and the Measurement of Bioelectric Events*. John Wiley, New York.
12. Geddes, L. A. (1973): Bioelectrodes. Part I: Recording bioelectric potentials. *Am. J. EEG Technol.*, 13:195–203.
13. Geddes, L. A. (1974): Bioelectrodes. Part II: The nature of electrode impedance. *Am. J. EEG Technol.*, 14:205–210.
14. Geddes, L. A. (1975): Bioelectrodes. Part III: The importance of amplifier input impedance. *Am. J. EEG Technol.*, 15:99–106.
15. Grass, A. M. (1949): Electrical characteristics of some types of electrodes. *Electroencephalogr. Clin. Neurophysiol.*, 1:255.
16. Grass, A. M., and Grass, E. R. (1977): *Electrode Maintenance and Infection Control in the EEG Laboratory*. Grass Instrument Co., Quincy, Massachusetts.
17. Hanley, J. W. (1981): A step-by-step approach to neonatal EEG. *Am. J. EEG Technol.*, 21:1–13.
18. Ives, J. R., and Gloor, P. (1978): Update: Chronic sphenoidal electrodes. *Electroencephalogr. Clin. Neurophysiol.*, 44:789–790.
19. Jones, D. P. (1951): Recording of the basal electroencephalogram with sphenoidal needle electrodes. *Electroencephalogr. Clin. Neurophysiol.*, 3:100.
20. Maclean, P. V. (1949): A new nasopharyngeal lead. *Electroencephalogr. Clin. Neurophysiol.*, 1:110–112.
21. Mavor, H., and Hellen, M. K. (1964): Nasopharyngeal electrode recordings. *Am. J. EEG Technol.*, 4:43–50.
22. Seaba, P., Reilly, E., and Peters, J. F. (1973): Patient discomfort related to measurement of electrode impedance. *Am. J. EEG Technol.*, 13:7–12.
23. Schoenfeld, R. J., Grekin, J. N., and Mehregan, A. (1965): Calcium deposition in the skin: A report of four cases following electroencephalography. *Neurology*, 15:477–480.
24. Tyner, F. S., and Knott, J. R. (1976): Amplitude asymmetries when using subdermal electrodes: Is accurate head marking sufficient? *Am. J. EEG Technol.*, 15:179–187.
25. White, J. C., Langston, J. W., and Pedley, T. A. (1977): Benign epileptiform transients of sleep. *Neurology*, 27:1061–1068.
26. Zablow, L., and Goldensohn, E. S. (1969): A comparison between scalp and needle electrodes for the EEG. *Electroencephalogr. Clin. Neurophysiol.*, 26:530–533.

Chapter 11

Electrode Placement

The development of clinical electroencephalography has evolved through the exchange of information and ideas between many different laboratories and workers. There was early recognition that this process would be facilitated if general agreement could be reached regarding the locations of the electrodes used in recording the EEG. The groundwork for formulating guidelines was laid out at the First International Congress of EEG in 1947. At the Second Congress, in 1949, a preliminary report was made which led to formal endorsement by the Fourth Congress (1957) and appeared as a part of the *Report of the Committee on Methods of Clinical Examination in Electroencephalography* (8). The system of electrode placement was called the "ten-twenty electrode system" and it is in wide use throughout the world. It has been formally endorsed by the American Electroencephalographic Society (1–4). The basic principles are:

1. Positions of electrodes should be determined by measurement from standard landmarks on the skull. Measurements should be proportional to skull size and shape, insofar as possible.
2. Adequate coverage of all parts of the head should be provided with standard designated positions. . . .
3. Designations of positions should be in terms of brain areas (Frontal, Parietal, etc.) rather than only in numbers, so that communication [will] become more meaningful. . . .
4. Anatomical studies should be carried out to determine the cortical areas most likely to be found beneath each of the standard electrode positions in the average subject. (8)

The locations of the electrodes of the ten-twenty system[1] are shown schematically in Fig. 11.1. Each electrode has a standard abbreviation, based on the brain area it represents. Odd-numbered electrodes are on the left and even-numbered positions are on the right.

The landmark anatomical points referred to by the Committee are shown in Fig. 11.2. These are (a) nasion, at the front of the head; (b) inion, at the back of the head; and (c) the left and (d) the right "preauricular points (felt as the depression at the root of the zygoma, just anterior to the tragus)" (8).

The inion and the nasion are, strictly speaking, skeletal points that cannot be demonstrated directly on a living subject. A close approximation of the inion is the occipital protuberance. Its location "can be felt as you run your finger up the back of the neck to the skull . . . [encountering] a depression with the ridge of the protruding inion just above it. If the location of the inion is not at first obvious . . . ask the patient to tilt his head . . . backward and forward while you try to feel the ridge" (6). The indentation between the nose and the forehead falls approximately over the anatomical (skeletal) nasion.

The preauricular points can be located readily by having the patient open the mouth slightly. By lightly running the finger up and down just anterior to the ear, the indentation of the zygoma is usually identified without difficulty.

By proceeding from these four landmarks, it is possible to establish locations for all of the electrode placements shown in Fig. 11.1.

In Fig. 11.3, the electrodes have been organized by lines, or rows, into anteroposterior (front to back) lines or planes. They also have been organized in transverse lines, or planes, crossing the head from left to right.

The anteroposterior (A–P) planes in Fig. 11.3 are identified as (a) the left parasagittal, (b) the sagittal (which is in the midline), and (c) the right parasagittal planes. The transverse planes are identified (from front to back) as (a) the frontal polar, (b) the frontal, (c) the central (coronal), (d) the parietal, and (e) the occipital planes. In Fig. 11.4, another line or plane is identified. This is a horizontal plane, defined by a circumferential line above the preauricular points.

Each electrode in the ten-twenty system shown in Fig. 11.1 can be located precisely after these planes have been established, based on the four anatomical landmarks described above.

[1] We would like to emphasize that the term "modified ten-twenty system" is often without meaning. If one deviates from the ten-twenty system, the new locations must be specified by measurements (7) and the placements are no longer the "ten-twenty electrode system."

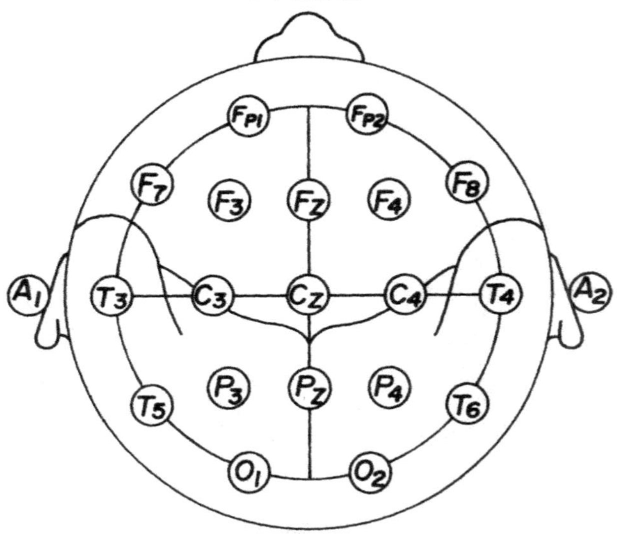

FIG. 11.1. Schema showing locations of electrodes in the ten-twenty system of electrode placement.

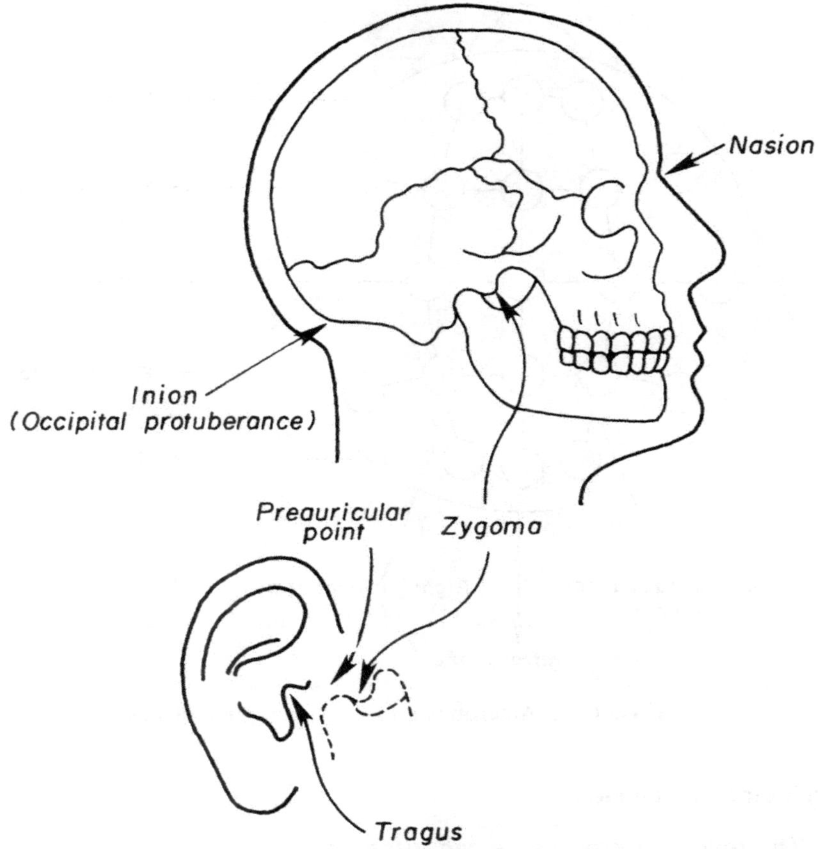

FIG. 11.2. Anatomical landmarks used to define primary measuring points in the ten-twenty system (see text).

TOOLS AND MEASUREMENTS FOR ELECTRODE PLACEMENT

The location of the electrode positions along these lines depends on careful measurements made by the technologist. Two basic tools are required: (a) a tape marked in millimeters, and (b) a nontoxic skin marking pencil. The tape should be narrow (no wider than 5 mm) to define better the lines between the primary reference points (the landmarks). Millimeter divisions improve the accuracy of locating the electrode positions. A retractable metal tape is the most satisfactory; it will not stretch, and it can be wiped clean after each use.

The pencil point should be kept sharp for precise marking. Having two contrasting colors on hand allows easy correction of any errors in measurements.

It sometimes is necessary to hold the patient's hair out of the way while measuring (9). A variety of clasps and hair pins are available that may be helpful, but much time is consumed in placing and removing clasps or pins, and a technologist may become overly dependent upon them.

A student's first attempts at measurement often are clumsy and can lead to discouragement. Nevertheless, with experience, the average technologist can accurately mark the head for electrode placement in 10 min or less.

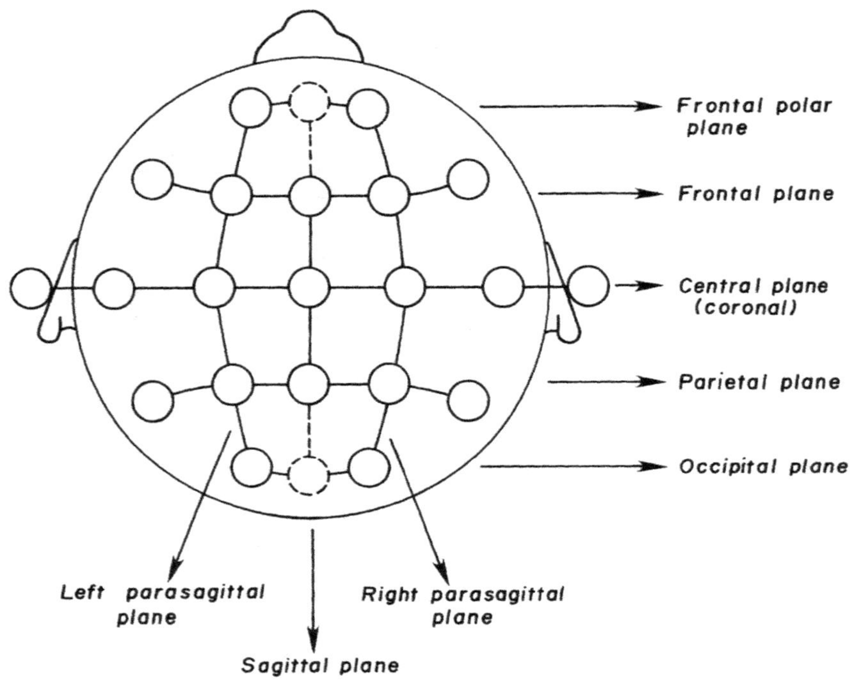

FIG. 11.3. Anteroposterior and transverse planes.

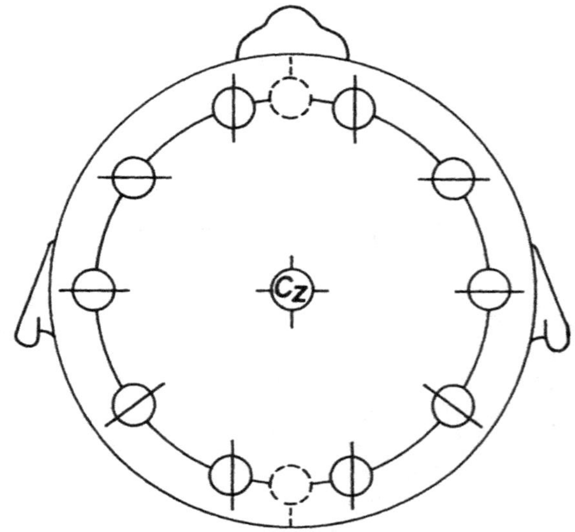

FIG. 11.4. Circumferential plane.

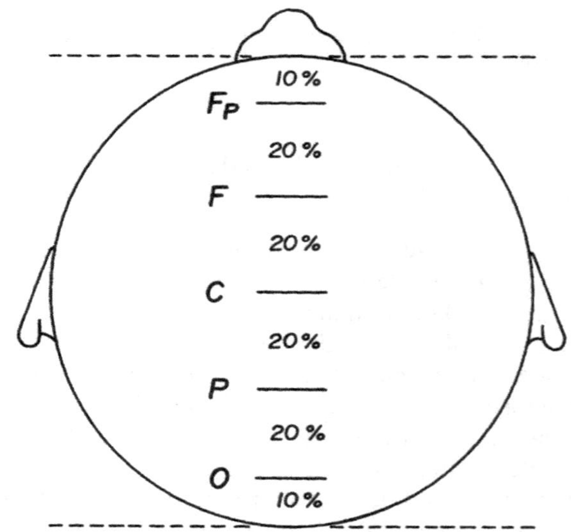

FIG. 11.5. *Step 1.* Measurement from nasion to inion along sagittal plane (see text).

Primary Placements

The following procedures can establish accurately and precisely the locations of the 19 primary scalp electrodes. The following steps should be carried out in the order in which they are discussed.

Step 1. (Fig. 11.5)

The sagittal line is measured from the nasion, over the top of the head, to the inion. A mark is made above the nasion, 10% of the total nasion–inion distance. This will fall on the frontal polar plane. Then, marks are made successively in a transverse direction at 20% of the nasion–inion distance until only 10% of the total distance remains. These lines will fall on the frontal, central, parietal, and occipital planes, respectively.

The central plane is 50% of the nasion–inion distance. The distance between the occipital plane and the inion will be 10% of the total distance. If it is not, a mistake has been made.

Step 2. (Fig. 11.6)

The distance from one preauricular point to the other then should be measured, going across the central plane as defined in step 1. Ten percent of the distance above the left preauricular point should be marked to establish the level of the left circumferential line (plane). Twenty percent above this plane, a mark is made indicating the left parasagittal plane. Twenty percent above this mark, where the central plane crosses the sagittal plane, a mark is made locating the placement of electrode C_z. Continuing 20% of the total distance to the right of C_z, a mark should be made locating the right parasagittal plane. Twenty percent below this, a mark is made which is at the level of the right circumferential line (plane). The remaining 10% of the total left to right preauricular distance should fall at the right preauricular point. If not, a mistake has been made.

It was on the basis of these proportional divisions, 10% and 20%, that the method of measurements was given its name: The ten-twenty system.

Step 3. (Fig. 11.7)

Step 3 locates other electrodes in the sagittal plane. The edge of the tape is placed at the nasion and inion and passes through C_z where it crosses the lines made earlier, defining the frontal and parietal planes. Marks are made establishing the positions for the F_z and P_z electrodes. The points Fp_z and O_z are marked where the tape and horizontal plane cross. Marking these latter two points is necessary to carry out the next two procedures.

Step 4. (Fig. 11.8)

The tape is placed at Fp_z and the distance to O_z is measured, passing through the left circumferential line established by the first measurement in step 2. Ten percent of the total distance along the line of the now-defined left circumferential plane is marked to indicate the location of the

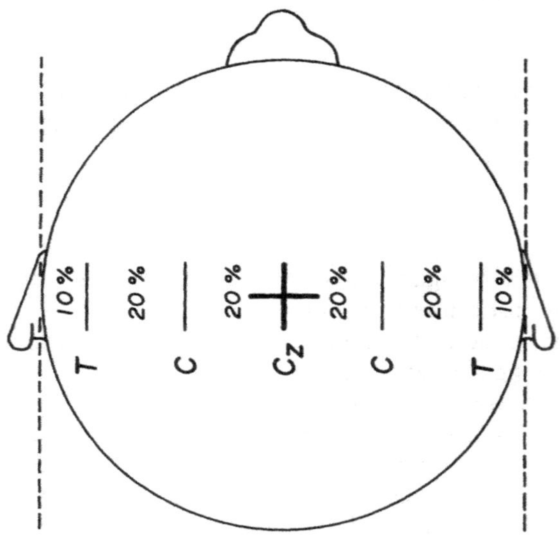

FIG. 11.6. *Step 2.* Measurement from left to right preauricular points along central (coronal) plane (see text). C_z is located.

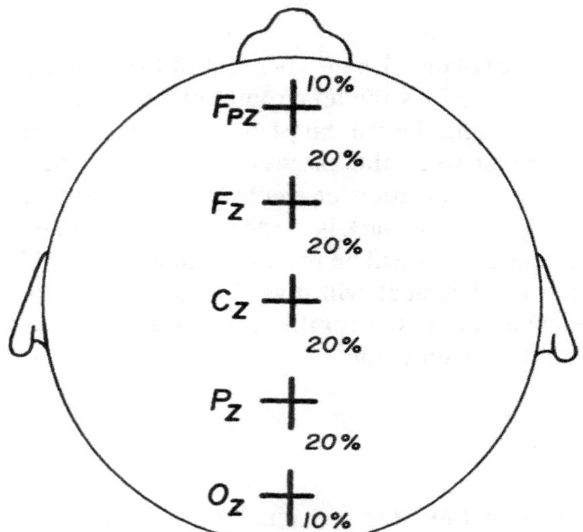

FIG. 11.7. *Step 3.* Location of Fp_z, F_z, C_z, P_z, and O_z on sagittal plane (see text).

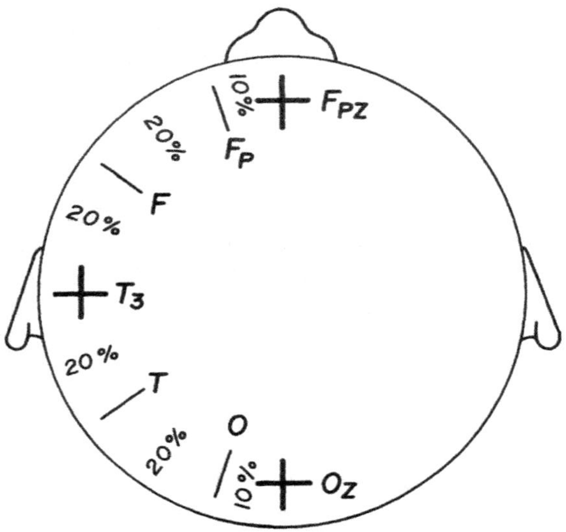

FIG. 11.8. *Step 4.* Measurement of left half of circumferential plane (see text). Electrode T_3 is located.

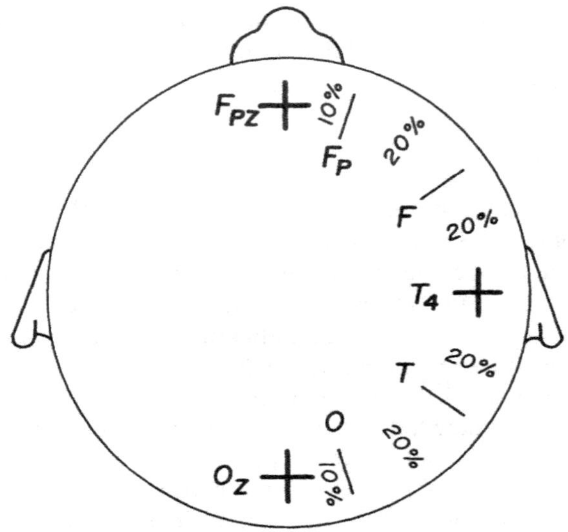

FIG. 11.9. *Step 5.* Measurement of right half of circumferential plane (see text). Electrode T_4 is located.

left frontal polar (Fp) plane. Twenty percent of the total Fp_z-O_z distance beyond the Fp mark defines the left frontal plane. Twenty percent of the Fp_z-O_z distance beyond the frontal plane (F), a mark is made as the circumferential plane crosses the previously marked line of the central plane. This defines the location of electrode T_3. Twenty percent (of the total distance) beyond T_3, a mark is made to define the lateral extremity of the left parietal plane. This will be used later to locate T_5. Twenty percent further (of the total distance) will give the location of the left occipital plane. Proceeding another 10% (of the total distance) should return to O_z. If not, a mistake has been made.

Step 5. (Fig. 11.9)

The procedures in this step are similar to those outlined in step 4, except that they are made over the right lateral surface of the head. They will establish a location for electrode T_4 where the line of the circumferential plane crosses the previously marked line of the central plane. The contralateral Fp, F, P, and O planes are located in the same manner as in step 4.

Step 6. (Fig. 11.10)

The tape is placed again on the point Fp_z, passing through electrode position T_3 and returning to position O_z. Where the circumferential line (defined by the edge of the tape measure) crosses marks of the frontal polar plane and the frontal plane, intersecting lines are drawn to define the placement of electrodes Fp_1 and F_7. Where the circumferential line crosses the parietal planes and occipital planes (see step 4), intersecting marks also are made. These establish the placements for electrodes T_5 and O_1.

The same procedures are carried out along the right circumferential line. These define the positions of electrodes Fp_2, F_8, T_6, and O_2. All interelectrode distances in the circumferential plane should be equal. If not, a mistake has been made.

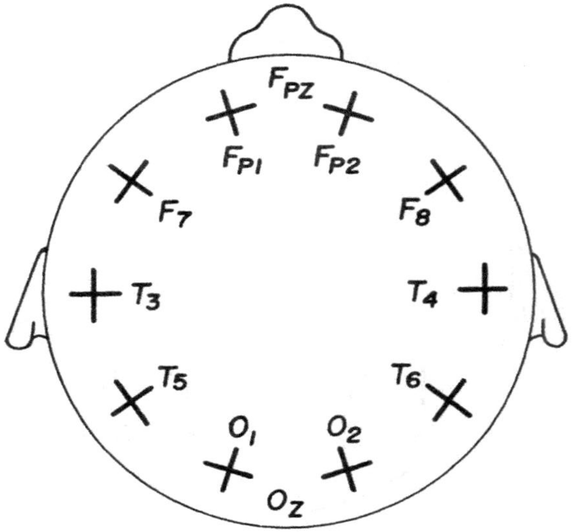

FIG. 11.10. *Step 6.* Location of Fp_1 and Fp_2, F_7 and F_8, T_5 and T_6, and O_1 and O_2 on circumferential plane (see text).

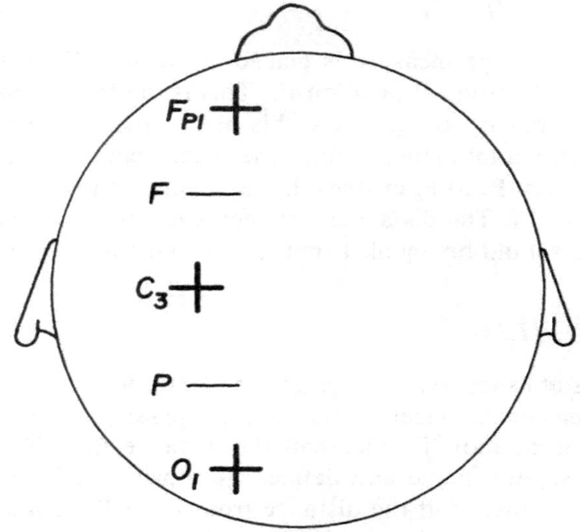

FIG. 11.11. *Step 7.* Location of C_3 and frontal and parietal planes on left parasagittal plane (see text).

Step 7. (Fig. 11.11)

In step 7, the left parasagittal electrode positions will be established. The tape is placed at position Fp_1 and passes along the line (established in step 2) of the left parasagittal plane, ending at position O_1. The total distance is measured. Twenty-five percent of the distance behind Fp_1, a transverse line is drawn, which will fall on the frontal plane. A further 25% (of the total distance) will cross the already established parasagittal plane. When this is marked, the position of electrode C_3 has been determined. Twenty-five percent of the total distance behind C_3, the parietal plane is marked. The remaining distance to O_1 should be 25% of the total Fp_1-O_1 distance. If not, a mistake has been made.

Step 8. (Fig. 11.12)

The same procedures are carried out along the right parasagittal line. This will establish the position of electrode C_4 and the frontal and parietal planes.

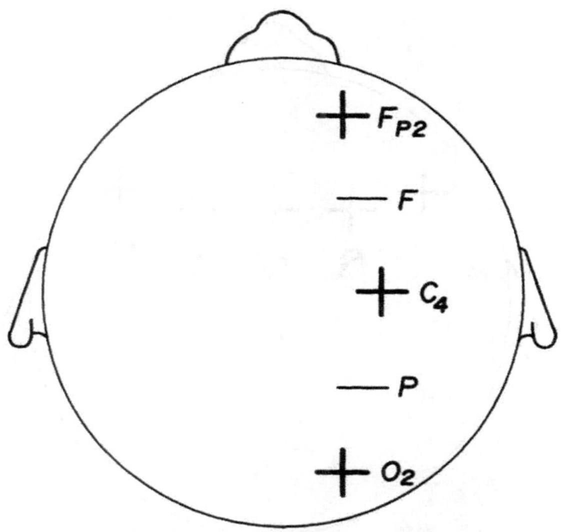

FIG. 11.12. *Step 8.* Location of C_4 and frontal and parietal planes on right parasagittal plane (see text).

Step 9. (Fig. 11.13)

In Step 9, the tape measure is placed at position F_7, passing through position F_z, and ending at position F_8. This is the frontal plane. One-half the distance from F_7 to F_z, where this plane crosses the previously defined left parasagittal plane, defines the placement of F_3. Similarly, half the distance from F_z to F_8 crosses the right parasagittal plane and defines the position of F_4. The distances between each electrode position in the frontal plane should be equal. If not, a mistake has been made.

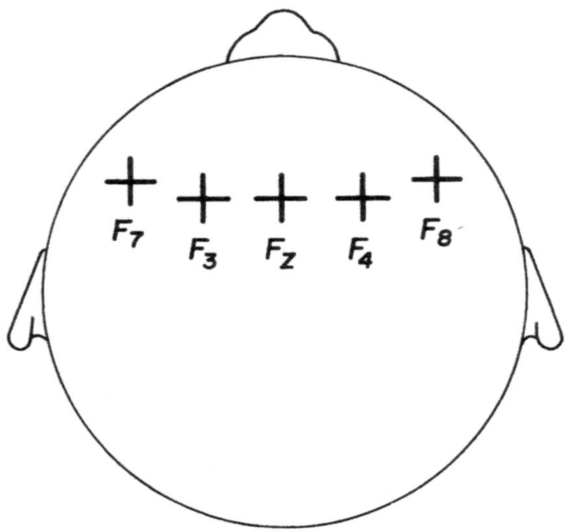

FIG. 11.13. *Step 9.* Location of electrodes on frontal plane (see text).

Step 10. (Fig. 11.14)

Step 10 establishes the position of the electrodes in the parietal plane. The tape measure is placed at position T_5, passing through position P_Z, and ending at position T_6. One-half the distance from T_5 to P_z crosses the left parasagittal plane and defines the position of the P_3 electrode. In the same manner, half the distance from F_z to T_6 defines the position of the P_4 electrode. Each interelectrode distance along the parietal line should be equal. If these conditions are not met, a mistake has been made.

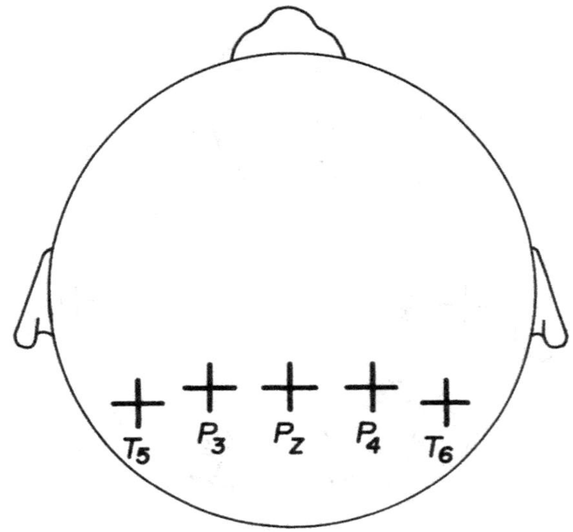

FIG. 11.14. *Step 10.* Location of electrodes on parietal plane (see text).

Two additional electrodes usually are placed on the lobes of the ears, left (A_1) and right (A_2), bringing the total number of conventional electrodes to 21.

Intermediate Placements

Provision is made in the ten-twenty system for electrodes in "intermediate positions (e.g., F_2, C_2, C_6, etc.) for special localization studies" (8). These are located in intermediate lateral planes with reference to the primary designators (e.g., F_3, C_3, and so forth). Examples in the central plane are illustrated in Fig. 11.15. Each intermediate position is determined by measuring one-half the distance between the primary positions.

Although there was no specific provision in the original ten-twenty system for intermediate electrode positions in the anteroposterior lines, such positions sometimes are necessary. We suggest that these be labeled as follows: For example, an electrode midway between Fp_1 and F_3 should be designated Fp_1' (Fp_1 prime). An electrode midway between C_3 and P_3

would be designated C_3'. This preserves the basic anatomical indexing of the original ten-twenty system.[2]

Jasper (8) regarded the choice of designators of electrode positions as using "traditional anatomical" terms. The central electrodes were regarded as "sensorimotor" in location. Jasper's report of the anatomical correspondence between measured scalp electrode positions and brain areas, based on studies of adults, stated that errors of ±1 cm could be expected. A schema of the scalp–cortical relationships is shown in Fig. 11.16.

[2] Sometimes frontal polar electrodes in neonates are placed above the measured points and designated as F_1 and F_2. Since these designators, in conventional ten-twenty usage, would refer to placements midway between F_3 and F_Z, and F_Z and F_4, respectively, ambiguity can easily occur. Designators Fp_1' and Fp_2' create no ambiguity.

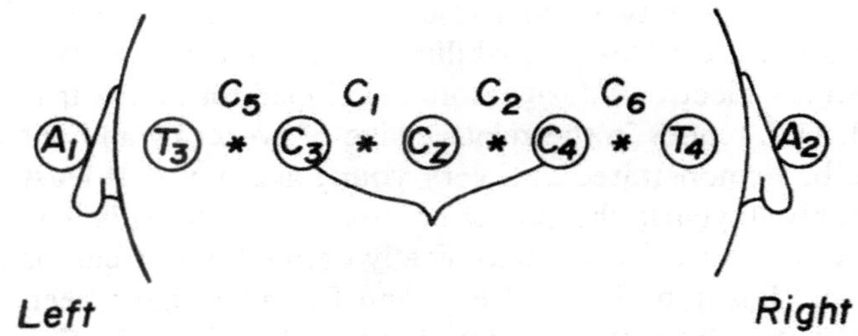

FIG. 11.15. Suggested intermediate electrodes for more precise localization, along the central plane. From Jasper (8).

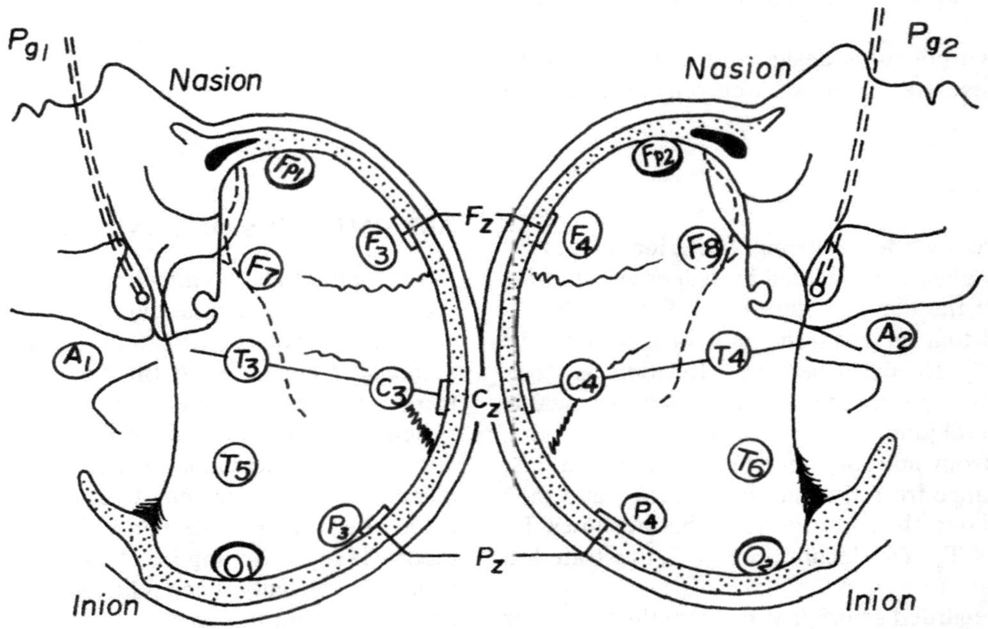

FIG. 11.16. Lateral view of left and right hemispheres showing the standard ten-twenty system electrodes projected on the surface of the brain. From Jasper (8).

When the ten-twenty system is used in recording the EEGs of very young children (neonates), variability in anatomical location occurs, and the ten-twenty electrode designators developed for adults may be imprecise (5,7). Differences in the relative size of posterior and anterior brain areas can be demonstrated at a very young age (up to at least 4 months, and probably 1 year); the posterior areas are relatively larger. Correspondence of brain area to anatomically defined points can be in considerable error. Positions Fp_1 and Fp_2, and F_7 and F_8 have been said to be relatively distant from the presumed cerebral surface (5). Consequently, different locations and numbers of electrodes are recommended by different authorities (7,11) when the EEGs of very small premature infants are recorded.

In addition to the scalp electrode positions arrived at by measurement, designators were originally assigned for pharyngeal electrodes: Pg_1 (left) and Pg_2 (right). In current terminology, these are referred to as nasopharyngeal (N–P) leads, although the positions on electrode selector systems usually are marked "Pg." (See Chapter 10 for further discussion of nasopharyngeal electrodes.)

Originally, there also were two positions designated as Cb_1 and Cb_2, called cerebellar electrodes. These are not used in current practice and have been omitted in this text.

Additional Electrode Placements

Although F_7 and F_8 usually are regarded as being "anterior temporal" electrode locations, they were originally designated by Jasper as "inferior frontal" and they do not lie over the temporal lobes (see Fig. 11.16).

Silverman (10) later proposed that an additional pair of electrodes be designated specifically T_1 and T_2. He described their location as "one centimeter above one third the distance from the external auditory meatus to the external canthus" (the lateral junction of the upper and lower lids). In practice, one draws a line from auditory meatus to outer canthus, determines one-third of the distance from the auditory meatus, and then locates a point 1 cm directly above this. On the left, this becomes T_1. On the right, the point becomes T_2. The location of T_2 is illustrated in Fig. 11.17.

Focal spike activity that was regarded as originating from the "anterior temporal" area in a majority of instances was reported to be somewhat better defined when recorded from T_1 and T_2 than when recorded from F_7 or F_8 (10).

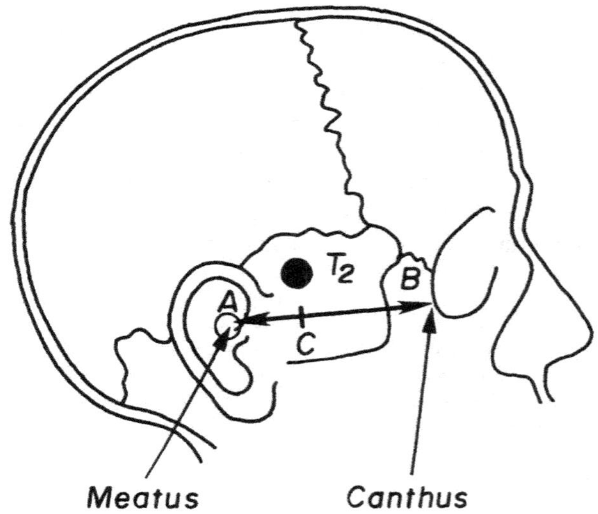

FIG. 11.17. Schematic diagram locating electrodes T_1 and T_2 (see text). A = External auditory meatus; B = outer canthus; C = 1/3 distance, A to B. From Silverman (10).

ASYMMETRIES OF PLACEMENT

True amplitude asymmetries of the EEG can carry much information. However, asymmetrical placement of electrodes can cause an amplitude asymmetry that is artifactual. Asymmetries of placement must be detected and corrected at the time of recording to avoid possible misinterpretation of amplitude differences at a later time.

Scalp lesions and head bandages sometimes require a deliberate alteration in the placement of electrodes. If it is necessary to change the placement of an electrode over one hemisphere, the corresponding electrode over the opposite hemisphere should be changed to maintain symmetry. If repositioning involves a change of considerable distance (such as may be the case when a bandage is in the way), it may be better to add an electrode on the contralateral side, matching the displaced electrode.

Whenever electrodes are placed in locations other than those established by the ten-twenty system, diagrams, notations, and measurements should be written on the EEG record to indicate the changes.

APPLICATION OF ELECTRODES WITHOUT HEAD MEASUREMENTS

It is rarely defensible to apply electrodes without actual measurement of the head. It could be justified if a patient has just had a seizure and an attempt is being made to evaluate EEG activity immediately thereafter. During bedside recordings, activity of the nursing staff or the close proximity of other equipment may make it difficult or impractical to make precise measurements. In other cases, it may not be permissable to turn the patient's head, and measurement is impossible.

In the instances just described, the objective usually is to determine the gross characteristics of, or the absence of, EEG activity, rather than its exact location. However, electrode placement without measurement, even under optimal conditions, can lead to errors in both the EEG record and its interpretation.

SUMMARY

The International Federation's ten-twenty system of electrode placement uses anatomical landmarks, defined anteriorly by the nasion, posteriorly by the inion, and laterally by the left and right preauricular points. From these landmarks, systematic grids can be drawn that locate 19 scalp electrodes. These locations are named in relation to the presumed underlying brain area.

Two additional electrode positions may be added to the ten-twenty locations for more exact definition of the anterior temporal areas. Deviations from the primary locations must always be described completely.

With practice and experience, accurate measurement procedures can be completed in about 10 min. Accurately placed electrodes lead to better evaluation of EEG data.

REFERENCES

1. American EEG Society (1980): 3. Minimum technical requirements for performing clinical electroencephalography. In: *Guidelines in EEG—1980*. American EEG Society, Tucker, Georgia.
2. American EEG Society (1980): 4. Minimum technical standards for EEG recording in suspected brain death. In: *Guidelines in EEG—1980*, American EEG Society, Tucker, Georgia.
3. American EEG Society (1980): 6. Minimal technical standards for pediatric electroencephalography. In: *Guidelines in EEG—1980*. American EEG Society, Tucker, Georgia.
4. American EEG Society (1980): 7. A proposal for standard montages to be used in clinical electroencephalography. In: *Guidelines in EEG—1980*. American EEG Society, Tucker, Georgia.
5. Blume, W. T., Buza, R. C. and Okazaki, H. (1974): Anatomic correlates of the ten-twenty placement system in neonates. *Electroencephalogr. Clin. Neurophysiol.*, 36:303–307.
6. Harner, P. F., and Sannit, T. (1974): *A Review of the International Ten-Twenty System of Electrode Placement*. Grass Instrument Co., Quincy, Massachusetts.
7. Heldström, B., Karlsson, B., and Müssbichler, H. (1963): Electrode placement in EEG of infants and its anatomical relationship studied radiologically. *Electroencephalogr. Clin. Neurophysiol.*, 15:115–117.
8. Jasper, H. H. (1958): The ten-twenty electrode system of the International Federation. *Electroencephalogr. Clin. Neurophysiol.*, 10:371–375.
9. Sannit, T. (1963): The ten-twenty system: Footnotes to measuring technique. *Am. J. EEG Technol.*, 3:23–30.
10. Silverman, D. (1960): The anterior temporal electrode and the ten-twenty system. *Electroencephalogr. Clin. Neurophysiol.*, 12:735–737.
11. Werner, S. S., Stockard, J. E., and Bickford, R. G., (1974): *Atlas of Neonatal Electroencephalography*, Raven Press, New York, p. 1.

Chapter 12

Polarity and Localization

The amplifiers used for EEG recording are differential amplifiers. Each channel is a recording of the difference in voltage between the electrode selected for Input Terminal 1 and the voltage at the electrode selected for Input Terminal 2 of the amplifier.[1]

When there is a voltage difference between the inputs, it follows that one electrode is either more negative or more positive than the other electrode. If there is no difference in voltage at the input terminals, the output will be zero. [See Knott (5) for further discussion.]

If Input 1 is $-100\ \mu V$ (with respect to ground) and Input 2 is $-50\ \mu V$ (with respect to ground), the potential difference between the two inputs is 50 μV. Input 1 is 50 μV more negative than Input 2. This will be reflected proportionately at the output of the amplifier. If the sensitivity is 5 μV/mm, the amplitude of the recorded EEG deflection will be 10 mm.

However, if Input 1 is $+100\ \mu V$ and Input 2 is $+125\ \mu V$, the difference is 25 μV. Input 1 is less positive than Input 2; Input 2 is 25 μV more positive than Input 1. If the sensitivity is 5 μV/mm, the deflection of the EEG recording pen will be 5 mm.

If the voltage at Input 1 is $-25\ \mu V$, and the voltage at Input 2 is $+25\ \mu V$, the difference is 50 μV. If the sensitivity is 5 μV/mm, there will be a 10-mm deflection of the EEG recording pen. This is the same voltage difference that produced a 10-mm deflection in the first example above. How can we distinguish between the conditions causing them? We need to be able to obtain information about the relative polarity of the voltage applied at either one of a pair of electrodes in relation to other electrodes. The EEG record is created by the continuous upward and downward movement of the galvanometer pen. Is it possible to relate the relative polarity at an electrode to the direction of movement of the pen, upward or downward? [See Knott (4,5) for further discussion.]

[1] The International Federation's Committee on Terminology (3) suggests that the terms "Input Terminal 1" and "Input Terminal 2" replace "G1" and "G2" which are common American terms. Used here, the term "input terminal" usually will be shortened to "input." G1 is equivalent to Input 1, and G2 is equivalent to Input 2.

Fortunately all EEG instruments, by international agreement, are designed so that when Input 1 is more negative than Input 2, the write-out, that is, the pen, moves in an upward direction. Further, when Input 2 is more negative than Input 1, the pen moves in a downward direction.

To complete the rules described above, when Input 1 is more positive than Input 2, the write-out moves in a downward direction, and when Input 2 is more positive, the write-out moves in an upward direction. [The international agreements (2,3) are given in the Appendix to this chapter.]

POLARITY SQUARE

These statements, based on international conventions, are schematically summarized in the Polarity Square (Fig. 12.1). This diagram illustrates four "up-down" rules and four "input" rules. These are:

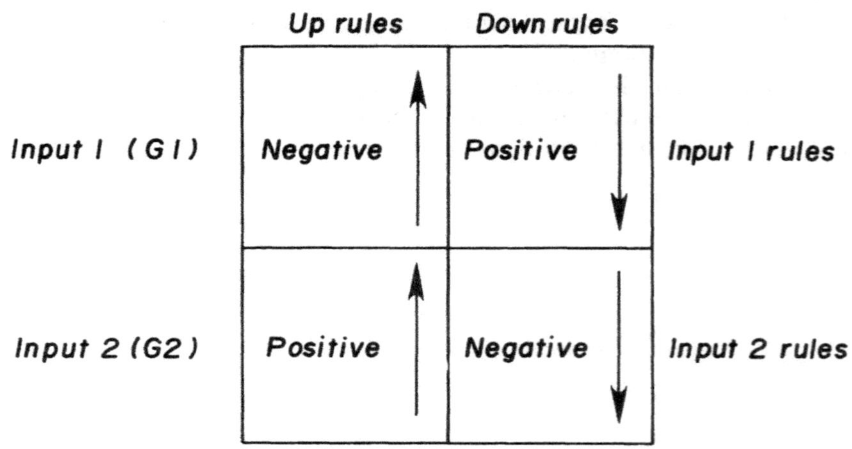

FIG. 12.1. Polarity Square. Summary of rules relating direction of EEG display and polarity of input voltage at each amplifier input.

Up—The pen goes up if Input 1 is negative or if Input 2 is positive.
Down—The pen goes down if Input 1 is positive or if Input 2 is negative.

These rules can be stated in another way:

Input 1—When Input 1 is negative, the pen goes up, but when Input 1 is positive, the pen goes down.
Input 2—When Input 2 is positive, the pen goes up, but when Input 2 is negative, the pen goes down.

An EEG amplifier is, by convention (see Chapter 5), represented by the symbol illustrated in Fig. 12.2. The inputs are conventionally designated so that Input Terminal 1 is represented by a solid line, and Input Terminal 2 by a dotted line (Fig. 12.3). The write-out of the recording pen is shown by a change in position of the line drawn to the right of the amplifier's output. It will be *up* or *down*, as seen in Fig. 12.4. The relative polarity of an input can be indicated by a plus (+) or minus (−) sign. The Polarity Square can be translated pictorially as shown in Fig. 12.5.

Given one amplifier with an upward display at one moment, t_1, and a downward display at another time, t_2 (Fig. 12.6), it is not possible to tell

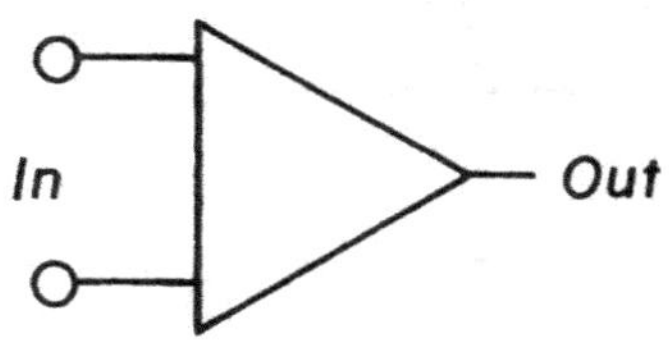

FIG. 12.2. Amplifier.

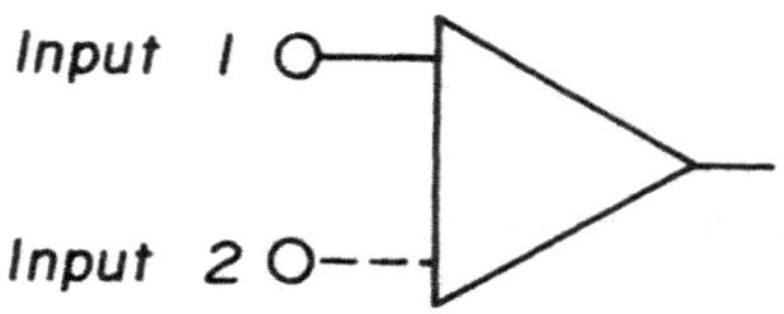

FIG. 12.3. Inputs 1 and 2.

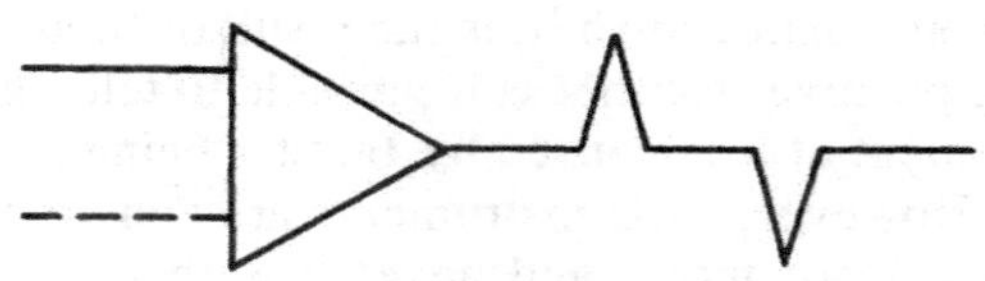

FIG. 12.4. Direction of display.

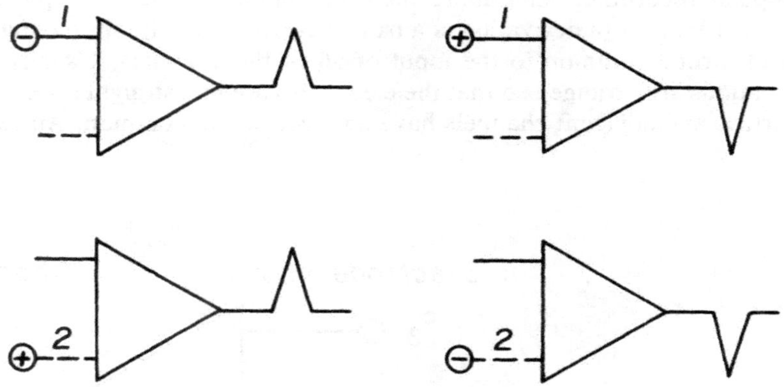

FIG. 12.5. Pictorial summary of Polarity Square (see Fig. 12.1 and text).

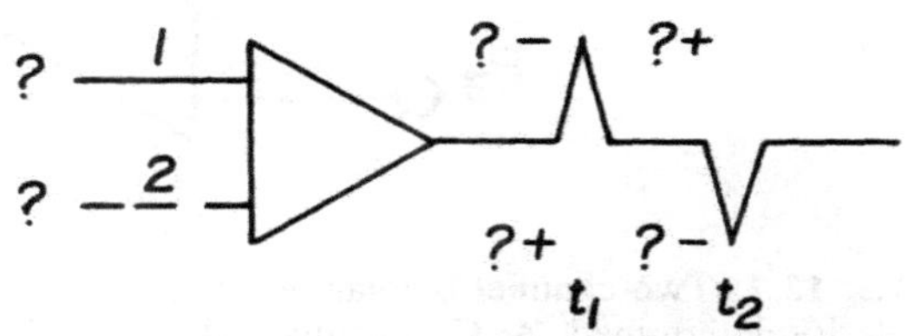

FIG. 12.6. Single amplifier with upward display at t_1 and downward display at t_2 (see text).

whether the upgoing deflection at t_1 is the result of Input 1 being negative or Input 2 being positive. Neither is it possible to tell whether the downgoing pen movement at t_2 is caused by Input 1 being positive or Input 2 being negative. However, EEG instruments are constructed with several channels, usually 16 or more, and never less than 8. The connections between electrodes on the scalp and the inputs of the amplifiers are arranged, according to agreed-upon conventions (3), to provide one or another of two types of EEG recordings: bipolar or referential.

BIPOLAR RECORDING

Bipolar recording, using more than one amplifier, uses multiple electrode derivations (a derivation is a pair of electrodes) without having any one electrode common to the input of all of the channels. Usually, the derivations are arranged so that the electrodes are in a straight line, called an array, and adjacent channels have an electrode in common. An example of multichannel bipolar arrangements is shown in Fig. 12.7, which is a simple two-channel bipolar array. The shared electrode is C_3, which is connected to Input 2 of channel 1 and to Input 1 of channel 2. Because of this arrangement, when a negative event occurs under or near electrode C_3, channel 1 has a downgoing movement of its pen and channel 2 has an upgoing movement of its pen (Fig. 12.7A). These outputs are predictable from the Polarity Square. We have localized a negative event at C_3.

If, however, C_3 becomes positive, the first channel has an upgoing deflection and the second channel's deflection is downgoing. This occurs because Input 2 of channel 1 is positive, and Input 1 of channel 2 simultaneously is positive (Fig. 12.7B).

Phase Reversal

In both examples, the pen movements are 180° out of phase. This is called phase reversal. When phase reversal involves adjacent channels in

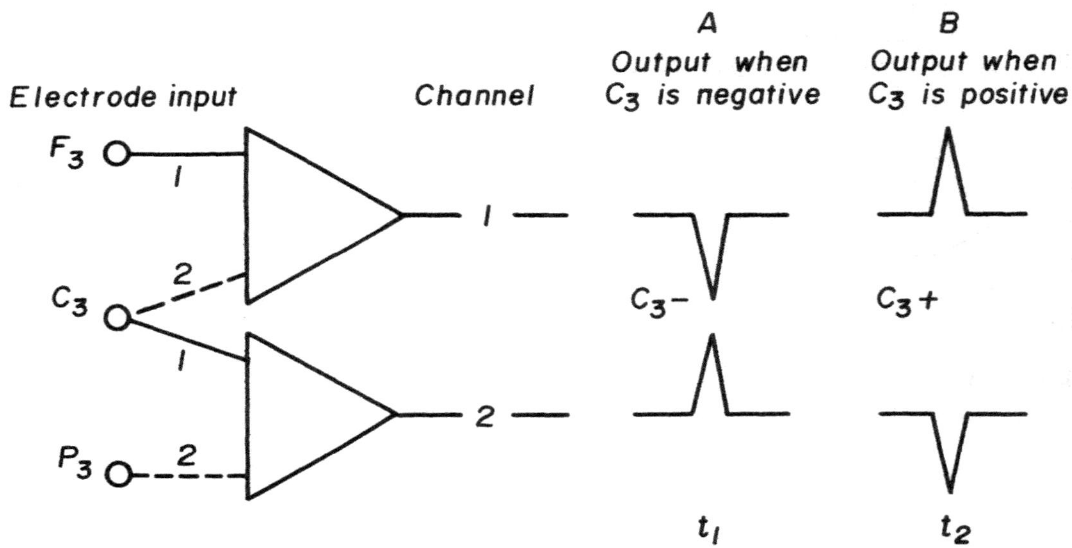

FIG. 12.7. Two-channel bipolar recording. When a distinctive EEG event occurs at the shared electrode, it can be localized and its polarity determined. **A:** C_3, negative. **B:** C_3, positive.

a bipolar array, it is because the shared electrode goes to opposing inputs, and the same electrical sign (positive or negative), because of instrumental convention, causes the opposing deflections to occur. This phase reversal provides a powerful perceptual clue that aids in identifying the surface area over which EEG activity occurs (1). It also aids in identifying the polarity of the activity. It should be emphasized that there is nothing abnormal about phase reversal. It can be of assistance in localizing both normal and abnormal activity (6).

REFERENTIAL RECORDING

Referential recording of the same EEG event would require three amplifiers, as shown in Fig. 12.8. In referential recording (sometimes improperly called monopolar recording), a different scalp electrode is connected to Input 1 of each amplifier, and a single common reference electrode is connected to Input 2 of each amplifier. In Fig. 12.8, the EEG is recorded from the same scalp electrodes as before. The left earlobe, A_1, is used as the reference, R. If a negative EEG event occurs at C_3 (time t_1) it will produce an upward deflection in channel 2 (Fig. 12.8A) because Input 1 of the second channel is negative. The other channels, because their inputs are not near the negativity, show no change. If a positive event occurs (time t_2), the output of channel 2 will deflect downward because positivity at Input 1 causes the display to go down. The other channels do not show any change (Fig. 12.8B).

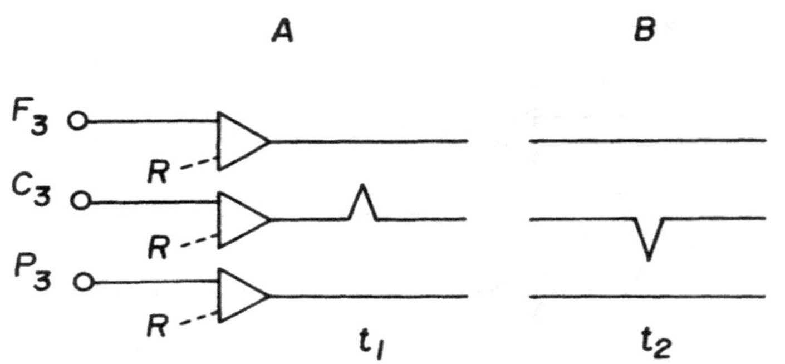

FIG. 12.8. Referential recording. A: Negativity at C_3 at time t_1. B: Positivity at C_3 at time t_2.

APPLICATION OF POLARITY RULES

These simple examples illustrate the fact that the same conclusions can be reached about an EEG event by the suitable use of either bipolar or referential recording. Both methods localized a negative and then a positive event at electrode C_3. These models illustrate the rules of polarity and the ways in which they can be used to localize and describe the characteristics of transient, or momentary, EEG activity. Many real EEG processes are, indeed, transient, but most EEG activity is more or less rhythmic.

Figure 12.9 illustrates the application of the polarity rules to the localization of rhythmic activity. In Fig. 12.9A, there is prominent rhythmic activity in channels 2 and 3. It is out of phase in these channels. The common electrode is C_3, which is connected to Input 2 of channel 2 and to Input 1 of channel 3. At time t_1, channel 2 is at peak upward amplitude and channel 3 is at peak downward amplitude. According to the polarity rules, this is explained by assuming that at time t_1, C_3 is more positive than F_3 and P_3. This is followed by decreasing positivity at C_3 and then by increasing negativity at C_3. At peak negativity (time t_2), channel 2 has a maximum downward amplitude and channel 3 has a maximum upward amplitude. The slowly changing surface polarity, shifting from positive to negative to positive, repetitively, is seen in the EEG as a slow rhythm. With referential recording (Fig. 12.9B), the activity is seen only in channel 3, which represents C_3.

The same rules apply to the demonstration of focal rhythmic activity and of focal transient activity. For simplicity, however, the following examples of the applications of polarity rules for localizing will employ models of transient events.

A fundamental characteristic of the differential amplifier is its failure to have any output when the voltages at its two inputs are equal. A model of this effect is shown in Fig. 12.10, which uses four electrodes and three amplifiers arranged in a bipolar array. In Fig. 12.10A, the EEG output at time t_1 shows a downgoing pen movement in channel 1 and an upgoing pen movement in channel 3. This is a phase reversal. There is no output in channel 2. How can these outputs be explained? First, note that C_3 is shared by channels 1 and 2, and P_3 is shared by channels 2 and 3. Using the Polarity Square as a starting point, the only logical explanation of the events seen in Fig. 12.10A is that the area represented by C_3 and P_3 has become transiently negative so that channel 1 goes down (Input 2

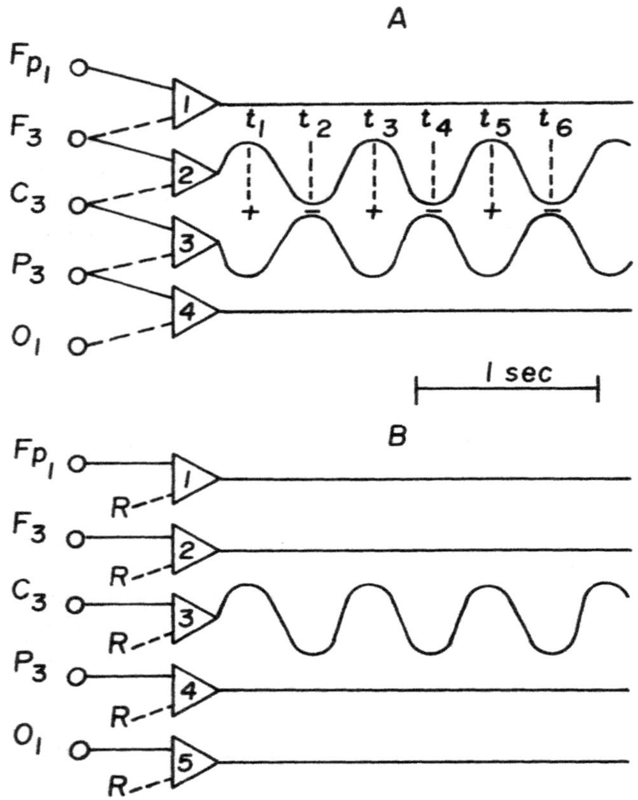

FIG. 12.9. A: Alternating negativity and positivity at C_3 at a frequency of 2 Hz explains the phase reversals in channels 2 and 3. B: The same activity with referential recording does not show phase reversal and 2-Hz activity occurs only in the channel connected to C_3.

negative) and channel 3 goes up (Input 1 negative). However, C_3 and P_3 are equally negative so that channel 2 has no deflection. This is an area of equipotential. At time t_2, this is an area of equipotential that is positive (Fig. 12.10B).

The same electrodes now are employed in a referential recording. The following events may be expected to occur if the assumptions made to explain Fig. 12.10A are correct. Figure 12.11 shows the derivations. The

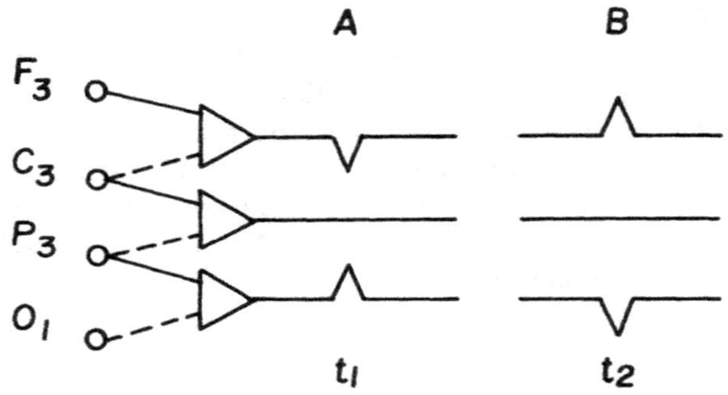

FIG. 12.10. A: Electrodes C_3 and P_3 are equally negative at time t_1. Since a differential amplifer amplifies only voltage *differences*, channel 2 has no response. The direction of deflection follows rules of the Polarity Square. B: At time t_2, electrodes C_3 and P_3 are equally positive. (See text for details.)

reference is A_1. Note that each electrode has an input to a single amplifier, via Input 1. Input 2 of each amplifier goes to a common electrode, in this instance chosen to be A_1, the left earlobe. At time t_1, C_3 and P_3 are negative, and the voltage of each is identical. There is no deflection in channels 1 and 4 because the negative event at C_3 and P_3 does not enter their inputs. The polarity of the event seen in Fig. 12.10A and its

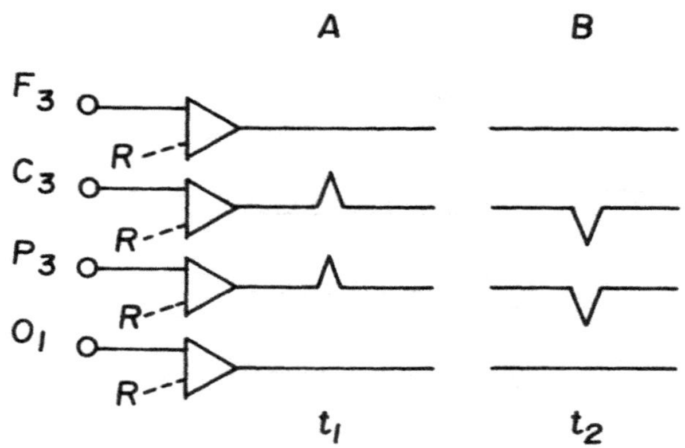

FIG. 12.11. Referential recordings of same events shown in Fig. 12.10A, B (see text).

equipotential status at C_3 and P_3 now have been demonstrated by both bipolar and referential recording.

Figure 12.11B shows the same event displayed in Fig. 12.10B, recorded referentially. The basic rules of the Polarity Square again lead to the conclusion that the areas represented by C_3 and P_3 have become transiently positive and, on the basis of the equal amplitudes of the deflections of channels 2 and 3, that this is an area of equipotential.

Fields

Transient focal EEG abnormalities that are negative at the surface of the scalp are called surface negative events. The events shown in Figs. 12.10A and 12.11A are surface negative. Figures 12.10B and 12.11B show surface positive events. By using either bipolar or referential derivations, it is possible to localize an EEG event to either a small or a large area of the scalp, called a field. The field can be described in terms of its surface polarity. In Fig. 12.12A the equipotential area deduced in Figs. 12.10 and 12.11 is shown as a series of concentric circles on the surface of the head. However, while C_3 and P_3 are equipotential, is it possible that another location within this area is at an even higher potential? Is there a more negative point midway between C_3 and P_3, while C_3 and P_3 are on equal potential lines and less negative?

These questions can be answered by adding three more electrodes to the array. Refer to Fig. 12.12B. One is placed midway between F_3 and C_3 and is labeled F_3'. Another is placed midway between C_3 and P_3, and it is labeled C_3'. The third electrode, P_3', is placed midway between P_3 and O_1.

Suppose that the transient negative event seen in Figs. 12.10A and 12.11A again occurs, as shown in Fig. 12.12A. With use of the additional electrodes (Fig. 12.12B), the event appears only in channels where inputs are connected to C_3, C_3', and P_3 (channels 2, 3, 4, and 5). Channel 2 ($F_3'-C_3$) and channel 3 (C_3-C_3') are in phase, but there is a larger amplitude in the C_3-C_3' derivation.

Channel 4 ($C_3'-P_3$) is 180° out of phase with channel 3, but their amplitudes are equal. The deflection in channel 5 (P_3-P_3') is in phase with $C_3'-P_3$ but of lower amplitude.

From these facts it can be deduced, using the Polarity Square, that there is maximal negativity at electrode C_3'. There is less negativity at C_3 and P_3. There appears to be no negativity extending to F_3' and P_3' as evidenced by no activity in channels 1 and 6. With respect to the questions raised earlier, we now know that there is a focus inside the field, and that C_3 and P_3 were not at the focal point. The field can be drawn schematically on the scalp, shown in Fig. 12.12C.

The circle inside the field on which C_3 and P_3 lie is an equipotential line, since no deflection appeared at the output of the amplifier to which they are connected. The small inner circle around C_3' represents the area of greatest negativity at the moment this event takes place. This is a map of the field of the negative event.

The field occurring in the region between electrodes C_3 and P_3 can also be viewed as a "bump of negativity" (Fig. 12.12C). The peak of the "bump" is at C_3', where the phase reversal occurs. Differences in voltage between C_3' and C_3 and between C_3' and P_3 are larger than between F_3' and C_3 and between P_3' and P_3. The differences in amplitude of the deflections in Fig. 12.11B are thus explained. The direction of the deflections is explained by the rules summarized in the Polarity Square: When Input 2 is more negative, the deflection is *down;* when Input 1 is more negative, the deflection is *up*.

The field can also be shown as a graph, with the voltage difference plotted against electrode location, as shown in Fig. 12.12D. This is another way to view the distribution of voltages.

A referential recording of the same events is displayed in Fig. 12.13. The same scalp electrodes were used as in Fig. 12.12. Point R at the extreme right of Fig. 12.13B is the voltage level of the reference electrode. It is assumed to have no activity related to the main event at C_3', C_3, and P_3. Again, the same conclusion is reached from both referential and bipolar recording. [See Osselton (8,9) for further discussion.]

Contaminated Reference

If the reference electrode is in the field of an abnormal EEG event, difficulties develop. Figure 12.14A diagrams such a situation. A focus is present at T_3, the left midtemporal area, with a wide field surrounding it, extending as far as F_7 and A_1. The voltage at A_1 is less than at T_3 and equal to the voltage at F_7. A referential recording is obtained, with A_1 as the reference. Figure 12.14B illustrates the connections of electrodes to the amplifiers and also the recorded EEG transient that occurs at time t_1. It shows six channels with a downward deflection, one channel with no deflection, and one channel with a small upward deflection. Review of the

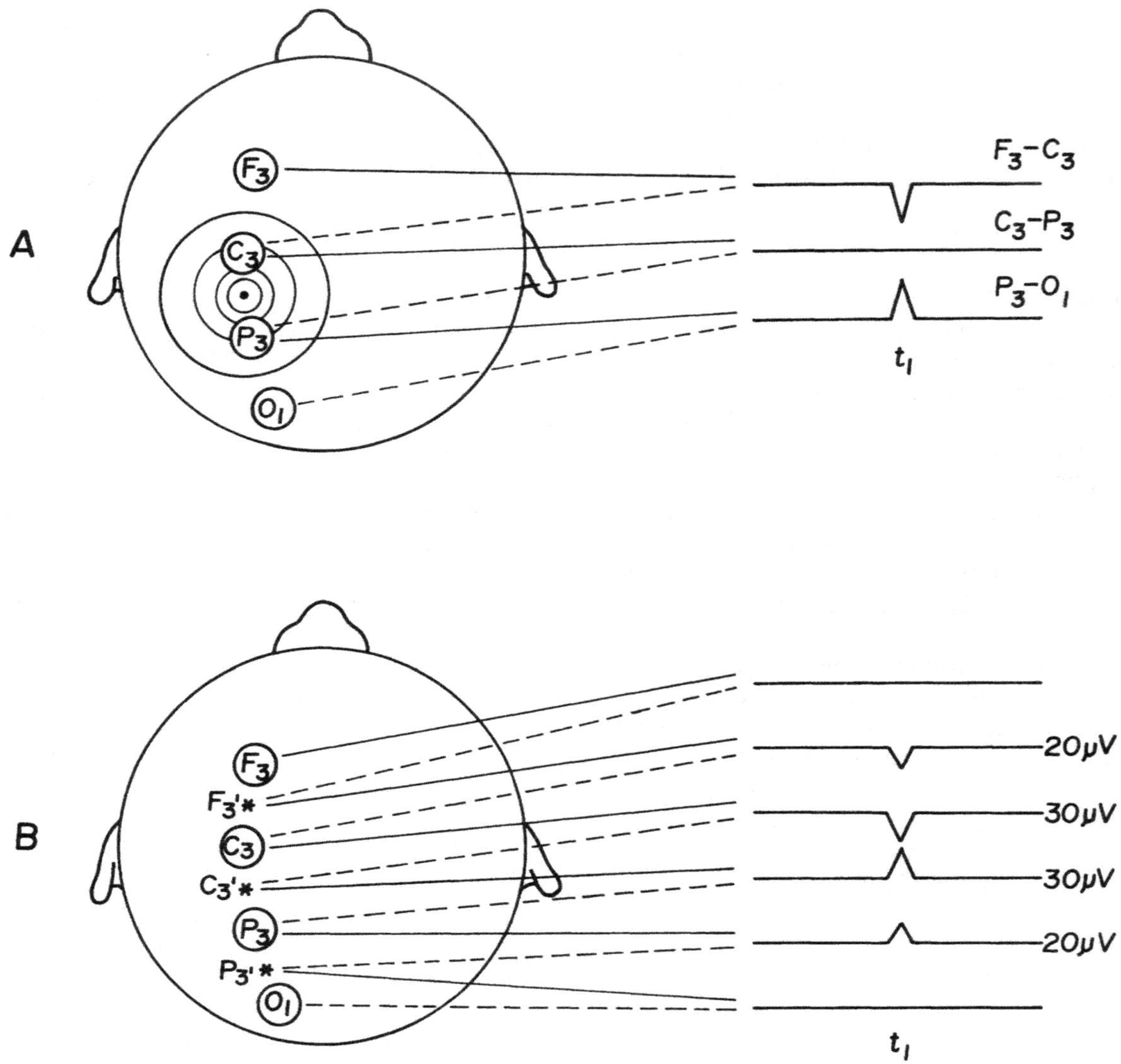

FIG. 12.12. A: Bipolar recording of large field with conventional ten-twenty electrode system. **B:** Recording of field with a larger number of intermediately placed electrodes. (*Contd.*)

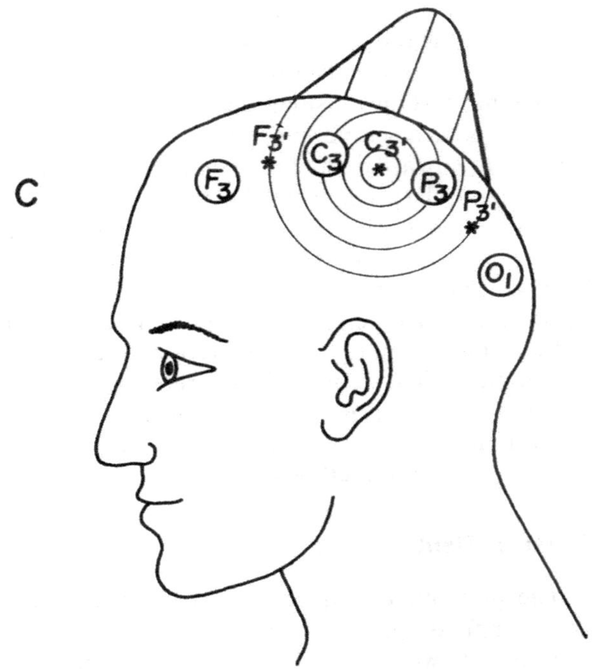

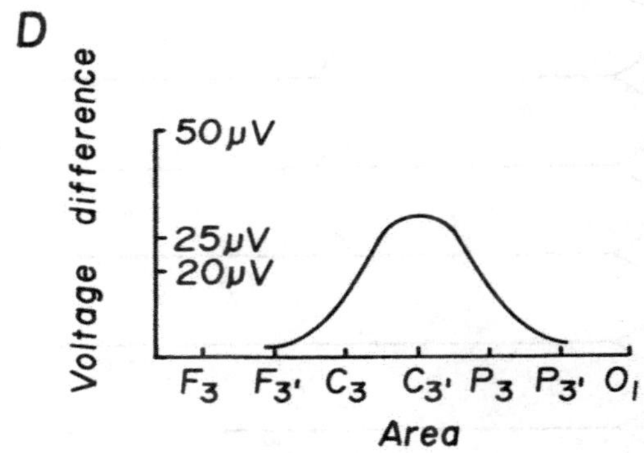

FIG. 12.12. (*contd.*) **C:** "Bump" of negativity across the field of **B. D:** Graphic representation of the field of **B** and **C.**

input connections reminds us that A_1 is common to all channels and that it goes to Input 2 of all channels.

These deflections therefore can be explained in the following manner. At time t_1:

1. T_3 is slightly more negative than A_1. T_3 goes to Input 1, causing an upward deflection (Input 1 negative, up).
2. A_1 is more negative than Fp_1, T_5, O_1, F_3, C_3, and P_3. Because A_1 is on Input 2, there is a downward deflection in all channels whose Input 1 is connected to these electrodes (Input 2 negative, down).
3. F_7 and A_1 are equipotential (no deflection).

This explanation can be tested in two ways. First, the reference going to Input 2 of all channels in Fig. 12.14B can be moved to a point far away from the field. For example, A_2 can be selected as the reference. In addition, the previous reference, A_1, can be connected to Input 1 of another channel, whose Input 2 is connected to A_2. When the same event occurs again, at time t_2, the output deflections shown in Fig. 12.14C will occur in the EEG. An upward deflection occurs in channels 2 and 3 because F_7 and T_3 go to Input 1 of those channels. The event is negative, and it is localized at those two positions. None of the other scalp electrodes is in the field, so there is no corresponding deflection in the channels to which they are connected.

In channel 9, the previous reference, A_1, is connected to Input 1, and A_2, the new reference, is connected to Input 2. The upgoing output at time T_2 indicates that A_1 has become negative. Its amplitude is equal to the amplitude of channel 2, the F_7-A_2 derivation, demonstrating that the two

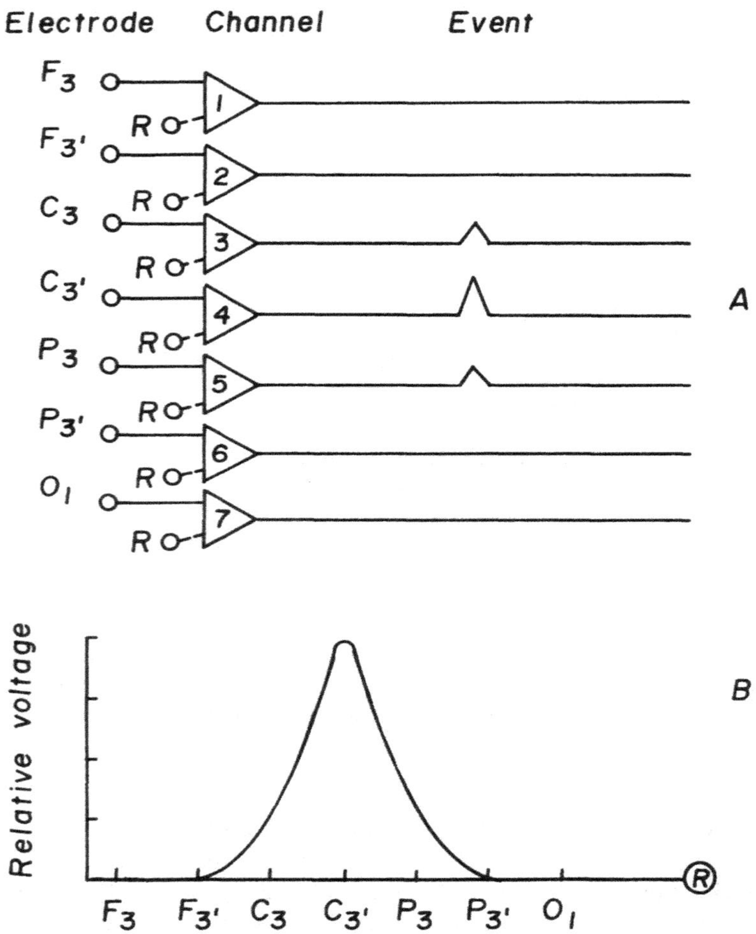

FIG. 12.13. **A:** Referential recording of same event, with same electrodes, as shown in Fig. 12.12B. **B:** Graphic representation of the field of A.

electrodes are on an equipotential line. The derivation T_3-A_2 has the highest amplitude, indicating it to be the most negative point being recorded.

The second test uses bipolar derivations. The electrode locations are shown in relation to the field in Fig. 12.15A. The derivations are shown in Fig. 12.15B. The event at t_3, similar to those at t_1 and t_2 of the earlier figures, yields the EEG shown in the third column of Fig. 12.15B. Channels 1, 2, 3 and 4, not in the field, show no deflection.

Channel 5 shows a small downward deflection because F_7 (Input 2) is slightly more negative than Fp_1 (Input 1). Channel 6 shows a larger amplitude downward deflection, since T_3 is more negative than F_7. Channel 7 shows a still larger upward deflection because T_3 (Input 1) is much more negative than T_5 (Input 2), which is outside the field.

Channels 9 through 13 give further confirmation: T_3 is more negative than A_1, and much more negative than C_3. A_1 and F_7 are equipotential but A_1 is more negative than T_5 (Input 1 negative, up).

Such involvement of a reference electrode is not uncommon. It is sometimes called a contaminated reference. Based on an understanding of the polarity rules, the alert technologist will recognize the signs, as first illustrated in Fig. 12.14B. The true state of affairs then should be demonstrated, using the methods shown in Figs. 12.14C and 12.15B.

Further Field Testing

The previous examples have described localizing procedures when a focus or field appears within the limits of a bipolar or referential array. Suppose, however, that a focus appears to be present at the end of an array, as shown in Fig. 12.16. The activity at time t_1 is in phase in channels 1 and 2, is higher in amplitude in channel 1, and is absent in channel 3. Therefore, F_3 and C_3 appear to be in a field of negativity. How can this be analyzed?

Based on the conventions summarized in the Polarity Square, F_3 must be much more negative than C_3, and C_3 must be somewhat more negative than P_3. There is no potential difference between P_3 and O_1. This analysis is graphically shown in Fig. 12.16. However, because F_3 is at the end of the line of electrodes, it is not possible to be certain that the focus actually is at that position. It is necessary to add a fifth electrode, anterior to F_3.

This is illustrated in Fig. 12.17. Figure 12.17A shows a bipolar array, using Fp_1 as the additional electrode. The inputs appear in Fig. 12.17B, and the outputs in Fig. 12.17C, which indicate that the greatest negativity must be at F_3, since the deflection in channel 1 is down, while in channel 2 it is up. Some negativity occurs at C_3. The deduced field is shown in Fig. 12.17D, with the assumed amounts of relative negativity at time t_1. Therefore, the information available in Fig. 12.16 was incomplete.

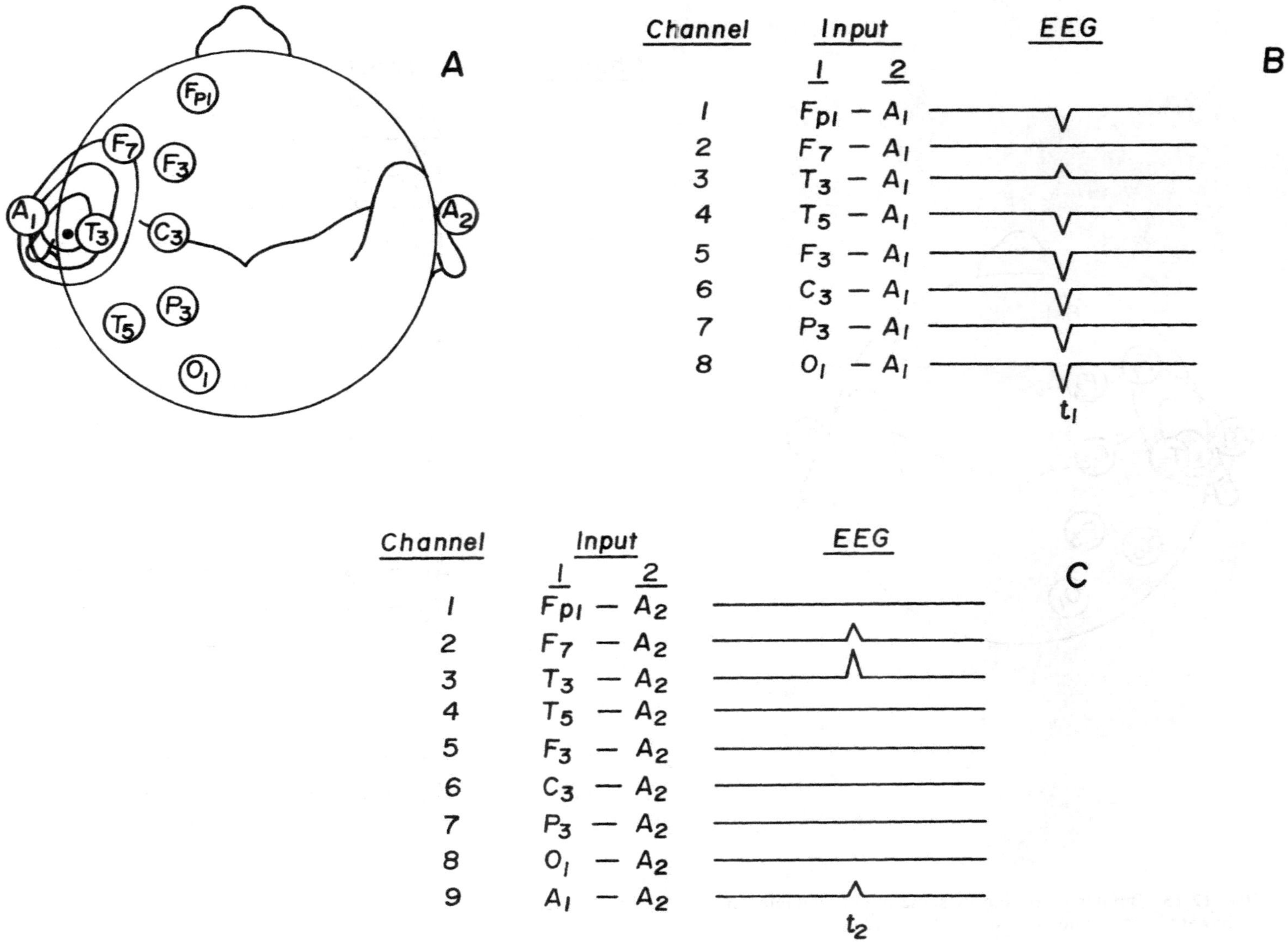

FIG. 12.14. Analysis of recording resulting when a reference electrode is in an active field. **A:** Schema of field relative to electrodes. **B:** Output of each designated channel when reference electrode is A_1 (see text). **C:** Output of each designated channel when the reference electrode is A_2. Compare with **B**. (See page 151 for details.)

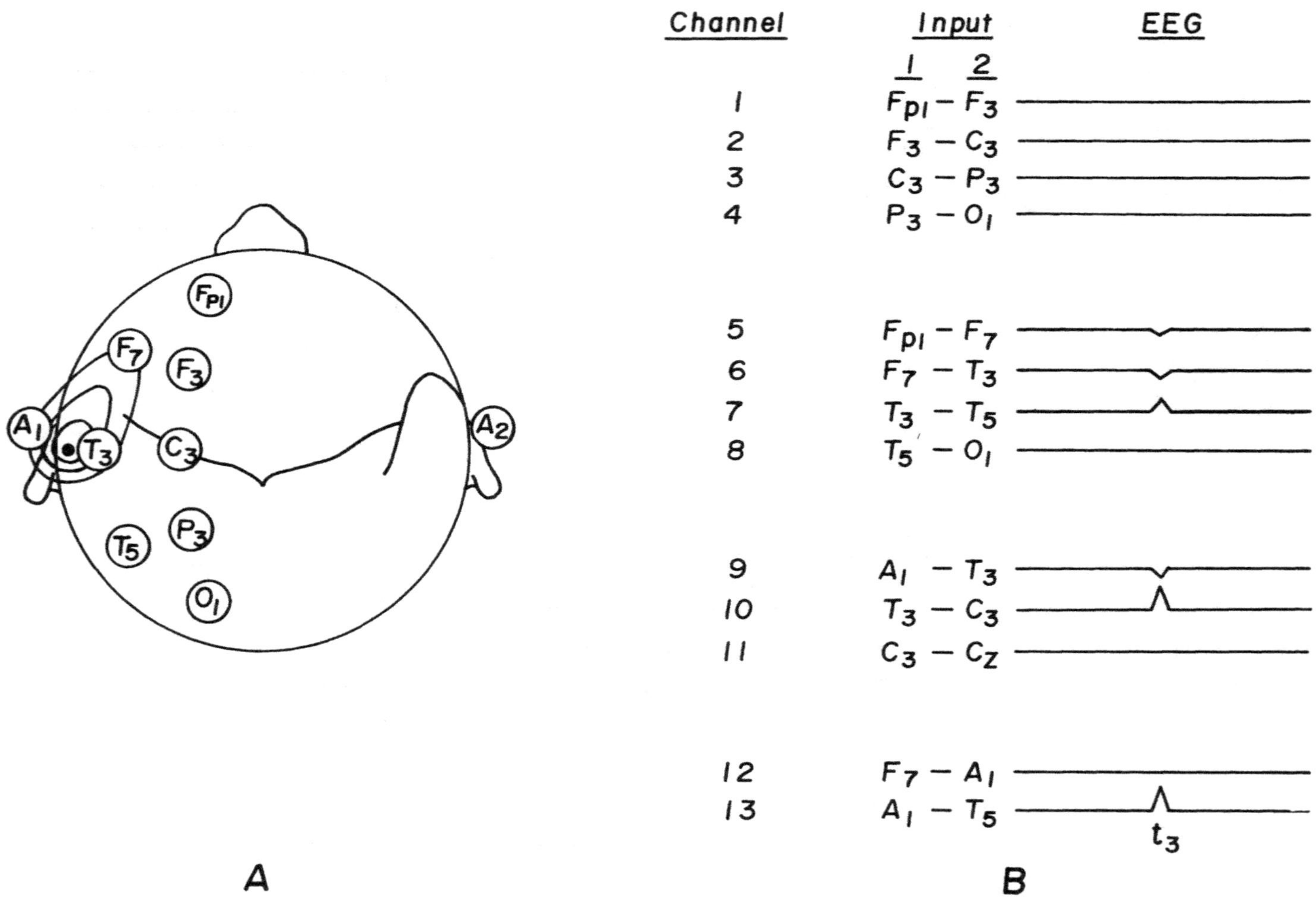

FIG. 12.15. Bipolar recording of same events depicted in Fig. 12.14. **A:** Field. **B:** Demonstration of focus at F_7, T_3, and A_1, with equipotential at F_7 and A_1. (See text for details.)

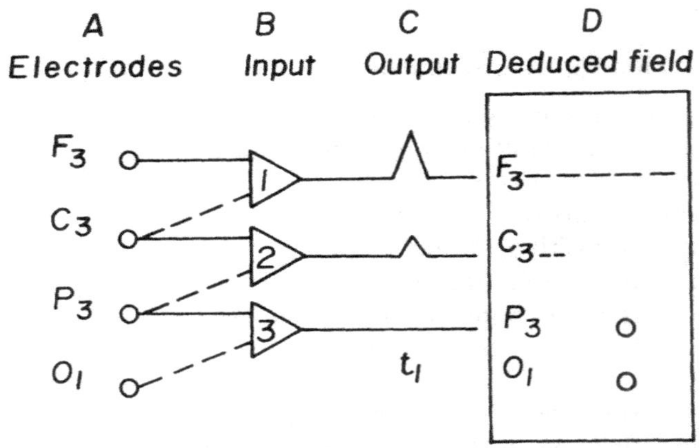

FIG. 12.16. A: Bipolar connections of electrodes F_3, C_3, P_3, and O_1. B: The channels. C: Upgoing EEG output at t_1. D: Diagrammatic display of the degree of relative negativity required to produce the transient response at t_1. F_3 is much more negative than C_3, and C_3 is more negative than P_3, but P_3 is not more negative than O_1.

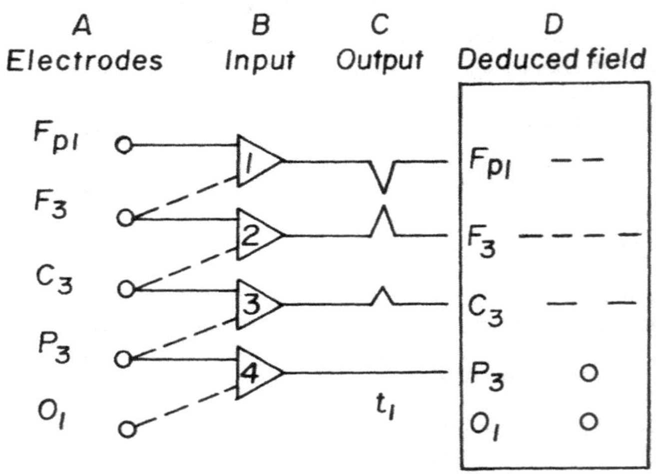

FIG. 12.17. A-C: Additional electrode Fp_1 used to resolve the ambiguity of Fig. 12.16. Electrode F_3 is more negative than Fp_1 and C_3. Electrodes P_3 and O_1 have no negativity. D: The relative negativity at t_1. (See text.)

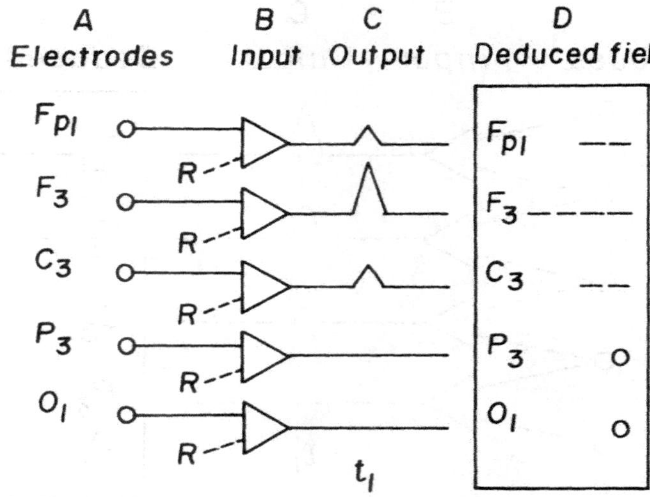

FIG. 12.18. A-C: Referential recording of the same event shown in Fig. 12.17. Electrode F_3 presents greater negativity then Fp_1 and C_3. The areas of P_3 and O_1 are not involved in this negative transient. D: The deduced field at t_1. (See text.)

Referential derivations will yield the same field as that deduced in Fig. 12.17, if the reference is inactive. Figure 12.18C presents the data and Fig. 12.18D, the analysis. Maximal negativity occurs at F_3, with less at Fp_1 and C_3; P_3 and O_1 show no simultaneous negativity.

Suppose that the extended bipolar array of Fig. 12.17 gave the information shown in Fig. 12.19C. The highest amplitude now is in channel 1 and is, again, at the end of the array. Since electrode Fp_1 is the most anterior electrode in the ten-twenty placement system, it can be assumed that this represents the focus, until proven otherwise. The deduced field is shown in Fig. 12.19D, based on the information available in Fig. 12.19A–C.

Confirmatory evidence may be found in a referential recording, assuming that the reference is inactive. Figure 12.20A–C presents the information and Fig. 12.20D shows the deduced field. This is similar to the field of Fig. 12.19.

Further models and discussions of these important rules can be found in Maulsby (7) and Osselton (8,9).

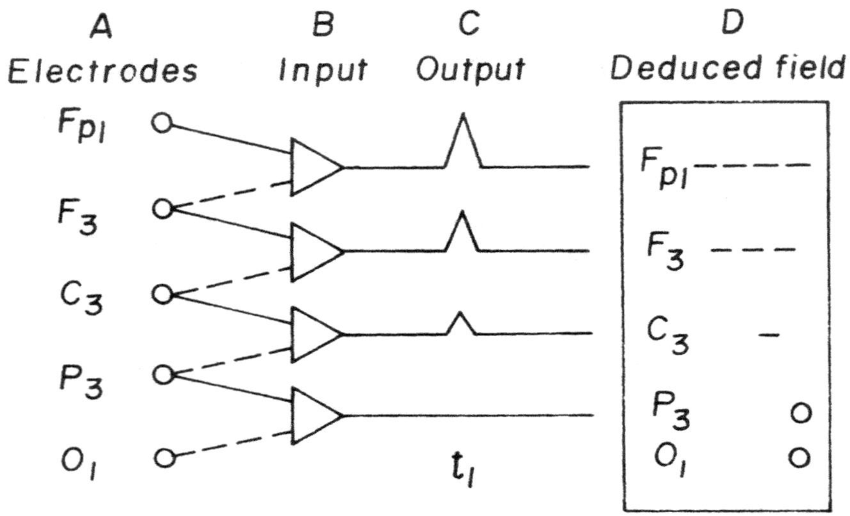

FIG. 12.19. Fp_1 is more negative than F_3. F_3 is more negative than C_3, and C_3 is more negative than P_3. P_3 and O_1 are at the same potential. (See text.)

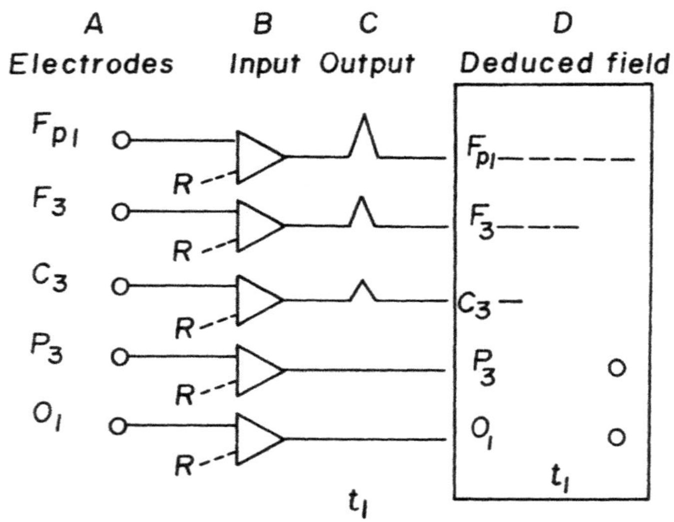

FIG. 12.20. **A-C:** Referential record of events shown in Fig. 12.18. **D:** Amplitude of deflection is proportional to relative negativity. (See text.)

SUMMARY

In this section we have seen that:

1. EEG instruments are constructed according to a convention that states that negativity at Input 1 of any channel causes an upward deflection of the pen of that channel.
2. Corollaries to this rule state that when:
   a. Input 2 is positive, the deflection is up.
   b. Input 2 is negative, the deflection is down.
   c. Input 1 is positive the deflection is down.
3. There are two types of input systems for multichannel EEG instruments:
   a. Bipolar (one electrode is common to two channels).
   b. Referential (one electrode is common to all channels and is usually connected to Input 2).
4. With bipolar recording, the usual localizing sign is phase reversal between adjacent channels having a common electrode in the maximum of the field of activity.
5. With referential recording, the usual localizing sign is maximum amplitude at the electrode located at the maximum of the field.
6. Surface polarity of EEG events can be determined, using the polarity rules, by either bipolar or referential recording.
7. Referential recording has an inherent weakness in that the chosen reference may be electrically active and introduce confusing information to all channels. Analytical procedures to identify this effect and techniques to demonstrate it were discussed.

APPENDIX

The Committee on EEG Instrumentation Standards of the International EEG Federation (2) specifies that "negativity at an electrode selected by the first of the pair of selector switches (*i.e.*, corresponding to Input Terminal 1) relative to an electrode selected by the second selector switch"—which corresponds to Input 2—"for the same channel results in an upward deflection on the write out."

The Federation's Committee on Terminology (3) defines a "polarity convention" in these words: "International agreement whereby differential EEG amplifiers are constructed so that negativity at the input terminal 1 relative to the input terminal 2 of the same amplifier produces an upward pen deflection." The Committee defines Input Terminal 1 as the input terminal "at which negativity, relative to the other input terminal, produces an upward pen deflection." Input

Terminal 2 is defined as the input terminal "at which negativity, relative to the other input terminal, produces a downward pen deflection."

REFERENCES

1. Adrian, E. E., and Yamagiwa, K. (1935): The origin of the Berger rhythm. *Brain,* 58:323–351.
2. Barlow, J. S., Kamp, A., Morton, H. B., Ripoche, A., Shipton, H., and Tchavdarov, D. B. (1978): EEG instrumentation standards (revised 1977): Report of the Committee on EEG Instrumentation Standards of the International Federation of Societies for Electroencephalography and Clinical Neurophysiology. *Electroencephalogr. Clin. Neurophysiol.,* 45:144–147.
3. Chatrian, G. E., Bergamini, L., Dondey, M., Klass, D. W., Lennox-Buchthal, M., and Petersén, I. (1974): A glossary of terms most commonly used by clinical electroencephalographers. *Electroencephalogr. Clin. Neurophysiol.,* 37:538–548.
4. Knott, J. R. (1961): Concerning electrode arrays. *Am. J. EEG Technol.,* 1:1–12.
5. Knott, J. R. (1969): Electrode montages revisited: How to tell up from down. *Am. J. EEG Technol.,* 9:33–45.
6. Magnus, O. (1961): On the technique of localization by electroencephalography. *Electroencephalogr. Clin. Neurophysiol.* Suppl. 19:1–35.
7. Maulsby, R. L. (1979): Basis for visual analysis: Polarity convention, principles of localization and electrical fields. In: *Current Practice of Clinical Electroencephalography,* edited by D. W. Klass and D. D. Daly, pp. 27–36. Raven Press, New York.
8. Osselton, J. W. (1966): Bipolar, unipolar and average reference recording methods. I. Mainly theoretical considerations. *Am. J. EEG Technol.,* 5:53–64.
9. Osselton, J. W. (1969): Bipolar, unipolar and average reference recording methods. II. Mainly practical considerations. *Am. J. EEG Technol.,* 9:117–133.

Chapter 13

Montages

A single pair of electrodes inputting an amplifier forms a derivation. As discussed under the topic of Polarity (Chapter 12), a single derivation without reference to another derivation provides only limited information about the EEG. However, if several derivations are assembled in a logical manner, a great deal of information can be obtained. It then becomes possible to arrive at conclusions about the sources and characteristics of various processes within the EEG recording.

The earliest electroencephalographers had only single channel instruments. This limitation led Berger (3,4) to believe that alpha activity was generated diffusely in the brain. His single derivation was from the frontal to the occipital area. Although he soon had two channels available for recording, he used the same basic derivation in each hemisphere. This gave him a very limited view of the brain's activity. Nevertheless, this two-channel recording used the first, even though primitive, EEG montage, enabling comparison of EEG activity of the two hemispheres simultaneously.

As the state of the art advanced so that more than two channels of recording became possible, the increase in information from the EEG expanded proportionately. It quickly became apparent that there are two basic methods of recording: bipolar recording and referential recording (see Chapter 12). Regardless of the method used, it also became obvious that multiple derivations can be displayed on multichannel equipment so that an orderly representation of the brain within the recording is possible. All that is required is an arrangement of derivations that place adjacent areas of the brain on adjacent channels of the EEG record. The electrode placement of the ten-twenty system readily encourages such electroanatomical displays.

ARRAYS AND MONTAGES

Within the ten-twenty system, the electrodes are arranged in rows of five, viewed either from front to back (longitudinally) or from side to side (transversely). A 4-channel, bipolar array[1] can be assembled by selecting a row of five electrodes and arranging the four derivations as shown in Fig. 13.1. Figure 13.1 schematically correlates area(s) of the brain, electrodes, EEG channels, recorded EEG activity, and the conclusion or interpretation based on the preceding information. In this figure, a negative event has been localized at electrode C_3.

The same EEG event can be viewed with a referential montage using five recording channels. Schematically, the process shown in Fig. 13.1, recorded with referential derivations, would appear as diagrammed in Fig. 13.2. The negative event is localized, again, at electrode C_3.

Each of these arrays provides an electroanatomical picture of the parasagittal areas of the left hemisphere. Each array is a building block from which larger views of the electrical activity of the brain can be constructed. The larger views are called montages. A montage is ". . . the process of combining several distinct pictures so that they blend with each other to form a composite picture" (20).

The American EEG Society's *Minimal Technical Requirements for Performing Clinical Electroencephalography* (1) state that "Sixteen channels of simultaneous recording of the EEG are encouraged. In no event should less than 8 channels be used" and that "To find the distribution of EEG activity, it is necessary to record simultaneously from as many regions of the scalp as possible. Inadequate simultaneous recording can lead to erroneous knowledge of the brain areas producing abnormality."

The Society's *Proposal for Standard Montages to be Used in Clinical Electroencephalography* (2) adds that (a) all of the 21 electrodes of the ten-twenty system should be used, (b) both bipolar and referential montages should be used, (c) bipolar derivations should run in straight and unbroken lines with equal interelectrode distances in each line, (d) derivations recorded from more anterior electrodes should be recorded above derivations from more posterior areas; and (e) the patterns of derivations forming a montage should be made "as simple as possible" so that they may easily be perceived and understood. It also was recommended that

[1] The word *array* is used here to indicate a sequential arrangement of electrodes that are recorded in adjacent channels of the EEG instrument. The sequential arrangements previously shown in Chapter 12 are arrays.

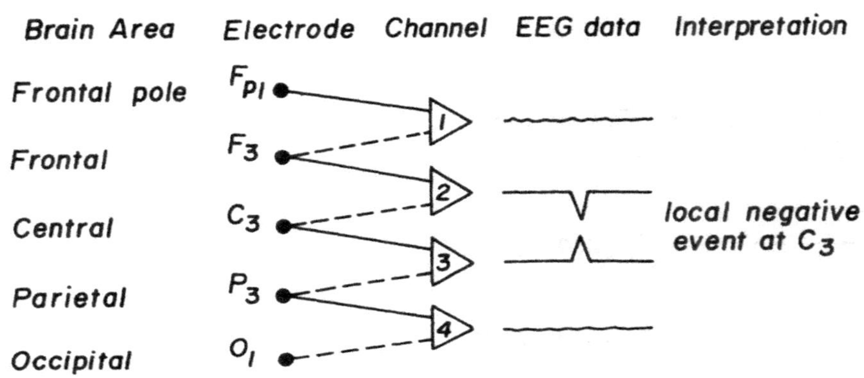

FIG. 13.1. Process leading from designated brain areas to interpretation of EEG data. Five of the ten-twenty electrodes are connected to four amplifiers. The outputs are shown as "Data." From the latter it is possible to localize a specific electrical event at electrode C_3.

derivations based on left hemisphere electrode placements be recorded on channels at the top of the record, above the derivations representing the right hemisphere. This is the most common procedure in North America, although many European laboratories (and a few in North America) record right above left.

These statements about the logic of designing EEG montages were drawn in large degree from the contributions made by the panel of a

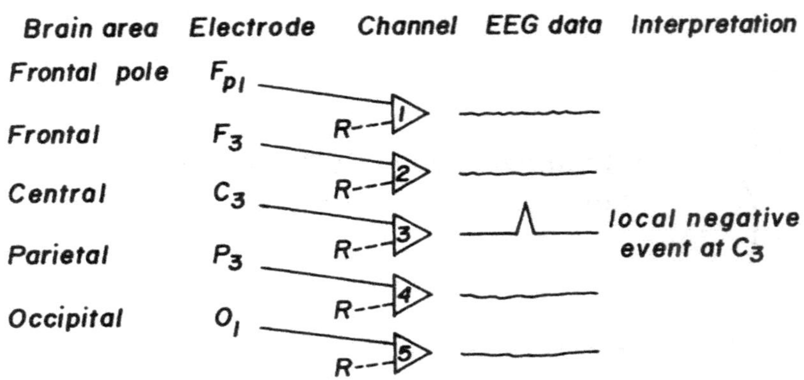

FIG. 13.2. The event localized in Fig. 13.1 can be localized by referential recording.

Symposium on EEG Montages, held in 1976 and sponsored by the American EEG Society and the American Society of EEG Technologists (7,9,10,12,13,15,18).

Assembling Bipolar Montages

There are two rules that may be followed for assembling bipolar montages. These are based on the direction in which arrays proceed (18). The electrodes can be organized into arrays or chains that proceed in a longitudinal, anterior-posterior (A–P; front to back) direction. They also can be organized in a transverse, left to right, direction. These organizational rules are diagrammed in Fig. 13.3. The American EEG Society's *Guidelines in EEG—1980* (2) refers to these as longitudinal bipolar (LB) and transverse bipolar (TB) montages, respectively. Notice that the temporal A–P arrays are based on portions of the circumferential, or horizontal, plane.

To organize these 21 electrodes into systematic montages, it is necessary to develop a shorthand system for making convenient reference to the arrangement of electrodes that has been chosen. One common system for representing a bipolar montage uses numbered arrows, as shown in Fig. 13.4A. Each arrow represents a derivation. The arrow starts from Input 1. The point of the arrow signifies Input 2. The pictorial method is convenient, easy to sketch, and readily comprehended. Beneath the pictorial system is the commonly used system of listing the electrodes in serial order: Fp_1-F_3 signifies a derivation from Fp_1 to F_3. Fp_1 inputs Input 1; F_3 inputs Input 2. Channel numbers are implied by the order of listing and may be omitted.

A referential montage may be similarly diagrammed or listed (Fig. 13.4B). It is not necessary to use arrows if the reference is clearly indicated.

Both methods are used commonly and will be interchangeably employed here. The pictorial method is easily perceived, particularly if the montage is "made as simple as possible." Listing electrode positions in serial order is space-saving. However, when many channels are used, this system loses clarity.

Figure 13.5 depicts an 18-channel bipolar montage. There are five chains or arrays. The arrays are displayed longitudinally, proceeding from left to right. All of the 19 scalp electrodes of the ten-twenty system are included.

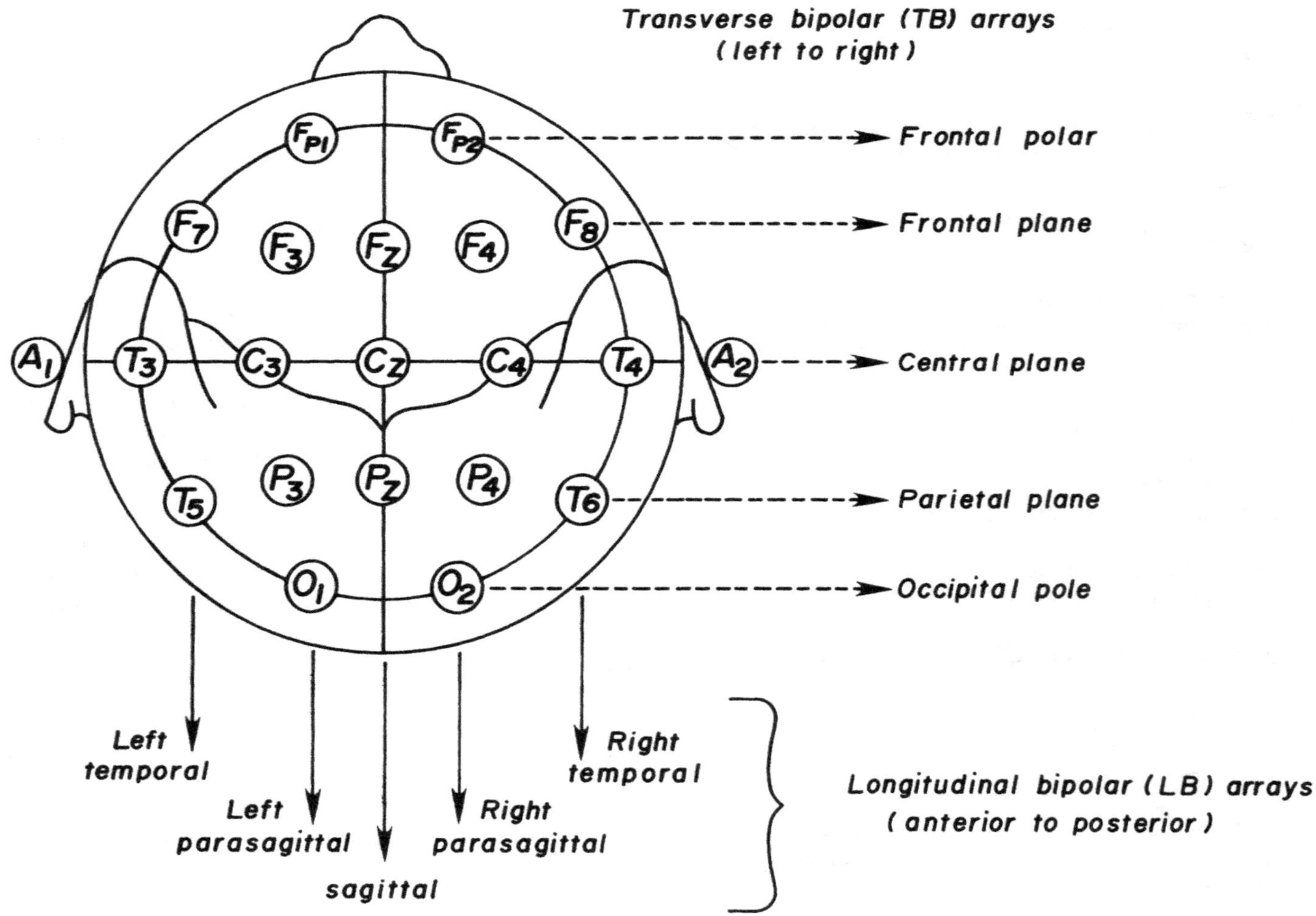

FIG. 13.3. Longitudinal and transverse bipolar arrays viewed as planes (see text for discussion).

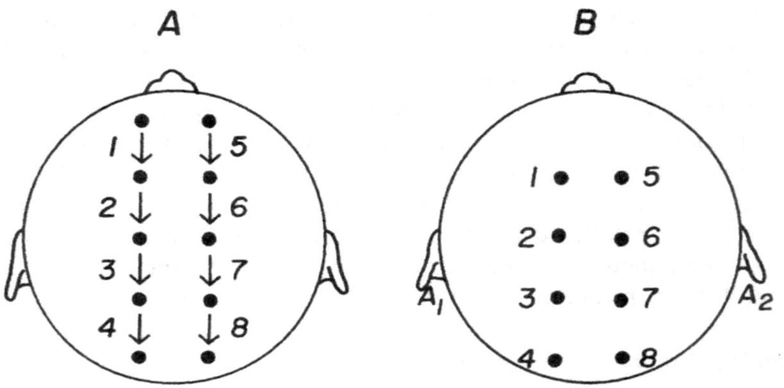

Longitudinal bipolar

Channel	Derivation
1	$F_{p1}-F_3$
2	F_3 C_3
3	C_3 P_3
4	P_3 O_1
5	F_{p2} F_4
6	F_4 C_4
7	C_4 P_4
8	P_4 O_2

Referential

Channel	Derivation	
1	F_3	A_1 (ipsilateral ear)
2	C_3	
3	P_3	
4	O_1	
5	F_4	A_2 (ipsilateral ear)
6	C_4	
7	P_4	
8	O_2	

FIG. 13.4. Organization of longitudinal planes into anteroposterior arrays. Notation systems may be diagrammed or written in as a conventional abbreviation. **A:** Bipolar. **B:** Referential. (See text for details.)

If only 16 channels are available, the two sagittal, or midline, derivations (F_z-C_z and C_z-P_z) can be omitted.

Transverse bipolar montages also are easily assembled from the ten-twenty electrode placements, as shown in Fig. 13.6. This transverse montage proceeds from left to right within each array. Anterior arrays are placed above more posterior ones. Only 16 EEG channels are required to display activity derived from all 21 electrodes of the ten-twenty system. It

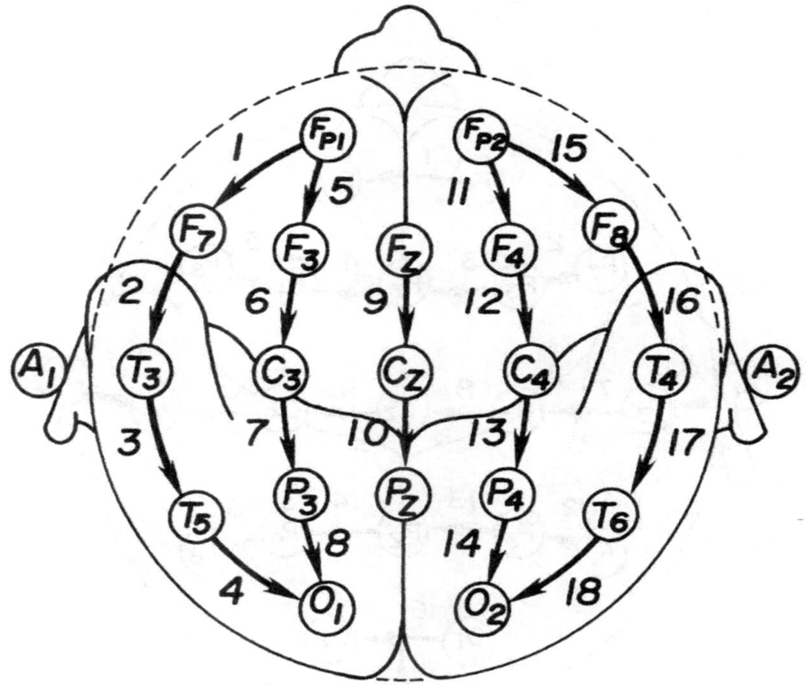

Channel	Plane
1 – 4	Left temporal
5 – 8	Left parasagittal
9 – 10	Sagittal
11 – 14	Right parasagittal
15 – 18	Right temporal

FIG. 13.5. An 18-channel bipolar montage displaying five anteroposterior planes in a left-to-right order (see text).

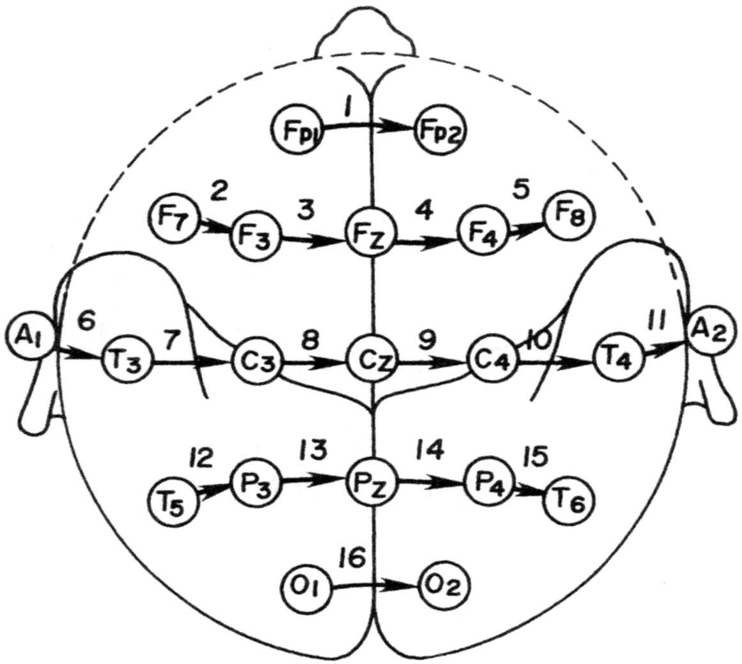

Channel	Array
1	Frontal polar
2–5	Frontal
6–11	Coronal
12–15	Parietal
16	Occipital

FIG. 13.6. A 16-channel transverse bipolar montage displaying five coronal planes arranged in anteroposterior order (see text).

should be noted that the derivations represented in channels 1 and 16 stand alone as single pairs. Sometimes these are called open-ended derivations, because they are not linked to another derivation by a common electrode. Therefore they cannot, on the basis of activity derived from the single pair alone, yield explicit information about what EEG processes occur under one of the electrodes. However, they are not isolated derivations. There are four in-line derivations in the array just posterior to channel 1 and four in-line derivations just anterior to channel 16. Activity from the open-ended derivations can be combined meaningfully with information from adjacent arrays to yield significant information.

Assembling Referential Montages

A referential montage is one in which Input 1 of each channel is connected to one individual scalp electrode and Input 2 of all channels is connected to a common reference electrode (see Chapter 12). The most direct translation from a bipolar to a referential display would use a longitudinal assembly, with left hemisphere derivations preceding those from the right. Such a montage is shown in Fig. 13.7. Like the bipolar montage of Fig. 13.5, it utilizes all 19 scalp electrodes of the ten-twenty system. However, it requires 19 channels for full display. If only 18 channels are available, either F_z or P_z must be omitted. When only 16 channels are available, all sagittal electrodes, F_z, C_z and P_z usually are omitted.

The five longitudinal arrays of this referential montage are defined by the blocks enclosed by dotted lines. Each represents an anatomically defined region of the brain: left temporal, left parasagittal, sagittal (midline), right parasagittal, and right temporal. Within each longitudinal row, the arrangement of electrodes (brain areas) is presented from front to back. These correspond to the planes of Fig. 13.3.

The choice of the reference point used in referential recording is critical (see Chapter 12). Many different reference points have been suggested. Many are in use, and there is no fixed or standard location. The most commonly used reference positons are A_1 and A_2. Left hemisphere derivations usually use A_1 as a reference; right hemisphere derivations use A_2.

Some electroencephalographers and technologists interconnect A_1 and A_2. If either A_1 or A_2 is electrically active because of the spread of a field from the adjacent temporal lobe, the reference is invalid. Sometimes either A_1 or A_2 can be the most active electrode; this occurs when the inferior midtemporal area of the brain is the focal region. If A_1 and A_2 are

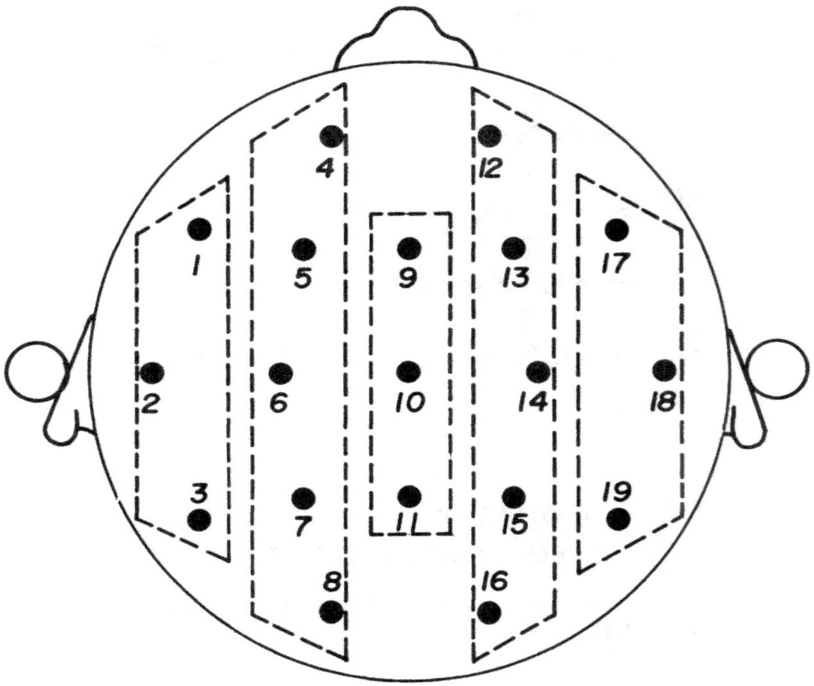

Channel	Reference
1 - 3	A_1 (ipsilateral ear)
4 - 8	A_1 (ipsilateral ear)
9 - 11	A_1 or A_2
12 - 16	A_2 (ipsilateral ear)
17 - 19	A_2 (ipsilateral ear)

FIG. 13.7. Organization of referential montages using anatomical logic similar to bipolar organization of Fig. 13.5.

interconnected when this occurs, it becomes difficult to untangle the puzzle of phase reversals and to discover the real source of the activity, which appears in all channels but is local to one.

Other reference points used are (a) the vertex (C_z), (b) the left and right mandibles, (c) the chin, (d) the nose, (e) the base of the skull below the inion, or (f) a high cervical location on the neck.

A C_z reference may be useful when there is an active temporal lobe process spreading to A_1 or A_2. However, when used in drowsiness and sleep, this reference will contribute high voltage sharp transients, or K complexes, (see Chapter 14) to all derivations. It is important not to confuse these vertex-generated transients with focal temporal activity. If both are present, each must be carefully identified.

The mandibles can be affected by spreading fields from the temporal areas in the same manner as A_1 and A_2. These fields have been known for many years. They first were described by Gibbs, et al. in 1948 (6). Spike activity originating in the anterior temporal lobe may be recorded from most of the face and jaw. This is dramatically illustrated by Gibbs and Gibbs in the *Atlas of Electroencephalography* (5).

The chin, as well as the mandibles, may be active because of glossokinetic potentials (see Chapter 16). The nose may be active for similar reasons, including its proximity to the eyes, which contribute massive potentials when they move.

Another reference point that sometimes has merit, especially when focal activity lies in the temporal areas, is the base of the skull or a high cervical (neck) point. This point may be very effective if there are no large signals in the occipital area or no activity is generated by neck muscles.

A noncephalic reference combining the neck and chest was first proposed by Stephenson and Gibbs (19) and has been revived recently by Ropper et al. (17). This requires the introduction of a potentiometer into the circuit to balance out EKG artifact (Fig. 13.8). It has been reported that EKG artifact can be satisfactorily reduced in 85% of patients over 18 years of age (17). However, depending on the resistance of the potentiometer used to balance out EKG artifact, there may be an appreciable impedance mismatch between Inputs 1 and 2. Even this noncephalic reference can sometimes be contaminated by focal discharges from the mesial surface of the temporal lobe. Care must be used in evaluating phase reversals involving nasopharyngeal derivations and scalp locations when this (or a cervical) reference is used.

The so-called average reference electrode was introduced by Offner (16) and Goldman (8). It is an adaptation of a method used earlier in EKG recording. The average reference is achieved by connecting all the scalp (Input 1) electrodes together through isolating or averaging resistors. The system is shown in Fig. 13.9. Each averaging resistor has a typical resis-

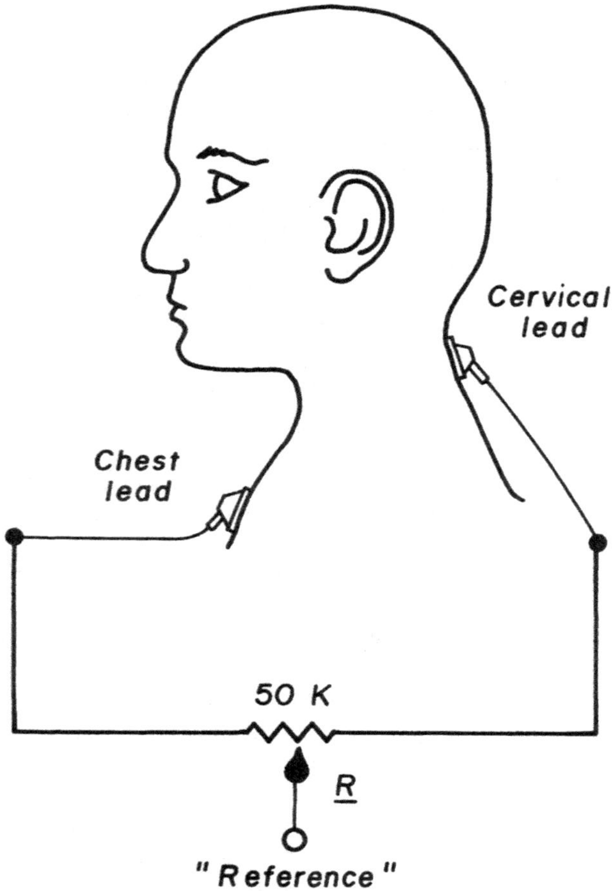

FIG. 13.8. Neck-chest reference. One lead is placed at cervical spine II, the other on the sternum. These are attached to opposite ends of a potentiometer (typical resistance suggested, 50 kΩ). By adjusting the moveable arm R, EKG can be virtually eliminated in the majority of instances.

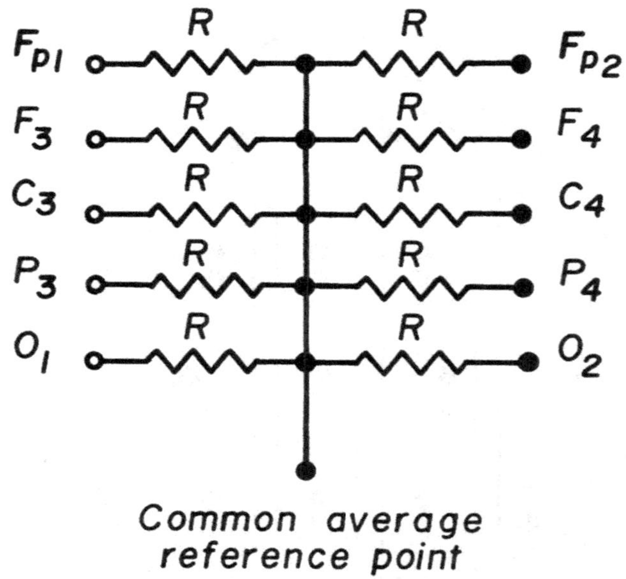

FIG. 13.9. Average reference to input 2 of each channel (simplified to use 10 electrodes). R = 1 MΩ.

tance of 1 MΩ. These resistors are in parallel between the scalp electrodes (where interelectrode resistance connects them) and Input 2. If 21 resistors with a resistance of 1 MΩ are in parallel, the resulting impedance of the average reference electrode is about 47 kΩ. If 16 resistors are used, the impedance will be about 62 kΩ.[2] This creates an exceedingly large impedance imbalance in the inputs of the EEG amplifiers, which in turn can lead to severe 60-Hz interference artifact in some locations, as well as possible changes in voltage representation of the EEG. Through the use of active electronic circuits rather than passive resistive circuits of the type shown, advances have been made in avoiding this impedance imbalance.

There also is the problem of the average reference becoming an active reference, as described earlier. If a very large voltage is introduced to the average by a single electrode, it will appear in all other channels in opposite phase to the signal in the channel to which the signal is focal. This is particularly troublesome when there is excessive eye movement. Contemporary instruments allow the technologist to disconnect from the av-

[2] These values are computed from the formula for resistors in parallel:

$$R = 1/(1/R_1 + 1/R_2 + 1/R_N).$$

erage any electrode with high voltage activity, thus avoiding or minimizing such artifacts.

OTHER MONTAGES OF PRACTICAL VALUE

Two basic multiple-channel, bipolar montages have been described: a longitudinal A-P montage and a transverse montage. At least two other bipolar montages are necessary to obtain clear localization of activity at those electrodes that are at the end of a chain. These electrodes are Fp_1 and Fp_2 and O_1 and O_2.

Circumferential Montage

A circumferential montage can be established, beginning at O_1 and initially proceeding in a posterior–anterior, clockwise, manner (i.e., going from left to right as the frontal pole is crossed). This is schematized in Fig. 13.10.

If there is a focus of, for example, 2-Hz activity at Fp_1, this circumferential montage will reveal the focus by local activity in channels 4 and 5. By virtue of the polarity convention, the 2-Hz activity will be out of phase in these channels. The usual longitudinal bipolar montage (Fig 13.5) will only show slow activity in channels terminating over Fp_1. Similarly, the transverse montage (Fig. 13.6) will show only slow activity in channels terminating over Fp_1, which in this case is a single channel, Fp_1-Fp_2. The astute technologist will know intuitively that a focus is at Fp_1, but phase reversal of 2-Hz activity at Fp_1 must be demonstrated for confirmation. It is clear that the selection of this circumferential montage would be made on the basis of information already available from the other two bipolar montages that have demonstrated 2-Hz activity only in derivations that include Fp_1. There is no ambiguity in the open-ended channel 1 slow activity of the transverse montage, since it already has been seen at Fp_1 on the A–P montage.

Suppose, however, that the initial information from the A–P montage suggested focal 2-Hz activity at electrode O_1. In the circumferential montage just reviewed, O_1 is effectively open-ended in channels 1 and 10. Detection of phase reversal would depend on comparing activity in channels that are separated by eight other channels. This can be perceived more easily in adjacent channels. Therefore, an alternate circumferential montage should be organized in an anterior–posterior direction, proceeding counterclockwise from Fp_1. The first ten channels are shown in Fig. 13.11.

Since the basic circumferential montage requires only ten channels, longitudinal derivations can be included if 16 or 18 channels are available. The remaining channels may be used to record complementary derivations in the parasagittal and sagittal planes. [See American EEG Society's *Guidelines in EEG–1980* (2).]

Transverse Triangular Montage

Another occasionally useful bipolar montage utilizes triangular arrays established in a transverse direction. One such array is diagrammed in Fig. 13.12, showing three derivations. Channel 1 has C_z on Input 1 and T_3 on Input 2. Channel 2 has T_3 on Input 1 and T_4 on Input 2. Channel 3 has T_4 on Input 1 and C_z on Input 2.

Note that the triangular array changes the rules pertaining to bipolar montages: First, it is not a straight-line array. Also, the last and first channels share a common electrode. Such an arrangement can, under certain conditions, lead to serious errors in interpretation, as will be discussed. A complete montage based on the building blocks of transverse triangles, sometimes called coronal triangles, (11,14), is shown in Fig. 13.13.

Since nine channels permit display of three coronal triangles, a 16-channel instrument will permit the addition of seven other derivations, six of which can sample the temporal areas in an A–P direction. These are shown in Fig. 13.14 as a continuation of the montage. The remaining channel can be used to observe an area of particular interest or as a monitor (e.g., for EKG). If drowsiness is intervening, a derivation from C_z to A_1 would serve as a monitor for K complexes (discussed in detail in Chapter 14).

The transverse triangular bipolar montage is of value in displaying low voltage sharp or slow activity in either temporal region that may be at or nearly at isopotential in longitudinal bipolar derivations (and in referential derivations involving an ipsilateral ear reference). An example of this is shown in Fig. 13.15.

In this figure there is a focus of activity midway between F_7 and T_3. Its field extends to include Fp_1 and T_5. As a consequence, the derivations Fp_1-T_3 and T_3-T_5 have relatively small differences of voltage. F_7 and T_3 are at isopotential. There will be quite low voltage activity seen in Fp_1-F_7 and T_3-T_5 and no activity seen in F_7-T_3. Recording from the triangular montages, the voltage differences between midline electrodes and the lateral electrodes F_7 and T_3 will be at maximum, since F_z and C_z

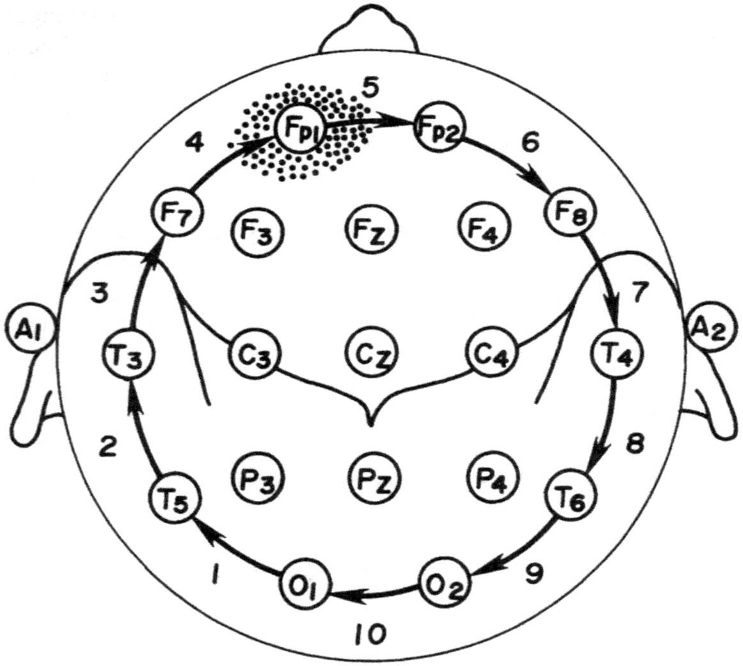

Channel	Electrodes	Data	Interpretation
1	$O_1 - T_5$		
2	$T_5 - T_3$		
3	$T_3 - F_7$		
4	$F_7 - Fp_1$		Left frontal focus
5	$Fp_1 - Fp_2$		
6	$Fp_2 - F_8$		
7	$F_8 - T_4$		
8	$T_4 - T_6$		
9	$T_6 - O_2$		
10	$O_2 - O_1$		

FIG. 13.10. Circumferential montage. Diagrammatic analysis of focal 2-Hz activity under electrode Fp_1. Map at left shows location of focus and connections of electrodes. O_1 is first electrode in the montage with input to channel 1, Input 1. The record is schematically shown in column labeled "Data" and is interpreted as showing a left frontal focus.

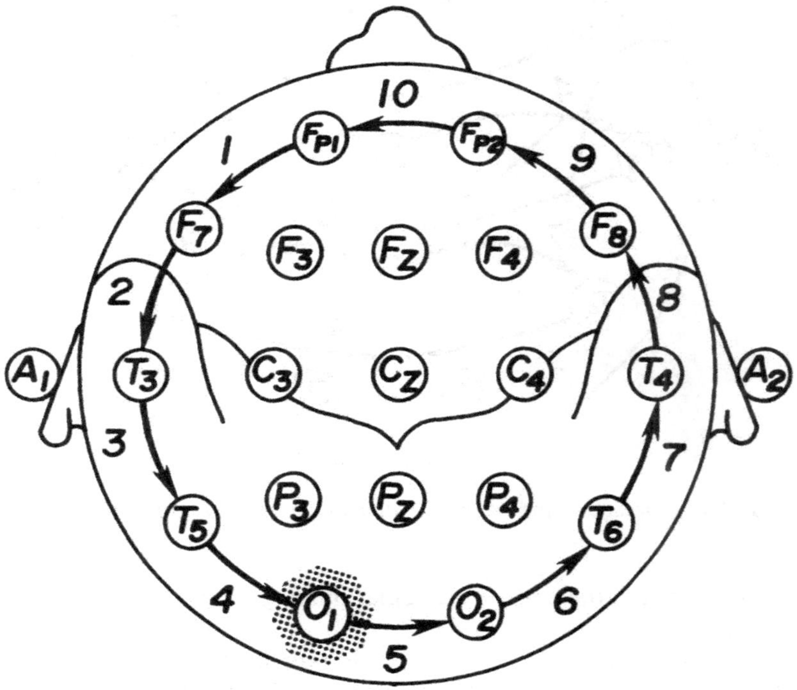

Channel	Electrodes	Data	Interpretation
1	$F_{p1}-F_7$		
2	F_7-T_3		
3	T_3-T_5		
4	T_5-O_1		Left occipital focus
5	O_1-O_2		
6	O_2-T_6		
7	T_6-T_4		
8	T_4-F_8		
9	F_8-F_{p2}		
10	$F_{p2}-F_{p1}$		

FIG. 13.11. Reversed circumferential montage used to localize posterior activity.

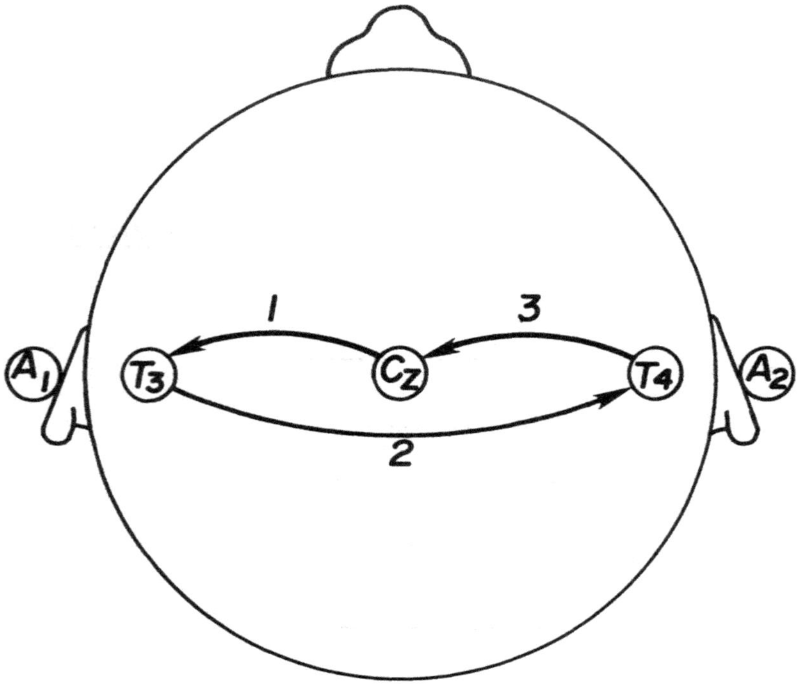

FIG. 13.12. Transverse triangular montage in coronal plane. Diagrammatic representation of inputs to channels 1, 2, and 3. (See text for discussion.)

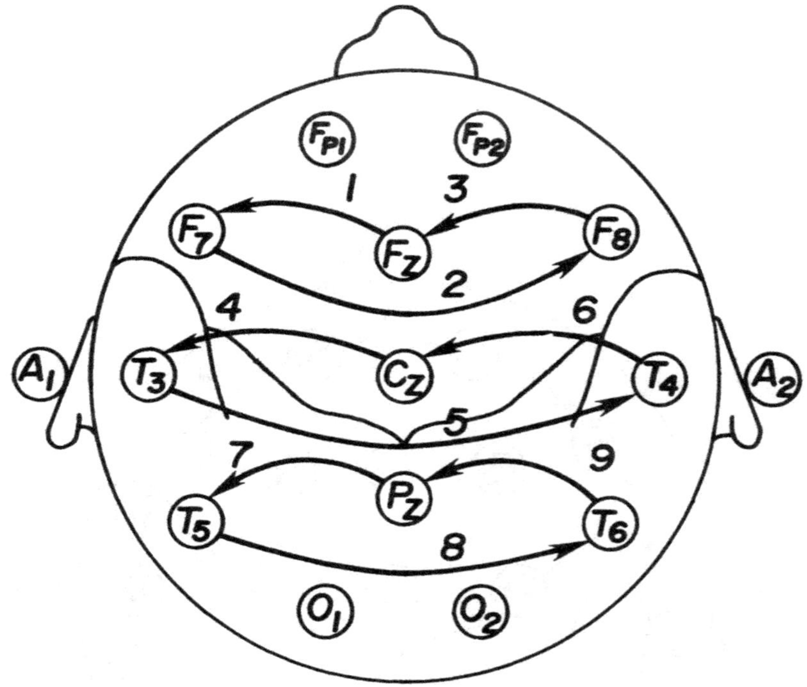

FIG. 13.13. Montage using triangles, displaying frontal, central, and parietal planes.

are entirely out of the field. Likewise, F_7-F_8 and T_3-T_4 will record the maximum voltage. Because of the configuration of the arrays, phase reversal will assist in localizing the focal activity. This set of montages acts to enhance activity that is less clearly seen in the AP temporal montage.

There is a serious danger inherent in the use of triangular montages (7). This is schematically analyzed in Fig. 13.16. Suppose that focal activity at C_3 (not included in the montage) equally affects T_3 and C_z. In consequence, the derivation C_z-T_3 does not record the activity. However, derivations T_3-T_4 and T_4-C_z both record it since T_4 is not in the field of the 2-Hz activity. Because T_3 goes to Input 1 of channel 2 and C_z goes to Input 2 of channel 3, the 2-Hz activity shows phase reversal between these channels. The electrode that is common to T_3 and C_z is T_4. In the usual analytic process, one would conclude that the 2-Hz activity originated at T_4, but in the case of triangular montages, this conclusion would be wrong.

The astute technologist never uses the triangular montage as a primary montage. The longitudinal and transverse bipolar montages and the referential montage will have been used earlier. The existence of the focal 2-Hz activity at C_3 therefore already will be known. The transverse or coronal triangles are inappropriate and the montage should not be used when a focus is present in this location. In the event that the C_3 activity is an intermittent spike, the simultaneous recording of the A–P temporal chains would establish that the spike was not originating at T_4, for it would not appear in the F_8-T_4, T_4-T_6 array. A parasagittal monitor, F_3-C_3, C_3-P_3, and so on, should be used to observe the activity directly.

This problem emphasizes three important principles about the selection

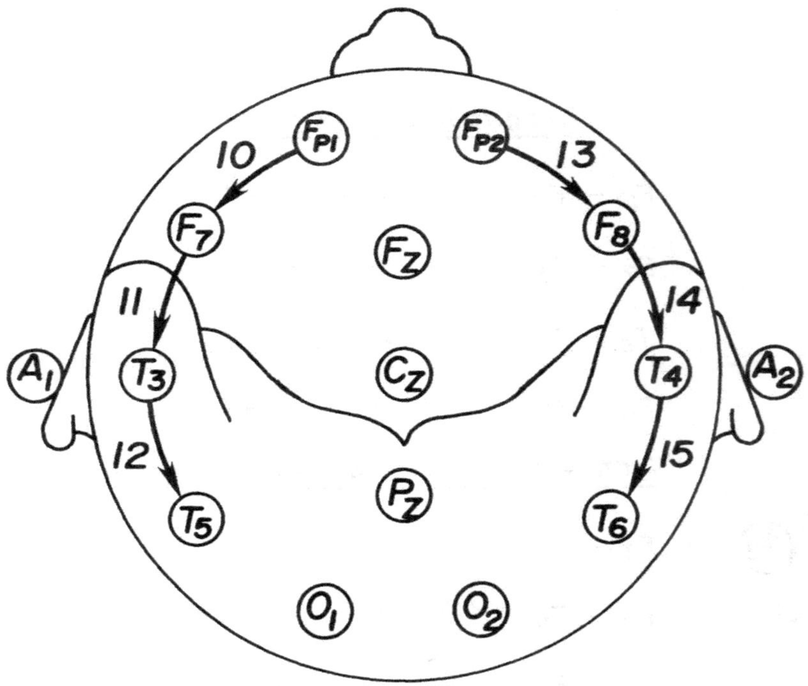

FIG. 13.14. Completion of full 16-channel montage used with coronal triangle derivations. (See text for discussion.)

of montages: (1) No montage should be used alone, in isolation from others. (2) Not all montages always should be used. (3) Some montages should be used only under special circumstances.

MONTAGES FOR 10 AND 8 CHANNELS

When fewer than 16 channels are available for the display of EEG activity, 8- or 10-channel montages can be derived from the larger 18-channel montages. However, 10- or 8-channel instrumentation sharply limits simultaneous views of the brain's electrical activity. If adequate sampling is accomplished, it is possible mentally to reassemble the information derived from several 8-channel montages and arrive at a composite equivalent to the information directly displayed by 16 or 18 channels. In the case of infrequently recurring focal activity, an abnormality will be missed if it occurs at a time when the montage sampling that area is not being utilized. In general, it is more difficult to record and interpret EEGs using 10- or 8-channel instrumentation.

The 10-channel montages listed in Tables 13.1 and 13.2 have been found to be useful.

Eight-channel instrumentation is still in common use although, fortunately, decreasingly so. Eight-channel instrumentation places severe restrictions on sampling and localizing. Nevertheless, with care and patience as well as knowledge and skill, entirely adequate recording can be performed. Tables 13.3 to 13.5 list useful groups of montages extracted from the basic sixteen- and eighteen-channel montages.

EFFICIENCY OF MULTICHANNEL RECORDING

Any one montage can be regarded as a camera with multiple lenses by which the electrical activities of the various areas of the brain are viewed. The completeness of the total view will depend on the number of electrodes used and the number of channels available for simultaneous recording. A greater number of electrodes and a larger number of channels will make it possible to take in a greater perspective. Fewer electrodes or channels act to diminish perspective. The clarity of the view will depend on the arrangements of the electrodes and the manner in which the derivations are displayed.

The efficiency of multichannel recording can be judged in part by evaluating the number of basic montages needed for an adequate view. Only three basic montages are needed when either 18- or 16-channel recording is used. Supplementary montages can be used for increasing the acuity of the viewing process. However, if only eight or ten channels are available, seven montages are required to provide minimal coverage. Alternate and supplementary montages may frequently be required to adequately display significant results. When using a small number of recording channels, it may not be possible to display events simultaneously at all critical locations.

Model Problem

To provide a further introduction to the use of montages, a model problem will be presented. It is based on a real clinical situation, but for

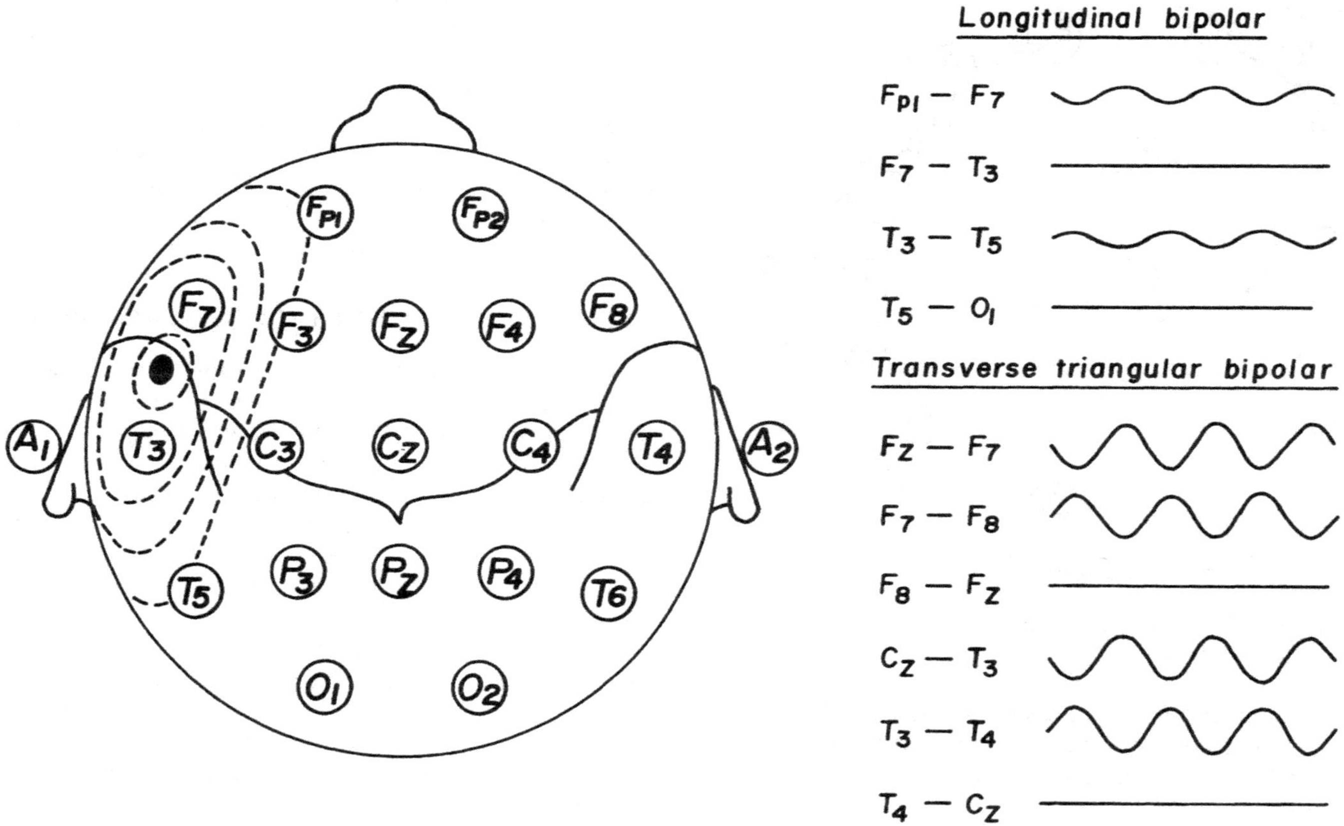

FIG. 13.15. (*Left*): A focus is present midway between F_7 and T_3, extending to Fp_1 and T_5. It does not extend to the midline. (*Right*): *Longitudinal bipolar derivations* recording across this field show a focus of low voltage activity equally involving F_7 and T_3. (The potential difference between T_5 and O_1 is negligible and not apparent against background.) *Transverse triangular derivations* show higher voltage focal activity at F_7 and T_3, easier to detect against background, because F_z and C_z are not in the field. Similarly, the activity of T_5 would be apparent in the parietal transverse plane, if included. (See text for further discussion.)

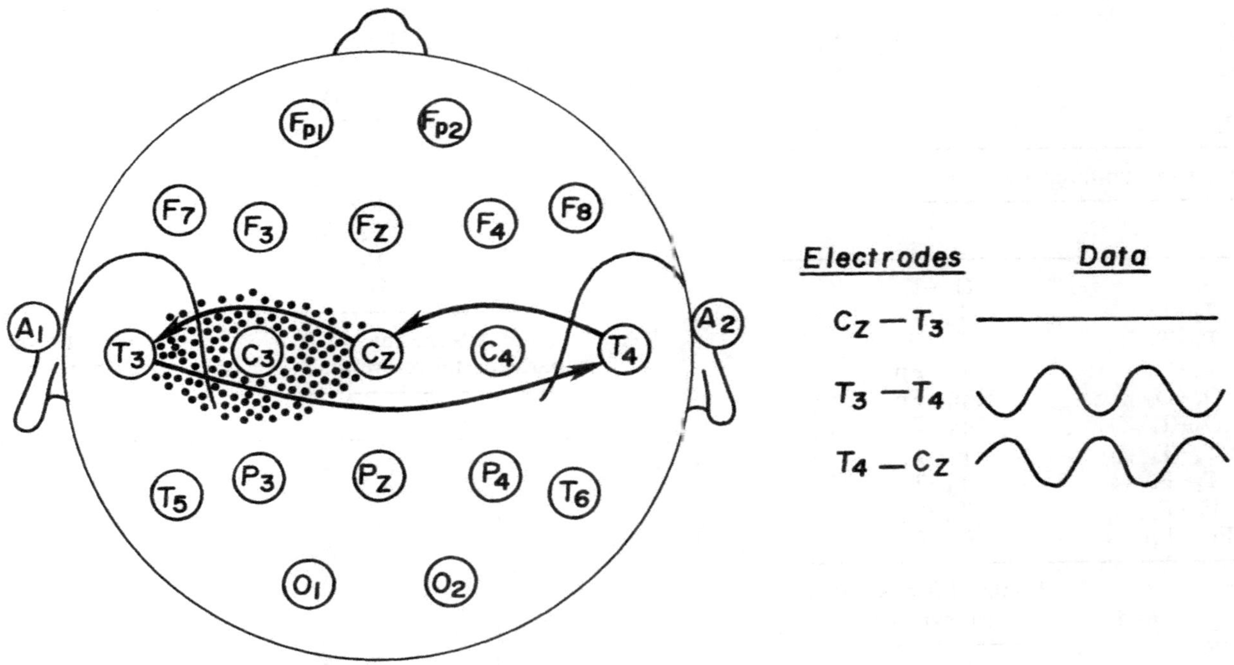

FIG. 13.16. A focus of 2-Hz activity exists at C_3. T_3 and C_z are at isopotential. T_4 acts, in effect, as a reference. Since T_3 is on Input 1 of channel 2 and C_z is on Input 2 of channel 3, there is phase reversal. (See text for discussion.)

TABLE 13.1. *Ten-channel bipolar montages*

Bipolar left-right (LB) temporal-sagittal[a] Channel		and	Bipolar left-right (LB) parasagittal-sagittal[a] Channel	
1	Fp_1-F_7		1	Fp_1-F_3
2	F_7-T_3		2	F_3-C_3
3	T_3-T_5		3	C_3-P_3
4	T_5-O_1		4	P_3-O_1
5	F_z-C_z		5	F_z-C_z
6	C_z-P_z		6	C_z-P_z
7	Fp_2-F_8		7	Fp_2-F_4
8	F_8-T_4		8	F_4-C_4
9	T_4-T_6		9	C_4-P_4
10	T_6-O_2		10	P_4-O_2

Bipolar circumferential Channel			
1	Fp_1-F_7	or	O_1-T_5
2	F_7-T_3		T_5-T_3
3	T_3-T_5		T_3-F_7
4	T_5-O_1		F_7-Fp_1
5	O_1-O_2		Fp_1-Fp_2
6	O_2-T_6		Fp_2-F_8
7	T_6-T_4		F_8-T_4
8	T_4-F_8		T_4-T_6
9	F_8-Fp_2		T_6-O_2
10	Fp_2-Fp_1		O_2-O_1

Bipolar TB anterior transverse[a] Channel		and	Bipolar TB posterior transverse[a] Channel	
1	F_7-F_3		1	A_1-T_3
2	F_3-F_z		2	T_3-C_3
3	F_z-F_4		3	C_3-C_z
4	F_4-F_8		4	C_z-C_4
5	A_1-T_3		5	C_4-T_4
6	T_3-C_3		6	T_4-A_2
7	C_3-C_z		7	T_5-P_3
8	C_z-C_4		8	P_3-P_z
9	C_4-T_4		9	P_z-P_4
10	T_4-A_2		10	P_4-T_6

[a] Recommended in the American EEG Society's *Guidelines in EEG—1980* (2).

TABLE 13.2. *Ten-channel referential montages*

Parasagittal referential[a] Channel		and	Temporal referential[a] Channel	
1	Fp_1-A_1		1	Fp_1-A_1
2	F_3-A_1		2	F_7-A_1
3	C_3-A_1		3	T_3-A_1
4	P_3-A_1		4	T_5-A_1
5	O_1-A_1		5	O_1-A_1
6	Fp_2-A_2		6	Fp_2-A_2
7	F_4-A_2		7	F_8-A_2
8	C_4-A_2		8	T_4-A_2
9	P_4-A_2		9	T_6-A_2
10	O_2-A_2		10	O_2-A_2

Alternating parasagittal referential[a] Channel		or	Alternating temporal referential[a]
1	Fp_1-A_1		Fp_1-A_1
2	Fp_2-A_2		Fp_2-A_2
3	F_3-A_1		F_7-A_1
4	F_4-A_2		F_8-A_2
5	C_3-A_1		T_3-A_1
6	C_4-A_2		T_4-A_2
7	P_3-A_1		T_5-A_1
8	P_4-A_2		T_6-A_2
9	O_1-A_1		O_1-A_1
10	O_2-A_2		O_2-A_2

[a] Recommended in the American EEG Society's *Guidelines in EEG—1980* (2).

In each instance, other references may be used and may be desirable.

TABLE 13.3. *Eight-channel bipolar montages*

Channel	Bipolar (LB) parasagittal[a]	and	Channel	Bipolar (LB) left–right temporal[a]
1	Fp_1-F_3		1	Fp_1-F_7
2	F_3-C_3		2	F_7-T_3
3	C_3-P_3		3	T_3-T_5
4	P_3-O_1		4	T_5-O_1
5	Fp_2-F_4		5	Fp_2-F_8
6	F_4-C_4		6	F_8-T_4
7	C_4-P_4		7	T_4-T_6
8	P_4-O_2		8	T_6-O_2

Channel	Bipolar anterior circumferential[b]	and/or when necessary	Bipolar posterior circumferential[c]
1	T_5-T_3		F_7-T_3
2	T_3-F_7		T_3-T_5
3	F_7-Fp_1		T_5-O_1
4	Fp_1-Fp_2		O_1-O_2
5	Fp_2-F_8		O_2-T_6
6	F_8-T_4		T_6-T_4
7	T_4-T_6		T_4-F_8
8	T_6-T_5		F_8-F_7

[a] Recommended in the American EEG Society's *Guidelines in EEG—1980* (2).
[b] Useful if there are foci at Fp_1 or Fp_2.
[c] Useful if there are foci at O_1 or O_2.

TABLE 13.4. *Eight-channel transverse bipolar montages*

Channel	Frontal–parietal transverse (TB)	and	Channel	Central transverse (TB)
1	F_7-F_3		1	A_1-T_3
2	F_3-F_z		2	T_3-C_3
3	F_z-F_4		3	C_3-C_z
4	F_4-F_8		4	C_z-T_4
5	T_5-P_3		5	T_4-T_6
6	P_3-P_z		6	T_6-A_2
7	P_z-P_4		7	F_z-C_z
8	P_4-T_6		8	C_z-P_z

These montages have features similar to 10-channel transverse bipolar montages.

TABLE 13.5. *Eight-channel referential montages*

Channel	Parasagittal referential[a]	and	Temporal referential[a]	or	Parasagittal referential alternating left–right[a]	and	Temporal referential alternating left–right[a]
1	F_3-A_1		Fp_1-A_1		F_3-A_1		Fp_1-A_1
2	C_3-A_1		F_7-A_1		F_4-A_2		Fp_2-A_2
3	P_3-A_1		T_3-A_1		C_3-A_1		F_7-A_1
4	O_1-A_1		T_5-A_1		C_4-A_2		F_8-A_2
5	F_4-A_2		Fp_2-A_2		P_3-A_1		T_3-A_1
6	C_4-A_2		F_8-A_2		P_4-A_2		T_4-A_2
7	P_4-A_2		T_4-A_2		O_1-A_1		T_5-A_1
8	O_2-A_2		T_6-A_2		O_2-A_2		T_6-A_2

[a] Recommended in the American EEG Society's *Guidelines in EEG—1980* (2).
In each instance, other references may be used and may be desirable.

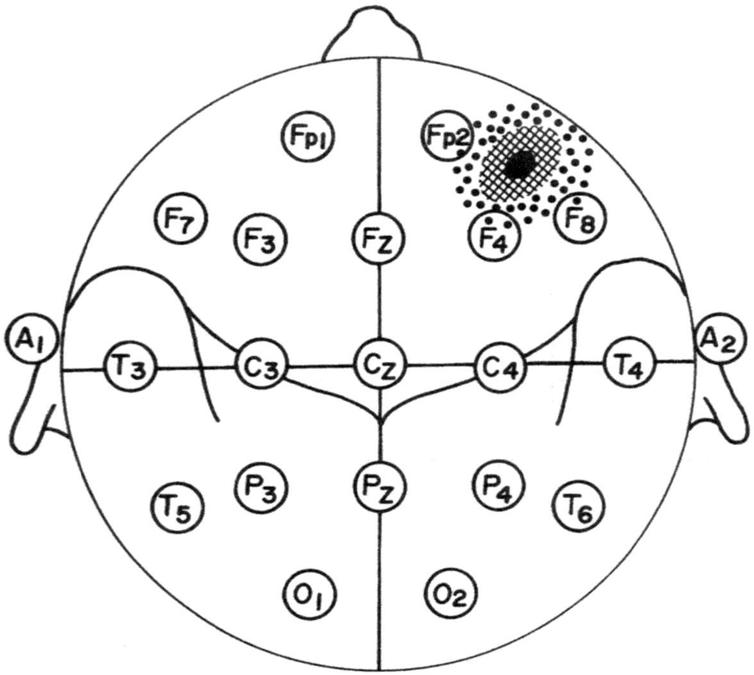

FIG. 13.17. Focus of 2-Hz activity maximal midway between F_8 and Fp_2 (*dense area*). Less involvement in *shaded zone;* still less involvement in *dotted zone*. (See text.)

clarity, schemas are utilized. The question is: Given a particular type of EEG field, what will appear on the record, when different montages are used?

Suppose there is a focus of 2-Hz activity midway between electrode F_8 and Fp_2, with equal spread of voltage to F_8, Fp_2, and F_4. How will this focus appear when 16-channel montages are used to display the record? A map of the field involved is shown in Fig. 13.17.

With the proposed 16-channel anteroposterior left, left, right, right montage, no 2-Hz activity will appear in the left hemisphere. In the right hemisphere, 2-Hz activity will be present equally at F_8, Fp_2, and F_4. This will be seen in the right parasagittal chain and in the right temporal chain, as shown in Fig. 13.18. From the data in Fig. 13.18, it is probable that there is an area of isopotential, including Fp_2 and F_4 and Fp_2, and F_8.

When a transverse montage is used, what appears in the anterior derivations can be seen in Fig. 13.19. When the circumferential montage is used, the display is as shown in Fig. 13.20. Channels 5 and 7 are out of phase because Input 2 of channel 5 and Input 1 of channel 7 simultaneously have the same polarities. In channel 6, they are equipotential. Channels 7 and 15 both show 2-Hz activity in phase because Input 1 of each channel becomes negative (or positive) at the same time.

When a referential montage (Fig. 13.21) is applied to this field, assuming the reference point is completely out of the 2-Hz field (e.g., a noncephalic, neck–chest reference), then the display will show no 2-Hz activity over the left hemisphere or over the midline. In the right hemisphere, it will be limited to Fp_2, F_4, and F_8.

The student can use this same field to analyze montages based on 8-channel instrumentation. It will be found that, using the relatively standard 8-channel montages shown above (Tables 13.3–13.5), it is not possible to display simultaneously the three involved areas in any single montage. On some montages, there will be an isopotential zone at the end of an array. It may prove difficult to synthesize the focus from the data provided by the seven standard montages. Some nonstandard montages therefore should be improvised. From the information made available by the standard series, such inventions should be straightforward. Good basic montages lead to easy improvisation (13). The ability to improvise in the face of necessity is the mark of a superior technologist.

A nonstandard, improvised, alternate montage might in this instance be based on referential procedures. A_1 would be an adequate reference. The montage shown in Fig. 13.22 would serve to demonstrate the focus. Some improvisation will be needed even with 10-channel instrumentation to demonstrate simultaneously the three areas of 2-Hz activity.

SUMMARY

In this chapter, some rules for constructing electrode montages have been presented. The basic unit in the display of EEG activity is formed by one pair of electrodes, called a derivation. Intermediate building blocks, called arrays, may be formed by using adjacent electrodes and recording channels. An array can depict the electrical activity of an anatomically defined region of the brain. A suitable combination of arrays can display an anatomically oriented record of the brain's electrical activity.

Bipolar montages utilize adjacent electrodes in the formation of their

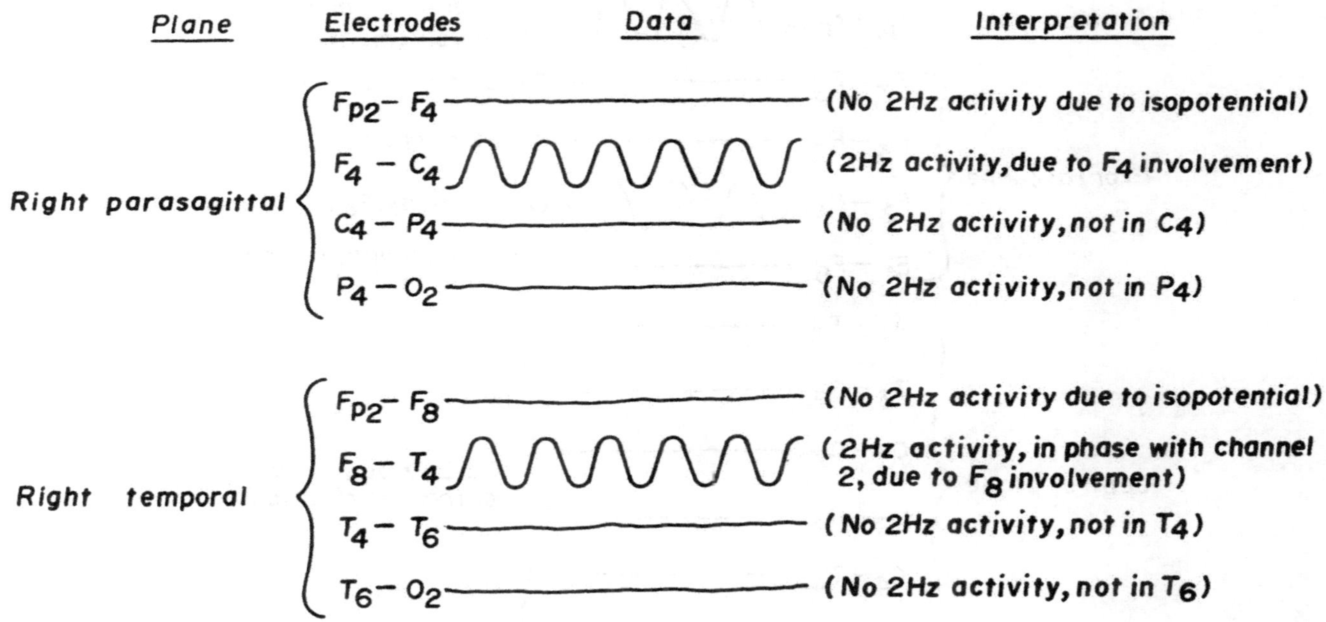

FIG. 13.18. Right hemisphere derivations of 16-channel A – P montage, including data and interpretation. (see text.) The term "isopotential" has the same meaning as "equipotential."

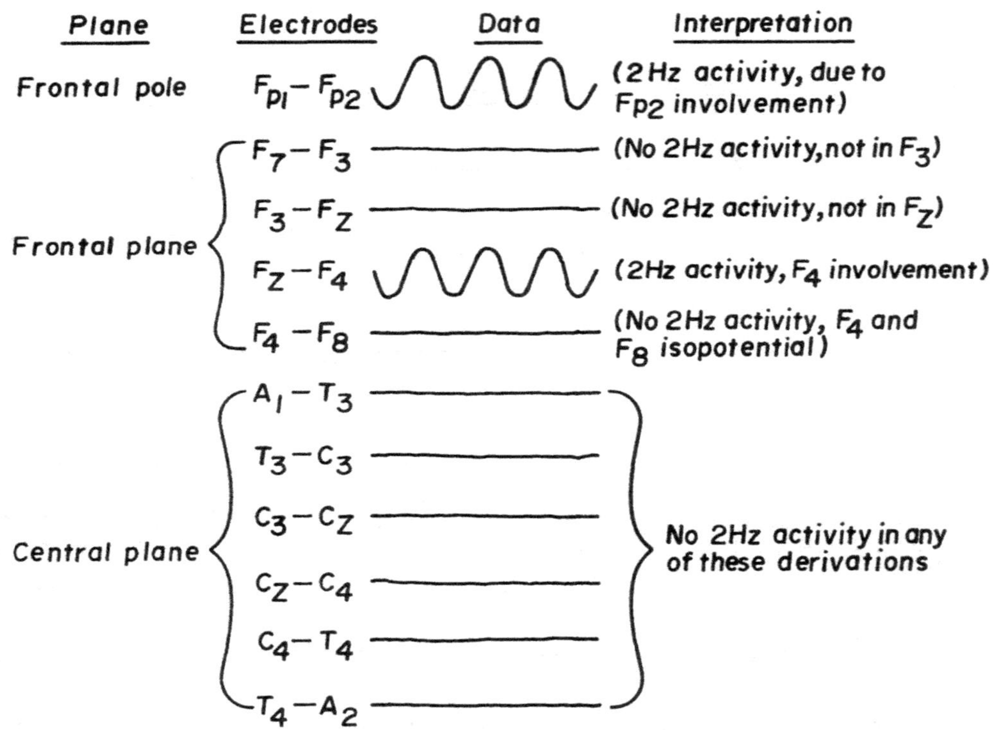

FIG. 13.19. Appearance in transverse bipolar montage of focal activity generated in Fig. 13.17. (see also Fig. 13.18 and text.)

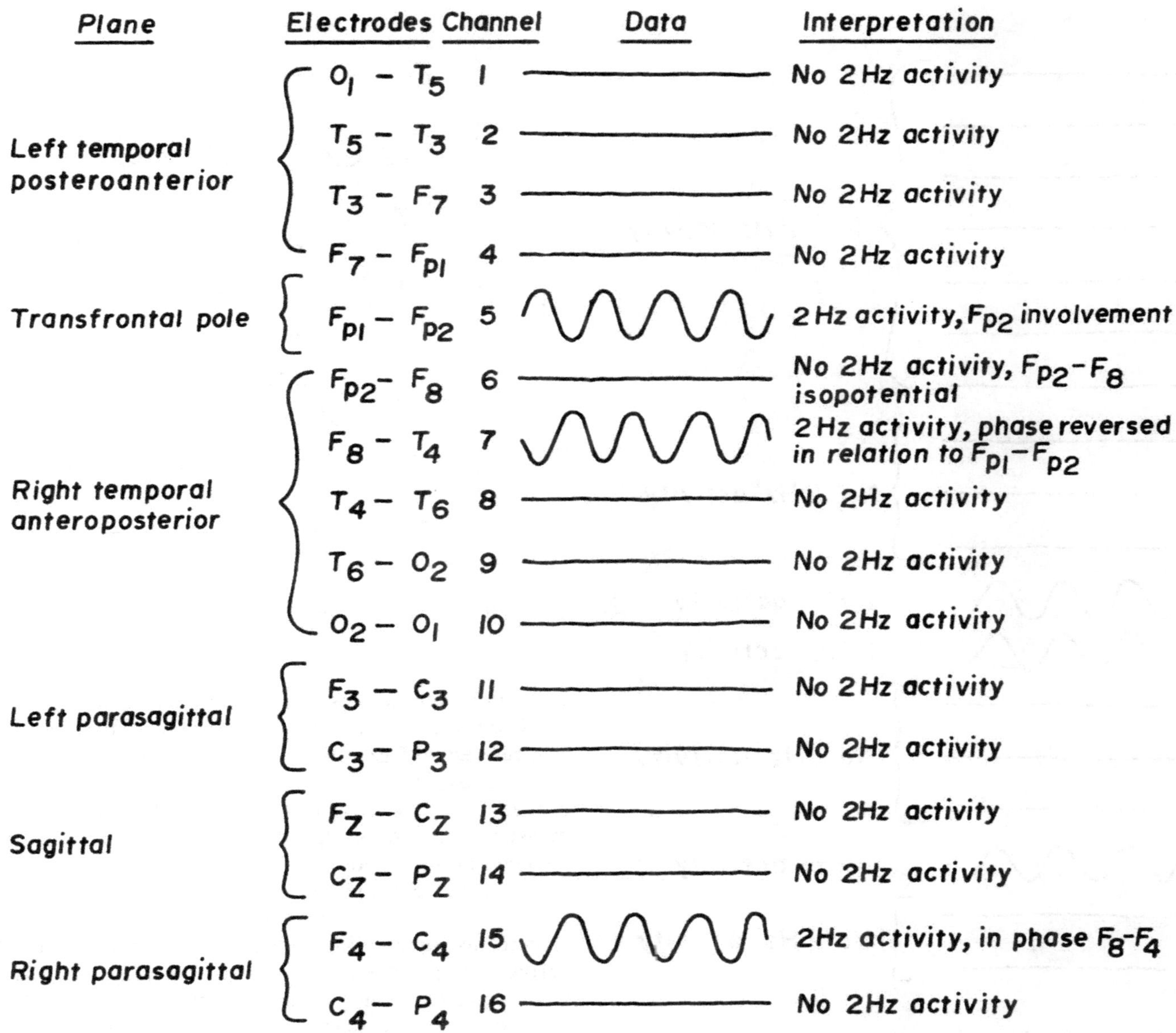

FIG. 13.20. A 16-channel circumferential montage, with 2-Hz activity at Fp_2. F_8-F_4 equipotential. Fp_2-F_8 and F_8-T_4 derivations phase reverse because of Fp_2-F_8 equipotential and their input connections to channels 5 and 7.

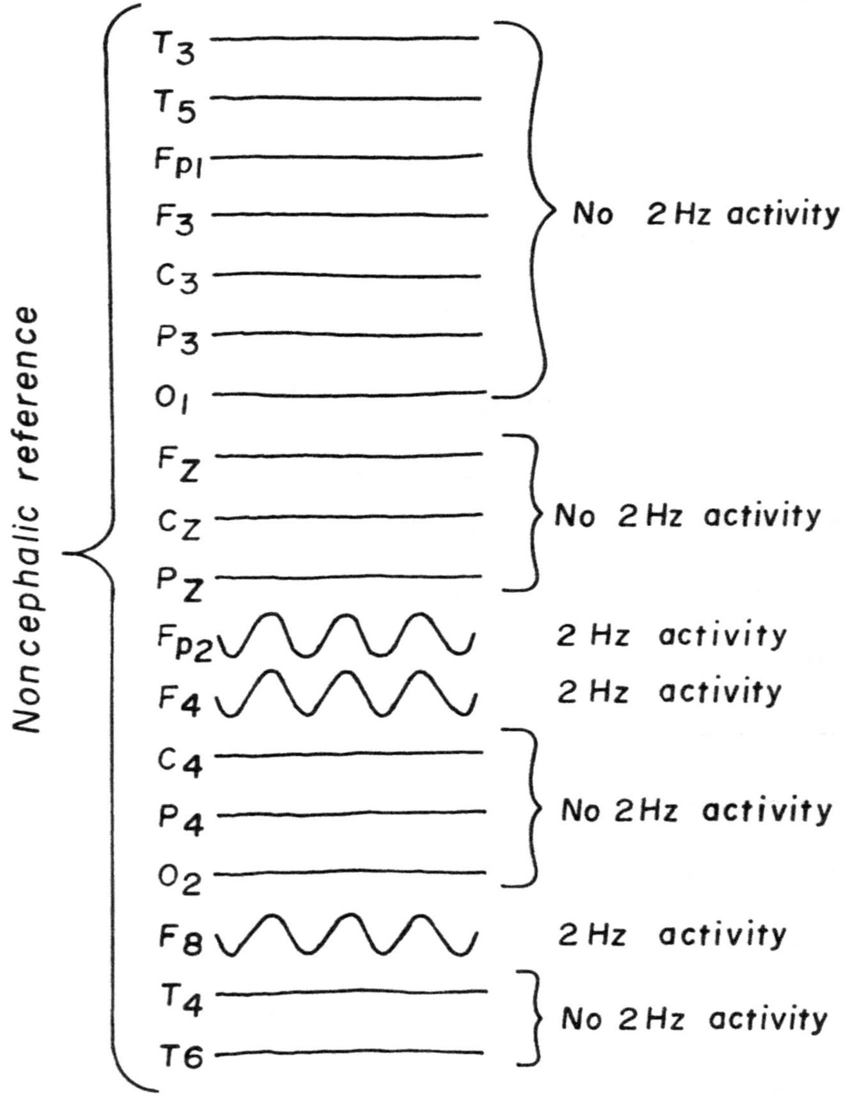

FIG. 13.21. An 18-channel referential montage. Same focus as Fig. 13.20. (see text.)

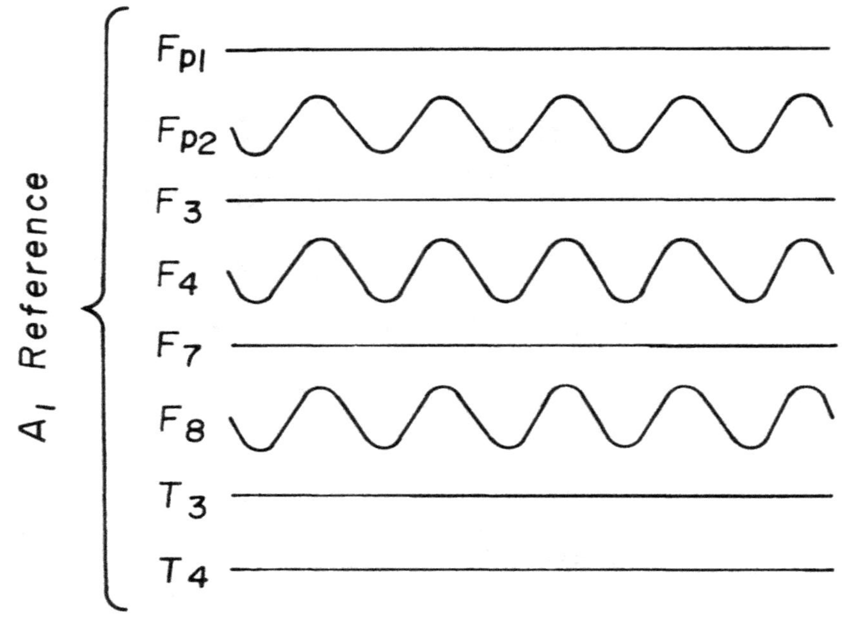

FIG. 13.22. Nonstandard, improvised alternate referential montage.

derivations and arrays. Using the polarity convention, it is possible to localize the origins and surface polarity of EEG activity.

A referential EEG montage uses one common electrode in every channel. It is assumed that this electrode has no significant input to the recorded EEG. Localization of activity then can be deduced by voltage measurements. As in the case of bipolar recording, polarity of an event also can be specified by using the polarity conventions. If the reference is active, however, localization and polarity may be difficult to deduce.

A basic series of practical montages was developed for 18- and 16-channel instrumentation. When fewer channels are used, montages can be derived that provide easily compared displays of EEG activity. However, while three basic montages will suffice for 18- or 16-channel use, seven montages are necessary for 10- and 8-channel applications. When 8-channel instrumentation is employed, supplementary montages are usually required.

The applications of various montages to several problems of localization demonstrate that bipolar and referential montages supplement each other.

REFERENCES

1. American EEG Society (1980): 3. Minimum technical requirements for performing clinical electroencephalography. In: *Guidelines in EEG—1980*. American EEG Society, Tucker, Georgia.
2. American EEG Society (1980): 7. A proposal for standard montages to be used in clinical electroencephalography. In: *Guidelines in EEG—1980*. American EEG Society, Tucker, Georgia.
3. Berger, H. (1929): Über das Elektrenkephalogramm des Menschen. *Arch. Psychiatr. Nervenkr.*, 87:527–570.
4. Berger, H. (1930): Über das Elektrenkephalogramm des Menschen. Zweite Mitteilung. *J. Psychol. Neurol.*, 40:160–179.
5. Gibbs, F. A., and Gibbs, E. L. (1952): *Atlas of Electroencephalography, Vol. II: Epilepsy*, p. 164. Addison-Wesley, Reading, Massachusetts.
6. Gibbs, E. L., Gibbs, F. A., and Fuster, B. (1948): Psychomotor epilepsy. *Arch. Neurol. Psychiatry*, 60:331–339.
7. Gloor, P. (1977): Application of volume conduction principles to montage design, *Am. J. EEG Technol.*, 17:5–20.
8. Goldman, D. (1950): The clinical use of the "average" reference electrode in monopolar recording. *Electroencephalogr. Clin. Neurophysiol.*, 2:211–214.
9. Harner, R. N. (1977): Recommendation for standard EEG montages. *Am. J. EEG Technol.* 17:105–114.
10. Henry, C. E. (1977): Relative merits of different montages for optimal display of EEG activity. *Am. J. EEG Technol.*, 17:21–51.
11. Henry, C. E. (1979): Optimal display of EEG activity. In: *Current Practice of Clinical Electroencephalography*, edited by D. W. Klass and D. D. Daly, pp. 179–220. Raven Press, New York.
12. Klass, D. W. (1977): Symposium on EEG montages: Which, when, why and whither. Introduction. *Am. J. EEG Technol.*, 17:1–4.
13. Klem, G. H. (1977): Montages from the standpoint of the EEG technologist. *Am. J. EEG Technol.*, 17:101–104.
14. Knott, J. R. (1976): *A Rationale for Developing Electrode Montages for 16, 8 and 10 Channel EEG Instrumentation*, 32 p. Grass Instrument Co., Quincy, Massachusetts.
15. Knott, J. R. (1977): Commonly used electrode montages in clinical electroencephalography. *Am. J. EEG Technol.*, 17:85–99.
16. Offner, F. F. (1950): The EEG as potential mapping: The value of the average monopolar reference. *Electroencephalogr. Clin. Neurophysiol.*, 2:215–216.
17. Ropper, A. H., Chiappa, K. H., and Grass, E. R. (1978): A practical non-cephalic reference electrode: The Stephenson-Gibbs non-cephalic system. *Clin. Electroencephalogr.*, 9:140–143.
18. Sharbrough, F. W. (1977): The mathematical logic for the design of montages. *Am. J. EEG Technol.*, 17:73–83.
19. Stephenson, W. A., and Gibbs, F. A., (1951): A balanced noncephalic reference electrode. *Electroencephalogr. Clin. Neurophysiol.*, 3:139–143.
20. *Webster's Third New International Dictionary* (1971): G. & C. Merriam Co., Springfield, Massachusetts.

Chapter 14

Classification of EEG Activity

The goal of clinical EEG is to make a useful diagnostic evaluation of a particular patient. Because the technologist views the ongoing EEG activity as it is recorded and selects the montages and makes changes in instrument controls to facilitate the display of the EEG, it is essential that he or she become familiar with and recognize the major features that appear in the ongoing record. On the basis of the features that do or do not appear, the record may be classified as normal or abnormal. However, a distinction must be made between normal and abnormal EEG *activity* and a normal or abnormal EEG *record*.

Electroencephalographers and technologists are surrounded by patients who are presumed to be ill. This presumption encourages the belief that any seemingly unusual characteristic that appears in the EEG record of a patient is an abnormality. It is necessary that properly designed investigations be carried out to establish whether particular EEG features are normal or abnormal.

NORMAL VERSUS ABNORMAL EEG ACTIVITY

Normal EEG activity is any of the many kinds of distinctive activities that, qualitatively and quantitatively, appear in the EEGs of large groups of persons known to have no complaints, no symptoms, no neurological or other disease, and no immediate relatives with neurological disease. These groups will be referred to as "healthy" or "control" groups. Any EEG activity observed in healthy groups in relation to age, gender, and state of the person (e.g., awake, asleep) is normal EEG activity.

Abnormal EEG activity is any of the many kinds of EEG activities that, qualitatively and quantitatively, do not appear in the EEGs of healthy groups but do appear in groups of persons defined by specific complaints, identifiable symptoms, or specific neurological or other disease in themselves or in close relatives. The latter groups will be referred to as "sick" or "patient" groups.

NORMAL VERSUS ABNORMAL EEG RECORD

A normal EEG record shows activity within ranges expected after study of healthy groups and does not show any activity, qualitatively or quantitatively, within the characteristic ranges of patient groups.

An abnormal EEG record qualitatively and quantitatively shows activities beyond the range expected in healthy groups, even though some, or perhaps nearly all, of the activity in the record may be normal.

To a considerable degree, the expressions "normal" and "abnormal" are defined negatively and in terms of each other.

GROUP COMPARISONS

Some EEG activities present in patient groups are, in varying degrees, seen in healthy groups. In some instances, there will be overlap of distinctive EEG characteristics between a healthy group and any chosen patient group. Since a great many patient EEGs are recorded, the healthy groups that are studied also must be very large. If an EEG pattern appears only in a very small number of patients (e.g., 5 in 5,000), then it is necessary to have a sufficiently large number of healthy subjects to allow for the pattern, if present, to appear in that group. Rarity of a pattern is not necessarily equivalent to abnormality.

The overlap of some EEG characteristics in healthy and patient groups can lead to diagnostic errors. If a record is called abnormal when there is a moderate overlap, the error may lead to a false-positive EEG diagnosis. If it is regarded as normal, the error may lead to a false-negative EEG diagnosis. It is important to remember that clear-cut, either-or, distinctions between normal and abnormal EEG activity and normal and abnormal EEG records are not always possible.

Comparison among patient groups without reference to healthy groups increases the possibility of false-positive and false-negative errors. Not only must healthy subjects be compared adequately with sick subjects, but many different, well-defined groups of patients with different illnesses must have their EEGs recorded and compared. Unless this is done, there is the danger that an EEG characteristic may be mistakenly believed to be associated with, for example, disease A, because it occurs three times more often in patients with that disease than in healthy subjects. When the EEGs of patients with disease B are investigated, however, the EEG pattern in question may appear equally as often as in disease A. Therefore, it has little diagnostic meaning.

Later investigations of healthy subjects sometimes have made it necessary to conclude that some EEG activities originally believed to be abnormal appear in control groups with sufficient frequency to regard them as normal variants. When qualitative patterns are involved, these sometimes have been called "patterns of uncertain diagnostic significance" (50).

Thus, over the course of time and as more adequate study has been made of healthy subjects, three categories of EEG characteristics have emerged: (1) normal activity, which appears in healthy persons, (2) abnormal activity, which appears much more often in patient groups, and (3) activity of uncertain significance, which appears in both healthy and patient groups.

A normal EEG record includes no abnormal activity, but it may contain patterns of uncertain significance. An abnormal EEG record may show a preponderance of normal activity, but it also shows abnormal activity that has such a small overlap with control groups that few false-positive EEG diagnoses will occur.

VARIABLES USED IN CLASSIFICATION OF EEG ACTIVITY

EEG activity is described in terms of several variables, each of which must be considered in relation to the patient's age and state. The expression "state" refers to the patient's level of responsiveness (e.g., alert, responsive, attentive, inattentive, relaxed, awake, asleep, stuporous, comatose, and so forth).

The EEG variables are, in one form or another, the basic descriptors used by most electroencephalographers (38,39,54,65,68). It should be stressed that they are electrographic, that is, they are derived from and described in terms of their EEG characteristics.

Further, EEG activity often is described in terms of its own context. What appears in the record at a specific point may be descriptively contrasted with what appears at an immediately preceding point. Major EEG patterns and changes in activity are often said to appear in or against a "background," which is the setting from which such (a change or pattern) is distinguished (10). Background activity can represent either normal or abnormal activity, and the EEG characteristic being described may itself be either normal or abnormal.

The following variables are used, sometimes quantitatively and sometimes qualitatively, to describe EEG activity. Not all terms are employed in the same manner by all electroencephalographers and technologists. The definitions given here are based on a review of common usage, and we have attempted to synthesize what appear to be general meanings.[1]

Frequency

Frequency refers to rhythmic repetitive EEG activity (in Hz) or the equivalent frequency (the inverse of the duration) of isolated single waves. Three terms are used relative to frequency:

1. *Rhythmic*. EEG activity consisting of waves of approximately constant frequency (Fig. 14.1).
2. *Arrhythmic*. EEG activity in which no stable rhythms are present (Fig. 14.2).
3. *Dysrhythmic*. The word *dysrhythmia* appears in many of the systems for classifying EEG activity. As used here (and by many American and English electroencephalographers) it refers to rhythms and/or patterns of EEG activity that characteristically appear in patient groups and are rarely or never seen in healthy subjects (Fig. 14.3). Thus, it has implications regarding not only specific frequencies but also morphology, which depends on mixtures of frequencies. The prefix *dys* comes from the Greek and means bad or difficult. Its use in the construction of medical terms is well-known. For example: dysplasia—abnormal growth or development; dyslexia—disturbance of the ability to read; dyspepsia—indigestion.

Voltage

Voltage refers to average voltage or peak voltage of EEG activity. Voltage values are dependent, in part, on the recording technique; closely spaced bipolar derivations yield lower voltages than widely spaced refer-

[1] We have drawn upon "A Glossary of Terms Most Commonly Used by Clinical Electroencephalographers" (10). However, we have modified definitions where we believe it would help to conform to common usage.

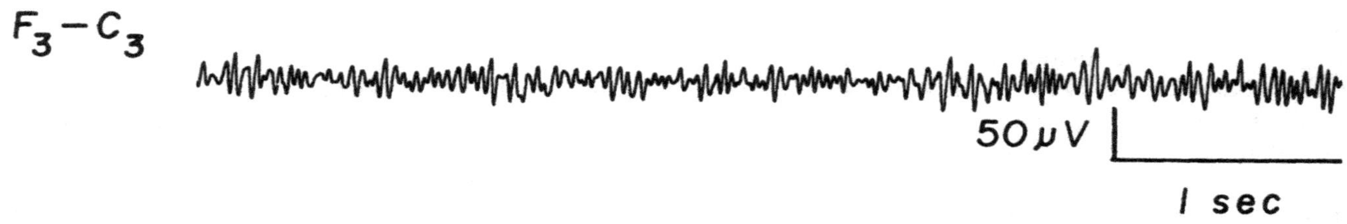

FIG. 14.1. Rhythmic beta activity.

ential derivations. EEG amplitude should be described in terms of the observed voltages and not as "low," "medium," or "high" amplitude. Amplitude alone has no quantitative meaning. A "high amplitude" EEG record will be obtained if 20-μV alpha activity is recorded with S = 1 μV/mm (a 20-mm deflection). The record will be "low amplitude" if S = 20 μV/mm (a 1-mm deflection). The voltage in either case is the same.

Three terms relating to voltage are:

1. *Attenuation* (synonyms: suppression, depression). Reduction of amplitude of EEG activity resulting from decreased voltage. When activity is attenuated by stimulation, it is said to have been "blocked" or to show "blocking" (see Fig. 14.4). If complete loss of EEG activity is implied, then the highest sensitivity available (1 μV/mm) must be used to demonstrate the loss.
2. *Hypersynchrony:* Seen as an increase in voltage and regularity of rhythmic activity, often within the alpha, beta or theta range. The term implies an increase in the number of neural elements contributing to the rhythm, but it is used here not in an interpretative sense but as descriptor of change in the EEG (see Fig. 14.5).
3. *Paroxysmal:* Activity that emerges from background with a rapid onset, reaching (usually) quite high voltage, and ending with an abrupt return to lower voltage activity. There is associated change in frequency and morphology. *The term does not directly imply abnormality.* Some normal activity has paroxysmal features (Fig. 14.6A). Much abnormal activity is paroxysmal (Fig. 14.6B).

Morphology (Wave-form)

Morphology refers to the shape of the waveform. The shape of a wave or of an EEG pattern is determined by the frequencies that combine to make up the waveform and by their phase and voltage relationships. Dawson and Walter (16) were the first to synthesize EEG patterns by mixing different sine wave frequencies and varying their voltage and phase relationships. This demonstration has been largely overlooked, although its importance in the practice of EEG seems obvious: Recording techniques should preserve as nearly as possible the original phase and voltage of component frequencies and thus avoid distortion of morphology.

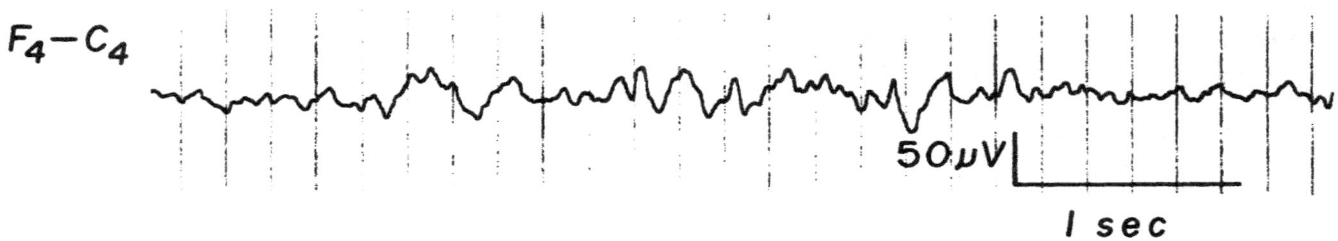

FIG. 14.2. Arrhythmic activity.

FIG. 14.3. Dysrhythmic activity with gross disturbance of frequency, voltage, and organization in a 6-month-old infant. HF = 70 Hz; LF = 1 Hz. Note: S = 30 μV/mm.

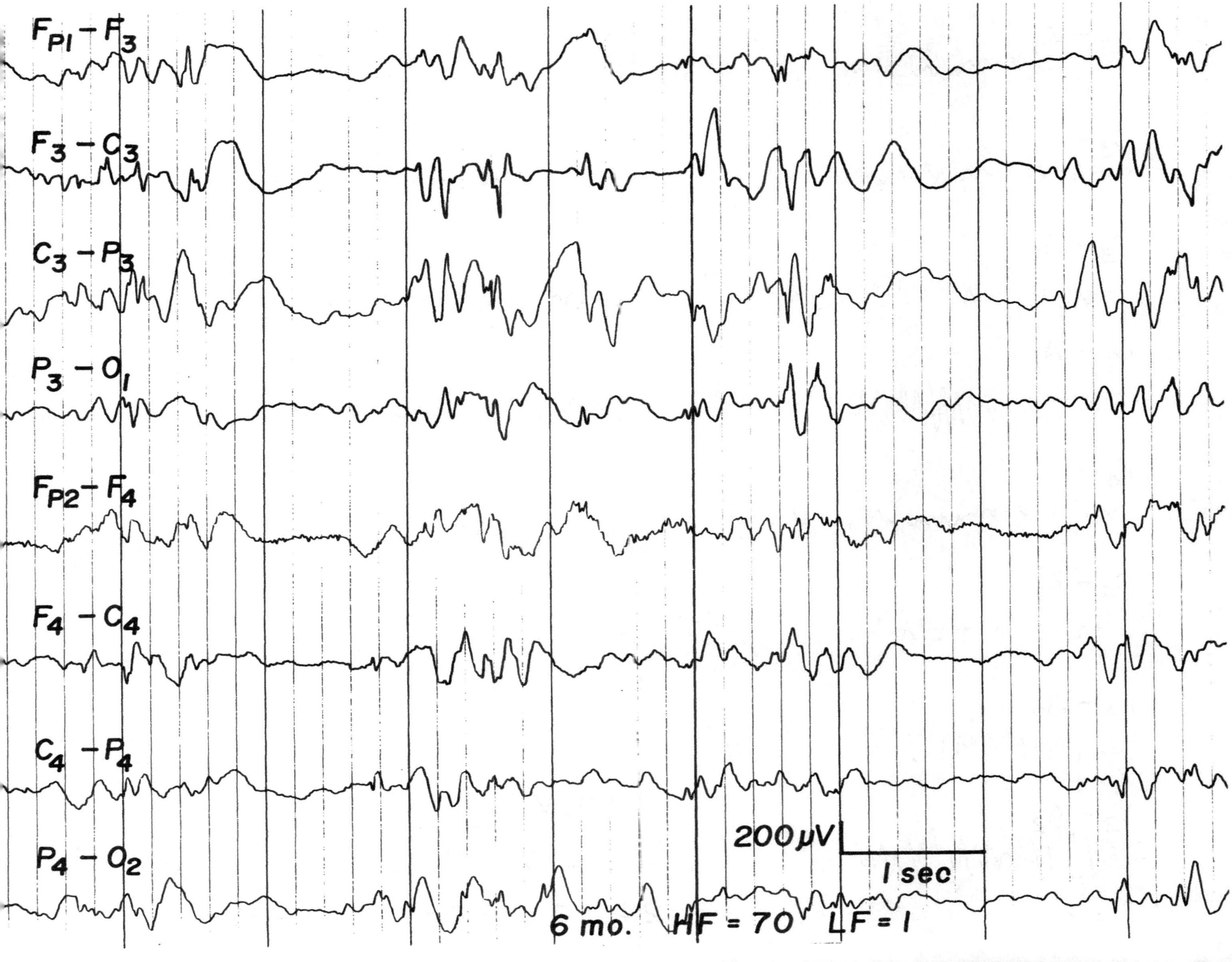

FP1 - F3
F3 - C3
C3 - P3
P3 - O1
FP2 - F4
F4 - C4
C4 - P4
P4 - O2
200 μV
1 sec
6 mo. HF = 70 LF = 1

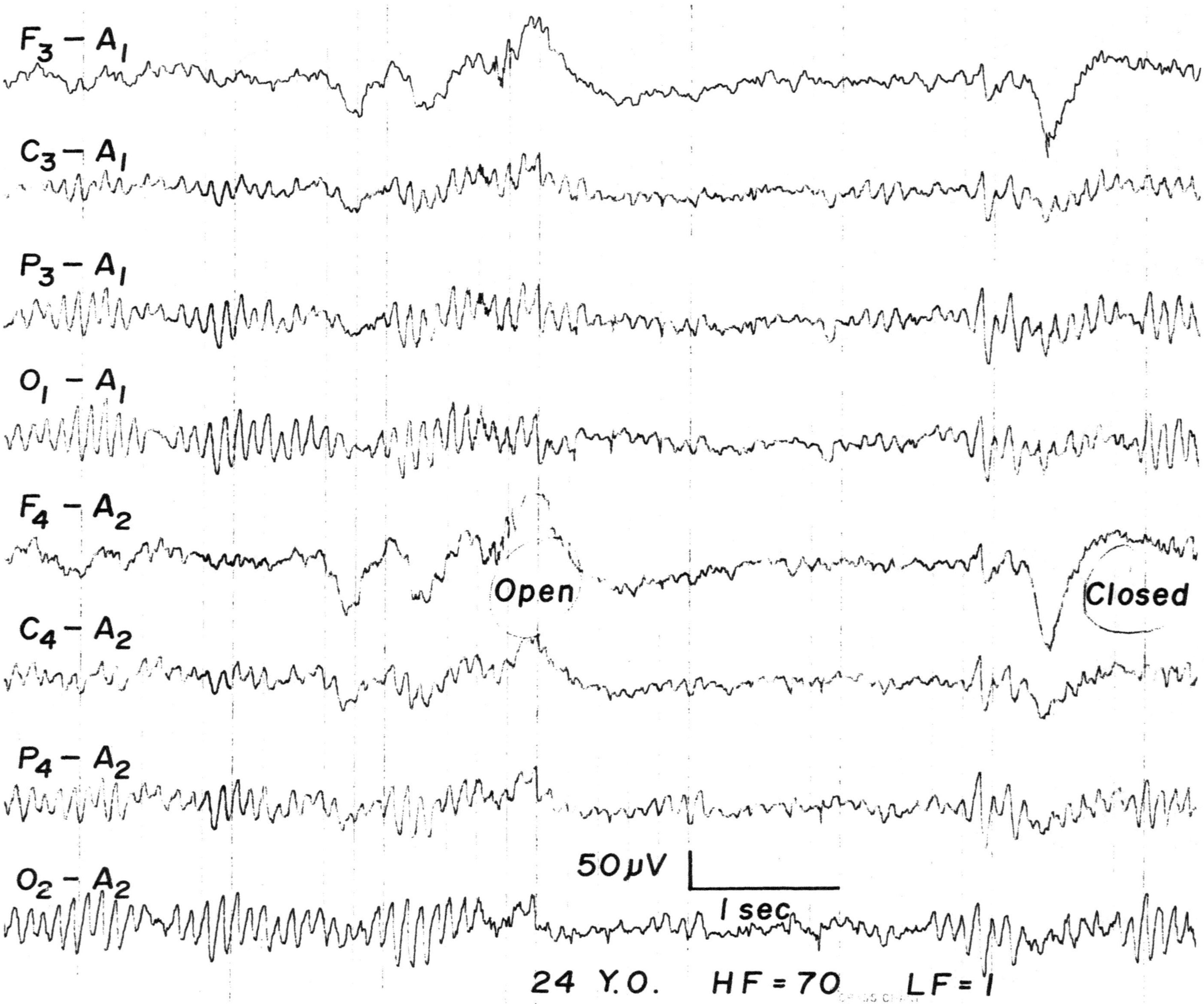
F3 – A1
C3 – A1
P3 – A1
O1 – A1
F4 – A2
Open
Closed
C4 – A2
P4 – A2
O2 – A2
50 μV
1 sec
24 Y.O. HF = 70 LF = 1

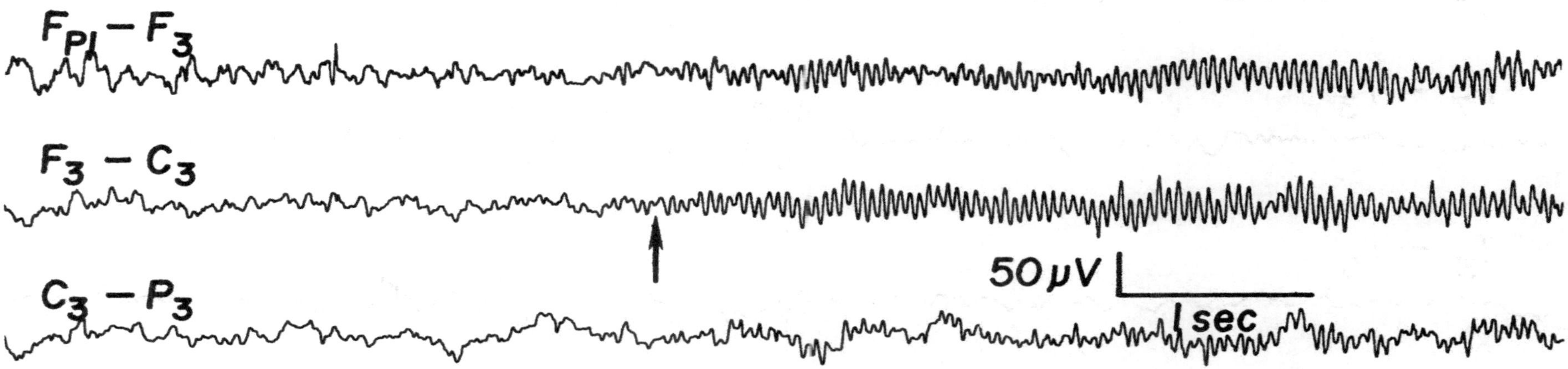

FIG. 14.5. Hypersynchronous 18- to 20-Hz activity beginning first at F_3-C_3 (*arrow*) and emerging from an arrhythmic background of less than 20 μV.

Surface polarity is described as the negative or positive polarity of a particular activity or waveform at a particular electrode location.

Terms relating to waveform include:

1. *Monomorphic*. Distinct EEG activity appearing to be composed of one dominant frequency (Fig. 14.7).
2. *Polymorphic*. Distinct EEG activity composed of multiple frequencies that combine to form a complex waveform (Fig. 14.8).
3. *Sinusoidal*. Waves resembling sine waves. Monomorphic activity usually is sinusoidal.
4. *Transient*. An isolated wave or pattern that is distinctly different from background activity (Fig. 14.9). (a) *Spike:* "A transient . . . with . . . a pointed peak and a duration from 20 to under 70 msec . . ." (10) (Fig. 14.10). (b) *Sharp wave:* "A transient . . . with . . . pointed peak and duration of 70–200 msec . . ." (10) (Fig. 14.11).
5. *Complex*. A sequence of two or more waves, not necessarily of the same frequency, with distinct form or pattern different from background activity, for example, (a) *spike-and-wave complex* (Fig. 14.12) and (b) *sharp-and-slow-wave complex* (Fig. 14.13).
6. *Biphasic* (*diphasic*). A wave or complex having two distinct components, one surface positive and the other surface negative (Fig. 14.14).
7. *Triphasic*. A wave or complex having three distinct components, such as negative—positive—negative or positive—negative—positive (Fig. 14.15).

Epileptiform pattern: According to the International Committee, an "interpretive term. Applies to distinctive waves or complexes, distinguished from background activity, and resembling those recorded in a proportion of human subjects suffering from epileptic disorders . . ." (10). The fact that this is an interpretive term should be stressed. It is not an *electrographic* term. For purposes of descriptive classification, it is preferable to use *only* electrographic terms and not to use terms implying clinical diagnostic specificity (37). Whenever the word is encountered, it should be placed in an electrographic frame of reference: Distinctive

FIG. 14.4. Alpha blocking elicited by eye opening in a 24-year-old subject. HF = 70 Hz; LF = 1 Hz.

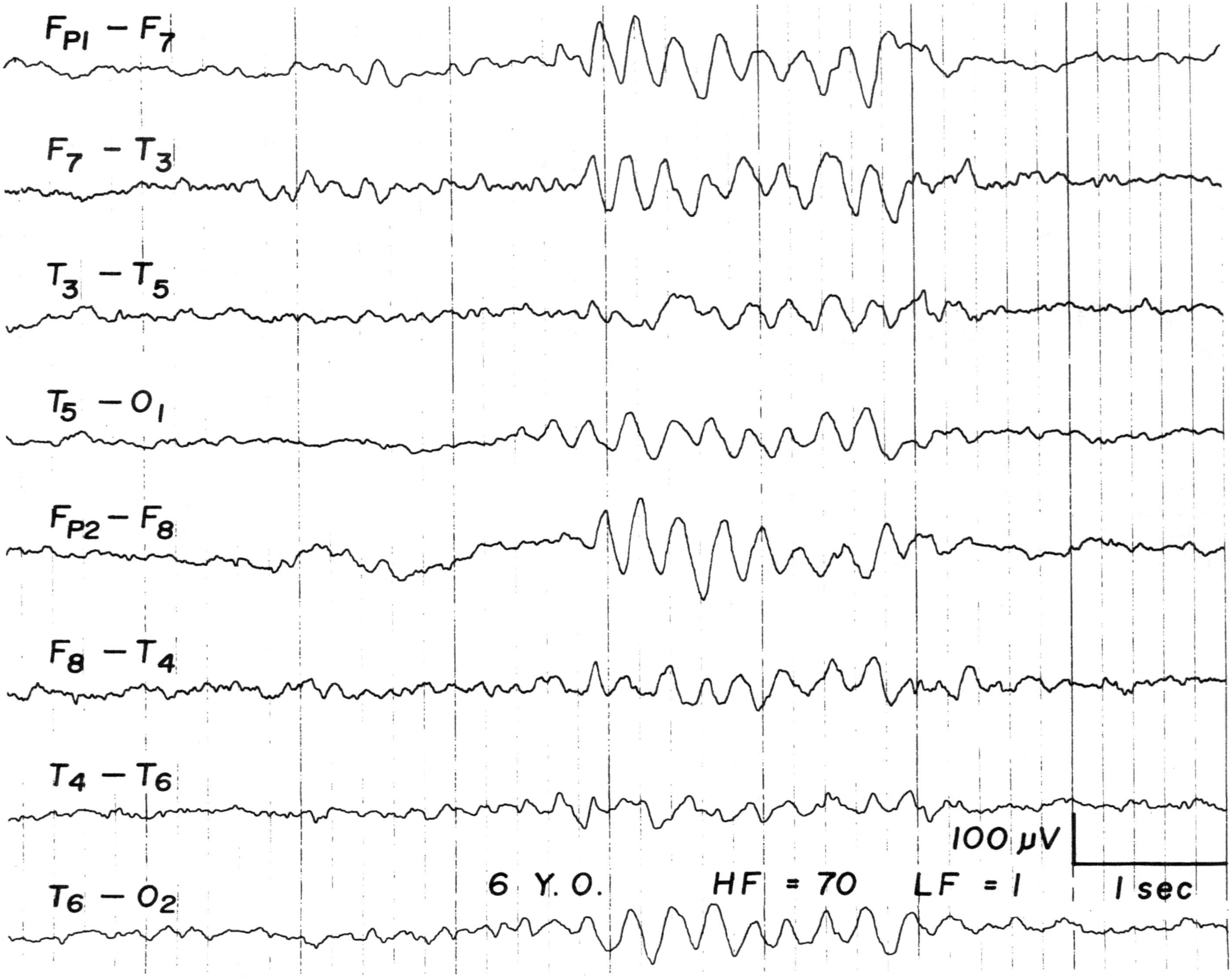

FIG. 14.6. A: Normal paroxysmal slow activity (3–4 Hz) during drowsiness in a 6-year-old child. (*cont'd.*)

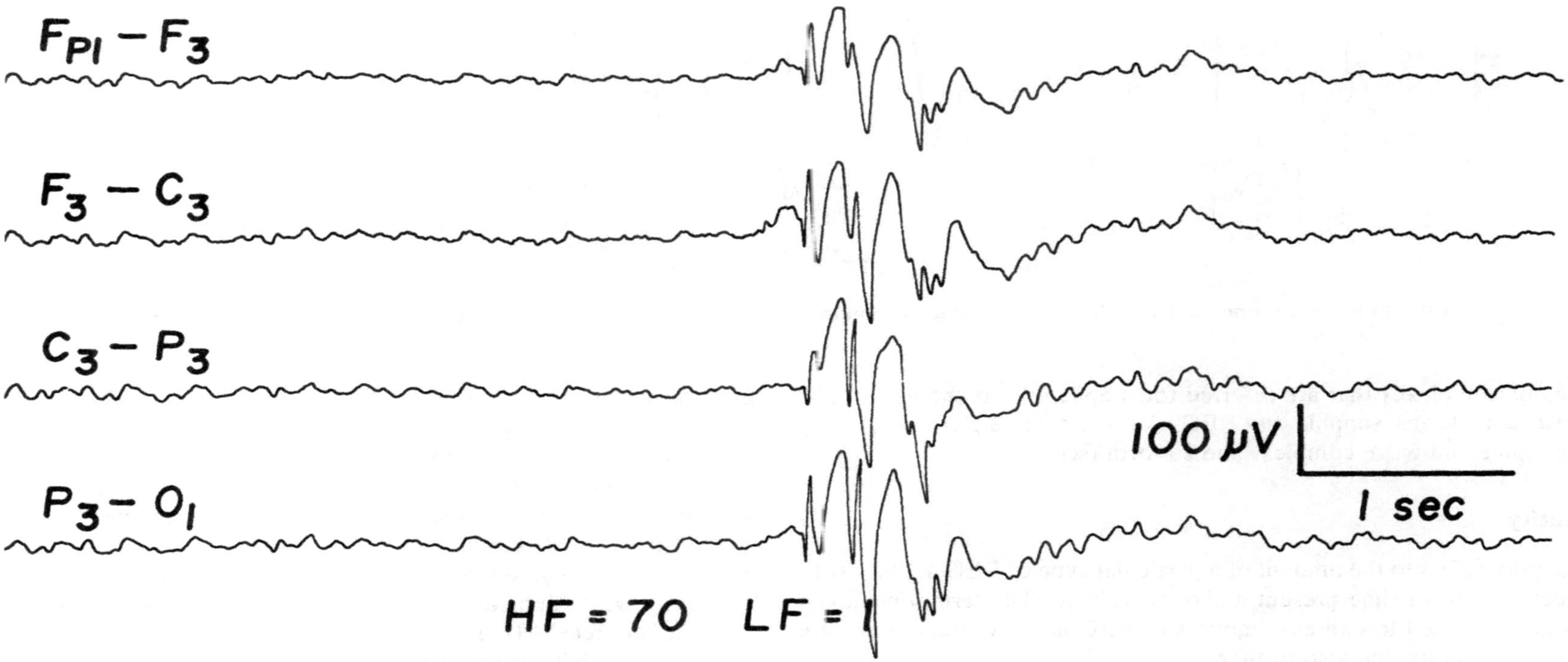

FIG. 14.6. (*cont'd.*). **B:** Abnormal paroxysmal activity consisting of spikes and waves. HF = 70 Hz; LF = 1 Hz.

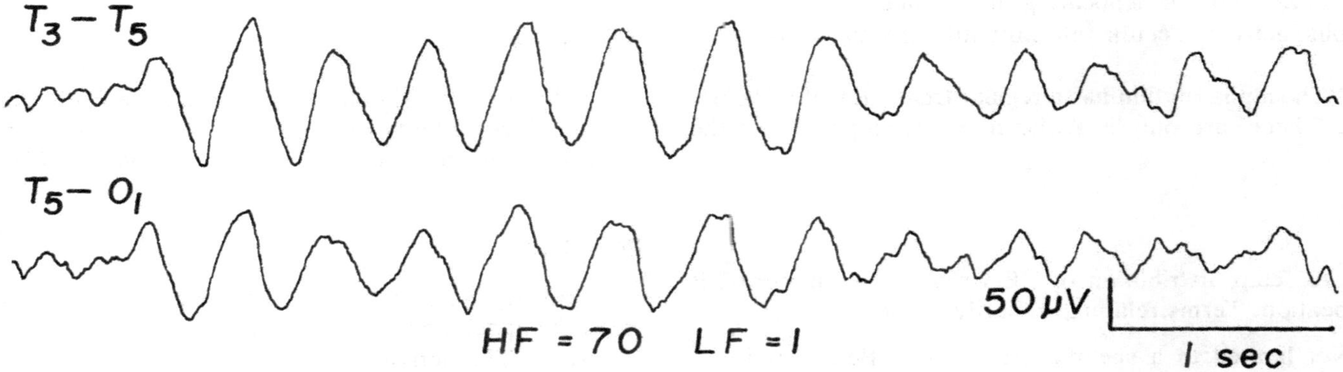

FIG. 14.7. Monomorphic 2.5-Hz activity. HF = 70 Hz; LF = 1 Hz.

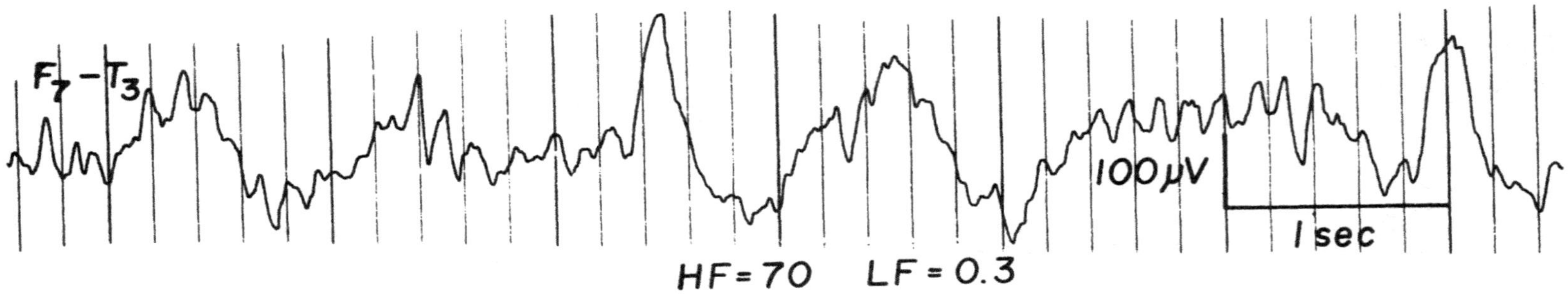

FIG. 14.8. Polymorphic activity. Multiple frequencies combine to form complex and varying waveforms. HF = 70 Hz; LF = 0.3 Hz.

waves or complexes that are referred to as epileptiform should be fully described in terms suitable for EEG classification [e.g., spike, sharp wave, spike-and-wave complex, and so forth (see 57)].

Quantity

Quantity refers to the amount of a particular type of EEG activity with respect to percent time present and/or to voltage. The term *abundance* sometimes is used to express amounts of EEG activity. Four terms are related to quantity and also to time:

1. *Continuous*. Occurring without interruption (e.g., "There is continuous alpha activity").
2. *Discontinuous* (*intermittent*). Appearing from time to time (e.g., "Rhythmic alpha activity occurs intermittently, in short trains or runs").
3. *Regular* (e.g., "The alpha rhythm has a regular frequency of 9 Hz").
4. *Irregular* (e.g., "There are only irregular frequencies present in the record").

Location

Location refers to scalp distribution of EEG rhythms or patterns; it implies cerebral location. Terms relating primarily to location are:

1. *Generalized*. Not limited to a specific area (e.g., "Beta activity is present in all areas") (Fig. 14.16).
2. *Lateral* (*lateralized*). Coming from one side (e.g., "Slow activity is present over the right temporal-frontal areas") (Fig. 14.17).
3. *Bilateral*. Coming from both sides (e.g., "Bilateral spike activity in the left and right anterior areas with foci at F_7 and F_8") (Fig. 14.18).
4. *Focal*. Coming from a local region (e.g., "Spike activity is present in the right frontal-central area") (Fig. 14.19).
5. *Symmetry*. Equal distribution of EEG activity over homologous head areas (e.g., "Alpha activity is seen symmetrically in the left and right occipital areas") (Fig. 14.20). Bilateral activity is symmetrical. Lateralized activity is asymmetrical. Activity may be asymmetrical because (a) it is generated only in one-half of the brain, or (b) it is attenuated in one-half of the brain.

Synchrony

Synchrony is the simultaneous appearance of rhythmic or morphologically distinct patterns over different regions of the head, either on the same side (unilateral) or on both sides (bilateral) (Fig. 14.20).

Periodicity

Periodicity refers to the distribution of patterns or elements in time (e.g., the appearance of a particular EEG activity at more or less regular intervals). The activity may be generalized, focal, or lateralized (Fig. 14.21).

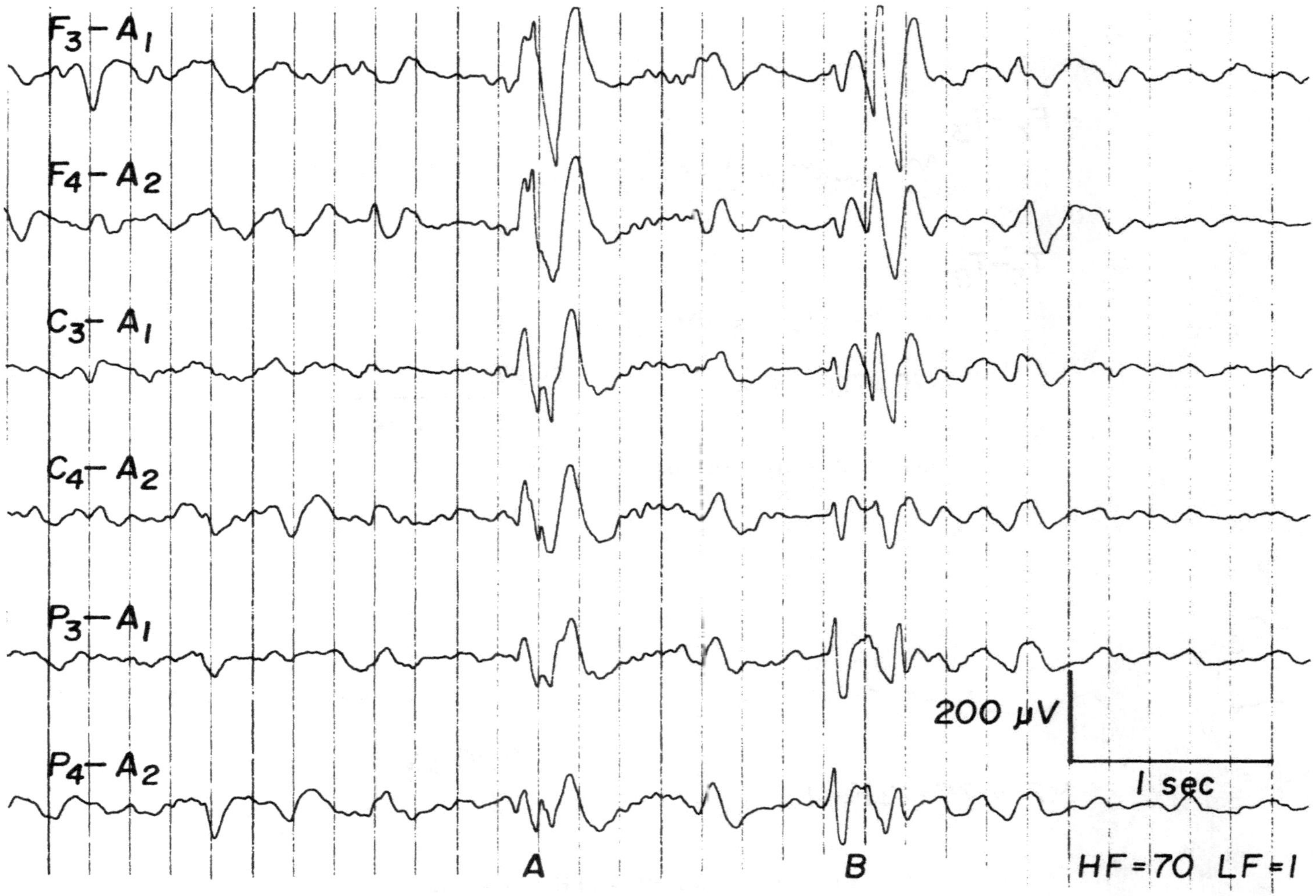

FIG. 14.9. Transient activity. Isolated waves at *A* and *B* appear as high voltage (>300 μV) waves. Background activity is composed of lower voltage (<150 μV) theta activity. HF = 70 Hz; LF = 1 Hz.

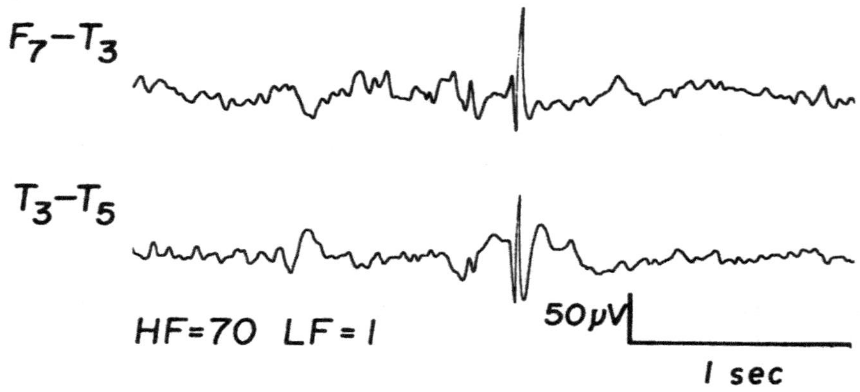

FIG. 14.10. An isolated spike. HF = 70 Hz; LF = 1 Hz.

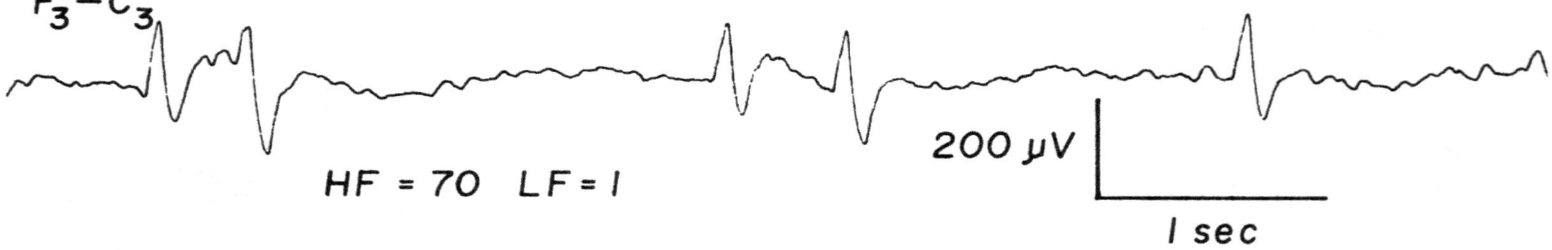

FIG. 14.11. Sharp waves. HF = 70 Hz; LF = 1 Hz.

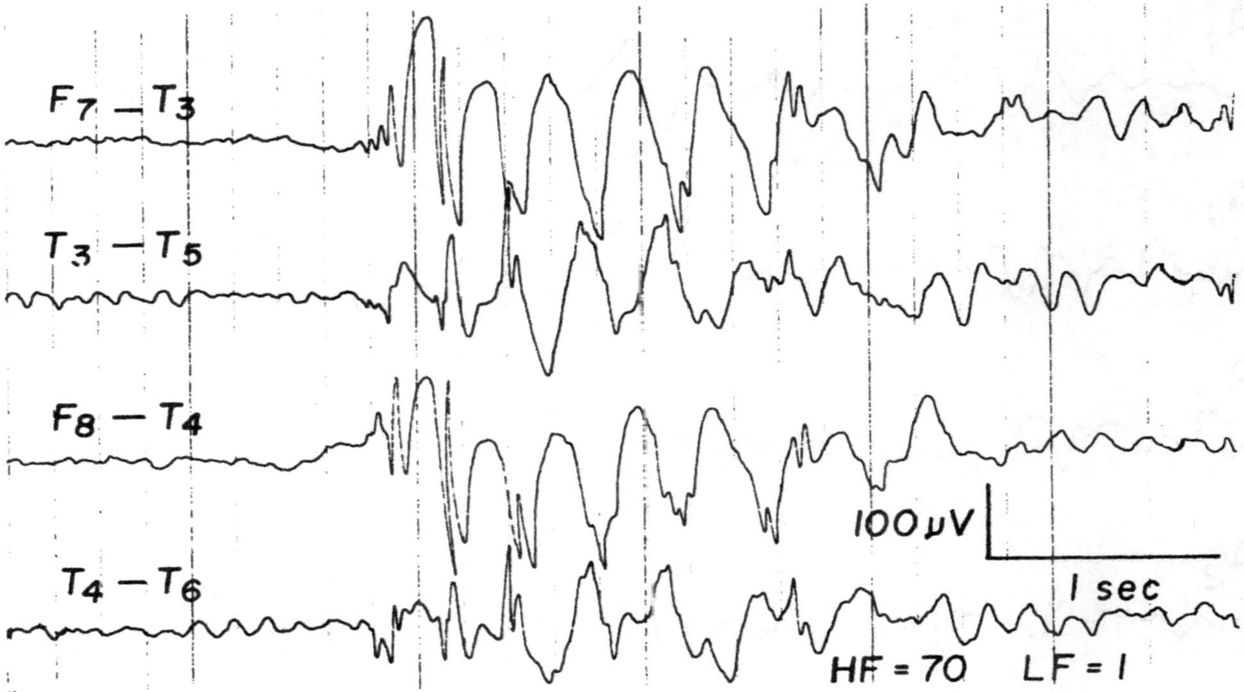

FIG. 14.12. Rhythmic 3-Hz spike-and-wave complex (a type of paroxysmal activity). HF = 70 Hz; LF = 1 Hz.

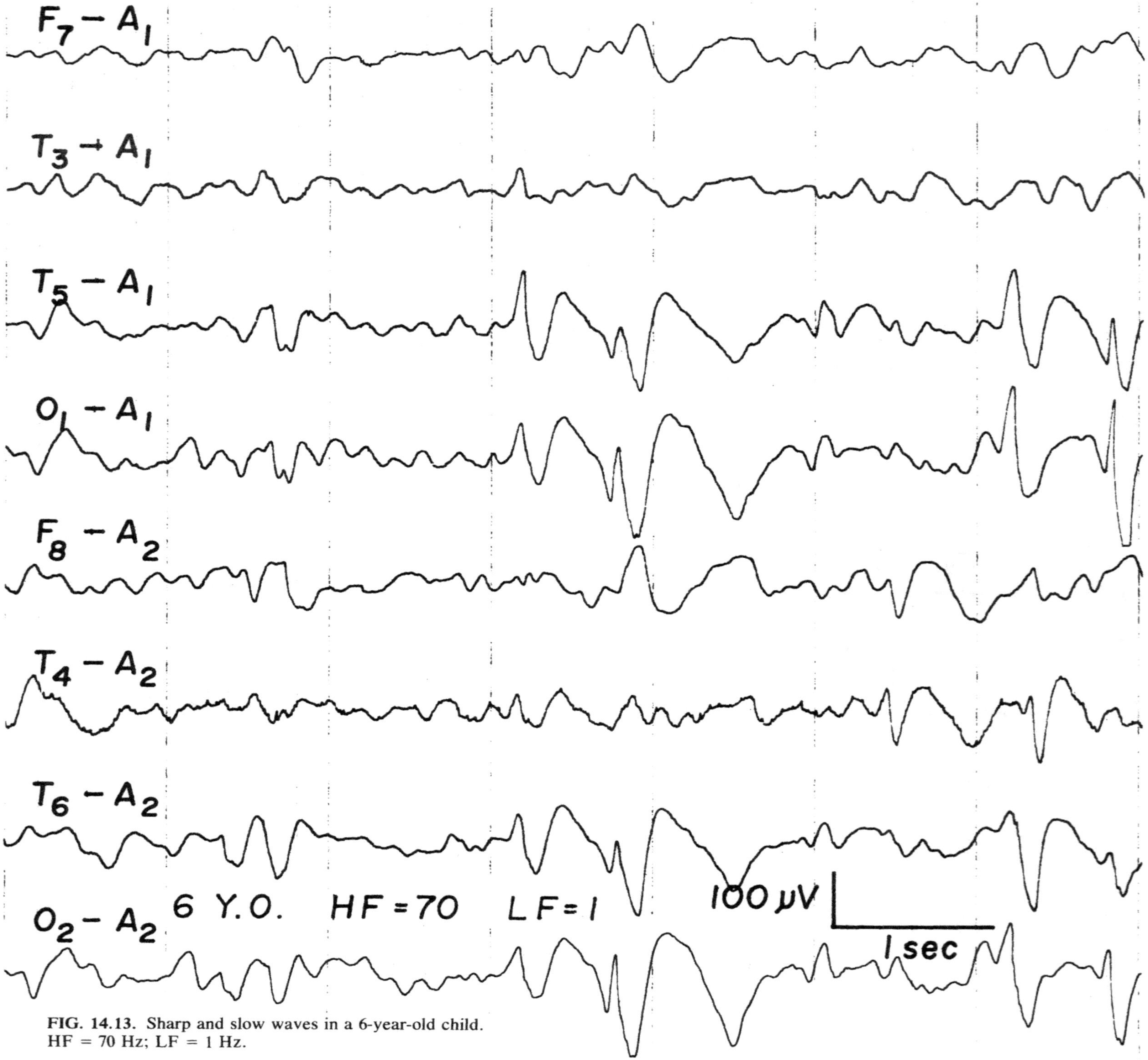

FIG. 14.13. Sharp and slow waves in a 6-year-old child. HF = 70 Hz; LF = 1 Hz.

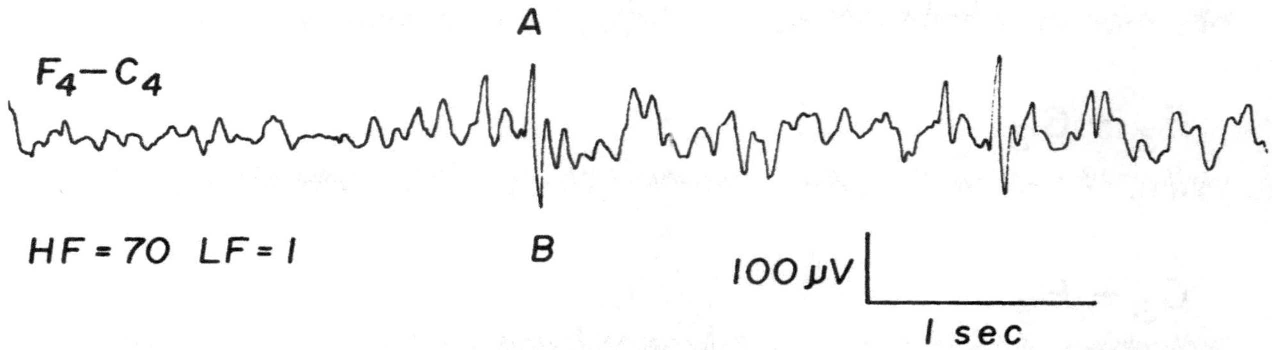

FIG. 14.14. Biphasic wave: F_4 is surface negative at (*A*) and surface positive at (*B*). HF = 70 Hz; LF = 1 Hz.

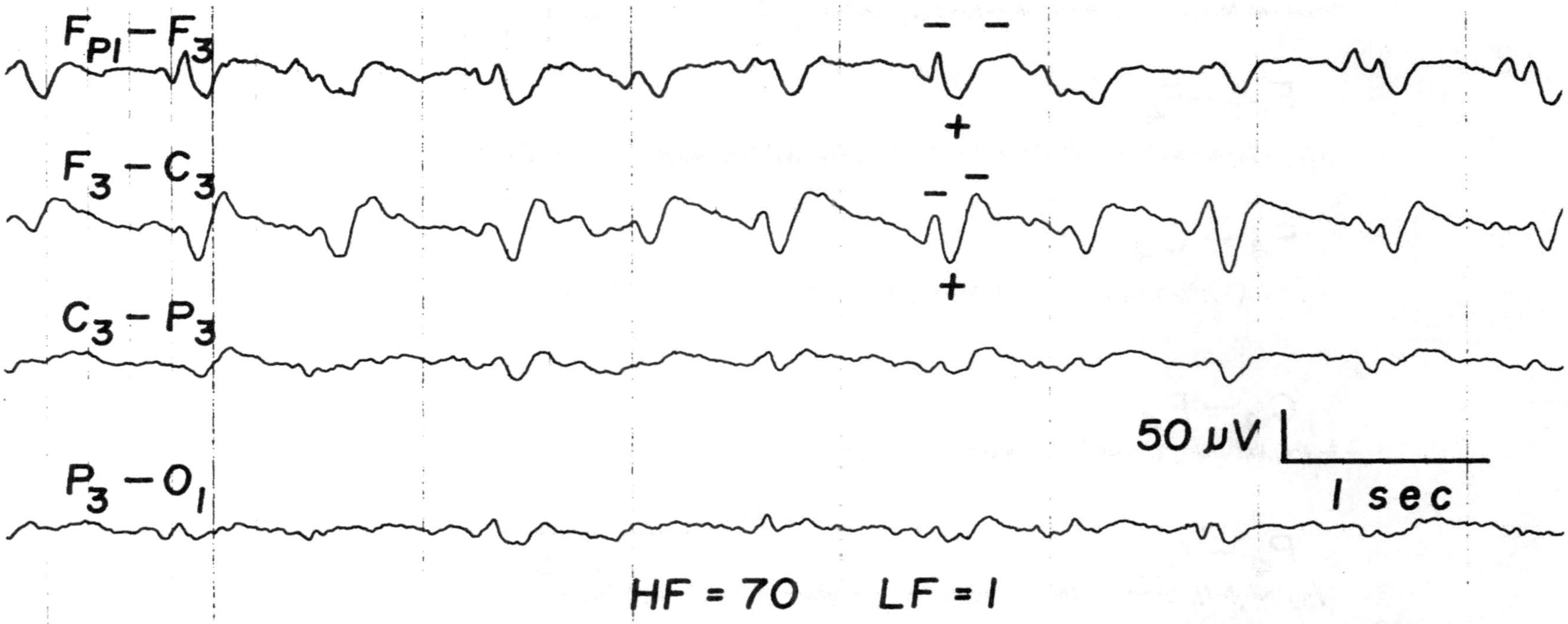

FIG. 14.15. Triphasic activity showing alternating negativity—positivity—negativity in anterior areas. HF = 70 Hz; LF = 1 Hz.

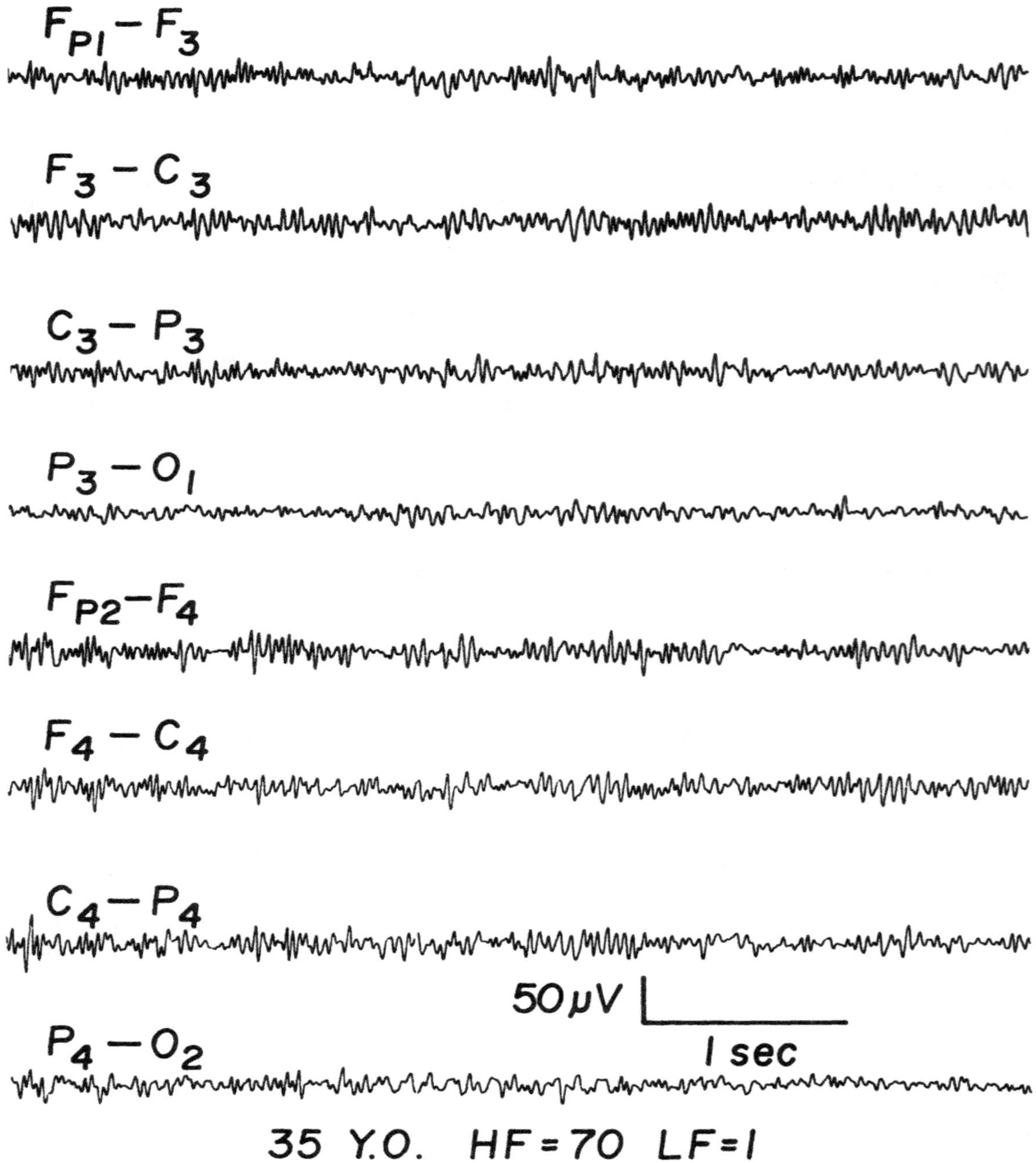

FIG. 14.16. Generalized beta activity in a 35-year-old subject. HF = 70 Hz; LF = 1 Hz.

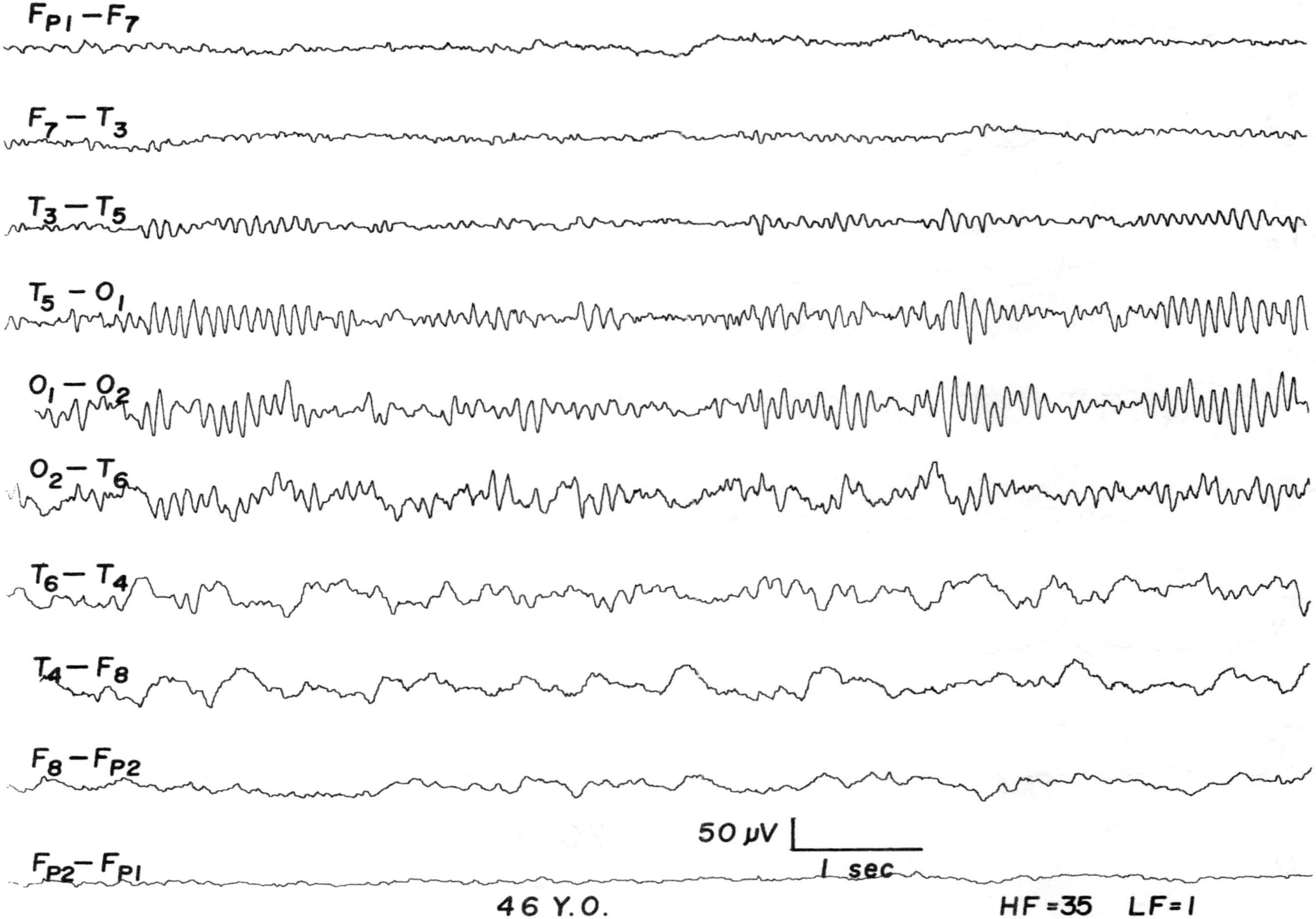

FIG. 14.17. Lateralized slow activity involving the right frontal and temporal areas with loss of background activity (alpha and beta) in a 46-year-old subject. HF = 35 Hz; LF = 1 Hz.

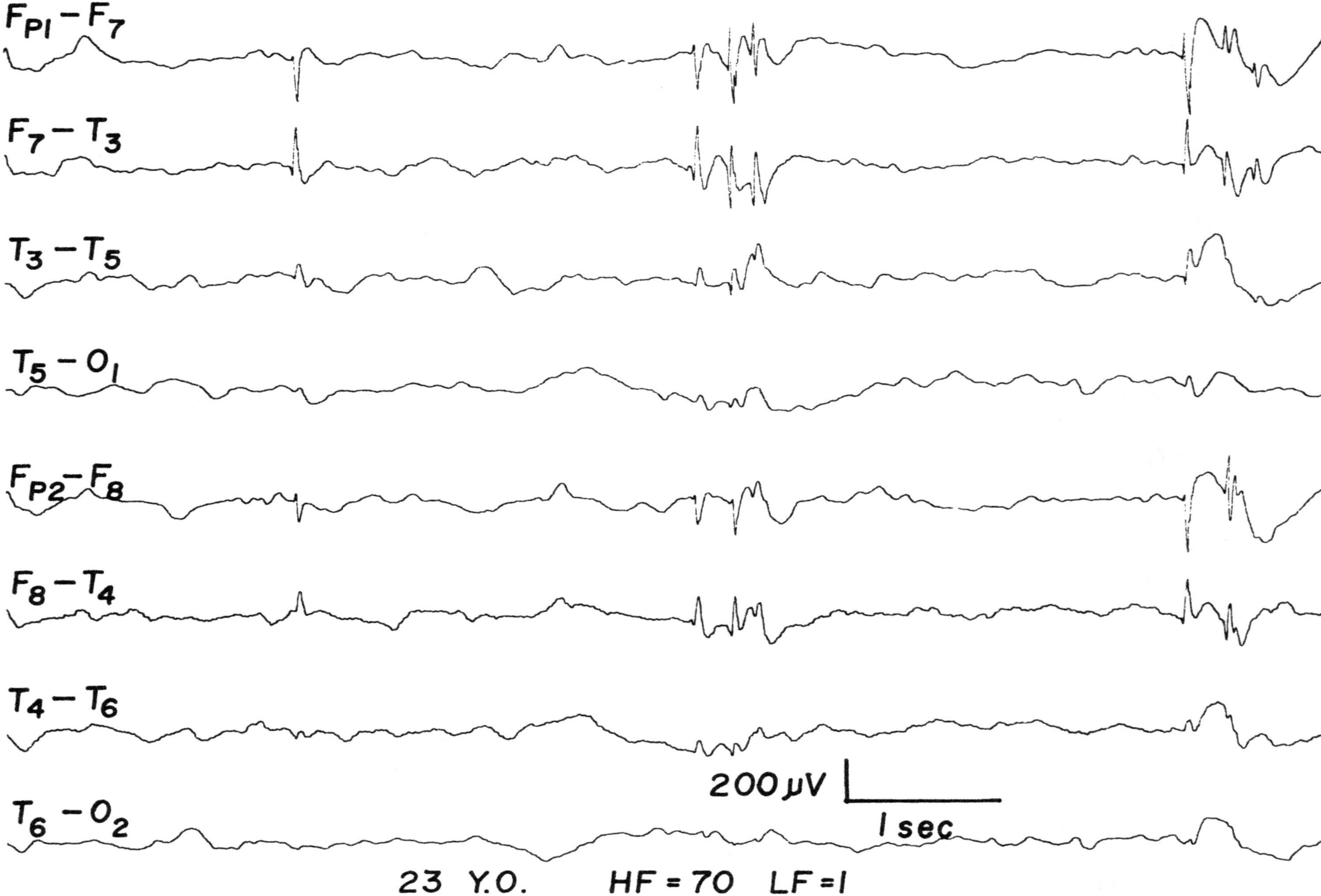

FIG. 14.18. Bilateral spike activity in a 23-year-old subject. HF = 70 Hz; LF = 1 Hz.

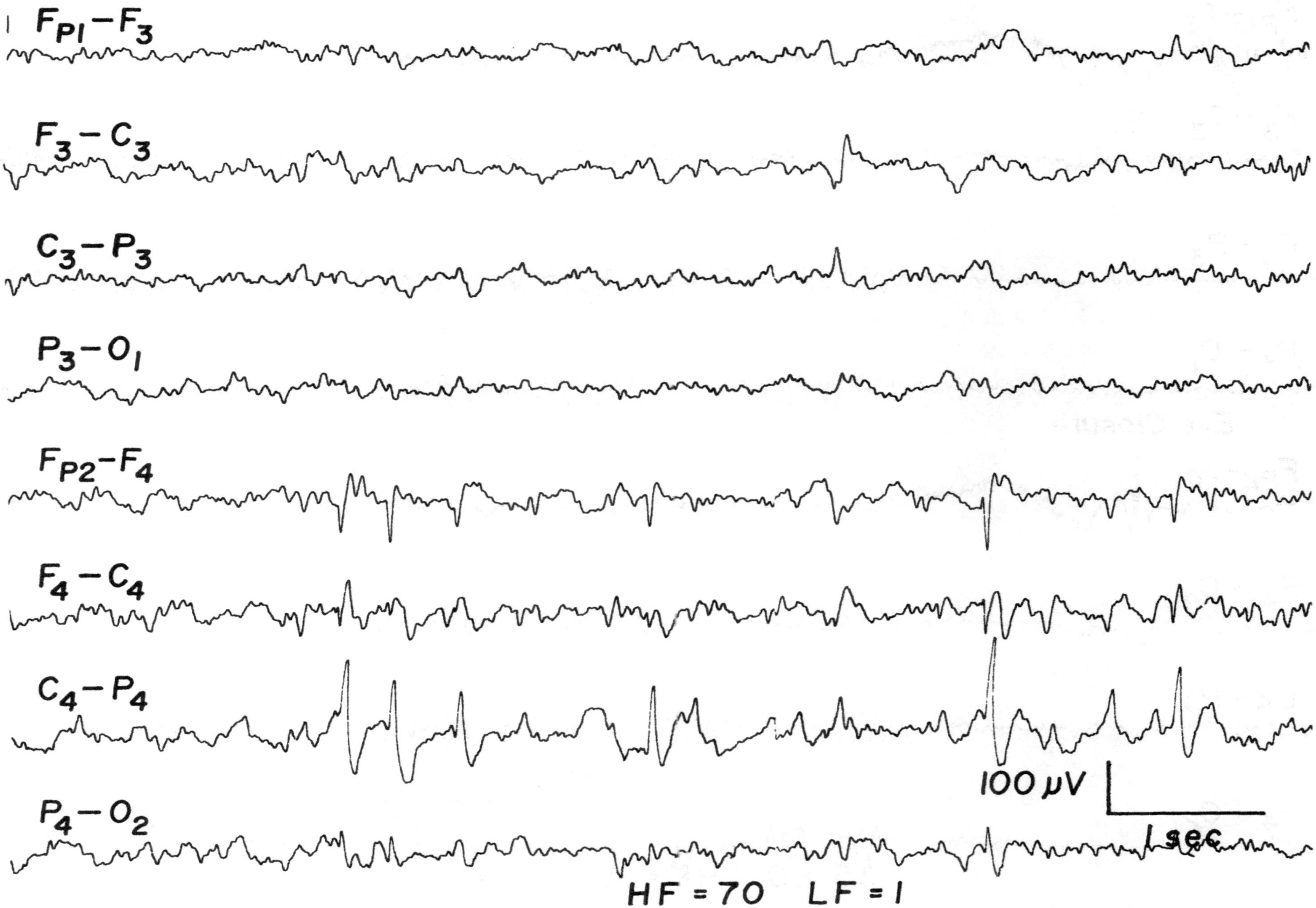

FIG. 14.19. Spike activity in right frontal-central areas. HF = 70 Hz; LF = 1 Hz.

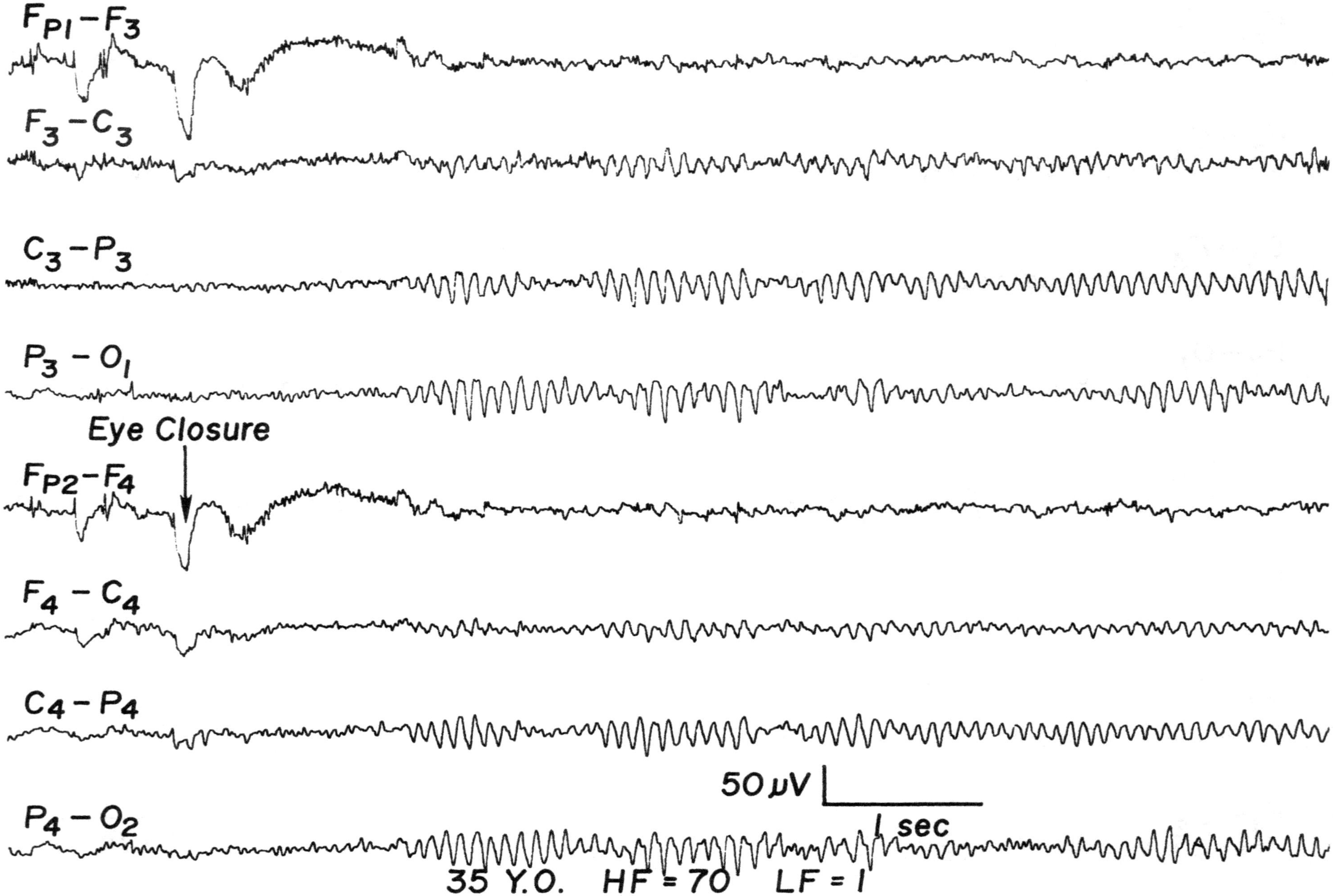

FIG. 14.20. Bilaterally synchronous alpha activity elicited by eye closure in a 35-year-old subject. Alpha activity also appears synchronously in occipital, parietal, and central regions of each hemisphere. HF = 70 Hz; LF = 1 Hz.

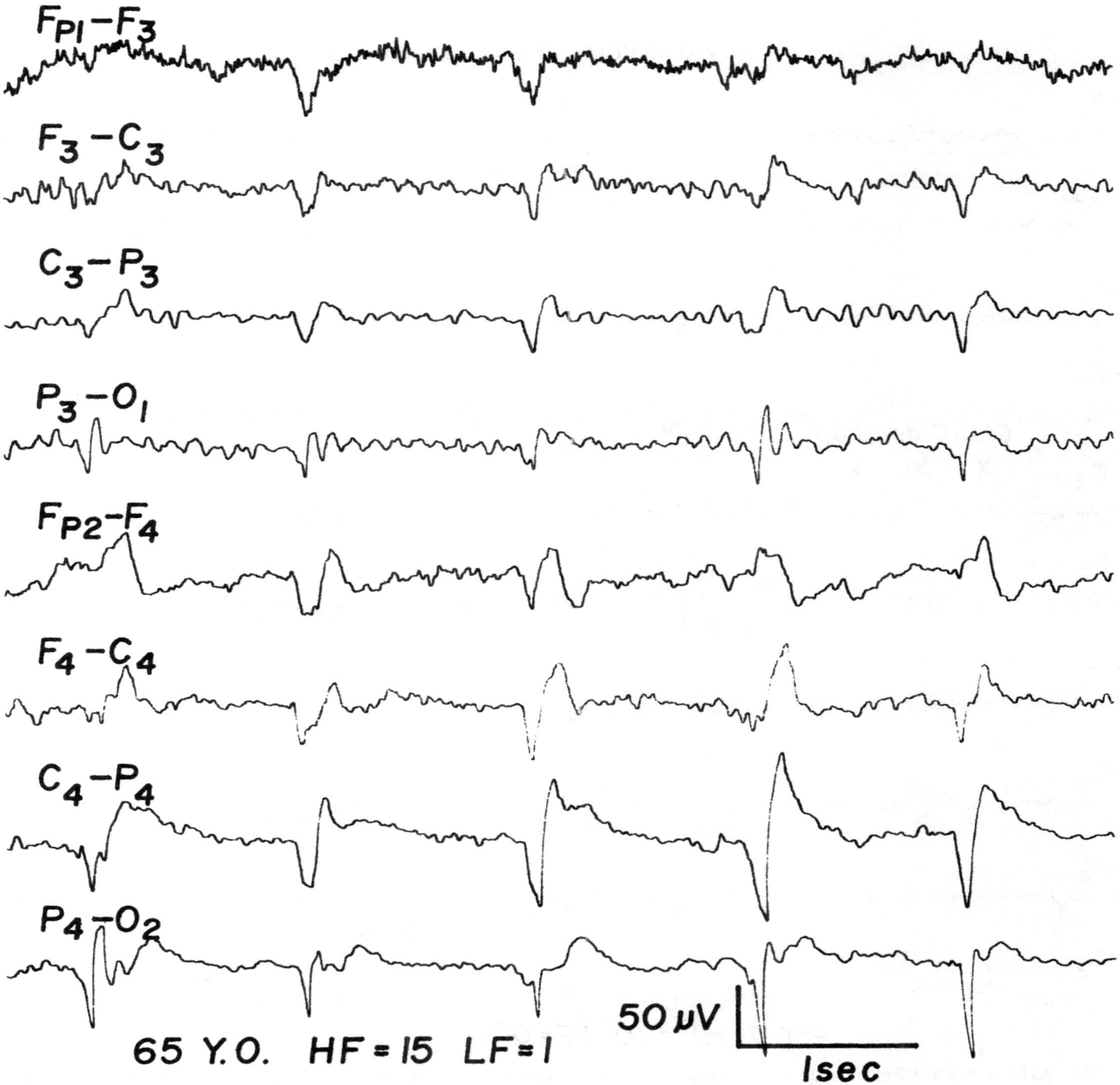

FIG. 14.21. Periodic sharp waves occurring approximately every 1⅓ sec throughout the recording in a 65-year-old man. HF = 15 Hz; LF = 1 Hz. Note that the periodic activity is asymmetrical; the distribution is greater over the right. Also note that there is attenuation of background activity over the right.

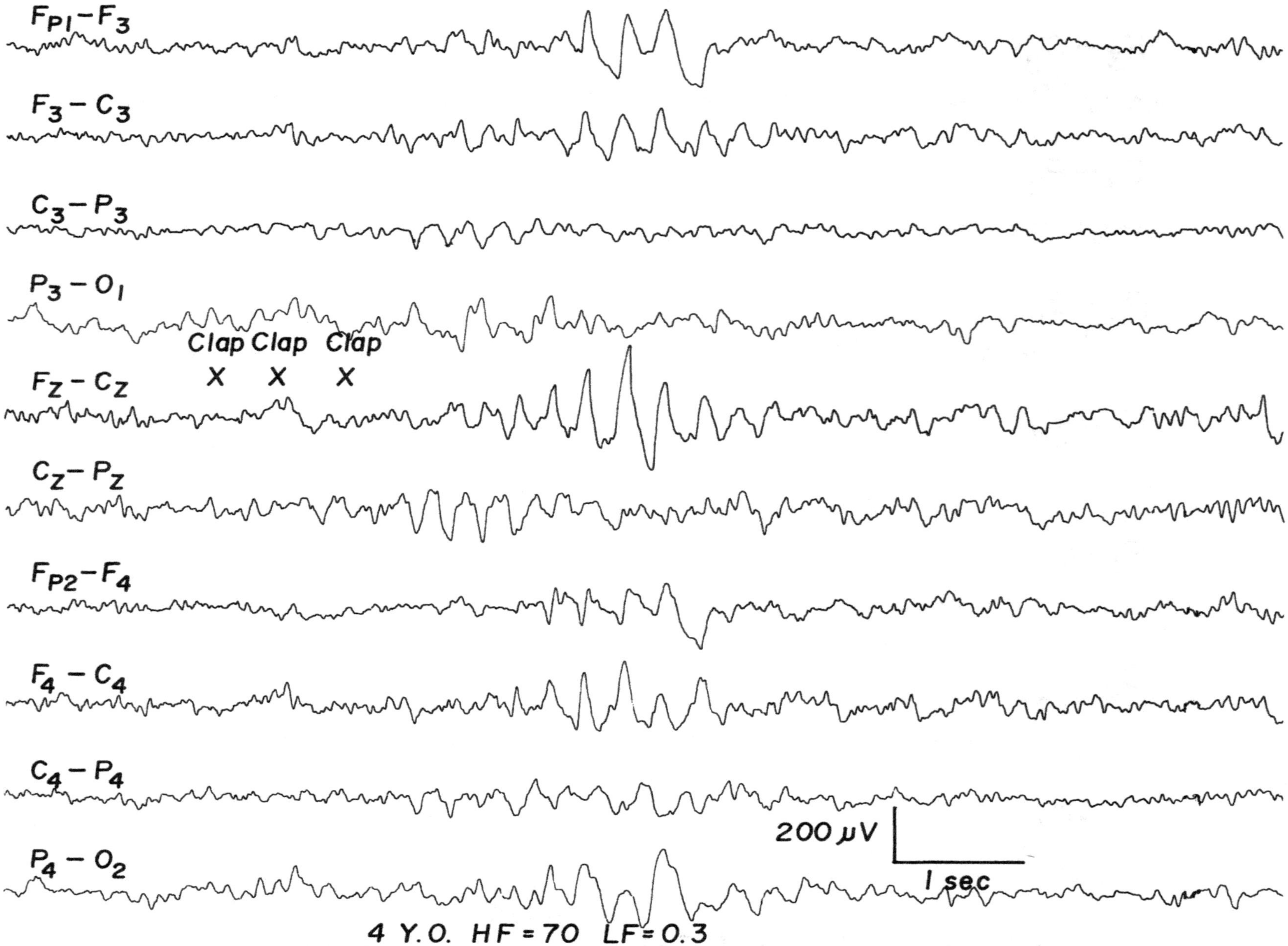

FIG. 14.22. Slow waves augmented in anterior regions by auditory stimuli during sleep in a 4-year-old child. HF = 70 Hz; LF = 0.3 Hz.

Reactivity

Reactivity refers to the reaction of the EEG to stimulation or to a stimulus-related change in morphology. Reactivity is a state-related term. An example of attenuation was presented in Fig. 14.4. Augmentation is shown in Fig. 14.22.

TYPES OF EEG ACTIVITIES

Types of EEG activities vary depending upon the age and the state of the individual. Consequently the following detailed analysis of activities will be subdivided, first to encompass ages that present systematic EEG findings, and second to contrast the normal extremes of state, waking and sleeping. Because the EEGs of adults are the least complex, in terms of variability from person to person, in both the waking and sleeping states, they will be discussed first. Elderly adults, however, do present minor changes in EEG characteristics, and they will be briefly discussed as a separate group. The EEGs of children show systematic age-related changes, both awake and asleep. They therefore are described separately. Finally, the EEG characteristics of the neonate are described, since they are the most complex, rapidly maturing and state-dependent of all groups.

The following review of EEG activities at various ages does not form a definitive atlas. A more thorough account of normal adult activity will be found in Chatrian and Lairy (11), of infants and children in Blume (6) and of neonates in Werner, Stockard and Bickford (76). References cited in the text should be consulted by the student interested in further details.

NORMAL EEG ACTIVITY IN ADULTS: AWAKE

Alpha Activity

The most easily recognized activity in the waking EEG of the normal, relaxed adult (20–60 years of age) whose eyes are closed is the alpha rhythm, prominent in the occipital region (see Fig. 14.20). It has a frequency ranging from 8 to 13 Hz, but averages 10 Hz (10). About 85% of healthy adults have an alpha frequency between 9.5 and 10.5 Hz (computed from Fig. 2 of ref. 38). Quantitative estimates of variability of alpha voltage indicate that in 28% of control subjects it is less than 20 μV; in 66% the average alpha voltage falls between 20 and 60 μV (66).

The amount (i.e., abundance) of alpha activity present in the waking EEG varies from person to person. This can be expressed as the percent time alpha is present, and subjects may be classified on the basis of this "alpha index" (14). About 11% of the healthy adult population has a more or less "non-alpha" record, sometimes called "low voltage fast" (31), with voltages typically between 10 and 20 μV, and without well-defined rhythmic alpha waves; some irregular alpha activity and other mixed frequencies are present.

Occipital alpha activity tends to be slightly asymmetrical. Usually, the activity shows a greater percent time and slightly higher voltage over the right hemisphere (13,60). The cause of the asymmetry is speculative.

Alpha activity is attenuated by stimulation, particularly visual stimulation. When the eyes are open, alpha activity tends to disappear (block) for varying periods of time. In most subjects, the alpha rhythm remains attenuated during the period of time the eyes are open; in others, it reappears after one or more seconds. A test for reactivity to eye opening should be carried out at some point during every EEG recording (see Fig. 14.4).

Alpha activity is also attenuated by increased vigilance or heightened attentiveness. In some persons, the rhythm may be fairly continuous, although it may disappear temporarily and then return. Some of these spontaneous non-alpha intervals may be related to mental activity (72).

Alpha activity is usually rhythmic and is sometimes referred to as sinusoidal. This does not mean that an alpha wave is a sine wave, only that it resembles a sine wave (and not always very closely). In most persons, it has no distinctive surface polarity. Rarely, there may be a surface negative, sharp, spike-like aspect to each cycle. This is normal.

"Alpha variants" are a mixture of an alpha rhythm and another rhythm that is usually half the frequency of the alpha rhythm. The slower activity is dominant, so that the typical alpha appears superimposed on it. The resulting activity is usually sharp and appears surface negative at the occiput. Alpha variants block with visual stimulation and in all respects act like alpha activity. They are regarded as normal.

Subjects with a faster than average alpha rhythm (11–13 Hz) sometimes have 14- to 16-Hz activity intermixed with the fast alpha activity (Fig. 14.23). If the 14- to 16-Hz activity attenuates coincidentally with the alpha rhythm and otherwise behaves like it, it is considered to be a "fast variant" of alpha activity. It is normal.

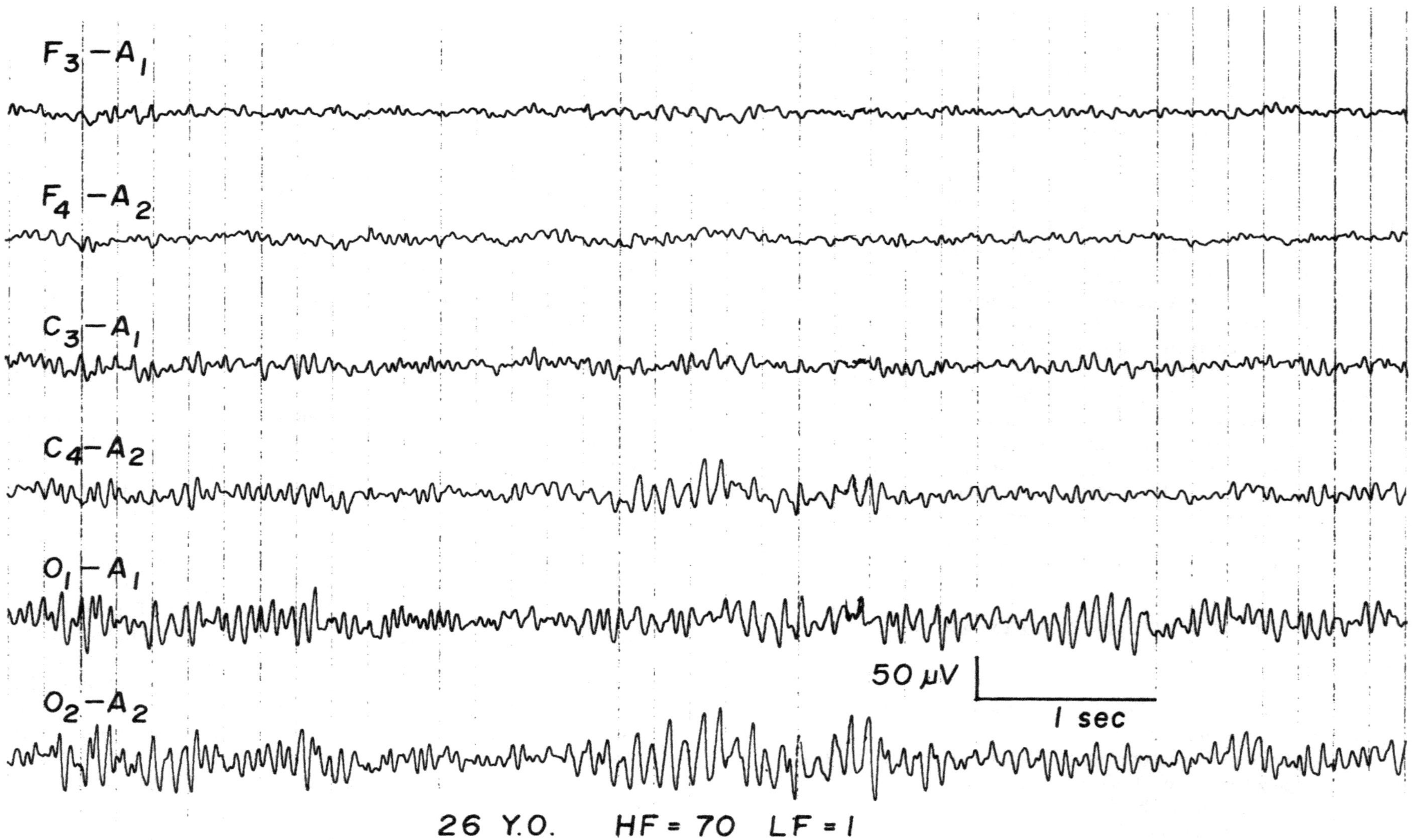

FIG. 14.23. Fast alpha variant and beta activity in a 26-year-old woman. HF = 70 Hz; LF = 1 Hz.

Beta Activity

Beta activity is defined as activity with a frequency faster than 13 Hz (10). Classically, it refers to more or less rhythmic activity in the 18- to 30-Hz frequency range (5). Occasionally, faster rhythmic activity may be seen. There is no distinguishing surface polarity (see Figs. 14.16 and 14.23). The voltage is not over 20 μV (13).

On the basis of observed distributions and reactivity of beta activity, it has been inferred (73,41) that there are three types: (a) generalized, (b) precentral and (c) posterior. It is commonly seen in the frontal and central regions.

The voltage of beta activity ranges from 5 to 20 μV (36). Beta activity, particularly the generalized type, is bilaterally synchronous. Central beta activity may show asymmetric features, and it may be reactive to movement-generated and proprioceptive stimuli, attenuating coincidentally with voluntary movement (36). The amount and voltage of beta activity is enhanced by commonly used tranquilizers such as diazepam as well as by barbiturates (24,41).

Theta Activity

Theta activity includes frequencies between 4 and 7 Hz (75). In the normal awake adult, a small amount may appear in the central, temporal, and parietal areas, but it rarely is rhythmic. It has been shown to be more prominent on the left side than the right in all age groups. When the incidence of theta activity in a group of 218 neurologically normal adults was studied, 34% showed asymmetric theta activity in the temporal areas (40), independently of central theta. Thirty-four percent of a group of 200 healthy young adult subjects had "traces" of 6- to 7-Hz theta activity in their waking EEGs (38). The voltage was reportedly less than 15 μV. In only 10% of subjects was voltage in the 15 to 25 μV range. If the amplitude of theta activity exceeds the alpha amplitude by 50% or more, it may have pathological significance (12). Temporal theta activity is shown in Fig. 14.24.

Mu Rhythm

The mu rhythm is a morphologically and topographically distinct activity seen in the central areas (Fig. 14.25). Its frequency is about 9 Hz but may range from 7 to 11 Hz (9). Although the frequency may be within the alpha range, it is not an alpha rhythm. First, its distribution is different. Second, it has a unique reactivity and typically is blocked by movement (fist clenching), by imagining a movement, or by tactile stimulation. The mu rhythm was first described in 1952 by Gastaut et al. (25,26), and named "rhythme rolandique en arceau." The arch-like morphology is its distinctive characteristic. The surface polarity of the sharp element is negative, and its voltage may range up to 80 μV. It is seen in about 19% of healthy adults, with a range of 0% to 34% (9).

The mu rhythm, while predominantly central, may appear in parietal derivations. It may be either bilateral or unilateral. If bilateral, it may appear independently in the left and right hemispheres. It may be fairly continuous, or it may appear intermittently. Asymmetry is not abnormal. When mu activity is seen in an EEG, it should be verified by testing its reactivity (i.e., blocking with movement of the opposite side of the body).

Activity of similar morphology and frequency, also with surface negative sharp elements, in the temporal areas has been called wicket spikes. It is quite rare, being reported in 0.8% of 4,458 cases (42,62).

Lambda Waves

Lambda waves were first described in 1951 by Y. Gastaut (27). They are sharp waves with an equivalent frequency of 4 to 6 Hz. The surface polarity is variable. They occur in the occipital areas when the subject intently scans a complex visual field with horizontal eye movements (Fig. 14.26). The illustration is of a typical subject. In some persons much more pronounced positivity occurs and in some subjects lambda activity cannot be demonstrated. Lambda waves are not seen when the subject's eyes are closed or if the eyes are opened in a dark room. They are normal and have no clinical significance.

Posterior Slow Waves Associated with Youth

Posterior slow waves of youth are composed of delta activity intermixed with activity of alpha frequency (Fig. 14.27). The combination of alpha and delta activity forms a pattern or complex that sometimes resembles sharp-and-slow-wave activity. These waves are maximal in the posterior head region, and their voltage may range from 75 to 150 μV.

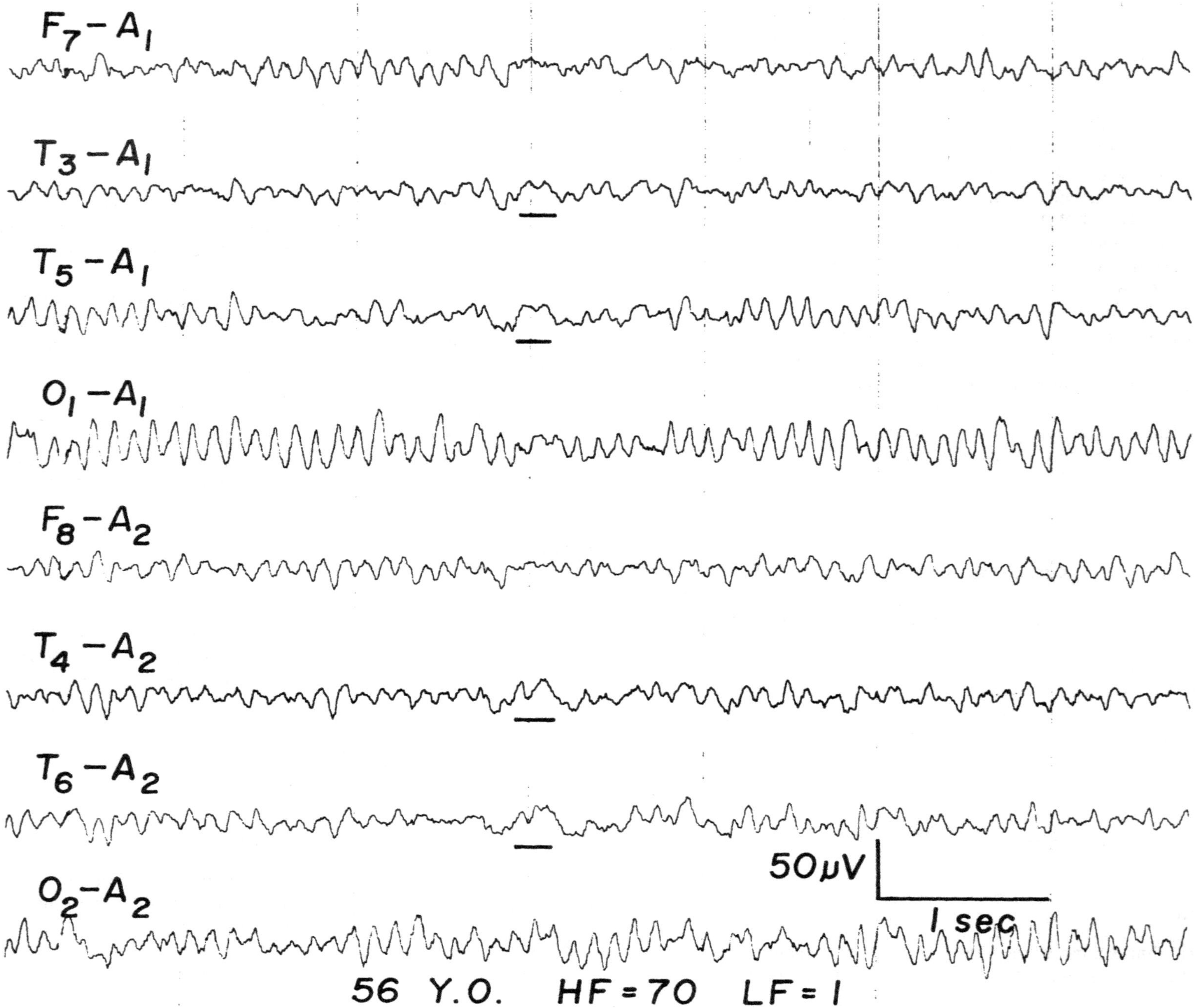

FIG. 14.24. Temporal theta activity in a 56-year-old awake woman. HF = 70 Hz; LF = 1 Hz.

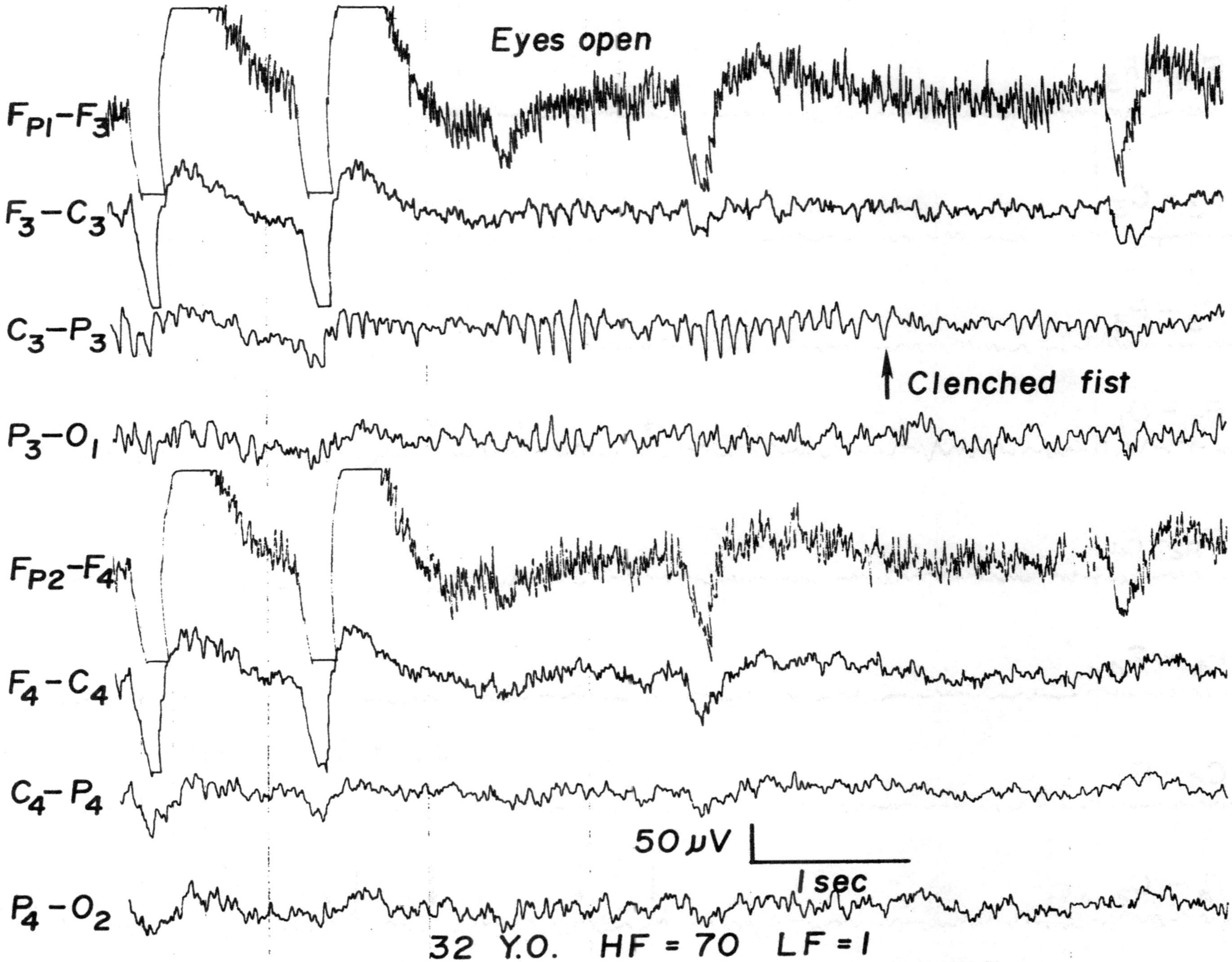

FIG. 14.25. Mu activity in central-parietal derivations. Note reactivity to fist clenching (arrow). Note that mu activity is present and alpha activity is diminished when eyes are open. HF = 70 Hz; LF = 1 Hz.

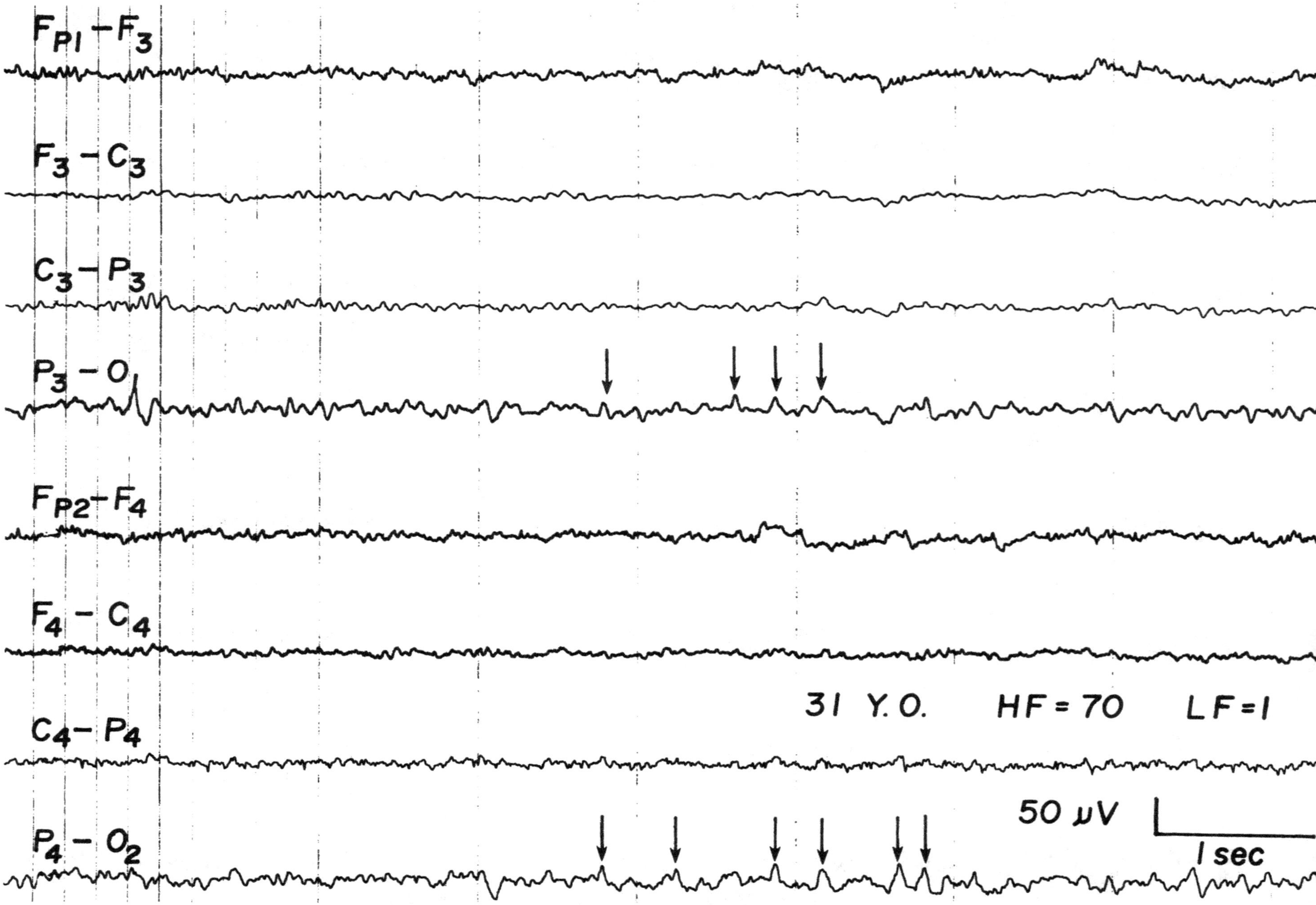

FIG. 14.26. Lambda activity (arrows) in occipital areas of a 31-year-old awake man. HF = 70 Hz; LF = 1 Hz.

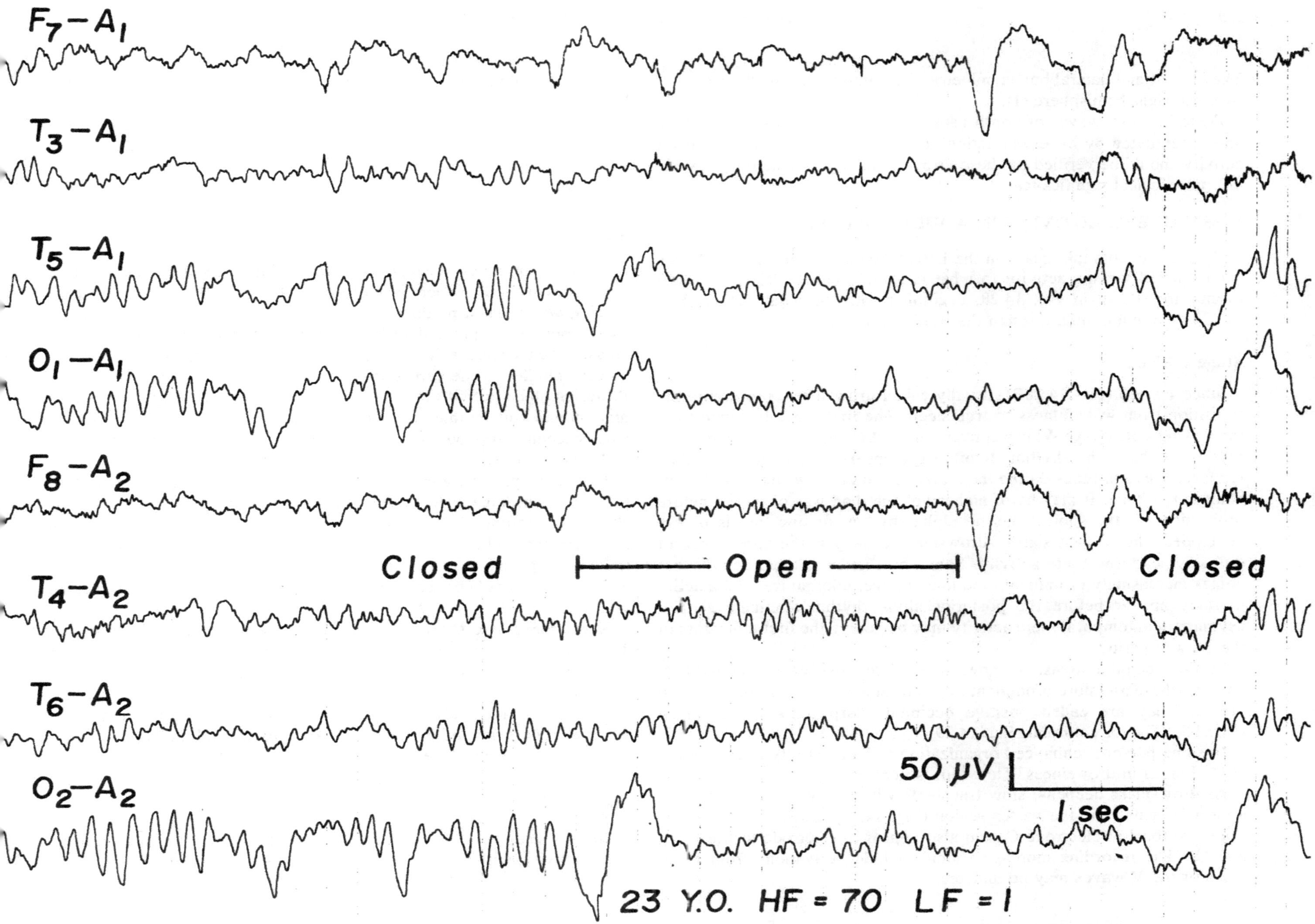

FIG. 14.27. Posterior slow waves of youth in a 23-year-old subject. Posterior dominance is clear; symmetry is variable. Both the slow and alpha components are attenuated when eyes are open. HF = 70 Hz; LF = 1 Hz.

They are often bilateral but asymmetric. The amplitude usually is greater over the right hemisphere (1).

Posterior slow waves of youth usually are attenuated by eye opening and accentuated by hyperventilation. They disappear in sleep. Their reactivity should be verified by these forms of testing. The activity is without pathological significance.

NORMAL EEG ACTIVITY IN ADULTS: ASLEEP

Dramatic events take place in the EEG when a person's state changes from relaxed waking activity to what is loosely called "sleep." These events are shown in Fig. 14.28, beginning with the awake state (Fig. 14.28A) and continuing through the five stages of sleep.

Stage 1 Sleep

Stage 1 sleep (Fig. 14.28B), usually called drowsiness, represents the transition from wakefulness to true sleep. The first typical change from the waking state (stage W) in a conventional EEG appears as a decrease in voltage of the alpha rhythm. It often disappears (attenuates) and then reappears several times during the initial period of drowsiness, with variability in voltage. It may be of higher voltage than was observed before drowsiness. If the subject has no alpha rhythm, or one that is poorly developed, the earliest sign of drowsiness usually is the appearance of diffusely scattered theta activity. Sometimes anterior theta activity becomes increasingly prominent, and low voltage, unorganized delta activity may appear before the posterior alpha rhythm attenuates. Also, asymmetrical temporal theta activity may be among the first indicators of the drowsy period.

In the occipital areas, a series of surface positive transients may emerge; these are more prominent in some subjects and may be absent in others. They are called positive occipital sharp transients of sleep (POSTS). They are normal (Fig. 14.29).

In some persons, enhanced organization of beta activity occurs in the central areas in drowsiness. This, too, is normal.

As drowsiness deepens, slow transients with a sharp surface element appear irregularly in the vertex region (Fig. 14.30). These are V waves. They are focal at electrode C_z and also appear at electrode locations C_3 and C_4. The recording montage should include derivations from these areas or the V waves may be undetected.

Coincidentally, slow lateral eye movements may be seen as very slow baseline shifts in channels whose derivations include F_7 and F_8.

All of the above changes, in various combinations, define Stage 1 sleep. It should be emphasized that there is much allowable variability among subjects and that not all of these changes occur in the order described in all persons in all periods of drowsiness.

Stage 2 Sleep

As sleep continues to deepen to Stage 2 (Fig. 14.28C), the next distinct change involves the appearance of a new, 11- to 15-Hz rhythm (typically 14 Hz), which has a predominantly central-vertex distribution. This activity appears in spindle-like bursts of rhythmic waves, which first increase, then decrease in voltage (Fig. 14.31). Hence, they are called "sleep spindles." The vertex sharp waves become more clearly defined. Posterior alpha activity is virtually absent. Theta activity is greater in amount and voltage than in Stage 1. In the temporal areas, theta activity may be asymmetric, but in most other regions, it is bilaterally symmetrical and synchronous.

The sleep spindles, appearing in bursts, are the principal EEG criteria that establish Stage 2 sleep. The duration of sleep spindle bursts is variable, ranging from 0.5 sec up to 2 or 3 sec; atypically, the duration may be much greater yet be normal. They are fairly symmetrical over the left and right hemispheres. The voltage of spindles may range up to 150 μV, although it is usually between 20 and 100 μV when measured in the central areas.

K complexes are sharp, slow waves, with associated spindle bursts. They are midline and predominantly central in origin and typically bilaterally symmetrical (Fig. 14.32). They are often seen as a response to an abrupt auditory stimulus, but they also appear spontaneously, without external stimulation. If a series of stimuli is given, the response may not occur to each stimulus. K complexes are normal, and they are a characteristic sign of Stage 2 sleep.

Stage 3 Sleep

Stage 3 sleep (Fig. 14.28D) differs quantitatively from Stage 2 sleep. Delta activity, with frequencies of 2 Hz or less, is present 20% to 50% of the time. Sleep spindles typically persist in this stage, although to a lesser

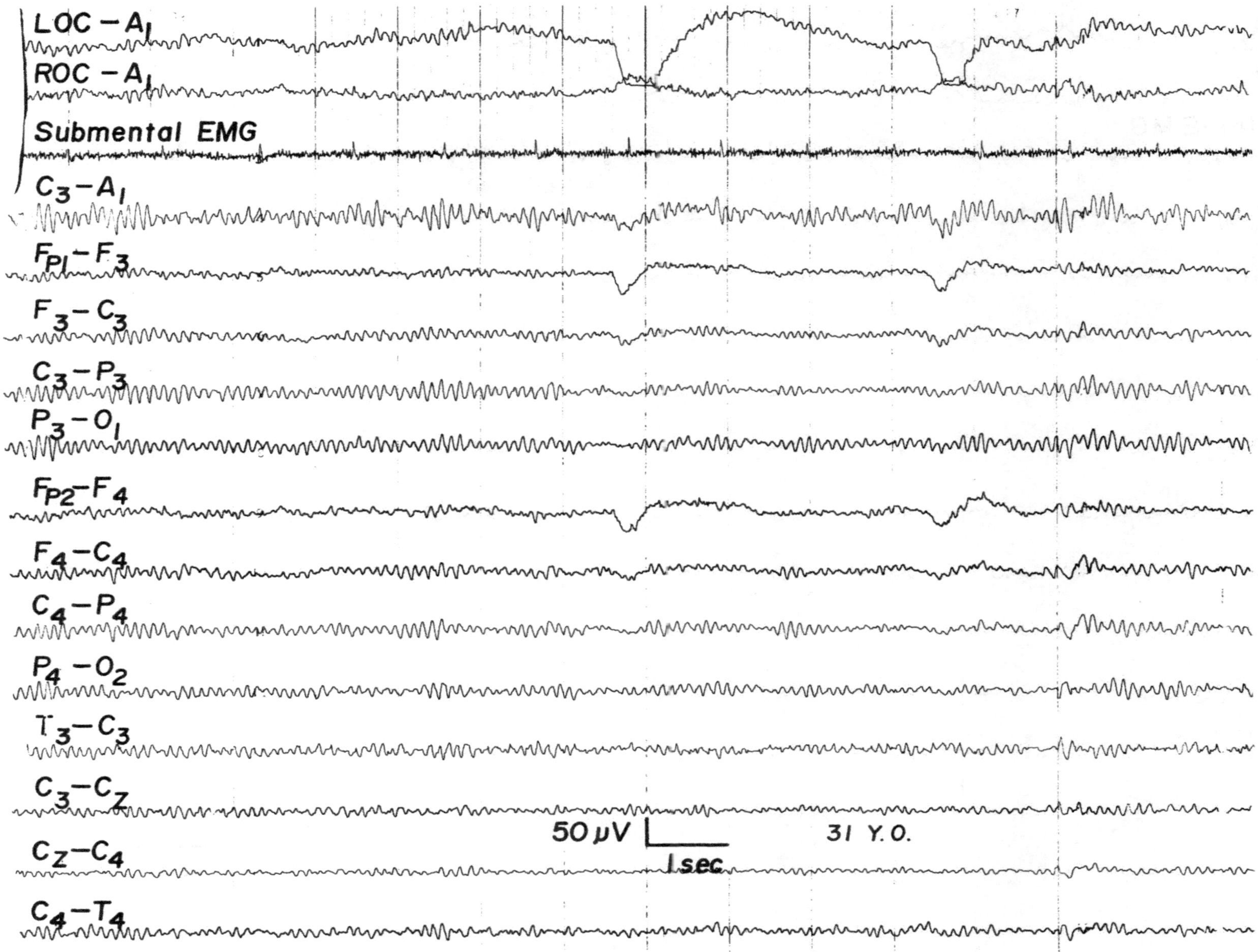

FIG. 14.28. A: Relaxed waking activity of a 31-year-old man with eyes closed. Note eyeblinks (channels 1 and 2). HF = 70 Hz; LF = 1 Hz. (*contd.*)

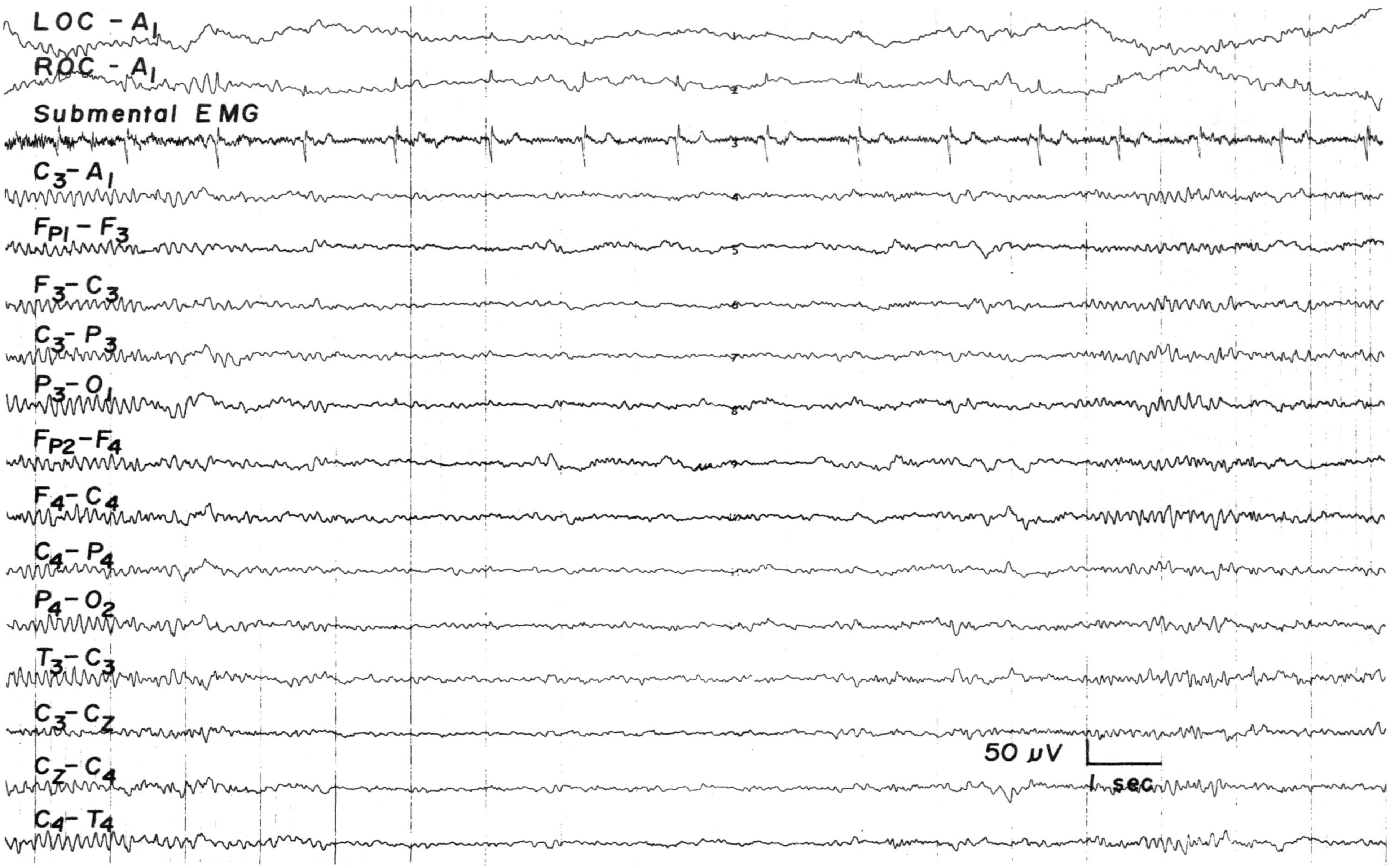

FIG. 14.28 (*contd.*). **B:** Stage 1 sleep. Decrease in voltage of alpha rhythm during drowsiness, with alpha activity disappearing and reappearing. Note spread of EEG activity into eye leads (channels 1 and 2). (*contd.*)

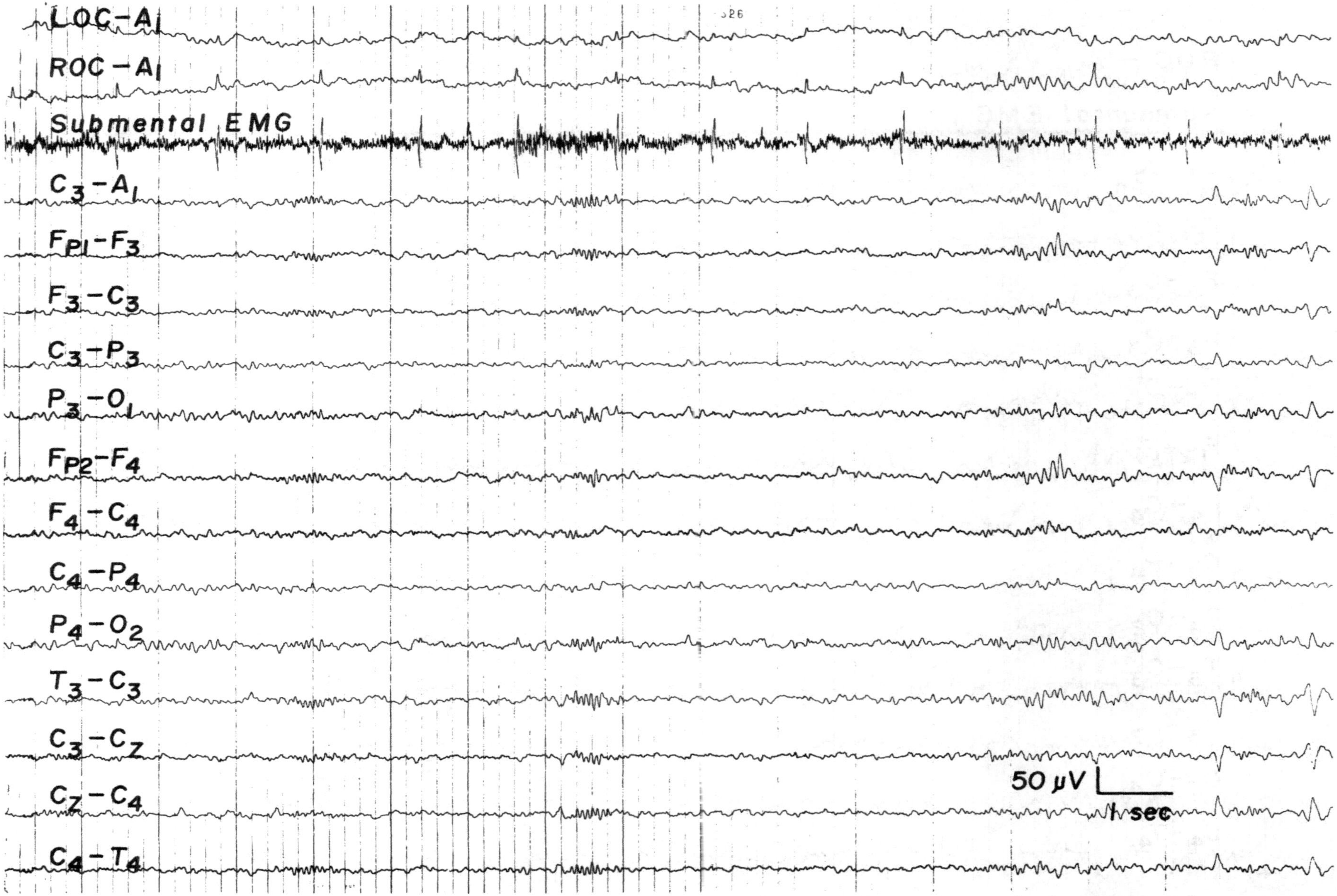

FIG. 14.28 (*contd.*). **C:** Stage 2 sleep. Appearance of 14-Hz central-vertex rhythmic activity and vertex sharp waves. (*contd.*)

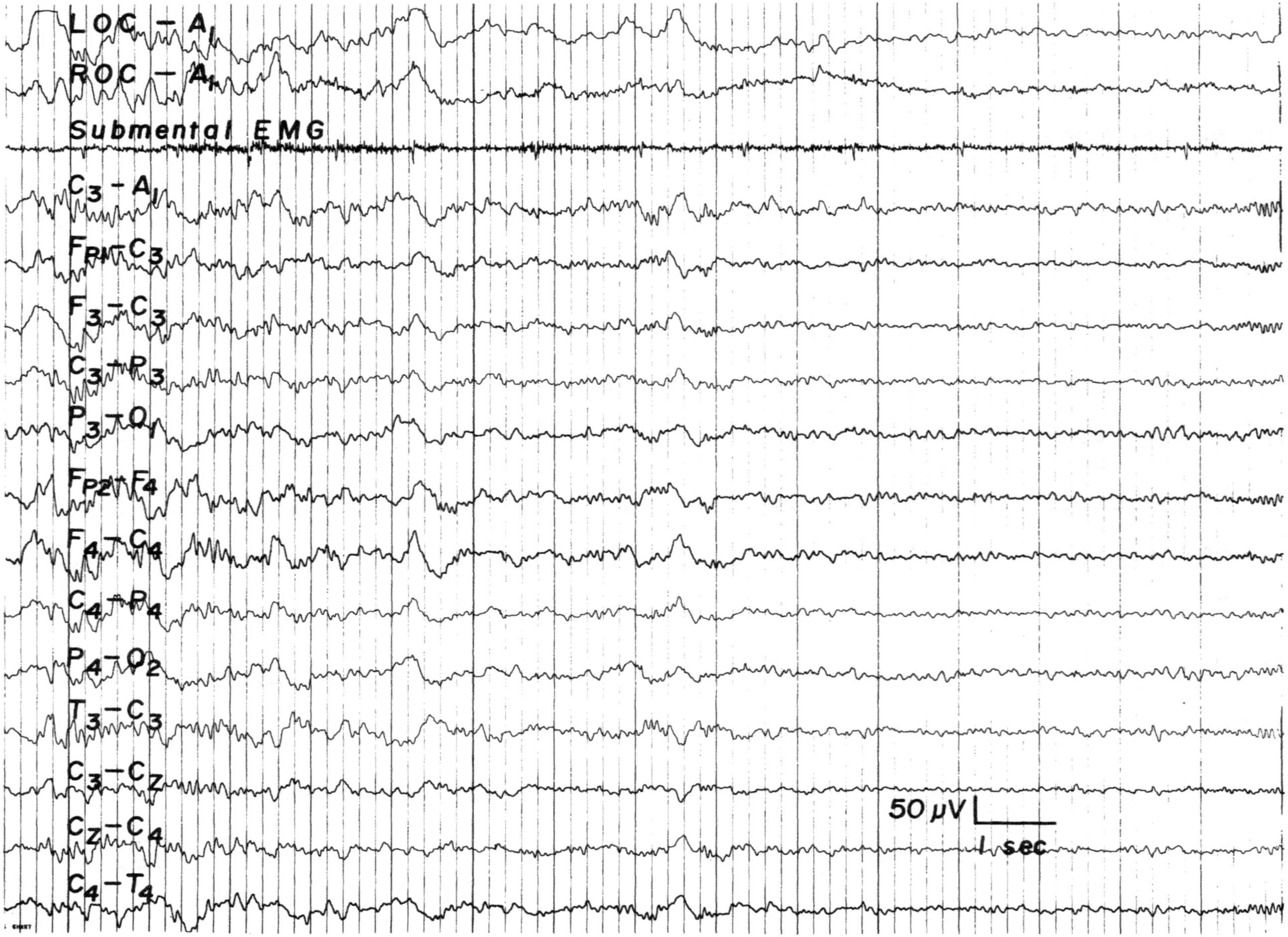

FIG. 14.28 (*contd.*). **D:** Stage 3 sleep. Presence of 2-Hz frontally predominant transients, with occasional bursts of 12- to 14-Hz spindles. (*contd.*)

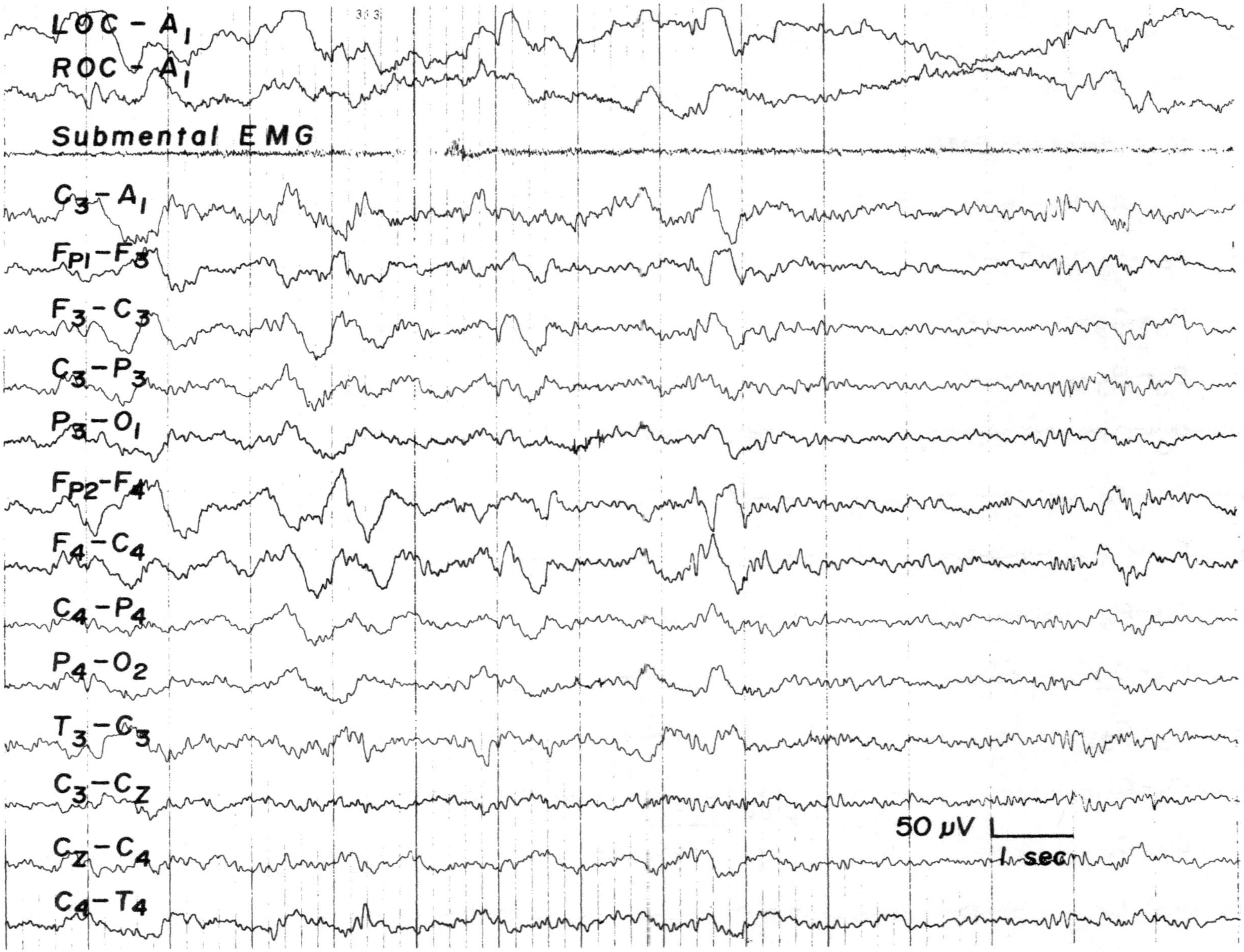

FIG. 14.28 (*contd.*). E: Stage 4 sleep. Anteriorally predominant delta activity present more than 50% of the time and with voltage greater than 75 μV. (*contd.*)

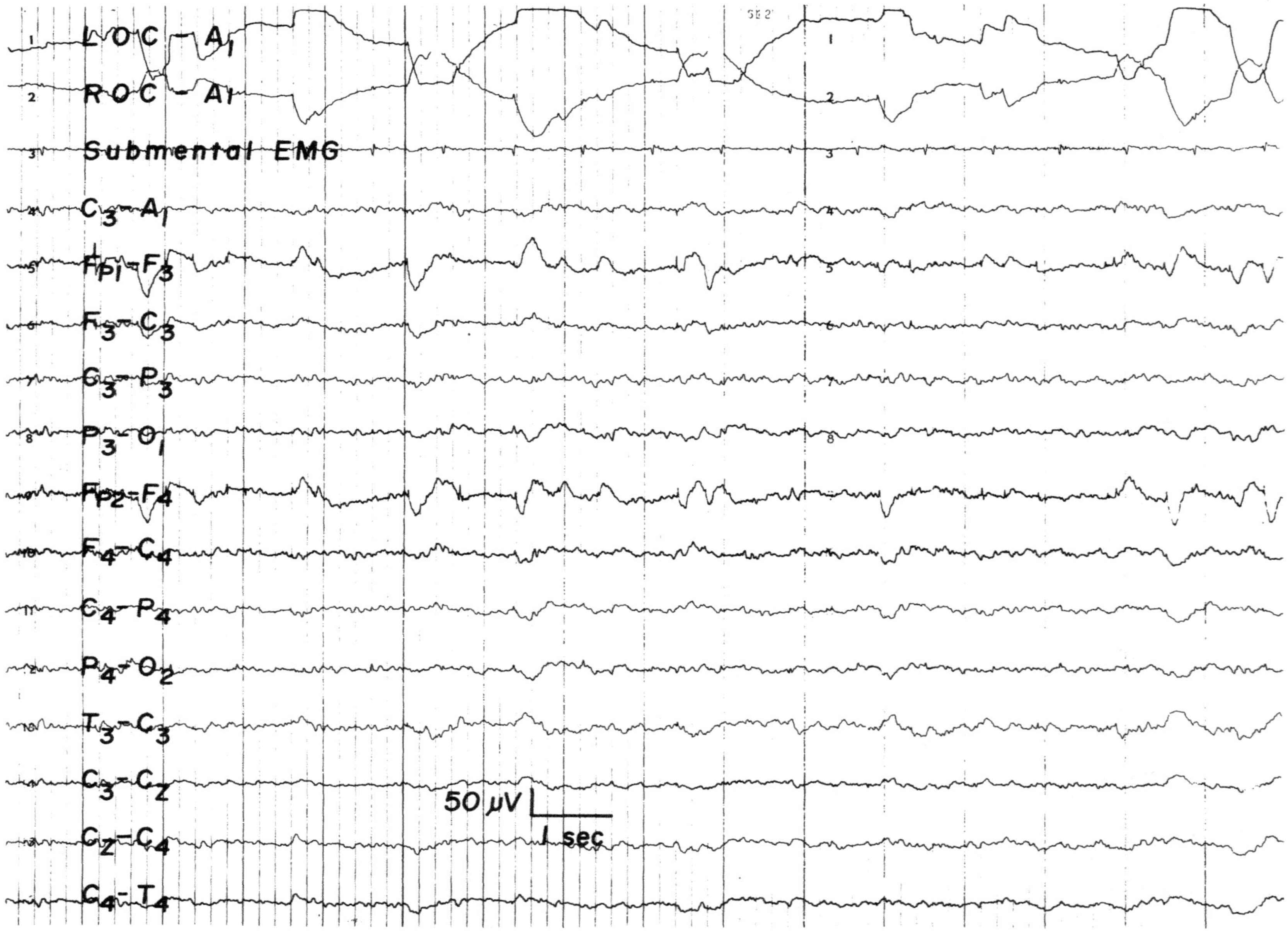

FIG. 14.28 (*contd.*). F: REM-stage sleep characterized by change in background activity, appearance of rapid eye movements, and decrease in muscle tone. Note the difference between appearance of rapid eye movements (F) and spontaneous eye blinks (A).

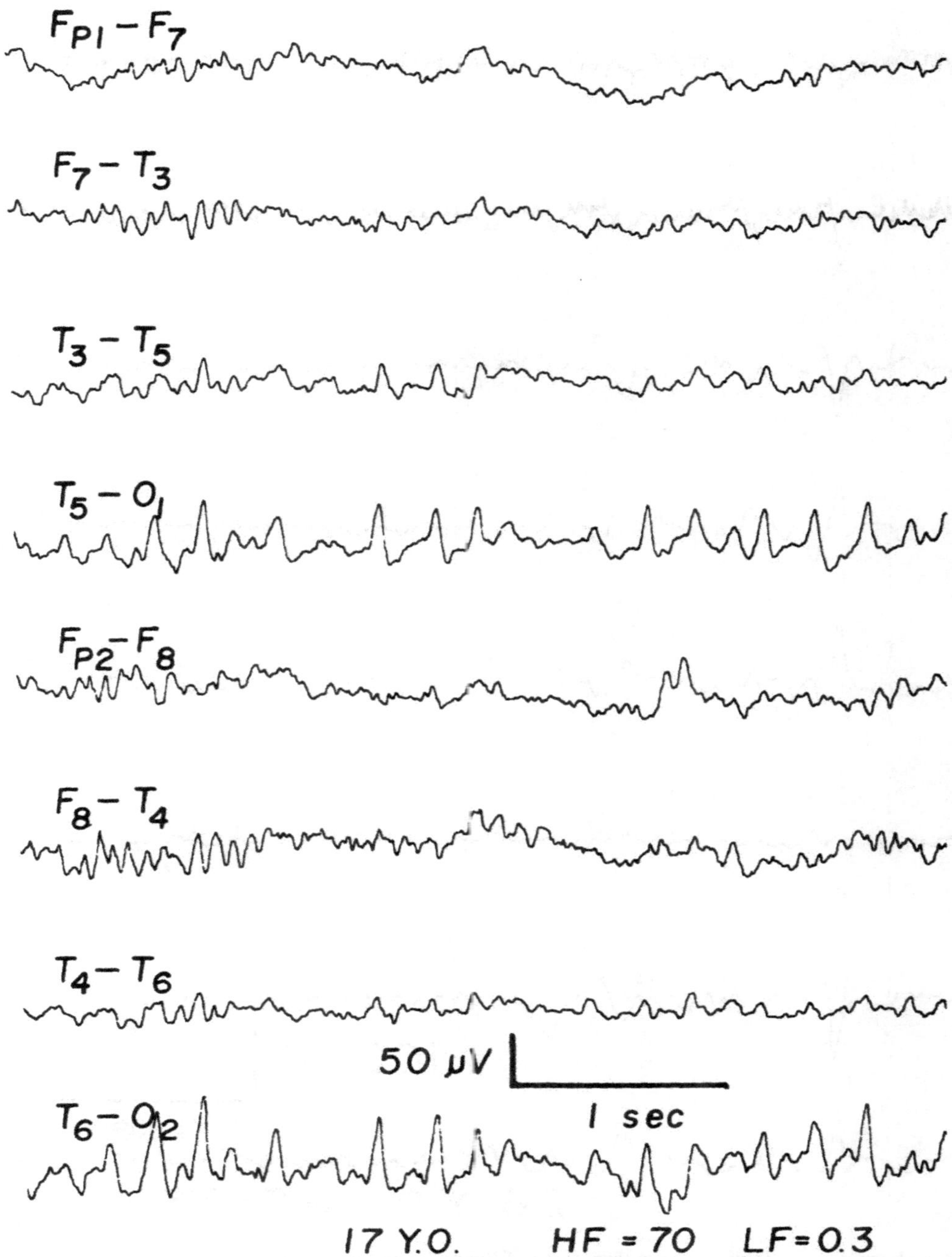

FIG. 14.29. Positive occipital sharp transients of sleep in Stage 2 sleep of a 17-year-old girl. HF = 70 Hz; LF = 0.3 Hz.

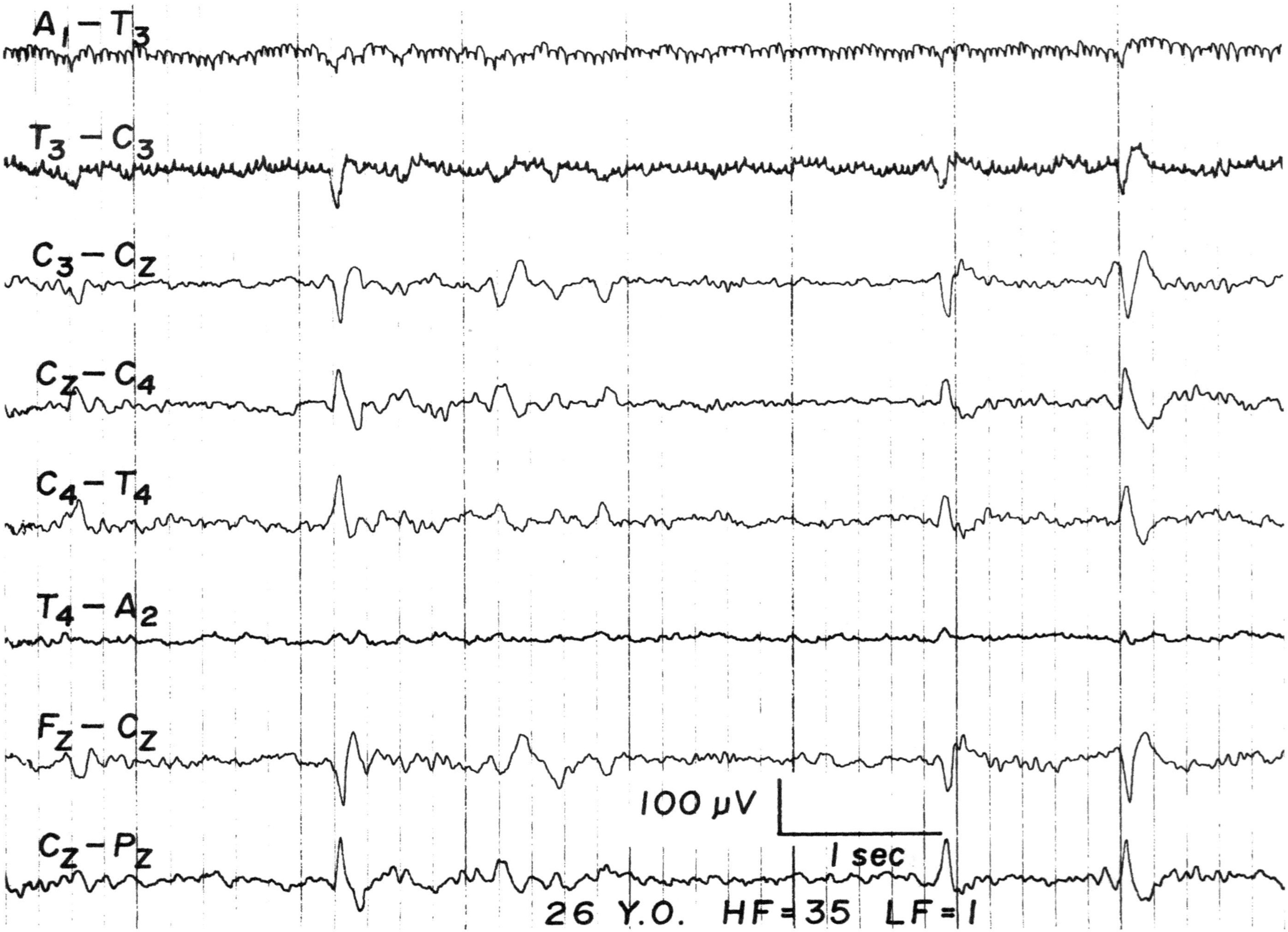

FIG. 14.30. Vertex sharp waves. Typical sharp transients of Stage 2 sleep in a 26-year-old subject. Note muscle activity (channels 1 and 2). HF = 35 Hz; LF = 1 Hz.

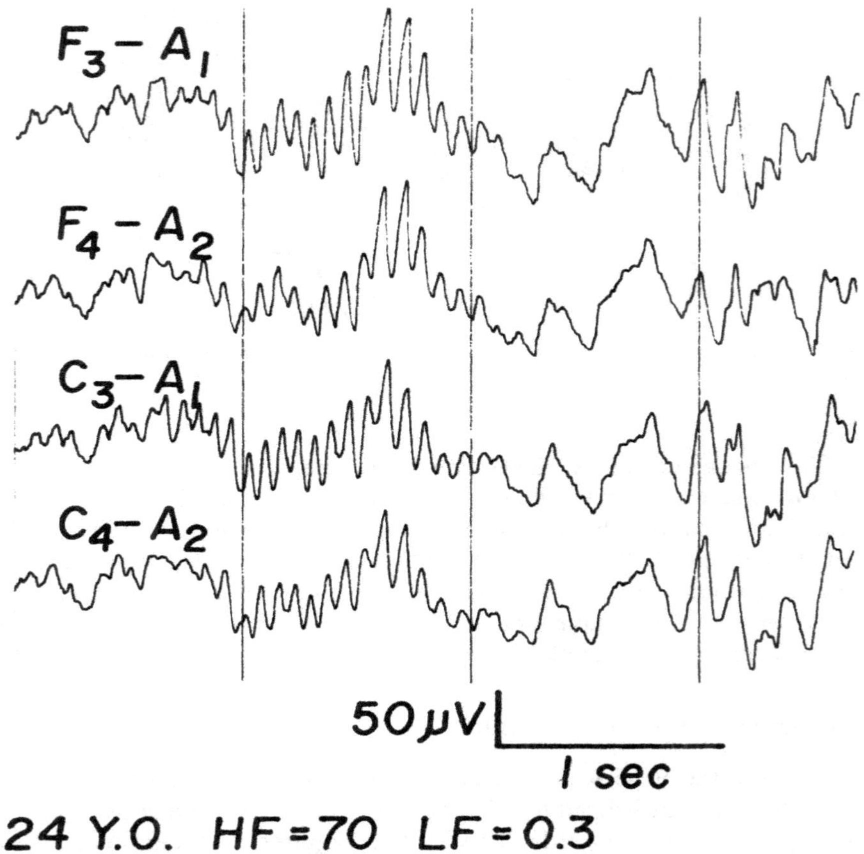

FIG. 14.31. Typical sleep spindles in frontal and central areas of a 24-year-old subject during sleep, starting as low voltage activity and increasing. HF = 70 Hz; LF = 0.3 Hz.

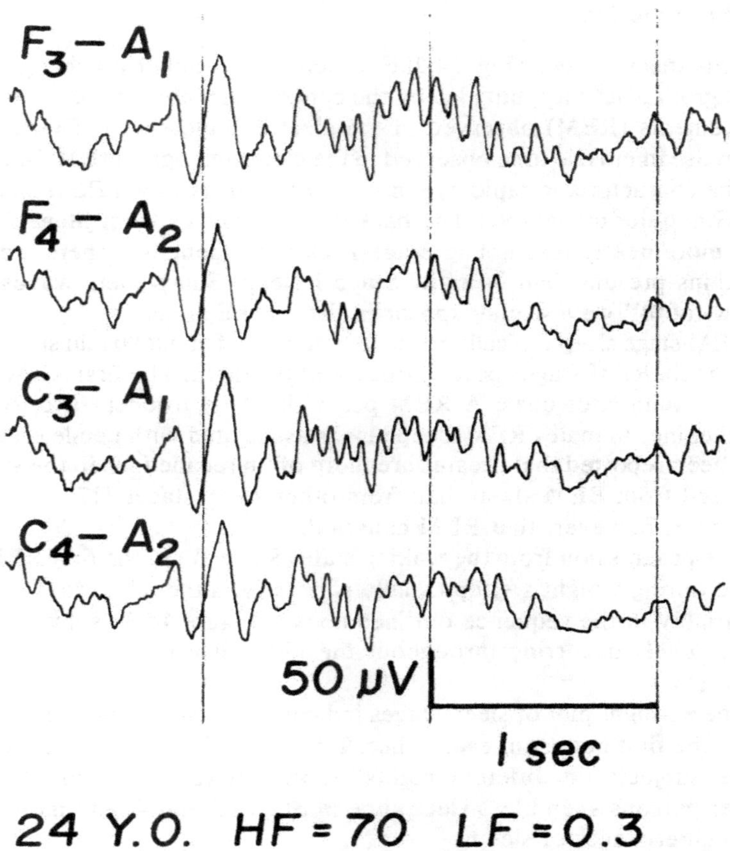

FIG. 14.32. K complex with sharp transient followed by spindle burst in a 24-year-old subject. HF = 70 Hz; LF = 0.3 Hz.

degree. K complexes also may persist. Frontal slow transients may appear.

Stage 4 Sleep

In Stage 4 sleep (Fig. 14.28E), delta activity is present more than 50% of the time, with voltage greater than 75 μV. This defines a further deepening of sleep. This stage may not be reached in all subjects on all occasions, especially during daytime naps. The sleep spindles usually are slower in frequency (e.g., 10 Hz rather than 14 Hz). Large regions of the brain appear to discharge synchronously, but there still is regional independence. The slow activity is typically maximal over the anterior areas, and sharper transients continue to be located centrally.

REM-Stage Sleep

This stage of sleep (Fig. 14.28F) is defined not only by a change in EEG background activity, but also by the concomitant appearance of rapid eye movements (REM) observed in the electro-oculogram (EOG) and by a decrease in muscle tone observed in the electromyogram (EMG). Because of the characteristic rapid eye movements, this is called *REM sleep*. The EEG is quite distinctive: The background changes from Stage 3 or 4 to one more nearly resembling Stage 1, although generally there are slower rhythms present than in initial Stage 1 sleep. Sharp theta waves, called "saw-tooth" waves, may appear in the central areas.

REM stage sleep typically recurs at intervals of about 90 min so that about five or six REM stages occur throughout the night. The first REM stage is shorter than later ones. A REM period is likely to occur shortly before awakening. In males REM sleep also is associated with penile erection. It has been reported that dreams are more often recalled when the subject is aroused from REM sleep than from other sleep stages (17). One should not infer, however, that REM causes dreams.

The progression from the waking state (Stage W) to the first REM sleep stage during a night's sleep usually is orderly, although it does not occur invariably in the sequence outlined above. Figure 14.33 shows changing sleep levels occurring throughout the night in a typical healthy young adult (51).

The all-night plot of sleep stages indicates that subsequent cycles differ from the first and from each other. Likewise, different subjects (and the same subjects on different nights) show different patterns of cycling. Older persons spend less sleep time in Stages 3 and 4, and more time in the lighter stages of sleep.

Sleep sometimes is categorically divided into two types, one represented by Stages 2, 3 and 4, called *slow wave sleep*, and one represented by faster and lower voltage activity (4–7-Hz theta activity and 13-Hz and faster beta activity) together with rapid eye movements, called *REM sleep*.

The total range of the levels described will not appear in daytime sleep recorded in the usual clinical EEG setting. The recording time is too short (typically, 10–30 min) to allow a patient to progress beyond Stage 2 sleep. Also, unless the patient has been deprived of sleep, daytime naps are usually self-limiting, and do not typically include Stages 3 and 4 or REM sleep. (Young children present exceptions to this general rule.) In the adult, REM sleep does not normally occur at sleep onset.

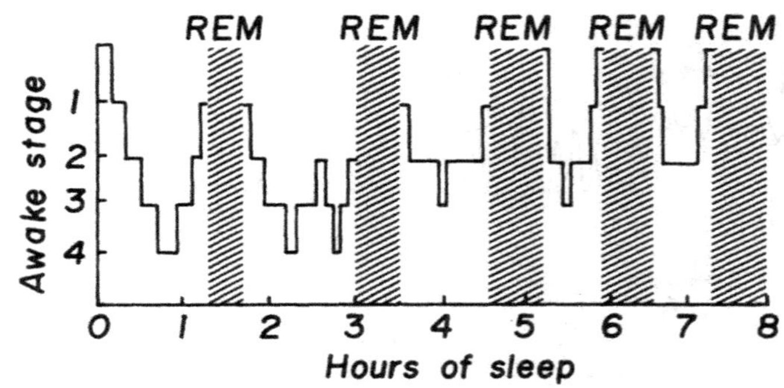

FIG. 14.33. The normal adult sleep cycle. [Redrawn from McGregor et al. (51), with permission.]

The above accounts of EEG changes in sleep are derived from observations made over many years by many investigators. The earliest detailed information about all-night sleep was provided in 1935–37 by Loomis et al. (47,48), who made the first graphic, minute-by-minute profile of all-night sleep levels. The identification of periodic rapid eye movements was not made for another 20 years (4). Further details of REM stage sleep and its possible relationship to dreams appeared in 1957 (17).

Techniques of Sleep Recording

Because the EEG was increasingly used to study patients with sleep disorders, a standardized terminology to describe and define sleep levels was published in 1968 (61). This system requires a specific technique, which includes recording from C_3 or C_4 to the contralateral ear. In addition, horizontal and vertical eye movements are recorded. Electrodes are placed at the outer canthus of each eye, 1 cm above on one eye and 1 cm below on the other eye. Both are referred to the same ear (A_1 or A_2). This derivation provides the electrooculogram (EOG), from which REMs are defined.

A measure of the level of background muscle tone is included, which is provided by electrodes placed over the submental muscle under the chin to record the EMG (using increased sensitivity). The respiratory rate and the heart rate may also be recorded. If REM stage sleep must be positively identified, it is essential that the EOG and EMG recordings be included with the EEG.

In the usual clinical EEG, it is not necessary to identify REM stage sleep, and non-EEG derivations are required only in special cases. EEGs can be classified at all other levels from data based on the usual clinical EEG montages, although it should be kept in mind that the most important information comes from the central and midline areas.

Application of the principles of sleep EEG to the problems met in clinical practice will be of assistance to the clinical technologist. Sometimes normal sleep EEG activity is confused with abnormal EEG phenomena; usually the confusion occurs when a change in the sleep stage has not been recognized by the technologist or the interpreter, e.g., slow activity of Stage 1 may be called abnormal because change from Stage W is not noted. In some patients, EEG abnormalities are more likely to occur during sleep and it often is necessary to allow the patient to progress from Stage W to Stage 2 without interruption, so that Stage 1 and Stage 2 can be seen in their normal context. In other patients, the intrusion of sleep can obscure clinically significant EEG activity. In such instances the patient may need to be kept alert. When alerting stimuli are delivered during the examination, they should always be identified on the EEG record so that reactivity can be assessed. In practice, the technologist must be able to recognize all levels of the awake-asleep cycle and carry out the EEG examination in a manner that will yield the greatest information.

In the ordinary practice of clinical EEG technology sleep EEGs are recorded during daytime naps. Such observations are to be contrasted with all-night sleep recordings, which include several non-EEG measures in addition to EOG and EMG. These are called *polysomnograms*. They are used to evaluate sleep disorders. (For further technical details see 69.)

EEG ACTIVITY IN THE ELDERLY

Certain EEG changes are associated with aging, but not all elderly persons show the same alterations. The four main types of changes are 1) decrease in frequency of the alpha rhythm, 2) increase in the amount of beta activity, 3) increase in diffuse slow activity, and 4) development of focal dysrhythmias (55).

Slowing of the alpha rhythm is probably the most characteristic change. This has been documented by serial recordings on the same patients, as well as by average alpha frequencies recorded from groups at different age levels (15,56). In addition to the change in frequencies, alpha activity may become less abundant and less reactive to visual stimulation (Fig. 14.34).

Beta activity exceeding 15 μV also increases with age and is greater anteriorly. It is seen more often in females (8).

Diffuse slow activity, seen as theta (4–7 Hz) and delta (1–3 Hz) activity, increases, particularly beyond age 75 (8). A pronounced increase in diffuse slow activity, however, probably is not a normal change, but is related to senility and intellectual deterioration, i.e., to a change from a healthy to a sick person.

Focal changes involve the appearance of localized theta and delta activity, amplitude asymmetries of more than 50%, and the development of focal spikes and/or sharp waves (7). Even in middle age, in the fifth decade of life, increases in temporal slow transients occur (40). There is a marked tendency for this focal slow activity to involve the left temporal area.

The elderly spend less sleep time in Stages 3 and 4 and relatively more time in Stages 1 and 2. The age-related focal slow changes are enhanced in Stage 1 sleep, but are less obvious in sleep Stages 2 and 3.

In general, EEG activity in the elderly does not change uniformly, but aging is a factor that must be considered in evaluating an individual's EEG record.

ABNORMAL EEG ACTIVITY IN ADULTS

We previously stated that a definition of abnormal involves a comparison of EEG characteristics observed in groups of patients with neurological or other diseases with those of healthy subjects. The following description of EEG elements is based on EEG samples drawn from various large populations of patients and on the same descriptive criteria used to classify normal EEG activity. For an EEG to be considered abnormal, one or more of the following conditions must be met.

1. The frequencies of basic rhythms are either faster or slower than established in a healthy group of the same age and state.
2. The voltage of a particular EEG activity (e.g., beta, theta, sleep spindles) is either higher or lower than the observed limits in healthy subjects of the same age and stage. It may be continuous, intermittent, or paroxysmal.
3. The locations of various EEG activities (i.e., the scalp distribution) are different than in control groups (e.g., alpha, beta, mu). One may ask: Is the activity in its usual location? Is it generalized (i.e., seen in all

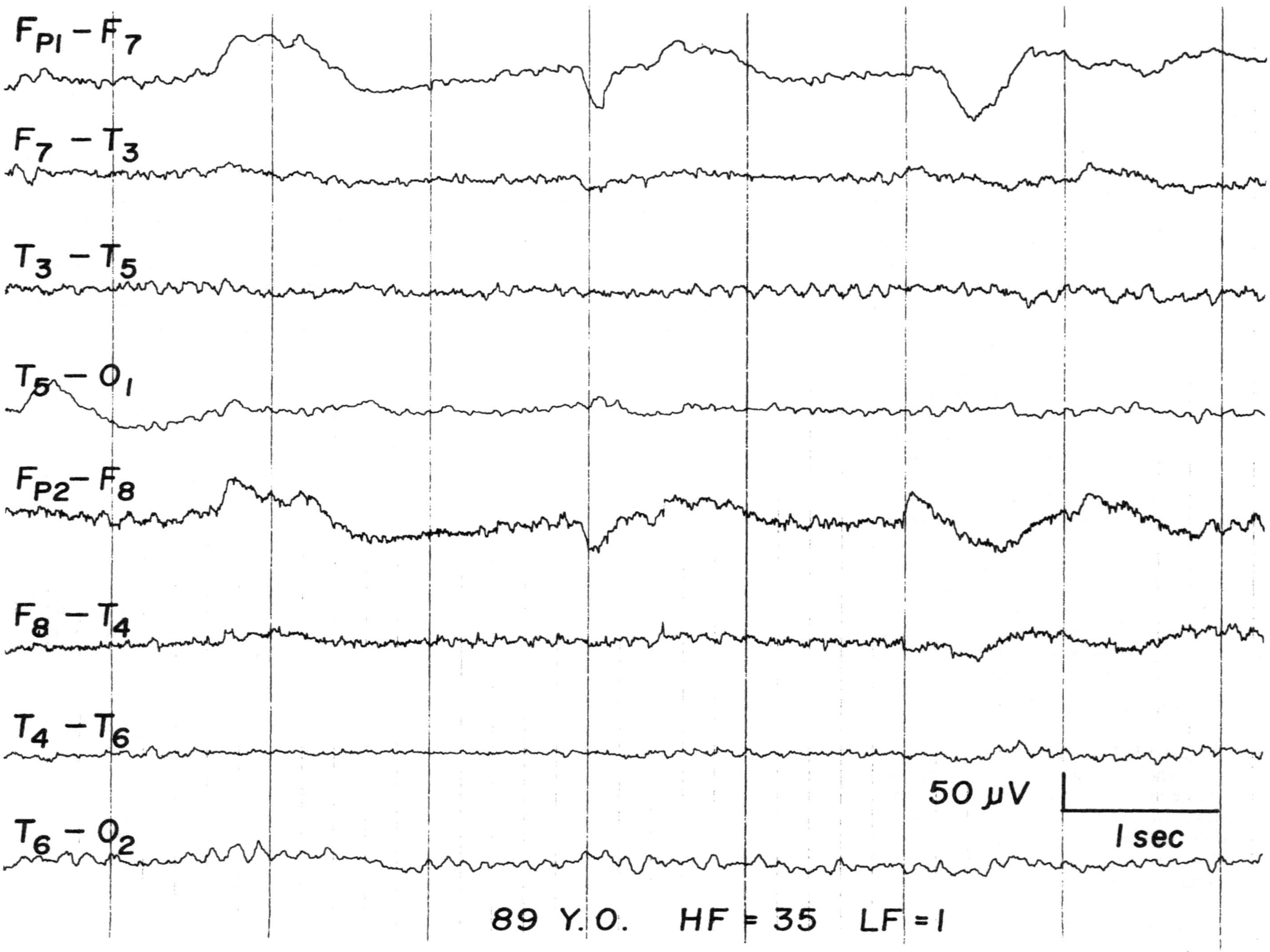

FIG. 14.34. 7- to 7.5-Hz posterior rhythm ("slowed alpha") in an 89-year-old awake subject. HF = 35 Hz; LF = 1 Hz.

areas)? Is it lateralized (i.e., asymmetrical and seen only on one side)? Is it focal (i.e., seen in a restricted area)?

4. Waveforms or patterns appear that have a morphology different than those encountered in a group of healthy subjects of the same age and state. The waveforms may have an unusual or distinctive surface polarity. They may be generalized, laterized, or focal. They may be continuous, intermittent or paroxysmal.
5. Distinctive elements with a periodic character, unusual for age and state appear. For example, a single slow wave of high amplitude may appear every 12 to 16 sec (i.e., periodically) or a high voltage, single, sharp transient with a duration of 150 to 200 msec may appear over one hemisphere every 1 to 3 sec. Usually they are paroxysmal in character.
6. Loss of reactivity to stimulation, or an atypical response occurs (e.g., stimulation produces a high voltage rhythmic discharge).

The question, then, is: How extensive is the deviation in frequency, voltage, morphology, quantity, location, synchrony, periodicity, and reactivity? The deviance may be rated on a 3-point scale: minimal, moderate, and extreme.

Specific Abnormal EEG Patterns

The word specific is used in two ways, which should be clearly distinguished. The first usage, as in "specific EEG patterns," means that a particular EEG pattern can reliably be distinguished from other EEG patterns. The second usage implies an EEG pattern that has specific clinical correlations. The term is not always used in the same way, and confusion can occur.

A specific pattern in the first sense might be a mu rhythm, distinguishable from an alpha rhythm by virtue of its location, its morphology, and its reactivity. Both of these activities are normal. On the other hand, there are many specific patterns that rarely are seen in healthy subjects and frequently are seen in various patient groups. These can be collectively assembled under the term "abnormal EEG patterns." It is in this sense that the term is used here. Whether any of these patterns has a unique or specific clinical meaning is not our concern at this point.

When the EEG characteristics of patient groups have been compared with those of healthy groups, the following have been found to be so overwhelmingly present in patient groups that they are usually regarded as being abnormal.

1. *Spikes* (focal or nonfocal) (see Fig. 14.10). (See p. 187).
2. *Sharp waves* (focal or nonfocal) (see Fig. 14.11). (See p. 187).
3. *Spike-and-wave complex.* Spikes followed by slow waves (10). The spikes may be multiple. The spike-and-wave complex is further defined by frequency:
   a. 3-Hz spike-and-wave (actually, 2.5–3.5 Hz) (see Fig. 14.12).
   b. Slow variant (<2.5 Hz).
   c. Fast variant (>3.5 Hz, may reach 6 Hz).
4. *Sharp-and-slow-wave complex.* Sharp wave rather than a spike. It is important to maintain this differentiation (see Fig. 14.13). The frequency usually is slow (1–2 Hz).
5. *Rhythmic hypersynchronous activity.* Rhythmic activity emerging from the background and appearing to be nonreactive. May be focal or generalized (see Fig. 14.5).
6. *Periodic discharges.*
   a. Periodic lateralized epileptiform discharges (PLEDS). Sharp and slow discharges occurring at an approximately periodic rate, usually <1/sec (Fig. 14.35).
   b. Periodic slow complexes. Usually, slow complexes or transients (may not always be of high voltage) occurring at approximately regular intervals (e.g., 3–20 sec) (Fig. 14.36).
   c. Burst-suppression activity. Characterized by bursts of slow activity (theta or delta) and/or spikes or sharp waves, with relatively long intervening periods of very low voltage activity (Fig. 14.37).
7. *Triphasic waves.* Waves "consisting of three components alternating about the baseline" (10), but in practice, more complex morphologies may be encountered (Fig. 14.38).
8. *"Alpha coma."* Defined by morphology, location, state of consciousness, and reactivity. Typically the "alpha" is seen as 9- to 10-Hz activity, which is central-frontal in location rather than occipital. It usually is nonreactive. It is associated with coma, often, but not always, following trauma (Fig. 14.39).
9. *"Spindle coma."* Defined by frequency, morphology, and state of consciousness. Usually, 12- to 14-Hz bursts distributed similarly to sleep spindles and seen in coma, sometimes posttraumatic (Fig. 14.40).

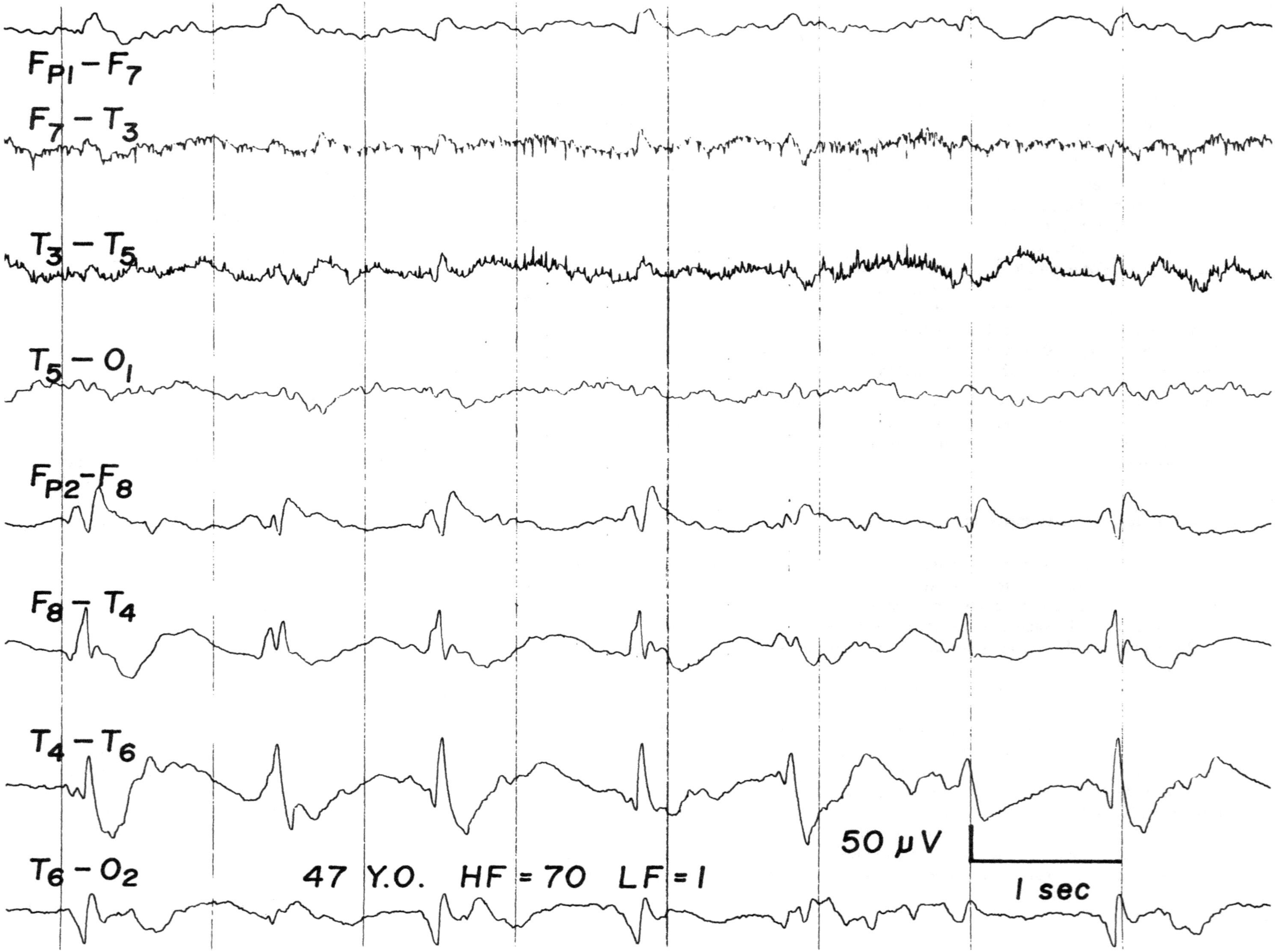

FIG. 14.35. Periodic lateralized epileptiform discharge (PLED) in a 47-year-old comatose patient. HF = 70 Hz; LF = 1 Hz.

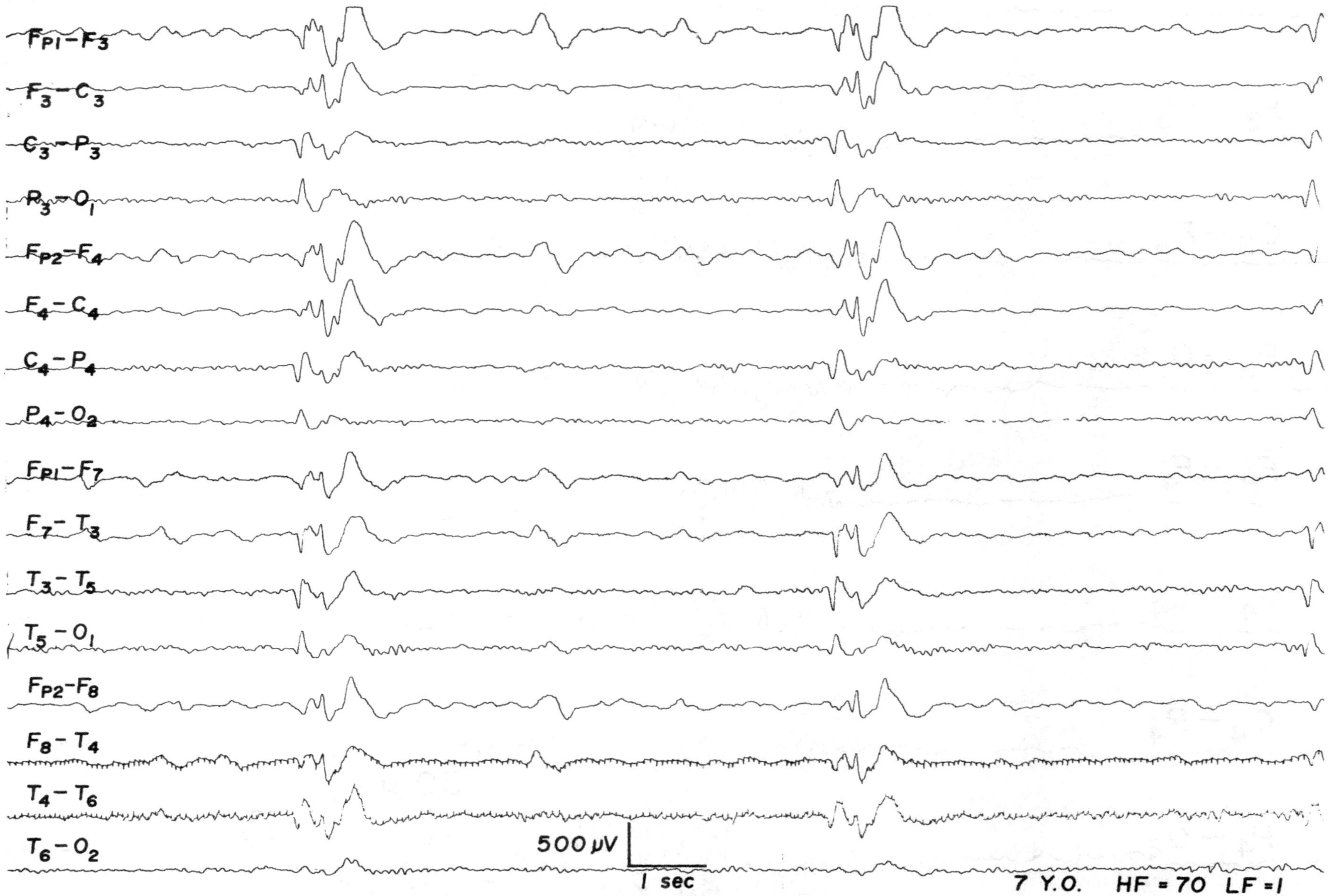

FIG. 14.36. Periodic slow-wave complex in a 7-year-old girl. Note partial preservation of alpha rhythm (about 9.5 Hz, 30–60 μV). HF = 70 Hz; LF = 1 Hz.

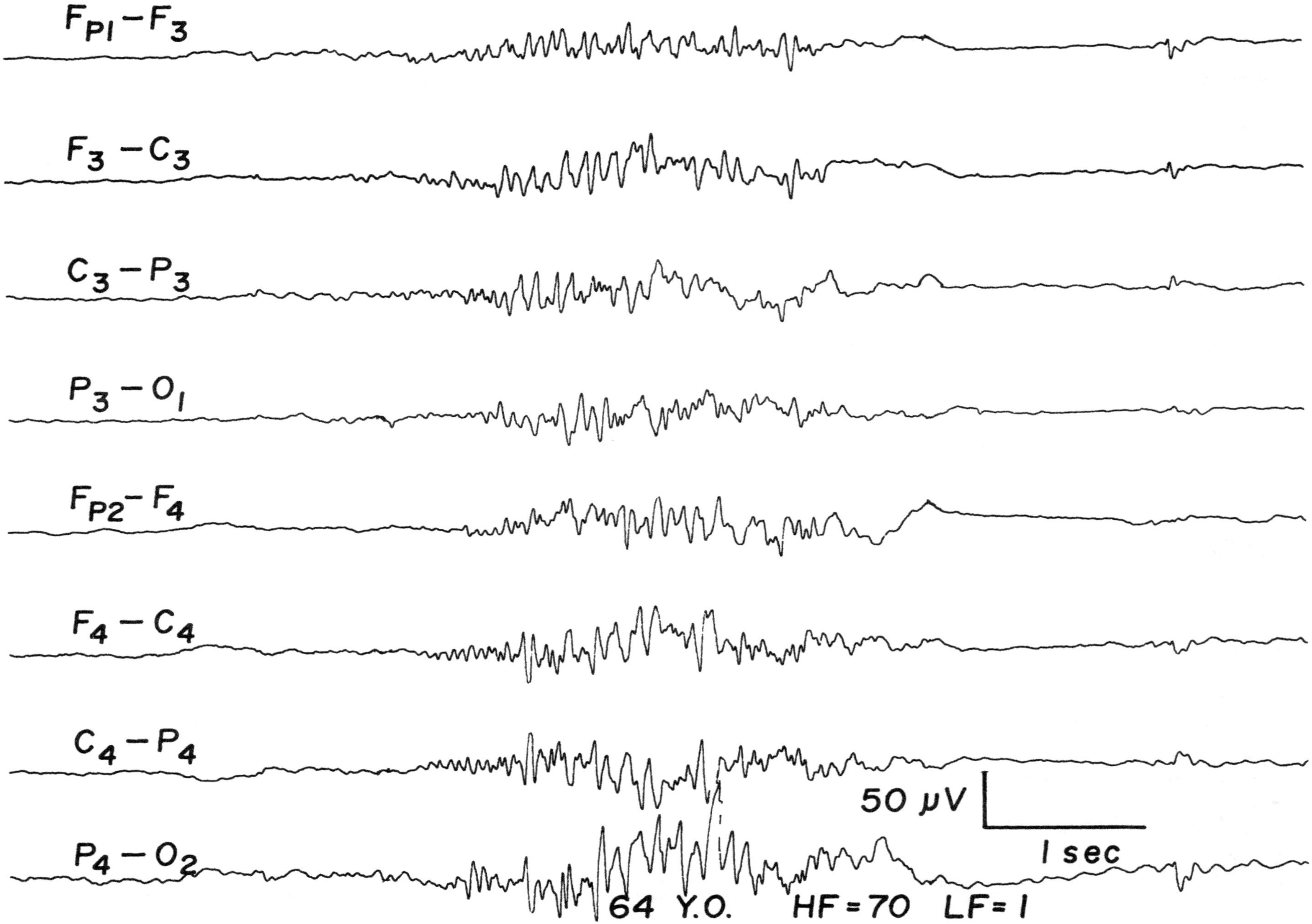

FIG. 14.37. Burst-suppression activity in a 64-year-old woman. HF = 70 Hz; LF = 1 Hz.

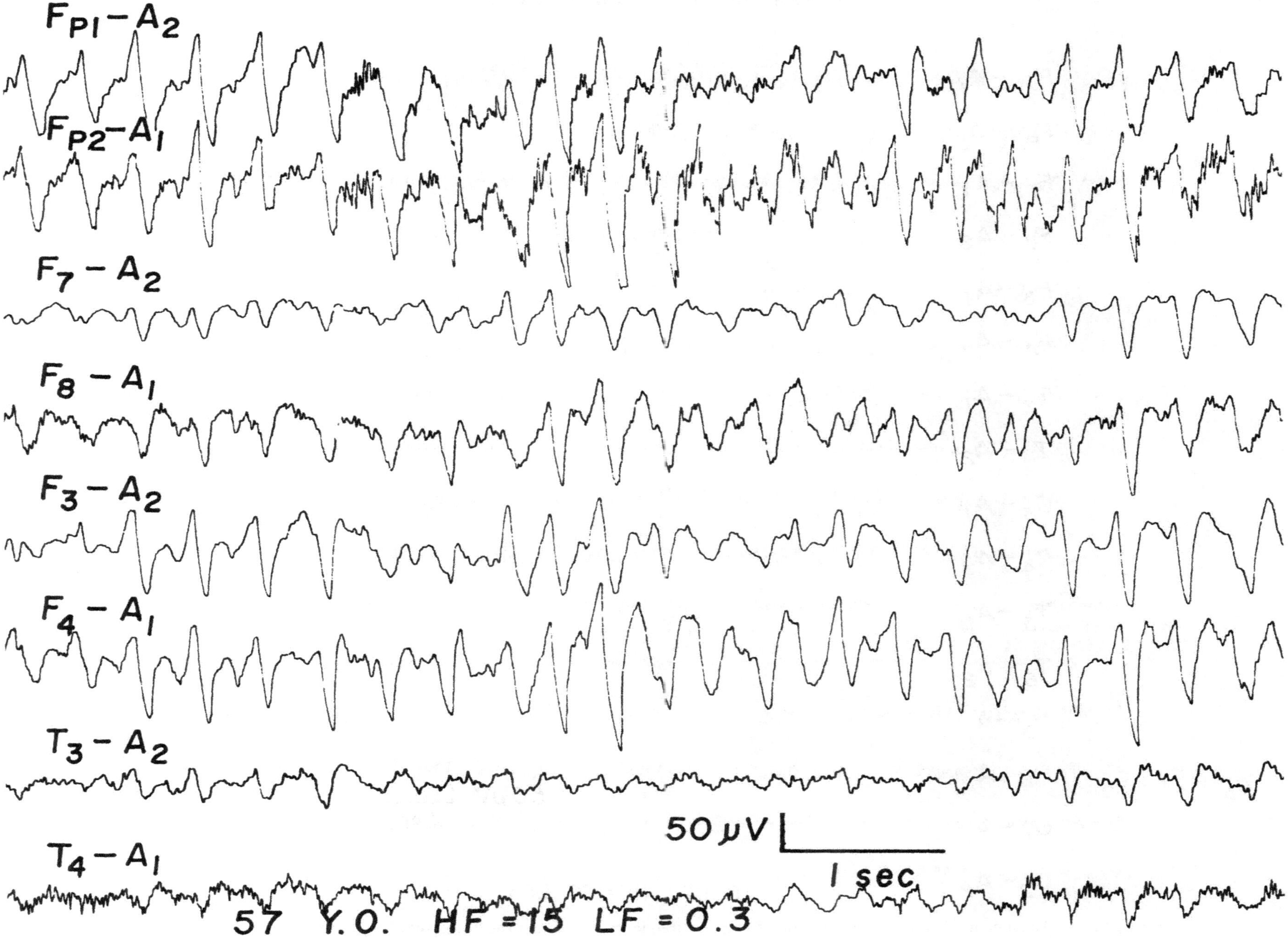

FIG. 14.38. Triphasic waves in a 57-year-old comatose patient. HF = 15 Hz; LF = 0.3 Hz.

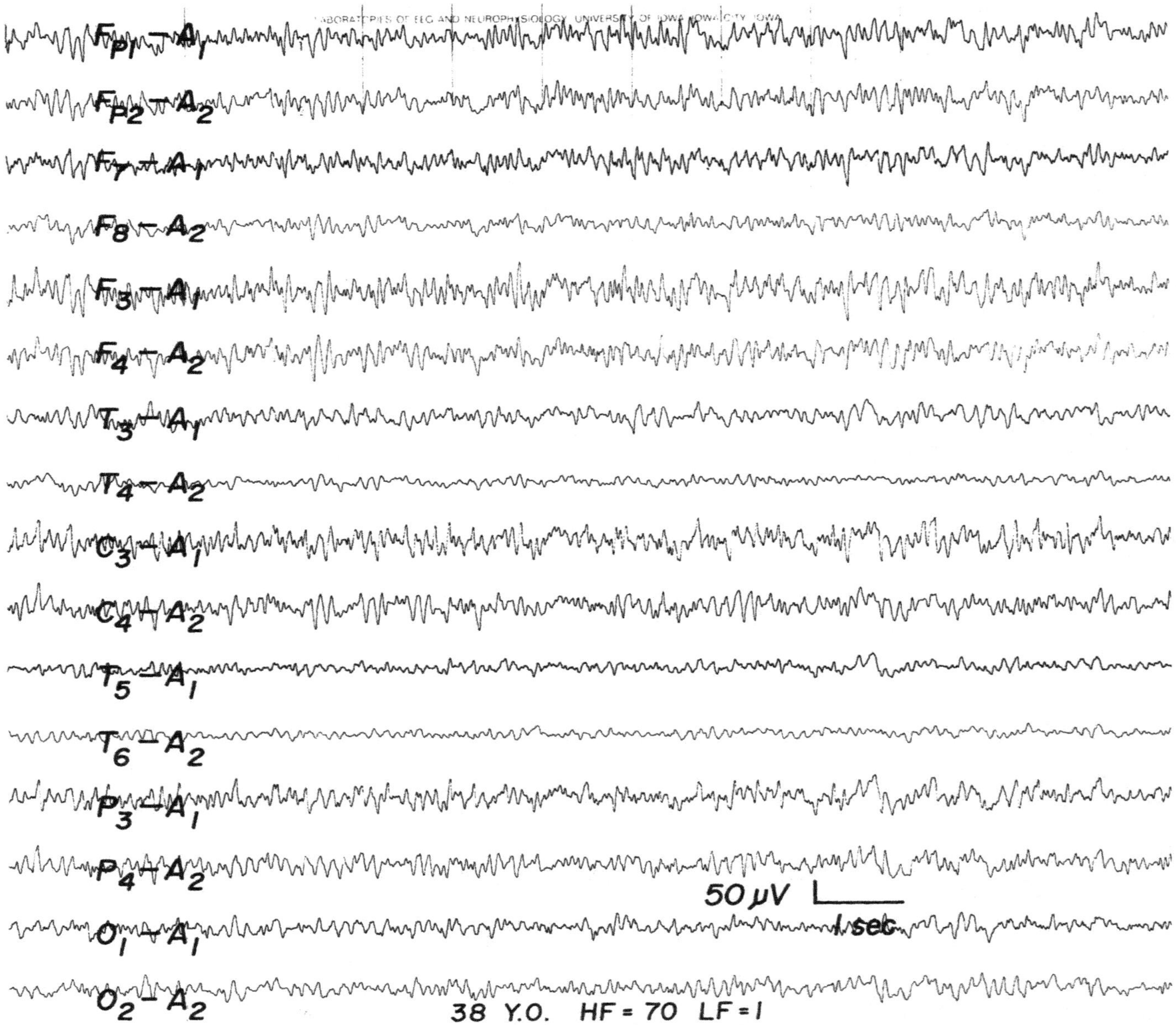

FIG. 14.39. "Alpha coma." Atypical distribution of "alpha" frequency in a comatose 38-year-old subject following cardiopulmonary arrest. HF = 70 Hz; LF = 1 Hz. (Courtesy of Elizabeth Meng, R. EEG T., and Margaret Gordon, R. EEG T., University of Iowa Hospitals, Iowa City, Iowa.)

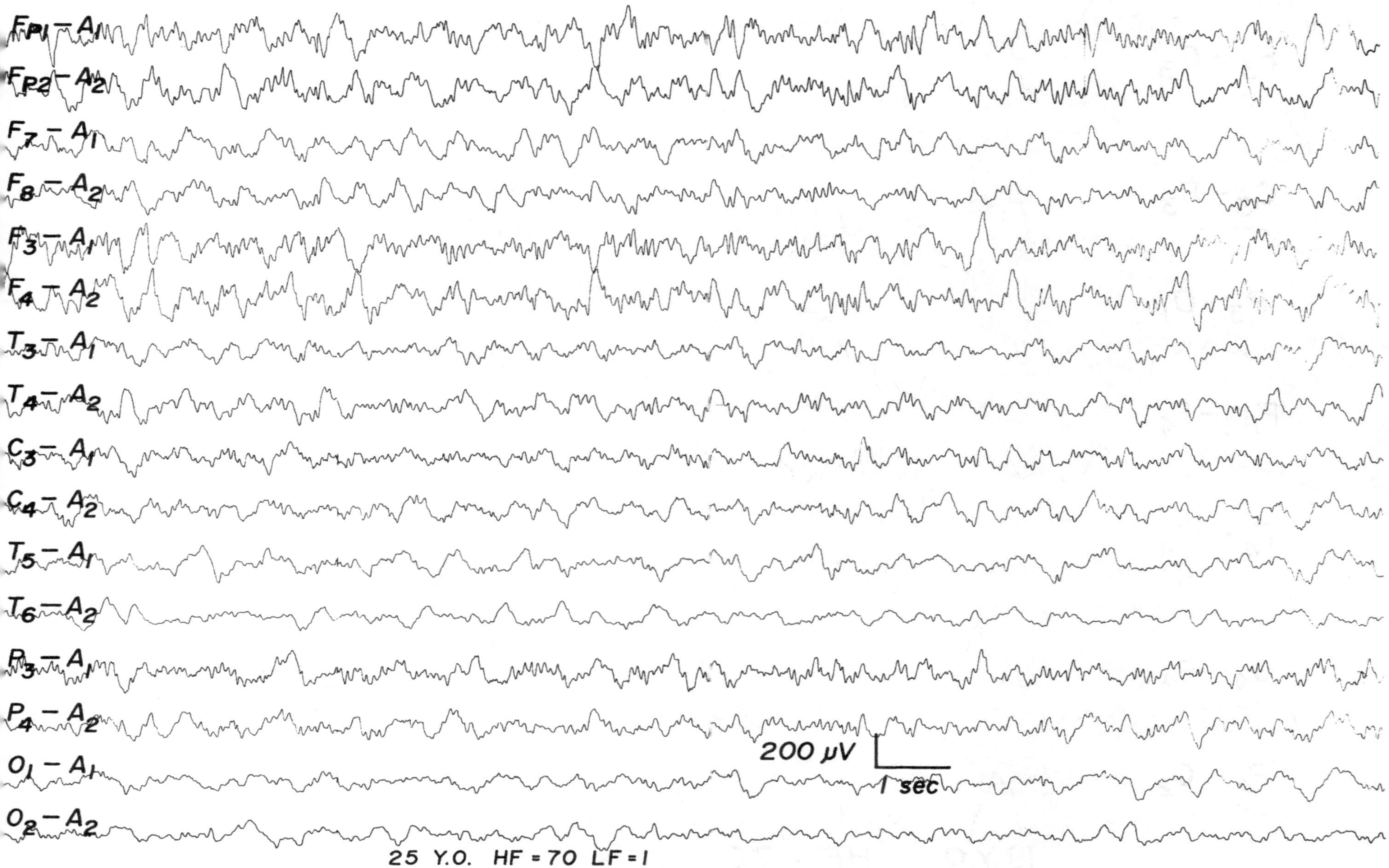

FIG. 14.40. "Spindle coma." Sleep-like patterns of 11- to 14-Hz anterior activity with slow transients and slow activity associated with coma following head injury in a 25-year-old subject. HF = 70 Hz; LF = 1 Hz. (Courtesy of Elizabeth Meng, R. EEG T., and Margaret Gordon, R. EEG T., University of Iowa Hospitals, Iowa City, Iowa.)

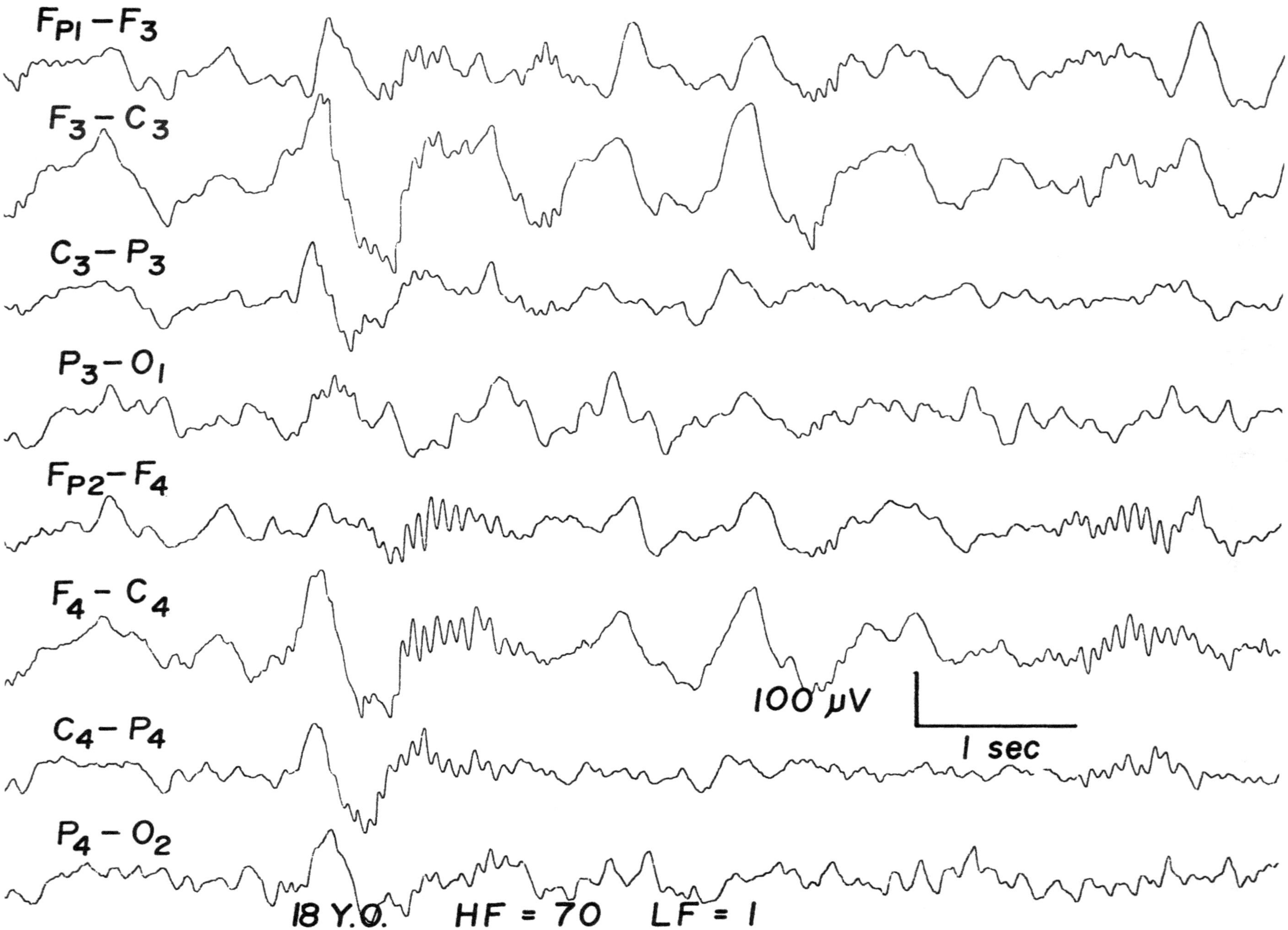

FIG. 14.41. Abnormal sleep activity in an 18-year-old woman. Sleep spindles (13–14 Hz) are seen over the right central-frontal region, but are virtually absent over the left side. This occurred consistently throughout sleep. HF = 70 Hz; LF = 1 Hz. (See page 234.)

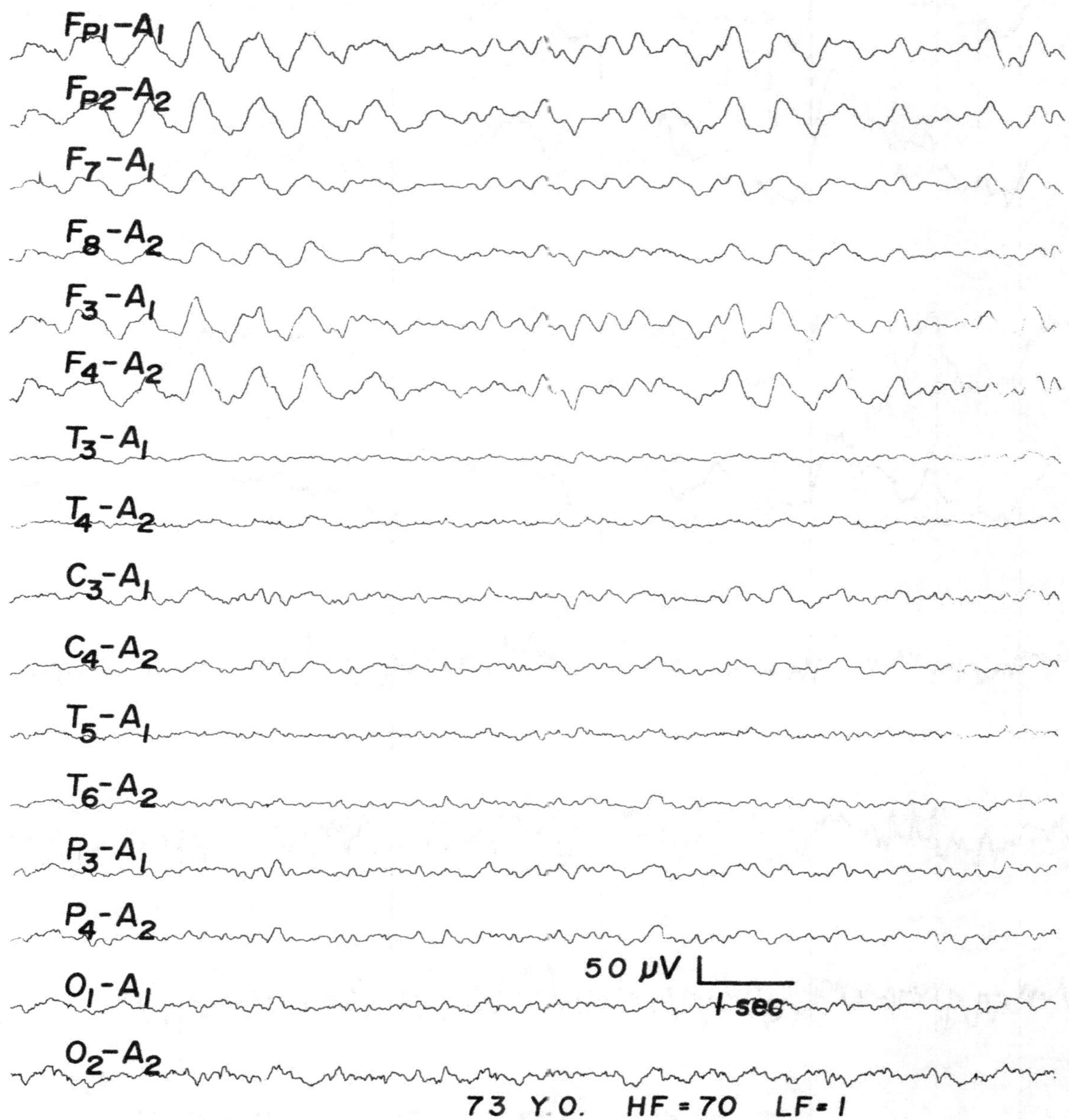

FIG. 14.42. Frontal, intermittent, rhythmic delta activity in a 73-year-old subject. HF = 70 Hz; LF = 1 Hz. (See text page 234.)

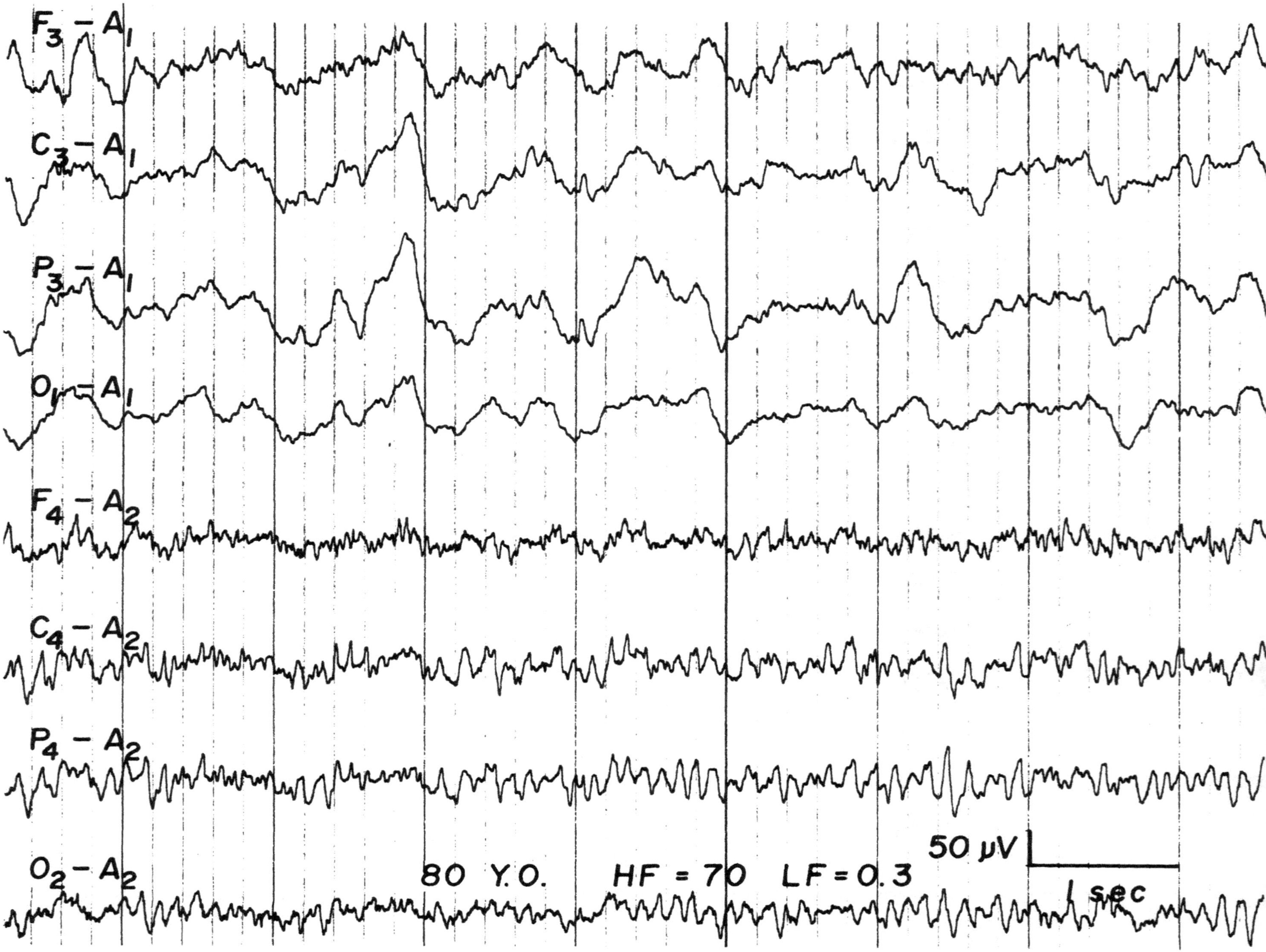

FIG. 14.43. Continuous, left hemisphere, polymorphic delta activity, posterior in P_3 and dominant in O_1, in an 80-year-old woman. Note loss of a background activity. HF = 70 Hz; LF = 0.3 Hz. (See text page 234.)

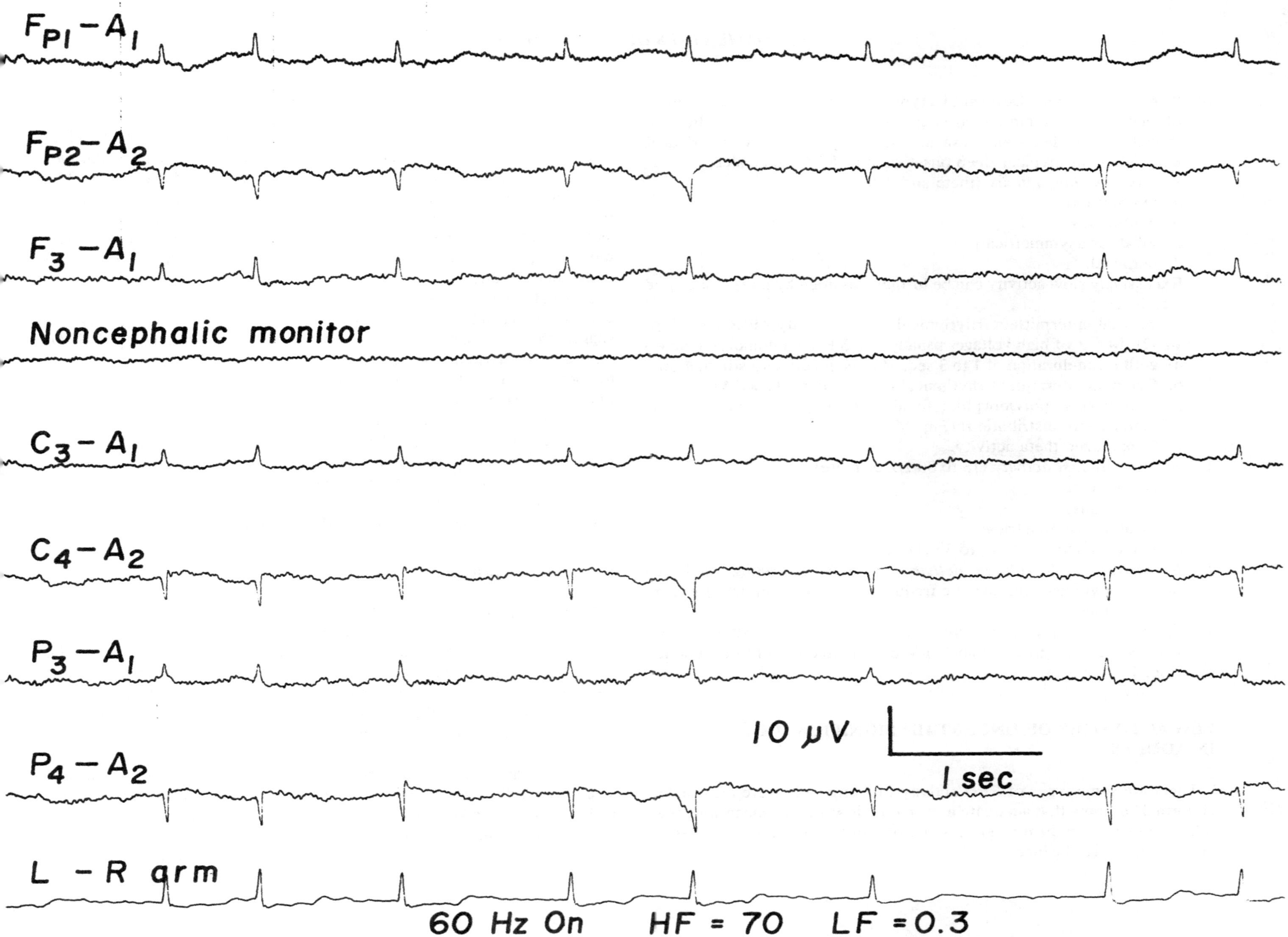

FIG. 14.44. Electrocerebral inactivity in a 69-year-old man following cardiac arrest. Referential montage with EKG monitor (L−R arm) and amplifier noise level monitor in channel 4. The apparent spikes are EKG artifact. S = 1 μV/mm; HF = 70 Hz; LF = 0.3 Hz; 60-Hz filter = on. (See text page 234.)

10. "*Abnormal sleep.*" Defined by atypical morphology for a given level of sleep [e.g., asymmetrical (Fig. 14.41) or no 14-Hz spindles, although K complexes and slow activity are present; asymmetrical K complexes, or atypical sleep onset such as REM-stage sleep].
11. *Excessively slow activity* (theta and delta activity).
    a. intermittent,
    b. continuous,
    c. focal (or asymmetrical),
    d. nonfocal.
    Excessively slow activity can be further classified by morphology and location:
    a. Frontal intermittent rhythmical delta activity (FIRDA) (Fig. 14.42). Bursts of high voltage, usually 2 to 3 Hz, monomorphic activity with mean duration of 1 to 3 sec. May be reactive to stimulation.
    b. Occipital intermittent rhythmical delta activity (OIRDA).
    c. Continuous, polymorphic, focal activity (e.g., asymmetrical, left hemisphere distribution) (Fig. 14.43).
    d. Generalized theta activity.
12. *Excessively fast activity* (13 to 30 Hz or more).
    a. intermittent,
    b. continuous,
    c. focal (or asymmetrical),
    d. nonfocal activity of 13 to 30 Hz or more.
13. *Excessively high voltage activity.* Activity exceeding published maximum voltages for specific frequencies or types of activity (e.g., sleep spindles).
14. *Electrocerebral inactivity.* Profound attenuation (e.g., suppression), with no activity greater than 2 μV attributable to cerebral function (Fig. 14.44).

EEG ACTIVITIES OF UNCERTAIN SIGNIFICANCE IN ADULTS

There are some types of EEG activity that originally were regarded as abnormal but, now that adequate information is available concerning their relative incidence in healthy groups, are presently considered of uncertain or no clinical significance.

Rhythmic Midtemporal Harmonic Discharge

Rhythmic midtemporal harmonic discharges were first described in 1952 and were called "psychomotor variant" (29). This is a specific pattern consisting of 4- to 7-Hz activity, "notched" by a faster wave. The superimposed faster frequency gives the pattern a sharp, surface negative, appearance. There typically is a harmonic relationship between the slower and faster frequencies (e.g., 4 Hz and 8 Hz or 6 Hz and 12 Hz). The morphology is determined by phase and voltage relationships between the component frequencies (16; see also 58).

This pattern has more recently been termed "rhythmical mid-temporal discharges" (RMTD) (44). Because of the notable harmonic features, we suggest that the name "rhythmic harmonic temporal discharges" (RHTD) be used. The harmonic structure distinguishes this pattern from "drowsy temporal theta." RHTD is maximal in the temporal regions and appears during drowsiness (Fig. 14.45).

Because this pattern first was seen in specific patient groups, the activity was originally thought to be associated with epilepsy and psychiatric disorders. However, it is so rare, both in patients and in healthy subjects, that most electroencephalographers now believe no specific pathological significance should be attached to it (50,58). It is not an epileptiform discharge and has no correlation with seizure disorders.

Small Sharp Spikes

Small sharp spikes (SSS) are surface negative fast transients that usually have a voltage between 30 and 50 μV, although it may reach 100 μV. They occur during drowsiness and sleep and are most prominent in the frontal and temporal regions. They often appear in nasopharyngeal derivations. They may occur, less conspicuously, in the parietal and occipital regions. Small sharp spikes can appear bilaterally and synchronously, but more commonly may involve one side or the other, shifting back and forth (Fig. 14.46).

Small sharp spikes also are known as "benign epileptiform transients of sleep" (BETS). This name was applied because the spikes resemble clinically significant spikes (i.e., they appear to be epileptiform), but they are not related to clinical disease (i.e., they are benign). They appear commonly in healthy subjects (78) and great caution should be used before

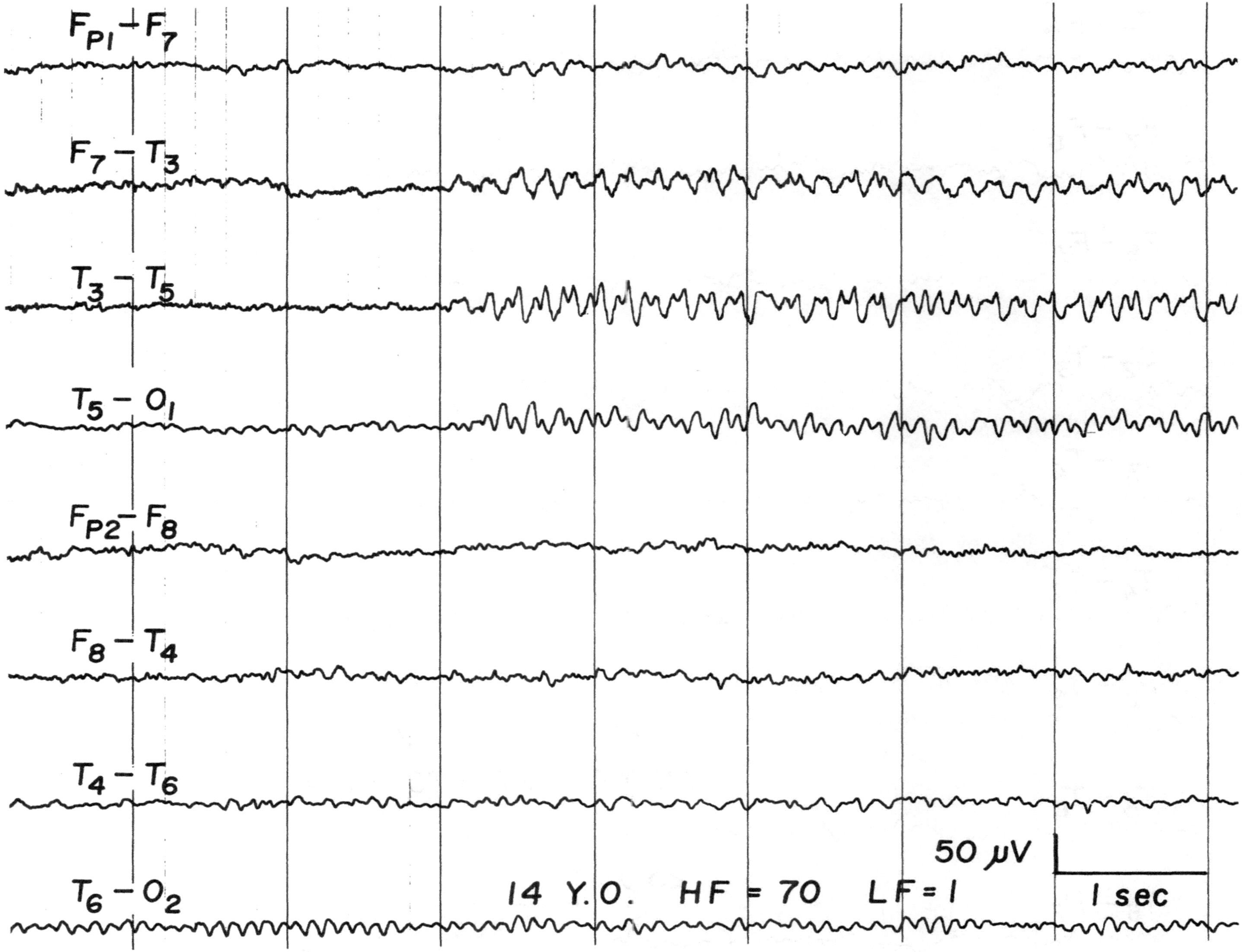

FIG. 14.45. Rhythmic harmonic temporal discharge in a 14-year-old subject. HF = 70 Hz; LF = 1 Hz.

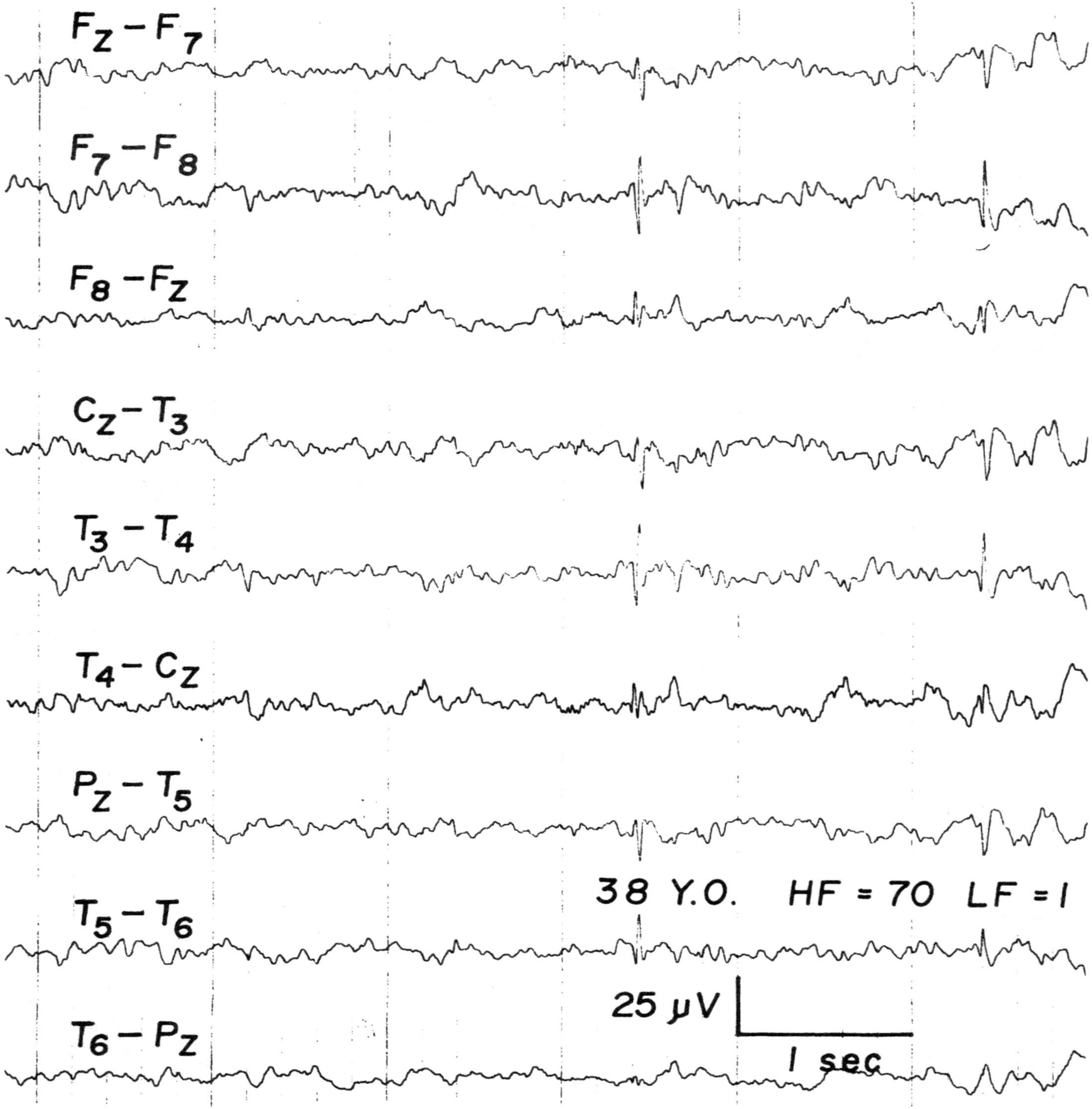

FIG. 14.46. Small sharp spikes, recorded with transverse triangular montage, in a 38-year-old subject. Note the relatively high sensitivity used. HF = 70 Hz; LF = 1 Hz.

they are regarded as abnormal (50,58), particularly if they are limited to nasopharyngeal derivations.

Six Per Second Spike-and-Wave Activity

The 6-Hz spike-and-wave activity is characterized by small spikes, usually no larger than 50 μV, followed by a low voltage slow wave (Fig. 14.47). These are rhythmic complexes that may range in frequency from 4 to 7 Hz and usually occur in bursts lasting less than 1 sec. In some cases, the bursts may be seen maximally in the anterior head regions, and in others they are maximal in the posterior regions. They appear in the awake state and sometimes are activated by photic stimulation. The occurrence of 6-Hz spike-and-wave activity is variably reported in different clinical groups. One group was said to show a 3.2% incidence (52). There was a 1.5% incidence in young adult volunteers, which increased to nearly 30% after activation by intravenous diphenhydramine (70). Although a correlation with seizures generally has not been clearly demonstrated, recent reviews suggest that an anterior location and a spike voltage above 45 μV is associated with seizures in 75% of cases, whereas lower voltage, posteriorly distributed activity is less clearly associated with seizures (36%) (34). Since the pattern appears in persons without seizures, it should not be regarded as having "epileptogenic significance" (58), and in some individuals it is a normal variant. Its "significance" appears to depend less on the specific pattern than on its location and voltage (and, perhaps, the patient's complaints).

Fourteen and/or 6-Hz Positive Spikes

The 14- and/or 6-Hz positive spikes are surface positive spike-like bursts that are most evident in the occipital and posterior temporal regions and, when present, usually are seen in drowsiness and early sleep. They may appear rarely in the awake state. They occur independently on either side of the head. They occur in runs of 14 Hz or 6 Hz, or in runs of both frequencies intermixed. The frequencies can vary from 6 to 8 Hz and 12 to 15 Hz (35) (Fig. 14.48 A,B).

The positive spike field sometimes extends into A_1 or A_2 and if care is not exercised, it can produce confusing results and erroneous conclusions (Fig. 14.48C).

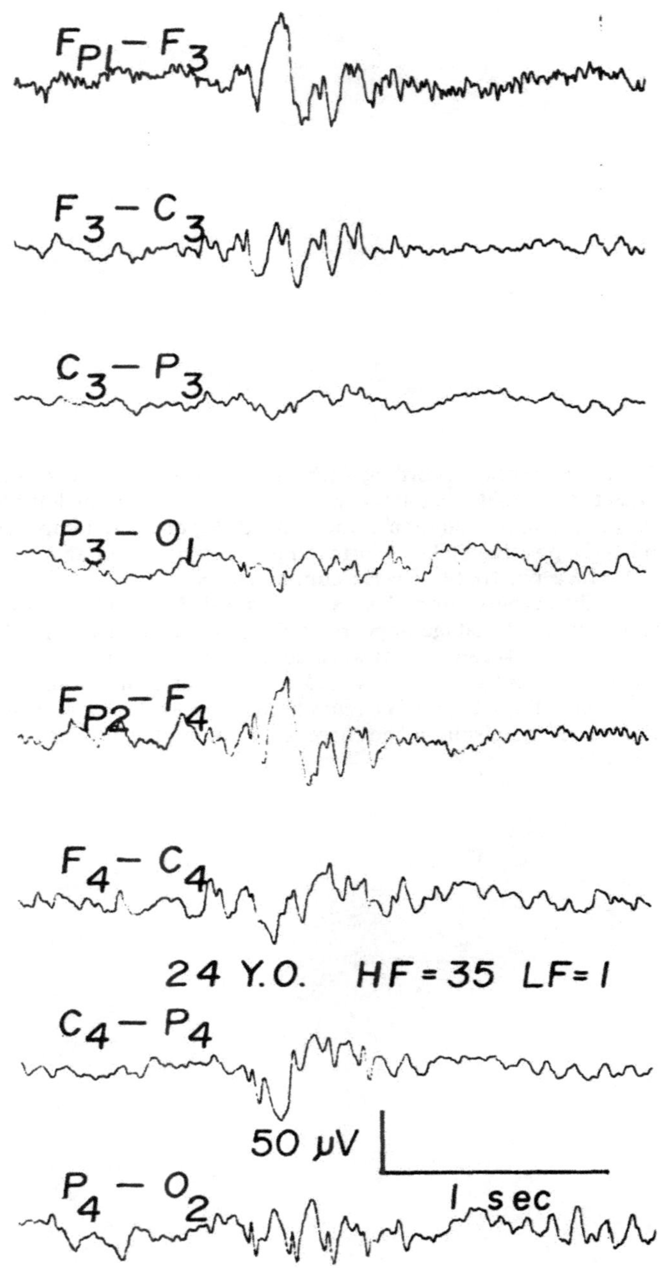

FIG. 14.47. 6-Hz spike-and-wave activity in a 24-year-old subject. HF = 35 Hz; LF = 1 Hz.

A

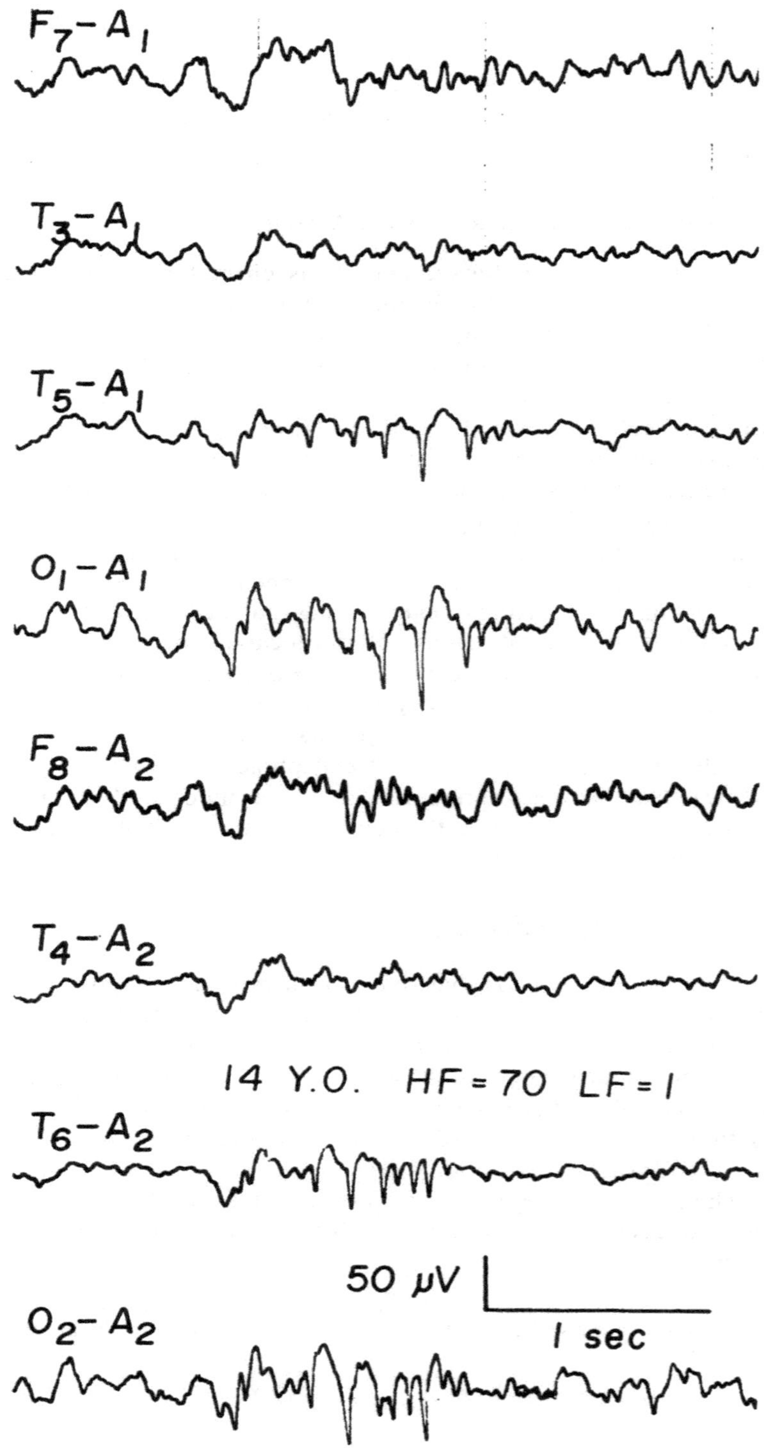

FIG. 14.48. A: Referential recording with 14- and 6-Hz positive spikes in a 14-year-old subject. Note that 6-Hz activity is most prominent in the left hemisphere and 14-Hz activity is more common in the right. **B:** Bipolar A-P temporal montage with 14- and 6-Hz positive spikes. Surface positivity of 14-Hz activity is clearly focal at T_6. Surface positivity of 6-Hz component is less clearly focal at T_5. **C:** 6-Hz positive spike activity during light sleep, recorded on contralateral ear reference montage. Maximal voltage appears at T_5. Positive spikes at T_3, T_5, and O_1 (Input 1 of channels 2–4) cause downward deflections. A_1 (contralateral ear reference) is also in the field of positivity and is on Input 2 of channels 5–8. The upward deflection in these channels occurs because Input 2 is more positive. O_2 is in the field of the left hemisphere and there is partial in-phase cancellation. HF = 70 Hz; LF = 1 Hz.

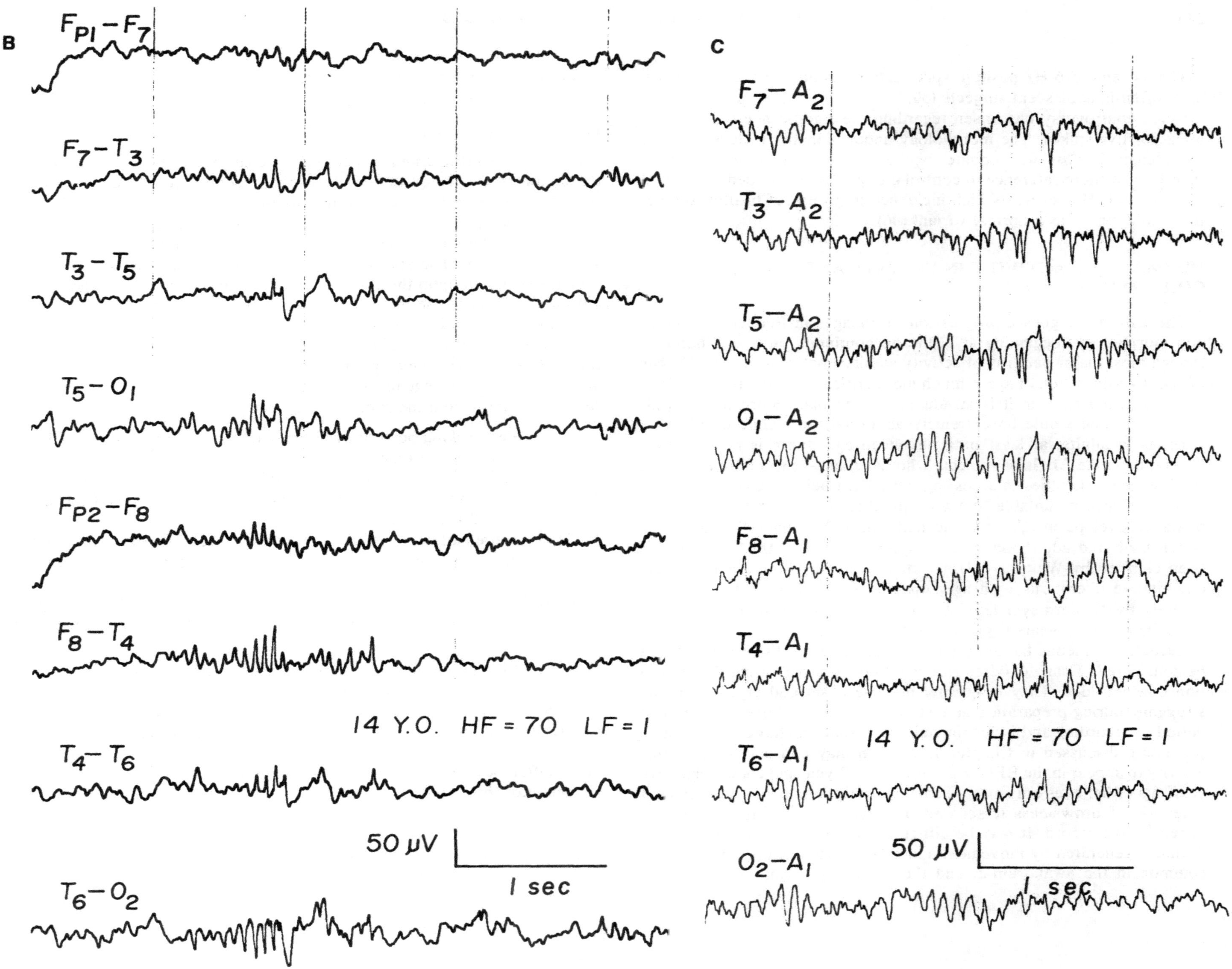
B
FP1 – F7
F7 – T3
T3 – T5
T5 – O1
FP2 – F8
F8 – T4
14 Y.O. HF = 70 LF = 1
T4 – T6
50 μV
1 sec
T6 – O2
C
F7 – A2
T3 – A2
T5 – A2
O1 – A2
F8 – A1
T4 – A1
14 Y.O. HF = 70 LF = 1
T6 – A1
50 μV
O2 – A1
1 sec

The 14- and/or 6-Hz positive spike activity is age-related, being seen most often in adolescent subjects (30).

Much controversy has arisen regarding the significance of 14- and/or 6-Hz positive spikes. The morphology unquestionably includes a spike-like element. Those who equate "spikes" with "epileptiform activity" therefore, without reference to control groups, have regarded this pattern as abnormal. However, its high incidence in groups of healthy subjects tends to define it as a normal variant (46).

NORMAL EEG ACTIVITY IN INFANTS AND CHILDREN: AWAKE

The EEG undergoes a progression of changes in frequency, voltage, and morphology, beginning at birth and continuing into adulthood, although most major patterns of activity stabilize between 15 and 20 years of age. Consideration of age is much more critical in evaluating the EEGs of young children than it is in adults. The normal record of an awake 2-year-old child would be extremely abnormal for a child of 10 years, whereas in adults, at least until advanced age, there is no noticeable difference in the EEGs of subjects who have an 8-year difference in age. At first, the difficulties in assessing the EEG tracings of young children may seem insurmountable, but with practice and experience, the technologist develops insight into the maturational changes that occur between birth and adulthood. The complex features of this process have been clarified by Walter's (74) narrative account of the qualitative and quantitative alterations with age, updated by Kellaway (38) and more recently by Niedermeyer (53). A detailed account of maturation of the EEG from 1 to 21 years is given in refs. 19 and 20.

Certain extraneous factors related to age influence the EEG and must be considered. Young children rarely are cooperative during the application of electrodes. They frequently become upset and cry. Crying and struggling during preparation almost always is carried over to the initial period of recording and is accompanied by rapid breathing (an activating procedure discussed in Chapter 15), which may cause slow frequency activity to appear in the EEG. Further, a 1- or 2-year-old child usually will close his or her eyes only after becoming drowsy, and slow activity characteristic of drowsiness (discussed in detail later in this chapter) will appear in the record. It may be difficult to obtain a true waking record. Artifacts generated by movement and other factors (see Chapter 16) are common in the awake child, and the technologist must constantly be aware of and evaluate the possible influence of the many variables that may alter or obscure the EEG.

Posterior EEG Activity

Perhaps the most dramatic age-related changes in the EEG occur in the dominant frequency of activity in the occipital area. These may be recognizable as early as 2 or 3 months of age, seen as rhythmic 3- to 4-Hz activity. At age 5 months, it may appear with a frequency of 5 Hz. At 1 year of age, the average posterior frequency is 6 to 7 Hz. It is reactive to visual stimulation. The appearance of dominant occipital activity of this type is dependent upon the child being awake and relaxed, with the eyes closed. The skill of the technologist will determine whether the activity can be recorded and its reactivity tested.

The classic and widely cited study of age and the posterior rhythm is that of Lindsley (43), which plotted dominant occipital waking frequency against chronological age in months and years. The data, based in part on serial recordings from the same children, showed that:

1. The earliest waking posterior rhythmic activity, at a frequency of 3⅓ to 4 Hz, occurs at 3 months of age.
2. There are individual differences in dominant frequency at all ages.
3. The increase in frequency with age is more uniform and rapid from age 3 months to 2 years than thereafter.
4. Some children attain occipital frequencies above 8 Hz, the lower adult alpha limit, at earlier ages than others (e.g., 4 years versus 9 years of age).
5. Posterior rhythms in some children, as observed by serial recording, may decrease in frequency from one year to the next, at least temporarily.

Figure 14.49 summarizes the change in mean frequency and voltage and also shows serial changes in frequency from four selected children.

Later studies of dominant reactive posterior activity (60) reported an average frequency of about 8 Hz by 2 years of age, which is somewhat earlier than in Lindsley's group. The difference in results probably reflects differences in technique, recording procedures, and mathematical treatment of the data.

Voltage of Dominant Posterior Rhythm

The voltage of occipital rhythmic activity also varies with age. In some infants, occipital rhythms increase in voltage up to 2 or 3 years of age. In

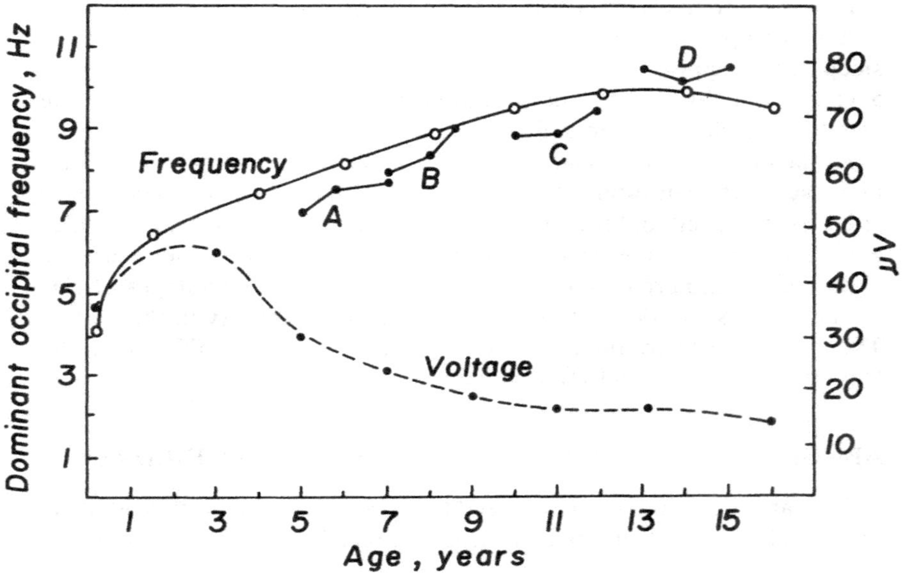

FIG. 14.49. Change in frequency (O——O) and voltage (●- - -●) of the dominant posterior rhythm with age (eyes closed). *Lines A–D* show annual change in dominant frequency in four healthy subjects. (Redrawn from Lindsley (43).)

general, there is a downward trend after the first year (43). The average voltage declines rapidly from age 3 to 5 years, and then levels off through adolescence. Petersén and Eeg-Olofsson (60) reported a somewhat later peak voltage. Beyond 12 years of age, compared with early ages, posterior voltage diminishes, although total voltage at 10, 11, and 12 Hz increases (32).

Asymmetries of voltage may be seen in children of all ages, but rarely does this exceed 20 μV. Usually, the voltage is higher over the right hemisphere (but is not specifically related to handedness) (60).

Attenuation of Posterior Rhythm

Like the alpha rhythm of adults, the predominant posterior rhythm in children tends to block (attenuate) on eye opening.

Posterior Slow Rhythms

Although the fundamental posterior rhythm increases in rate from early childhood until maturity, there usually are intermingled slow waves. These different frequencies combine to form polymorphic waves with sharp elements. These have been called slow fused transients (38). They are most prominent between ages 6 and 12 years. They are analogous to the posterior slow waves associated with youth in the adult and are seen up to 65% of the time in older chldren. Posterior 1- to 5-Hz activity decreases from 1 to 29 years of age (32). Slow alpha variant activity (described in adults) may also be present in childhood. It blocks on eye opening.

Other Posterior Activity

Lambda activity may appear in children (38), and it may be asymmetrical. Also, in children, eye blinks may be preceded or followed by sharp slow waves (77). Whether this activity is related to lambda activity is perhaps speculative.

Central EEG Activity

Quantitative observations of the EEG in the central areas of the infant and child (67) show that rhythmic central activity can be recorded at birth, the mean frequency being 7.1 Hz. The frequency and voltage of this activity gradually increases with age. It is independent of the posterior rhythms.

Another type of activity that may occur in the central areas of children as early as 3 to 5 years of age is mu activity. The number of children showing mu rhythm increases with age (60). Central and temporal theta may be evoked in infants by emotional stimuli (49).

Anterior EEG Activity

Beta activity shows age-related increases (73) and it is in general more prominent in anterior than posterior areas.

Rhythmic 6- to 7-Hz theta activity may also be seen in the anterior regions as early as 3 to 5 years of age (60).

NORMAL EEG ACTIVITY IN INFANTS AND CHILDREN: ASLEEP

Sleep patterns in children are highly age dependent and show qualitative and quantitative characteristics distinctly different from those of adults.

One of the major differences in the sleep EEG of full-term infants (40 weeks gestational age) compared with older children and adults is that newborns spend about 50% of sleep time in the REM stage. There is REM onset of sleep, rather than slow wave onset, as in adults. Indeed, in newborns, there may sometimes be difficulty in distinguishing wakefulness and drowsiness and sleep. Therefore, the sleep patterns of newborns will be considered separately, and this discussion will deal with children older than 1 month of age.

One of the characteristics of true adult sleep, Stage 2, is the sleep spindle. This activity generally does not appear in infants until sometime between 6 weeks and 2 months of age, although a few rudimentary spindles may occur at about 1 month of age. In one series, all of 17 full-term infants showed sleep spindles by the age of 9 weeks (22).

One of the characteristics of sleep spindles in infants is the development of sharp surface negativity in the central and parietal regions. This is shown in Fig. 14.50. They may be seen in children from 6 to 24 months of age. It is a normal characteristic. If surface negativity persists beyond 2 or 3 years of age, it probably represents immaturity rather than abnormality.

The K complex, another indicator of Stage 2 sleep, also appears at about 4 to 6 months of age. Diffuse slow activity may be present in the newborn child during early REM sleep. It tends to become more characteristic of non-REM sleep after 3 to 4 months of age.

After about the fifth month, and certainly up through the sixth year, Stage 1 sleep is characterized by bursts of high voltage slow activity with a frequency range of 3 to 5 Hz, usually appearing predominantly in the frontal and central regions. An example of this activity is shown in Fig. 14.51. The voltage may reach 200 μV. The bursts may be brief, or they may last for several seconds or several minutes. This activity or pattern sometimes is called "continuous hypnogogic hypersynchrony" (38). Activity with the same characteristics may be seen on arousal from sleep, and it is commonly observed when young children are awakened from an afternoon nap. This slow activity is normal both on initial drowsiness and on awakening. It may appear infrequently in healthy adults in relation to either sleep onset or arousal (28).

In some young children, fast activity in the 20- to 30-Hz range, with a voltage of up to 30 μV, may develop in late Stage 1 and early Stage 2 sleep. It first appears at 7 or 8 months of age and disappears about age 4 or 5 years. Usually, it does not continue to be prominent after the sleep spindles are clearly established.

At the earliest ages, symmetry of EEG activity in sleep is poor, but it increases with maturation. In the first year of life the appearance of sleep spindles in the left and the right hemisphere often is asynchronous. However, the percent time present and the amplitude will on the average be about equal. Children's daytime naps progress to deeper stages of sleep than do adults', as defined by abundance of slow activity in their EEGs. The full range of variations that may appear in the sleep EEGs of children can only be appreciated after extensive experience.

ABNORMAL EEG ACTIVITY IN INFANTS AND CHILDREN

The same descriptive criteria used to classify EEG activity in adults are employed in the description and classification of EEG activity in children.

Specific Abnormal EEG Patterns

1. *Generalized 3-Hz spike-and-wave complex*. This morphologically distinct pattern is extremely abnormal, and it does not appear in healthy children (29). It may or may not be related to clinical absence seizures. Figure 14.52 (A and B) shows a 10-sec burst of 3-Hz spike-and-wave activity accompanied by a clinical absence attack. The 3-Hz spike-and-wave activity may appear in the waking EEG; it is augmented in sleep. Although only lighter stages of sleep are seen, in the usual daytime EEG recording the greatest increase of generalized spike-and-wave activity is in sleep Stages 3 and 4. It is seen least in REM-stage sleep (63,64). In many instances, the morphology of the 3-Hz pattern changes in sleep. The frequency, or repetition rate, becomes irregular and the spike element becomes multiple.
2. *Sharp-and-slow-wave-complex*. Made up of alternating sharp waves (duration, 70–200 msec) and slow waves (duration, 350–450 msec), with a repetition rate of about 1.5–2.5 Hz. The peak age range for its occurrence is 2 to 6 years (6). Usually, the discharges are bilaterally symmetrical, although they occasionally may shift in location.
3. *Hypsarrhythmia*. Distinguished by 0.5- to 3-Hz multifocal, asyn-

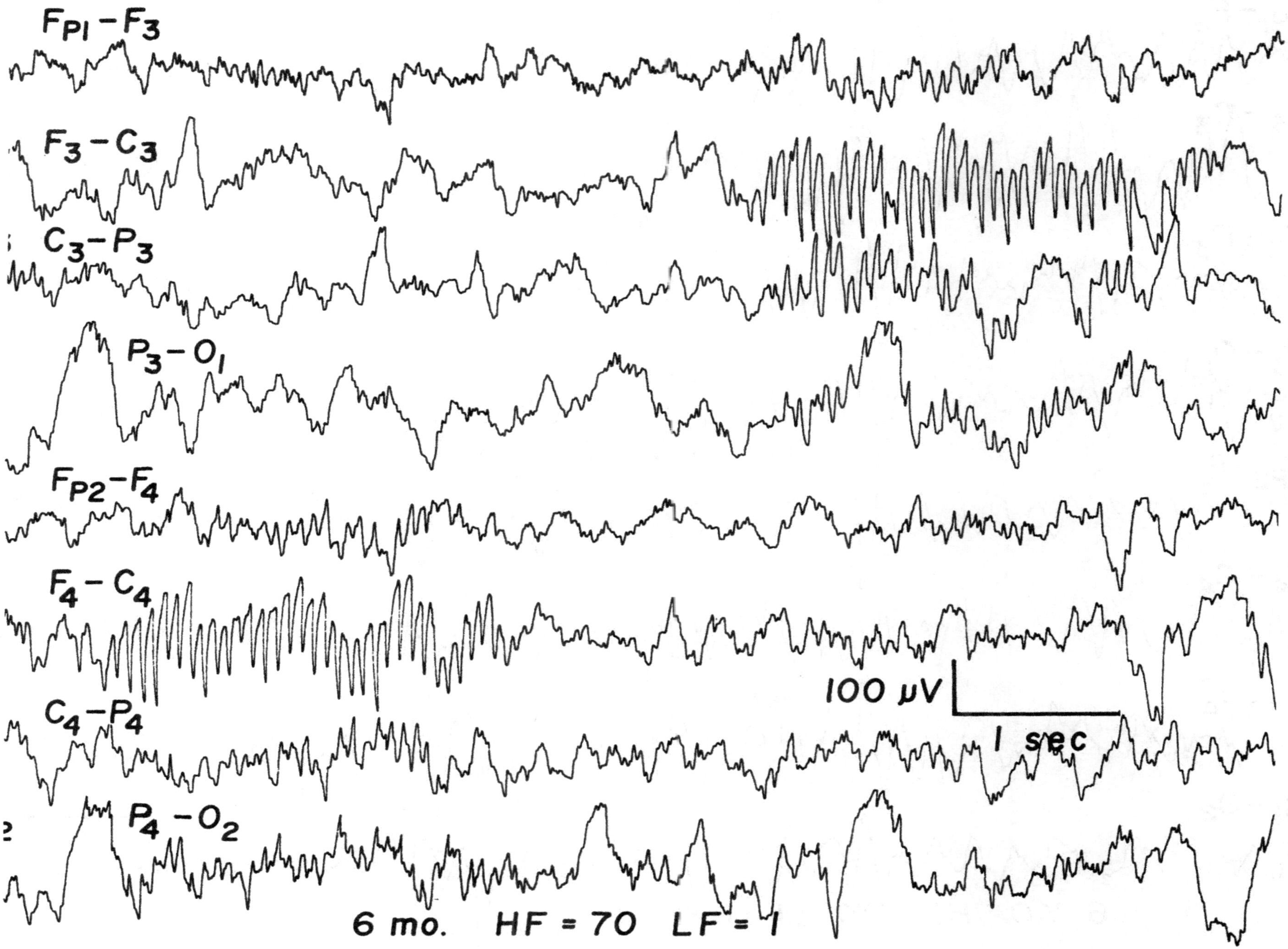

FIG. 14.50. Negative sleep spindles of stage 2 sleep in a 6-month-old girl. HF = 70 Hz; LF = 1 Hz.

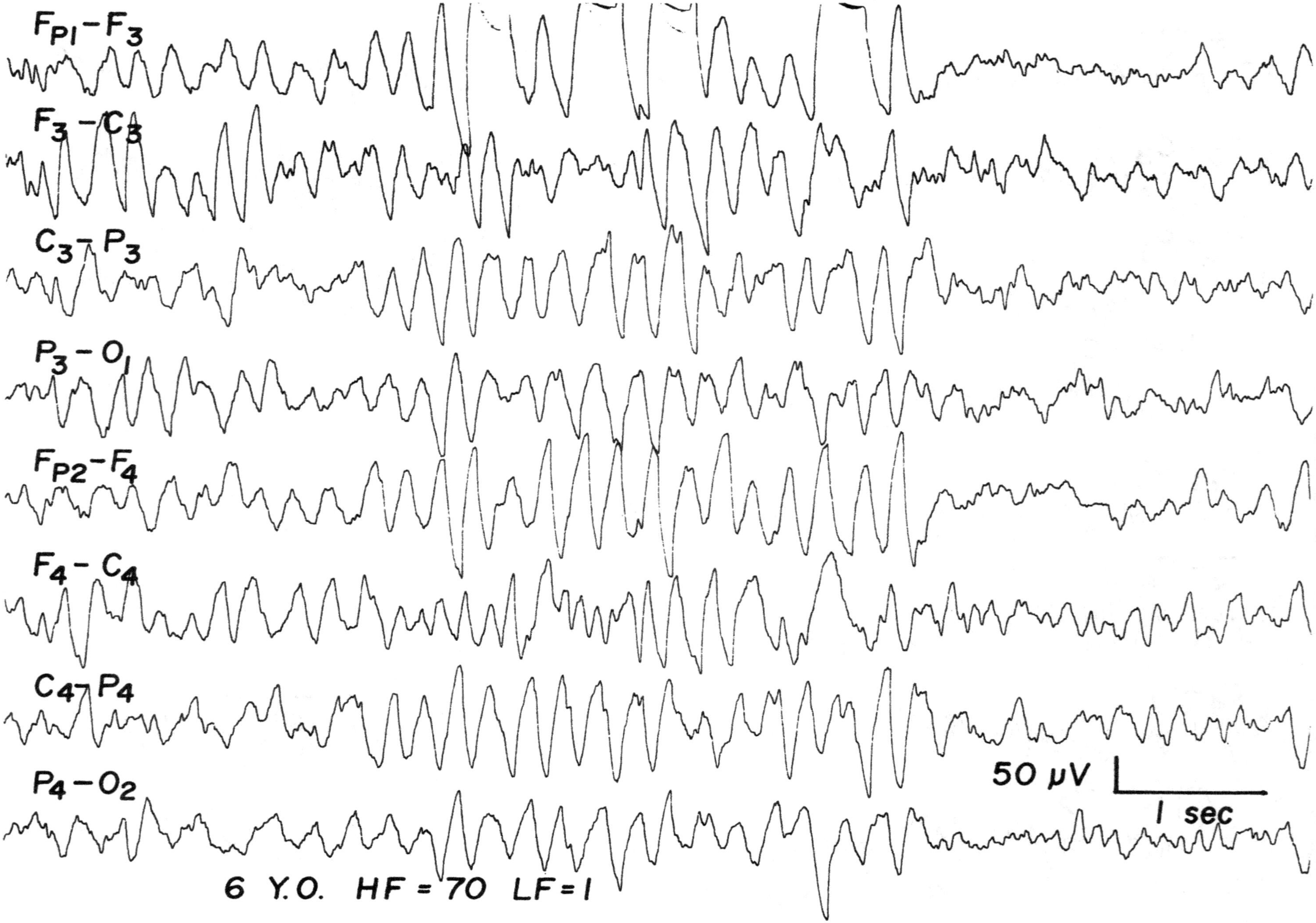

FIG. 14.51. Hypnogogic slow activity in a 6-year-old child, characteristic of drowsiness and arousal in young children, particularly between 2 and 10 years of age. HF = 70 Hz; LF = 1 Hz.

chronous spikes and sharp and slow waves, all of excessively high voltage ranging from 300 to >2,000 μV (Fig. 14.54 A and B). There sometimes are brief intervals of attenuation (decrementing). Hypsarrhythmia predominantly occurs between the ages of 3 months and 5 years. It is not seen in healthy children.

4. *Rolandic spikes.* High voltage spikes with a following slow wave (Fig. 14.53). They appear principally at central and midtemporal electrode locations. They should be distinguished from the V waves of sleep. Rolandic spikes are sharper and laterally distinguished, whereas V waves are focal at C_z.
5. *Anterior temporal spikes (and sharp waves).* Located at F_7 and/or F_8 (and T_1 and/or T_2); this differentiates them from Rolandic spikes.
6. *Multiple independent spike foci.* Defined as focal spikes seen in "3 non-contiguous electrode positions with at least one focus in each hemisphere" (6). They do not occur in healthy children.
7. *Periodic phenomena.* Recurring bursts of unusual activity (e.g., spikes, slow waves, sharp waves, high voltage complexes) that are fairly constant in morphology. They may be focal, lateralized, or generalized. They do not appear in healthy children. (See Fig. 14.36 for an example of periodic slow complexes.)
8. *Focal slow activity.* Focal slow activity, either delta or theta, can result from a brain lesion or local inflammation. If there is a coincident loss of background activity, especially beta activity, in the focal area, the significance may be more certain.
9. *Extreme spindles.* Recognized by their exceptionally high voltage (200–400 μV) and abundance. They are virtually continuous (29). They are seen primarily in children below the age of 9 years. This rare pattern is not seen in healthy children.
10. *Absence of spindles.* In otherwise clearly defined Stages 2 and 3 sleep, an absence of spindles is abnormal. Consistent asymmetries of spindles and V waves are also abnormal.

EEG ACTIVITY OF UNCERTAIN SIGNIFICANCE IN INFANTS AND CHILDREN

Because of the great variability of slow activity in children during drowsiness and after arousal from sleep, all nonspecific slow bursts during these periods should be regarded as normal variants. They continue to occur, although less commonly, throughout the adolescent years (28).

Related to this hypnogogic slow activity is a morphological pattern formed by the slow elements combined with such background activity as spindles or beta waves, which can simulate a poorly formed spike-and-wave complex (Fig. 14.55). This pattern is regarded as normal (6,38,58) and is differentiated from true paroxysmal spike-and-wave activity by the fact that it appears essentially as an isolated morphological entity, whereas clinically significant spike-and-wave discharges increase as drowsiness deepens and sleep ensues.

The aforementioned 14- and 6-Hz positive spikes are not categorically abnormal (18) and are regarded as normal variants.

NORMAL EEG ACTIVITY IN NEONATES

Assuming that the birth of the child occurred at term (38 to 40 weeks after conception), a neonate is an infant less than 1 month of age. A fairly large number of infants are born prematurely and consequently are immature. It is necessary to define several key terms in order to evaluate the EEGs of neonates (45).

1. *Gestational age (GA).* The time in weeks from conception (computed from the mother's last menstrual period to the infant's birth).
2. *Conceptional age (CA).* Gestational age plus the time in weeks since birth.
3. *Premature (PT) infant.* One born before 38 weeks GA.
4. *Full-term (FT) infant.* One born 38 to 40 weeks GA.
5. *Newborn period.* First 4 weeks after term.
6. *Infantile period.* Between 5 and 12 weeks postterm.

Historical Perspective

Although neonatal EEGs were recorded as early as 1936, and EEGs of premature infants were described in some detail as early as 1962, a more widespread appreciation of their complexity and the rapid maturational changes that occur has emerged only within the last 10 to 15 years.

FIG. 14.52. (*Overleaf*) **A:** Onset of paroxysmal 2.5-Hz spike-and-wave discharge during a clinical absence attack in a 12-year-old patient. Patient is slightly drowsy, with decreased alpha. **B:** Continuation of spike-and-wave discharge. Patient opened eyes coincidentally with termination of spike-and-wave paroxysm (*open*). Eyes were opened and then closed spontaneously (*close*). Alpha activity is fully restored and patient is awake. HF = 70 Hz; LF = 1 Hz. (See page 242.)

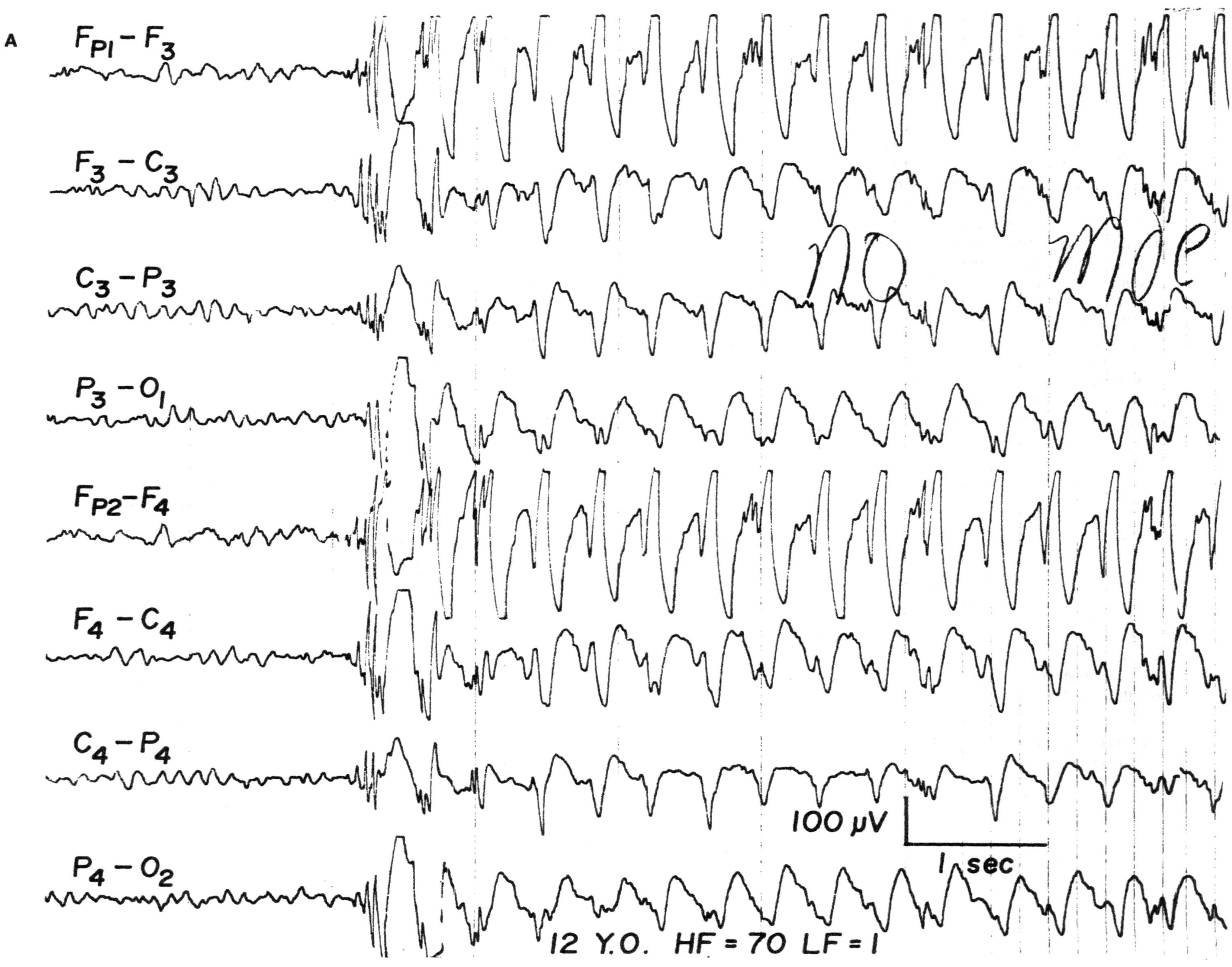

A
FP1 - F3
F3 - C3
C3 - P3
P3 - O1
FP2 - F4
F4 - C4
C4 - P4
P4 - O2
100 μV
1 sec
12 Y.O. HF = 70 LF = 1

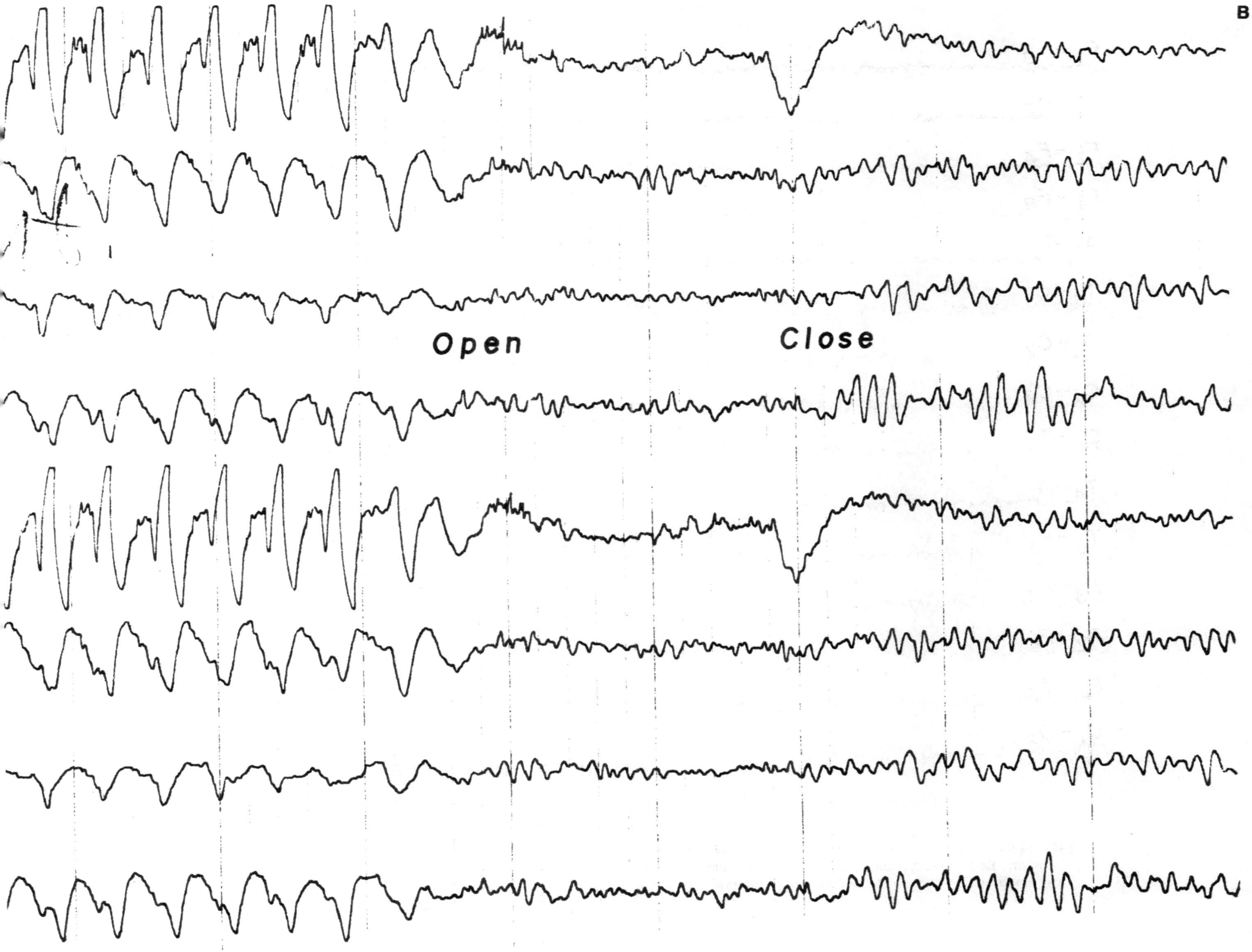
B
Open
Close

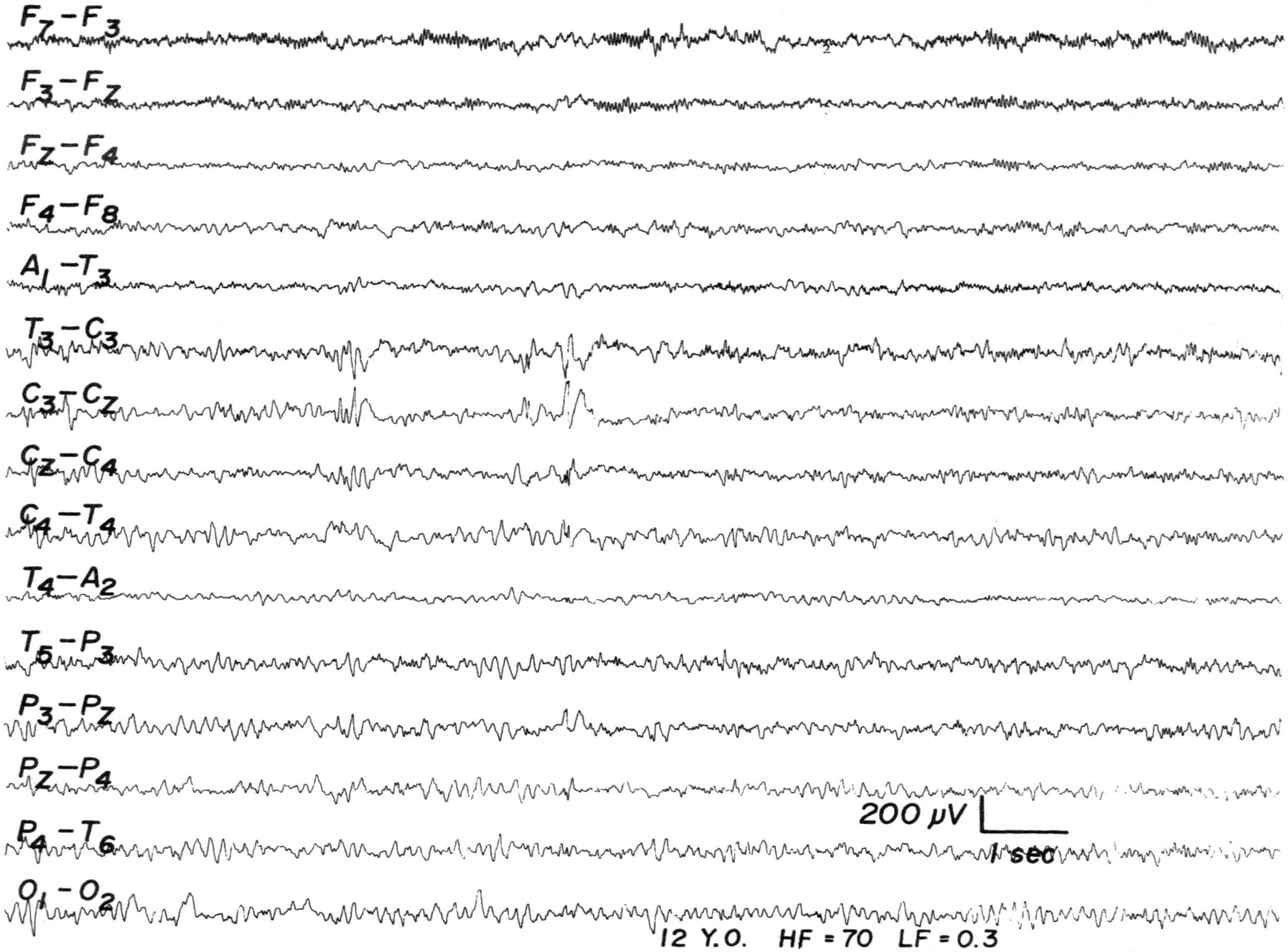

FIG. 14.53. Rolandic spikes in a 12-year-old child. HF = 70 Hz; LF = 0.3 Hz. (See page 245.)

FIG. 14.54. A: Hypsarrhythmia with paroxysmal spike bursts (400-μV peak) and sharp and slow waves (1,000-μV peak) in a 6-month-old infant. **B:** Hypsarrhythmia with paroxysmal sharp and slow waves exceeding 2,600 μV (2.6 mV) in a 10-month-old infant. The "low amplitude" waves in the decrementing intervals are 100 μV or greater. HF = 70 Hz; LF = 1 Hz. (See page 245.)

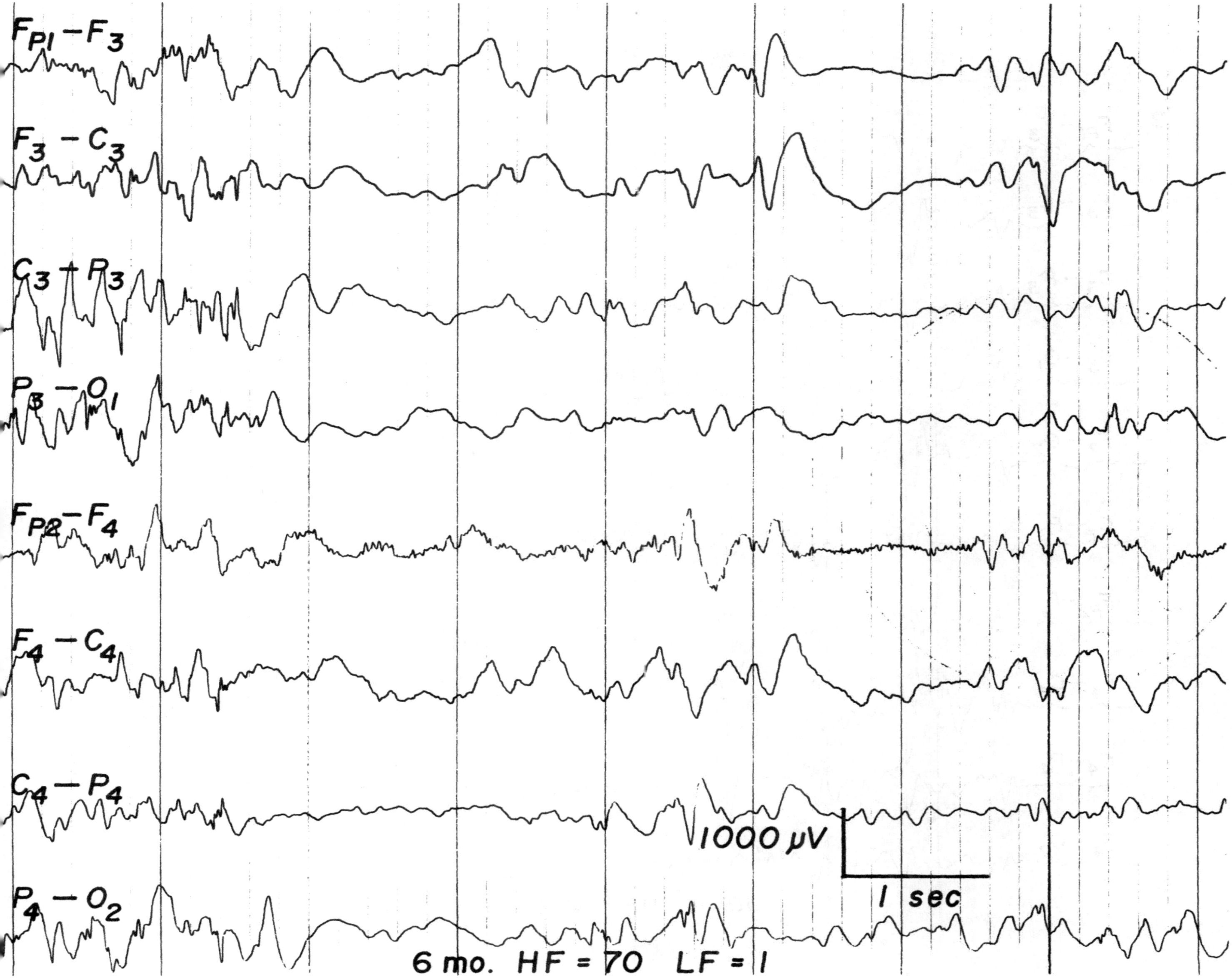

A
$F_{P1}-F_3$
F_3-C_3
C_3-P_3
P_3-O_1
$F_{P2}-F_4$
F_4-C_4
C_4-P_4
P_4-O_2
1000 μV
1 sec
6 mo. HF = 70 LF = 1

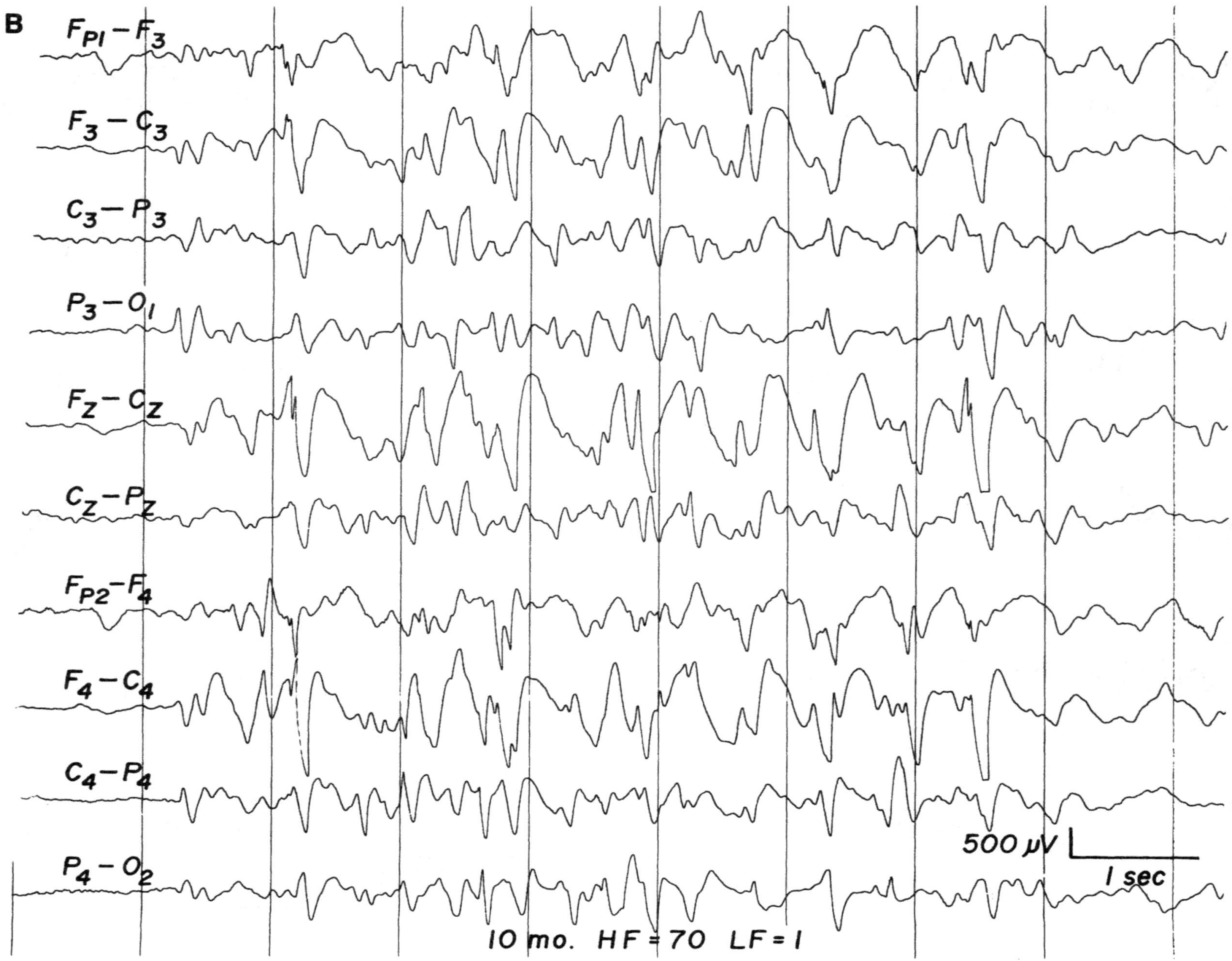
B
$F_{P1}-F_3$
F_3-C_3
C_3-P_3
P_3-O_1
F_Z-C_Z
C_Z-P_Z
$F_{P2}-F_4$
F_4-C_4
C_4-P_4
P_4-O_2
500 µV
1 sec
10 mo. HF = 70 LF = 1

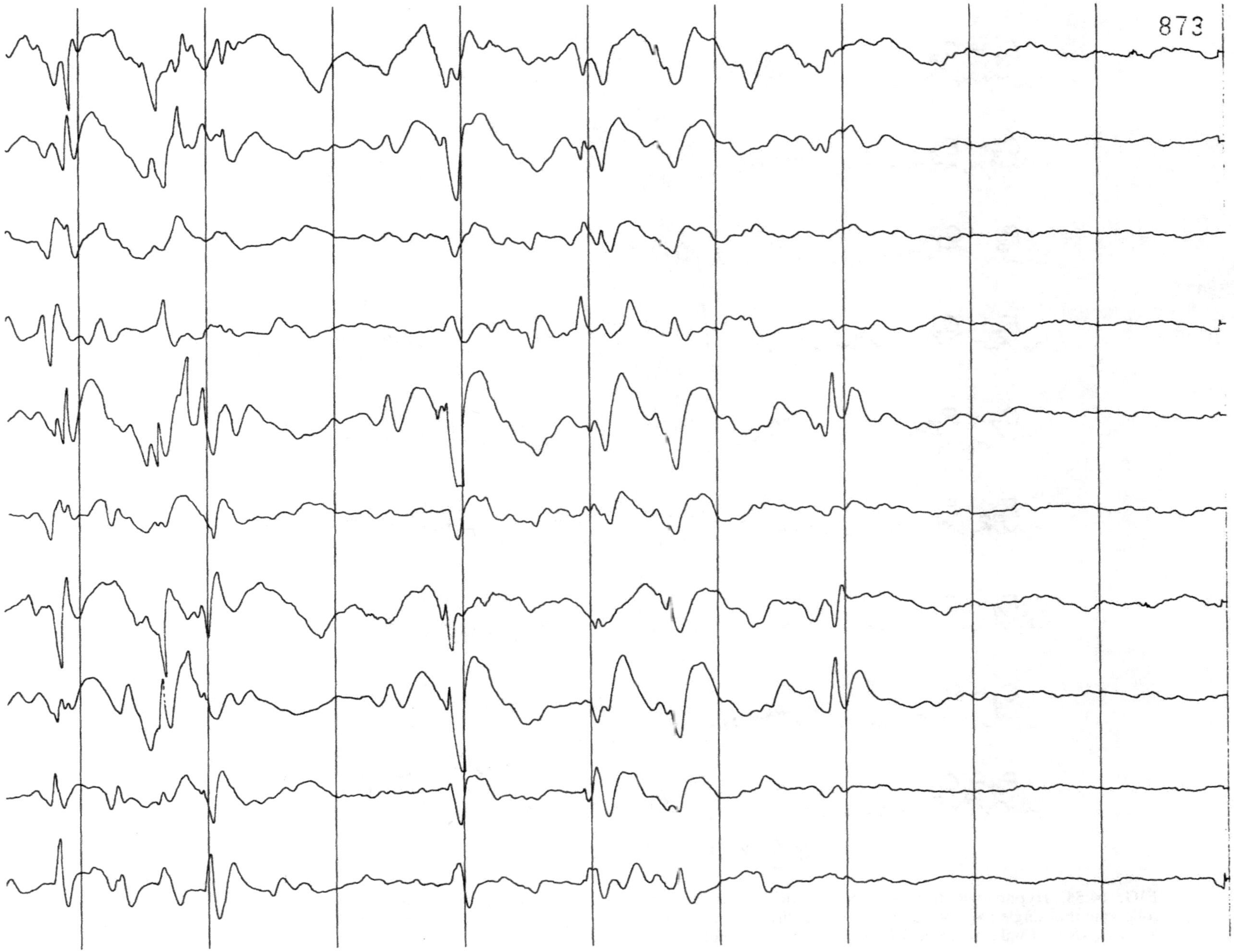
873

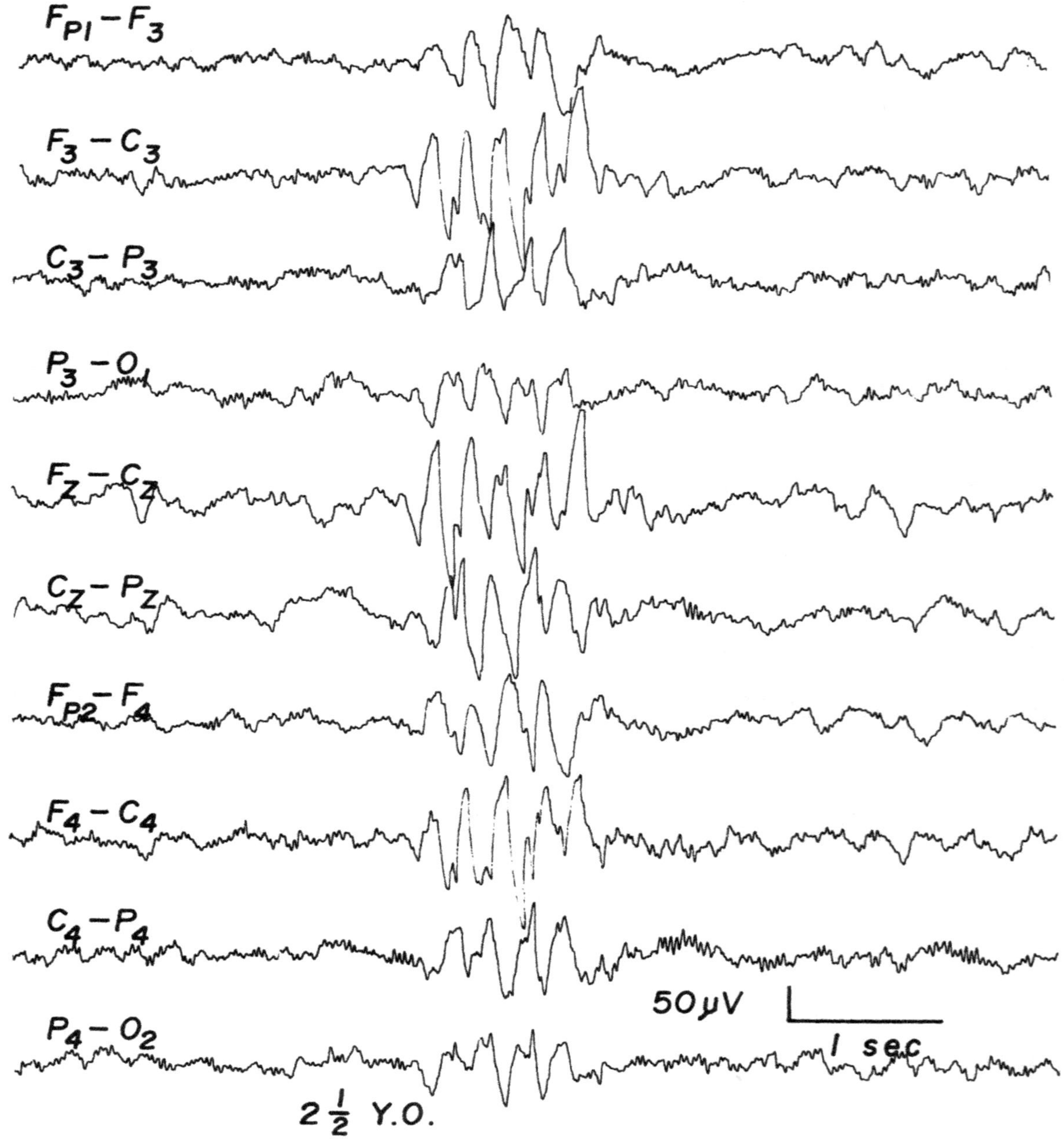

FIG. 14.55. Hypnogogic hypersynchrony with sharp elements in a 2½-year-old child. This is not abnormal. The sleep activity following this single paroxysmal event was entirely normal, as was the record before and after sleep. (Courtesy of K. McPeck, R. EEG T., Tufts-New England Medical Center Hospital, Boston, Massachusetts.)

Perhaps one reason for the lack of recognition of characteristic features of the neonatal EEG was the early preoccupation with waking occipital rhythms. Another reason was failure to recognize sleeping-waking differences in newborns and, until 1964, the inability to differentiate two primary types of sleep, REM and non-REM.

It now is clear that neonatal EEG is a subspecialty in its own right, requiring a somewhat different technology as well as a different set of guidelines for evaluation of the record. Even though an EEG technologist may be experienced in adult EEG techniques, additional training is required for successful recording of neonatal EEGs (71). The technologist must become thoroughly familiar with premature and full-term infants and their behavior as well as with standard procedures in newborn nurseries and neonatal intensive care units. There are many technical details involved in recording neonatal EEGs (33). These include meeting problems of electrical interference, electrical safety, measurement of the head for electrodes, electrode application and clean-up, in addition to special recording procedures.

Neonatal States

It is necessary to have a complete account of the moment-to-moment changes in the infant's state during the recording. As in adults, state is defined in terms of behavioral reactivity and in sleep additional physiological observations are included. The presence or absence of REMs is determined by recording the electro-oculogram (EOG). The tonic level of certain postural muscles is recorded by means of the electromyogram (EMG). In the infant, respiration is another key measure and heart rate (recorded as EKG) often is included. The moment-to-moment observations of spontaneous movements and reactions to external stimuli are facilitated by placing the infant as closely as possible to the technologist and the EEG instrument.

An experienced neonatal EEG technologist (33) has described the observation process as follows: "The technologist's eyes should be focussed upon the baby 99.9% of the time and the hand should be making continual observation notations. This point cannot be overemphasized. The presence or absence of eye movements, color changes, body movements (subtle and gross), facial grimaces, hiccoughs, sucks, smacking movements, patting or touching, noises made by the baby or near the baby should all be carefully, meticulously documented on the EEG . . . care should be taken that they are written at the exact moment of observation. . . ."

It is on the basis of these annotated behavioral observations and the simultaneously recorded physiological measures that the state of the infant is determined. The EEG data then are evaluated in relation to the infant's state. Neonatal states have been described and discussed by many investigators (21,45,59,71,76); the following is a composite statement:

1. If the eyes are open and alert, the child may be considered *awake*.
2. If the eyes remain closed for an extended time (more than 1 min) the child may be considered *asleep*.
   a. *Active sleep* (*AS*). Characterized by REMs (usually primarily horizontal), irregular breathing, frequent movements, smiling, grimacing, sucking, irregular respiration and brief periods of apnea (cessation of breathing), decreased tonic EMG level from facial and neck muscles.
   b. *Quiet sleep* (*QS*). No REMs, but there may be isolated eye movements, regular respiration, heart rate slower than in the awake state, little body movement except occasional startle or brief jerks, tonic level of EMG activity (neck, face) typically higher than in active sleep.
   c. *Transitional sleep* (*TS*). Sometimes called indeterminate sleep. The behavioral and physiological information provides a mixture of active sleep and quiet sleep signs. It occurs between active sleep and quiet sleep or vice versa. It is not well understood.

The sleep cycle (awake—active sleep—quiet sleep—awake) of neonates typically is 60 min. A complete EEG examination requires that the recording include an entire cycle. Further details of sleep stages in infants can be found in Anders et al. (3).

Techniques of Neonatal Recording

Technical considerations in recording EEGs in neonates include the use of ten-twenty placements, with a full set of 21 electrodes (2). The F_p

electrodes may be moved slightly above the positions determined by the usual measurement (see Chapter 11). These then should be designated F_{P1}' and F_{P2}'. Preferred attachment is by collodion (2,33,59,76). However, when ventilation is poor (e.g., the infant is confined within an isolette), an adhesive electrode cream should be used. This avoids unnecessary exposure of the infant to the fumes of collodion and acetone (33).

If the infant's head is very small in diameter, typically less than 30 cm, a lesser number of electrodes may be used (2,33,71). If fewer than 21 electrodes are initially applied, it may sometimes be necessary to add others to localize individual EEG characteristics.

Electrode impedances must be as low as possible and should range from 3 to 5 kΩ. Instrument controls should provide a wide pass band, 0.3 to 70 Hz. Sensitivity should be adjusted to provide easily measured data; 7 μV/mm usually is appropriate. If high voltages are encountered, going beyond the dynamic range of the setting, sensitivity of 10 or 15 μV/mm may be used. If the voltage is exceptionally low, sensitivity of 2 μV/mm may be required.

A paper speed of 15 mm/sec is used in many neonatal EEG laboratories. This allows periodic activity to be compressed and more readily perceived. Some of the figures illustrate this technical feature.

The EEG should be scheduled for a feeding time. First, the electrodes should be applied. Second, the infant should be fed and the diapers changed; this will encourage sleep. Then the recording may be started. The recording period must be long enough to include a complete waking-sleeping cycle, as described above. A "20-min EEG recording" cannot provide adequate information for a worthwhile EEG interpretation. Attempts to record the EEG in a hungry, fretful infant will be fruitless. There are no short cuts (33).

The EEG instrument should have at least 16 channels (2,33,71), and 18 channels provide even more useful information. Eight channels are not adequate (21,71). At least 16 channels are needed because three, and often four, channels are required for physiological monitoring (EOG, EMG, EKG, respiration). The montage should include all of the basic ten-twenty electrode positions, and the montage should remain unchanged throughout the recording to provide a continuous evaluation of EEG and the infant's state (33).

The basic rule that montages should be organized in straight-line arrays should be followed. Using the same logic that was applied to adult montages (see Chapter 13), the 18-channel, longitudinal bipolar montage shown in Table 14.1 is quite practical.

TABLE 14.1. *Suggested 18-channel, longitudinal bipolar montage for neonatal EEG recording*[a]

Channel	Electrode placement
1	Oculogram (left to right outer canthus)
2	EMG (submental muscle)
3	EKG (left to right arm)
4	Respirogram (nasal thermistor or chest respirometer)
5	F_7-T_3
6	T_3-T_5
7	$F_{P1}-F_3$
8	F_3-C_3
9	C_3-P_3
10	P_3-O_1
11	F_z-C_z
12	C_z-P_z
13	$F_{P2}-F_4$
14	F_4-C_4
15	C_4-P_4
16	P_4-O_2
17	F_8-T_4
18	T_4-T_6

[a] If modified F_P placements are used, these may be designated $F_{P1'}$ and $F_{P2'}$ (see Chapter 13). The voltage in the $F_{P1'}-C_3$ and $F_{P2'}-C_4$ derivations will be reduced because of the decreased interelectrode distance.

If only 16 channels are available, either the midline array ($F_z-C_z-P_z$) can be omitted or, alternatively, the EKG channel can be omitted, together with F_z-C_z. This will provide some, even though incomplete, sampling of midline activity. It is strongly recommended that at least one derivation including C_z be retained.

Infants who are referred because of sleep apnea should have both nasal and thoracic respiratory monitors included.

After a satisfactory, completely annotated recording is obtained, the infant's head should be thoroughly cleaned. Hanley (33) has outlined the necessary procedures. The scalp and hair should be absolutely clean before the child is returned to the nursery.

EEG Activities Unique to Neonates

The EEG activity observed in neonates, PT and FT, has a terminology of it own, because there are no equivalent patterns in the EEGs of older infants, children, and adults. Much of the early research in the field of neonatal EEG was carried out in France, and a few of the patterns unique to this age range continue to carry French names.

The following descriptive classifications are based on summaries of the work of many investigators (21,22,45,59,71,76). The reader should refer to these references for further details and discussion.

1. *Delta brushes.* Named for their appearance (45,76), and forming a morphologically unique pattern: low-voltage, fast (10–24 Hz) activity superimposed on bursts of single or multiple delta waves with a frequency of about 1 Hz (Fig. 14.56). Their abundance (i.e., the number per 1 min or 5 min) is a function of conceptional age (45). They appear most clearly in quiet sleep at 33 to 34 weeks of age. They disappear shortly after term (40 weeks CA).
2. *Frontal sharp transients.* Biphasic (negative–positive) frontal sharp waves, either bilateral or unilateral (Fig. 14.57); may shift laterally. The French name *encoches frontales* is occasionally used in English-language literature (71). They disappear by 8 weeks in full-term infants (45).
3. *Other sharp transients.* Infrequently occurring sharp wave transients, surface negative and without a stable focus, may occur usually in quiet sleep, especially after 38 weeks CA (Fig. 14.58). Surface temporal positive spikes also may occur normally (Fig. 14.59). However, if frequently present or if observed in repeated recordings they are abnormal. Generalized low voltage activity may occur at 37 to 40 weeks CA, in association with REM sleep (Fig. 14.60).
4. *Anterior slow activity.* The term "slow dysrhythmia" often is used by those who follow the French nomenclature. Since the activity is normal, it is not *dys*rhythmic by our earlier definition. This activity occurs principally in quiet sleep. It appears as bursts of 2- to 4-Hz activity, up to 200 μV. Sharp transients may be associated with these bursts. The morphology is variably mono- or polymorphic (71,76).
5. *Theta bursts.* Sharp, 4- to 7-Hz activity, 50 to 100 μV. Maximal incidence occurs at 29 to 31 weeks CA.
6. *Delta activity.* Dominant in the posterior areas, with frequencies of 0.5 to 1.5 Hz and amplitudes up to 300 μV. Appears between 29 and 31 weeks CA, develops into delta brushes, and disappears after 33 weeks of age (71).
7. *Periodic patterns* (in neonatal EEG terms, "discontinuous background").
   a. *"Tracé alternant."* Semiperiodic bursts of 1- to 3-Hz, 50- to 100-μV, delta and theta activity, 2 to 5 sec in duration, separated by lower amplitude (20–50 μV) intervals of mixed frequency activity (Fig. 14.61). The interburst interval ranges from 3 to 10 sec. This pattern is seen predominantly in quiet sleep of healthy full-term infants (45,59,76) and disappears by 7 weeks (45). With increasing age it is replaced by more or less continuous slow wave activity. It is normal and should not be confused with burst-suppression activity.
   b. *"Tracé discontinu."* Appears in quiet sleep of premature neonates. Similar to tracé alternant, but the interburst intervals are longer and the voltage between bursts is lower. The periodic bursts may be mixtures of delta activity and delta brushes (71). It also is normal and should not be confused with abnormal periodic activity.

The EEGs shown in Figs. 14.57, 14.58, 14.61, and 14.62 were recorded sequentially from a neonate of 38 weeks CA (37 weeks GA) and show spontaneous changes in background activity and waveform morphology during one sleep cycle.

Figure 14.57 is early REM sleep with predominantly slower waves. In a transitional period (Fig. 14.58), sharp elements, some of them paroxysmal, become prominent. REMs again occur (Fig. 14.60), but with a low voltage intermittent background. When quiet sleep is reached with regular respiration and no REMs, the tracé alternant pattern evolves (Fig. 14.61). Attenuation of background activity, caused by auditory stimulation, occurs during quiet sleep (Fig. 14.62).

Neonatal EEGs, like adult EEGs, are evaluated in terms of concordance with the on-going behavioral state. By 35 weeks CA, in healthy premature infants, there should be close agreement between the EEG criteria of sleep level and the behavioral variables (59).

EEGs also are evaluated with respect to synchrony between hemispheres. Bilateral symmetry is well established in adults and older children, but it is variable in neonates. By term, 80% of high voltage bursts in the EEG are bilaterally synchronous (59).

ABNORMAL EEG ACTIVITY IN NEONATES

Neonatal EEG abnormality is defined not only by the infant's clinical status at the time of recording but also in terms of its past history (e.g., anoxia) and its final outcome. Lombroso (45) divides neonatal abnor-

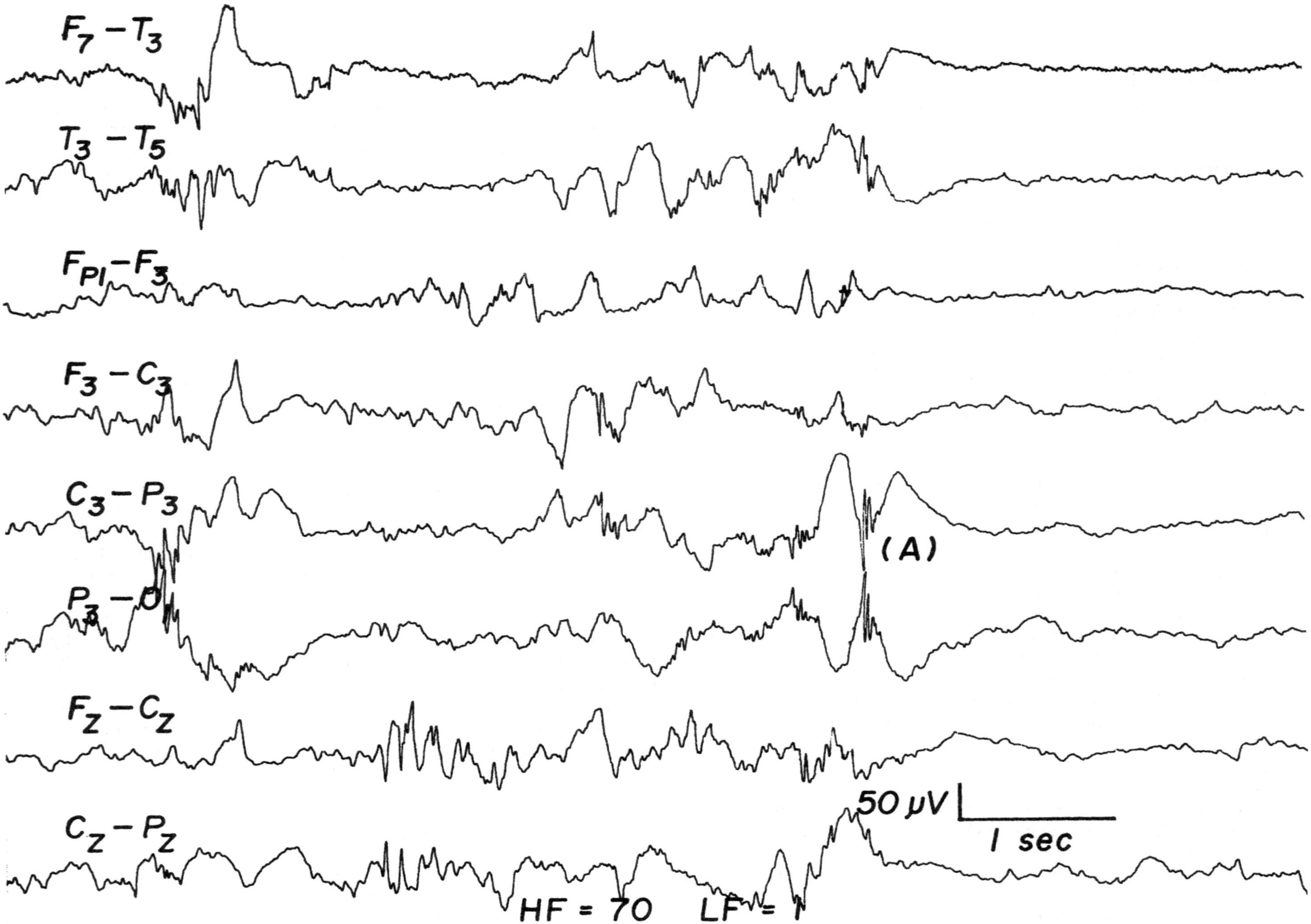

FIG. 14.56. Delta brush (*A*) in a premature infant (37 week gestational age, 38 weeks conceptional age). HF = 70 Hz; LF = 1 Hz. (This and the following neonatal figures were obtained with the assistance of K. McPeck, R. EEG T.)

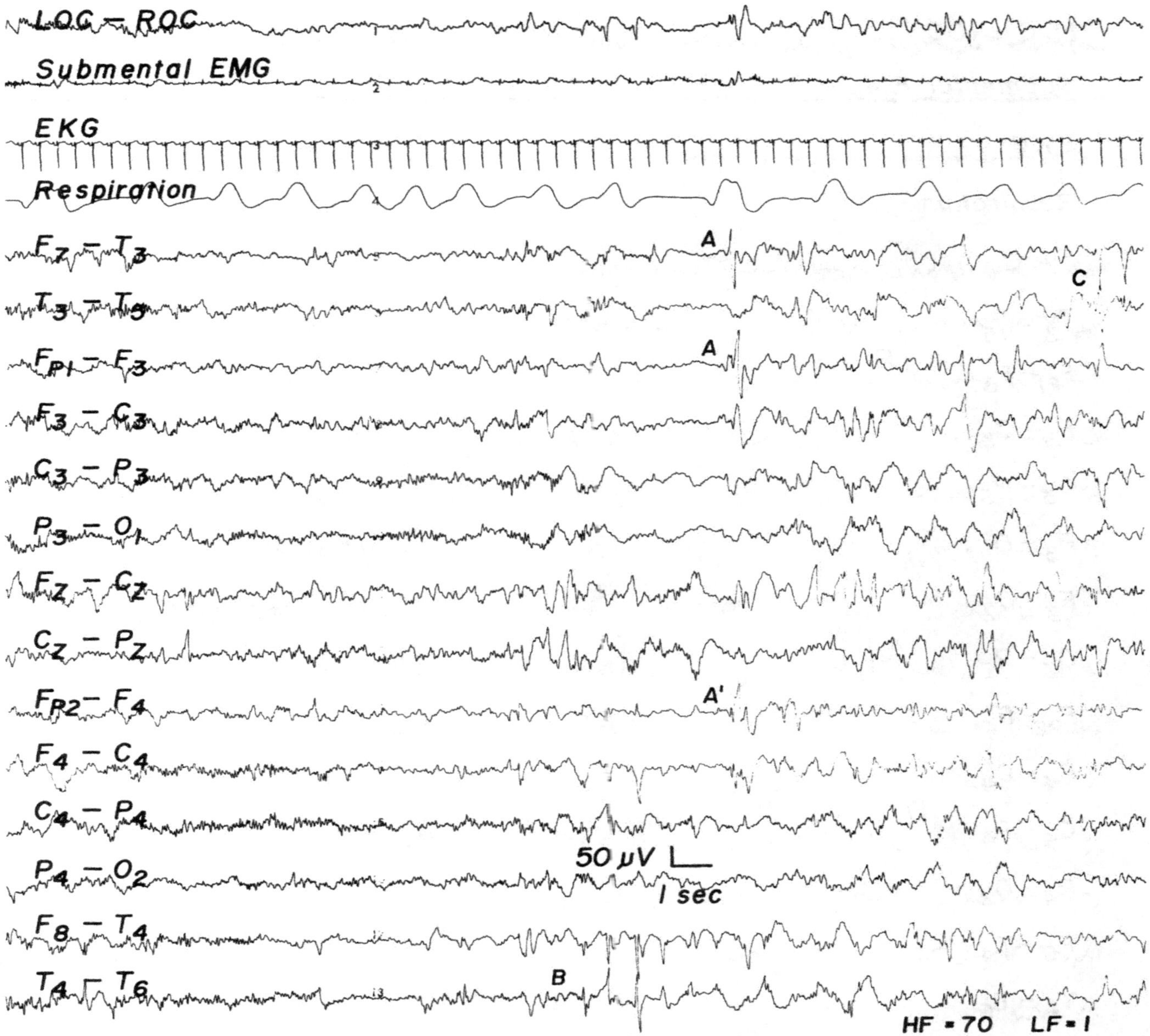

FIG. 14.57. REM sleep. Defined by loss of EMG activity, irregular respiration, and slow EEG background activity in a premature infant (37 weeks gestational age, 38 weeks conceptional age). Left frontal sharp transient (*A*), lower voltage, slightly different morphology in right frontal sharp transient (*A′*), right midtemporal negative spike activity (*B*), and left midtemporal negative spike activity (*C*). HF = 70 Hz; LF = 1 Hz. In this Fig., and all others including submental EMG, the sensitivity in the EMG channel is 3 times that of the EEG.

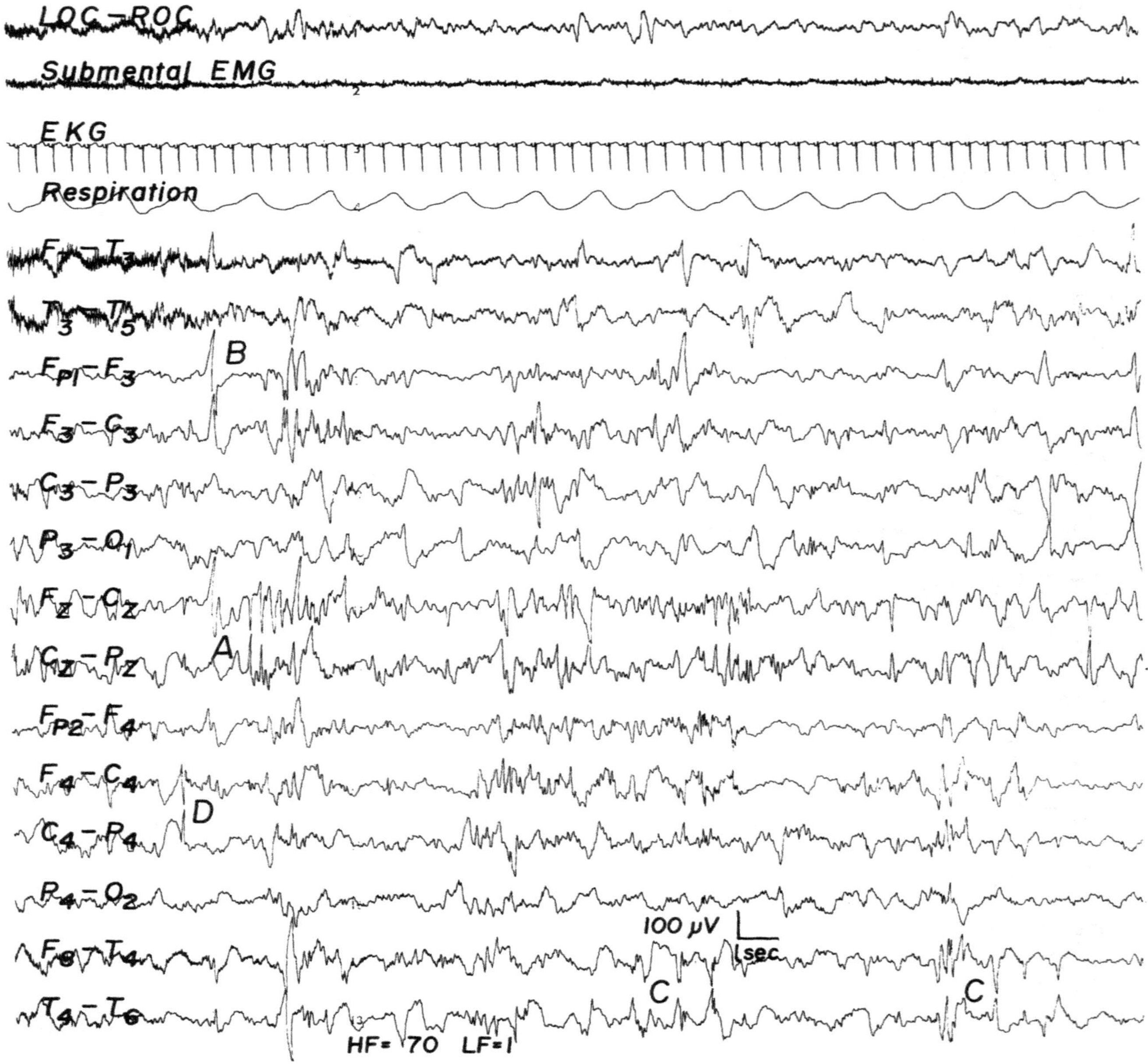

FIG. 14.58. Transitional sleep (between a REM period and before quiet sleep) in a premature infant (37 weeks gestational age, 38 weeks conceptional age). Note the very active midline. C_z negative spiking (*A*), left frontal sharp transients (*B*), right midtemporal negative spikes (*C*), and right central negative spike (*D*). HF = 70 Hz; LF = 1 Hz.

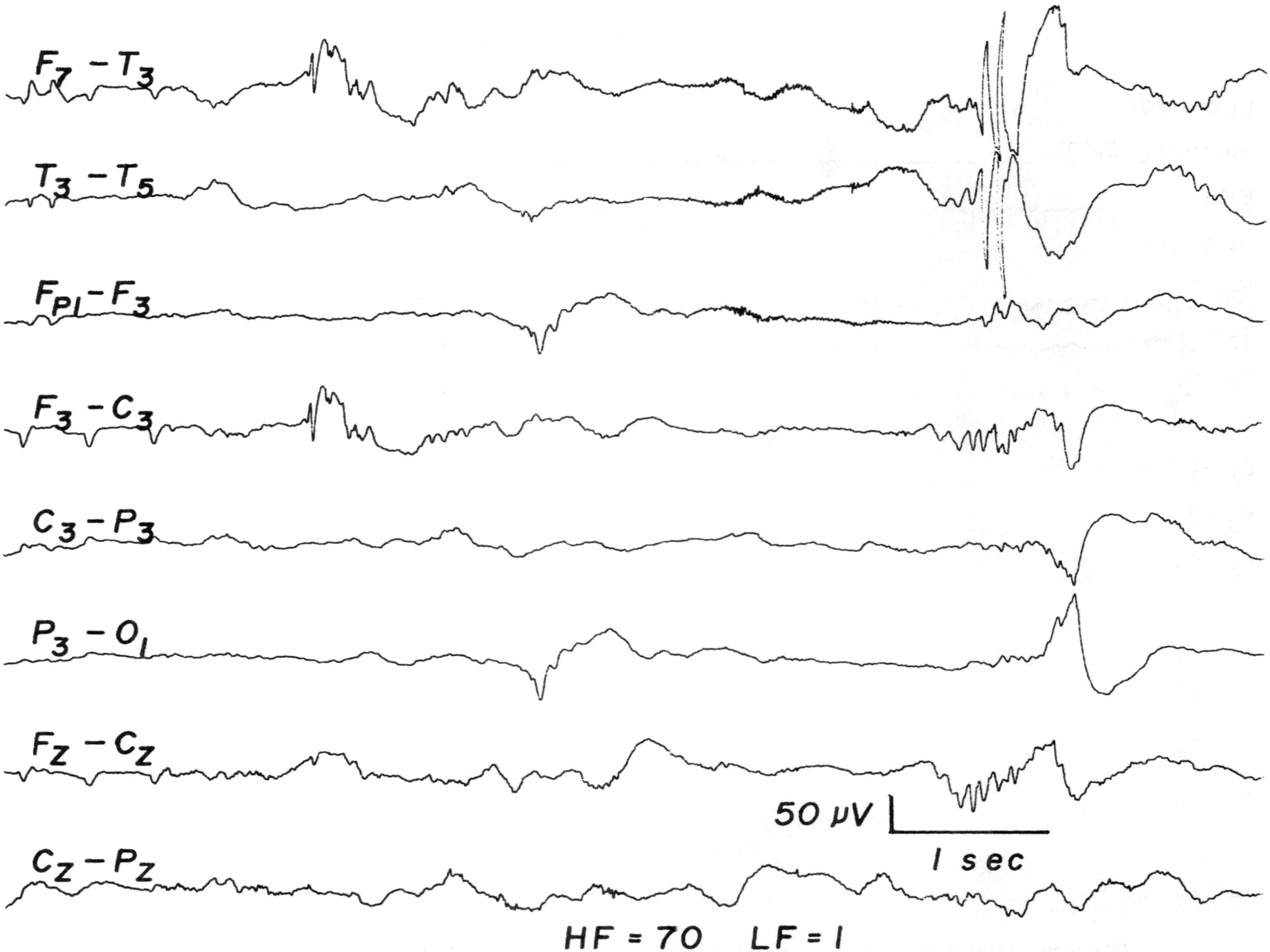

FIG. 14.59. Positive temporal spike in a premature infant (31 weeks gestational age, 32 weeks conceptional age). HF = 70 Hz; LF = 1 Hz. This is a portion of the montage shown in Table 14.1, limited to show left hemisphere and midline activity.

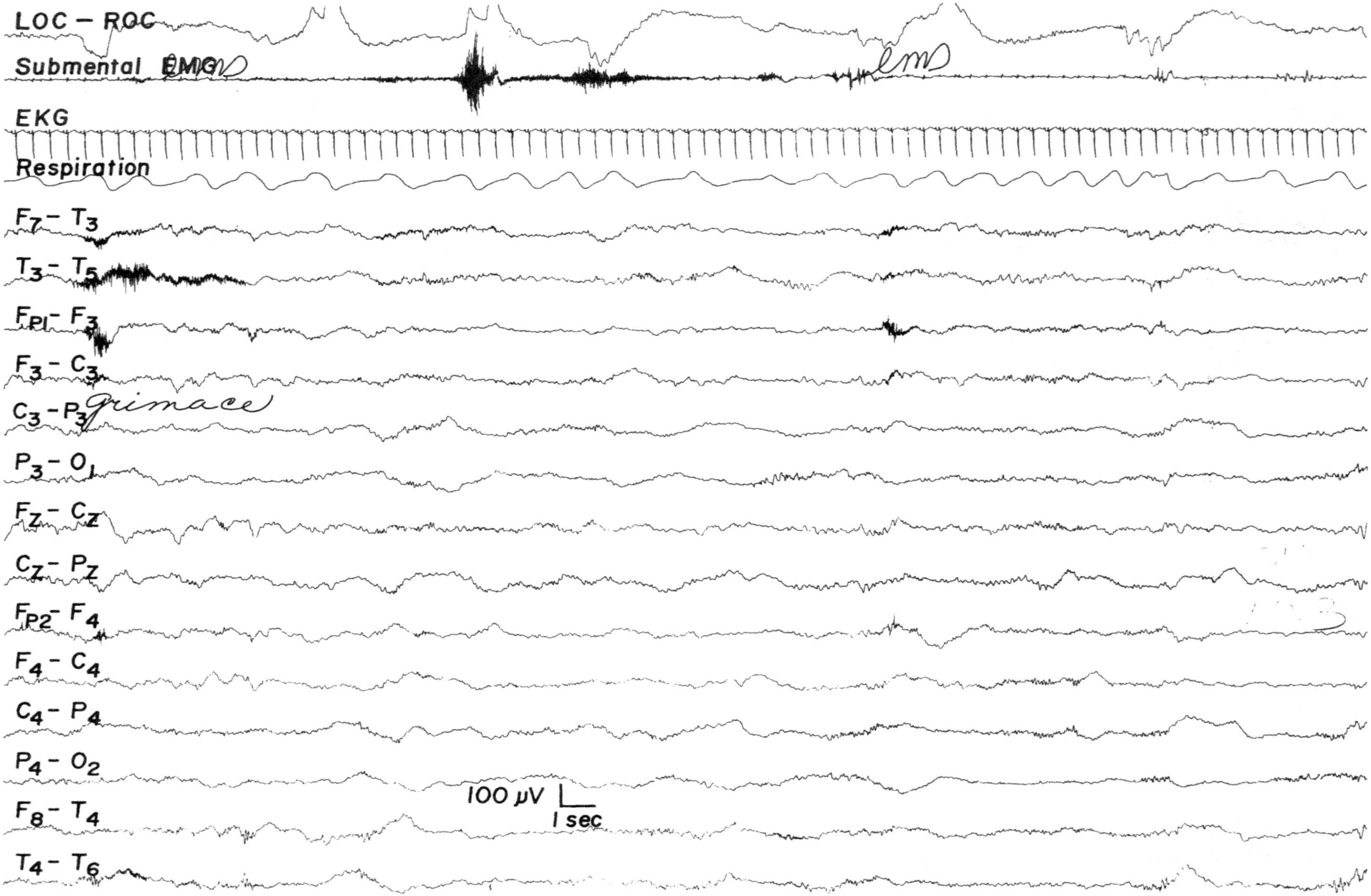

FIG. 14.60. REM-stage sleep. Defined by oculogram, technologist's notes, loss of EMG background tonic activity, and irregular respiration, with associated low voltage, irregular EEG activity. Note occasional phasic EMG activity.

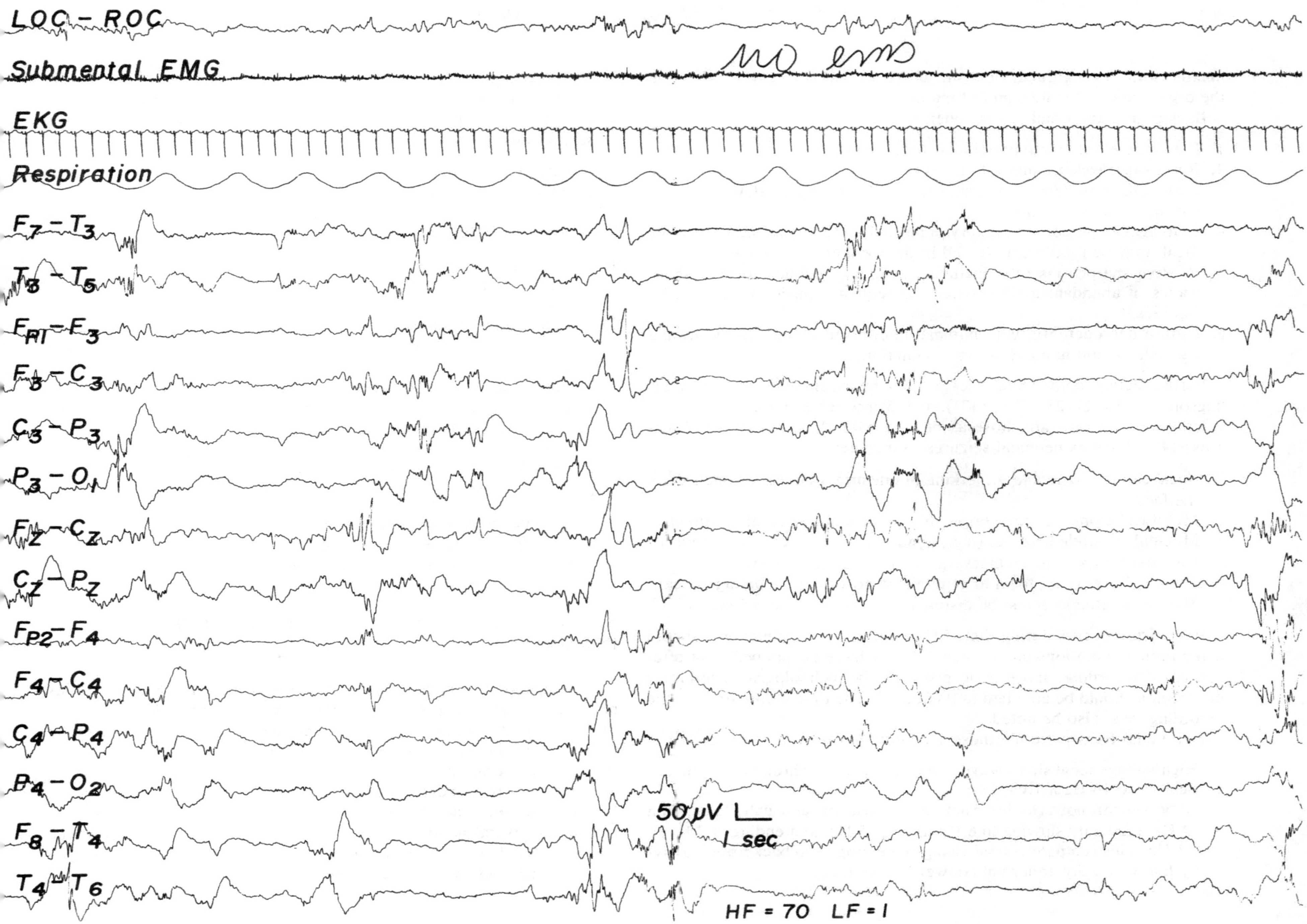

FIG. 14.61. Tracé alternant (quiet sleep). Tonic EMG (channel 2); regular respiration (channel 4). Technologist noted no eye movements. Note EEG activity in EOG channel. HF = 70 Hz; LF = 1 Hz.

malities into "background" and "ictal" types and adds abnormalities in the organization of states, and of maturtion.

Background abnormalities include:

1. Electrocerebral inactivity (similar to adult type).
2. Burst-suppression (similar to adult type).
3. Low voltage pattern, less than 5 to 30 μV, during all states and persisting 2 weeks or more.
4. Left-right amplitude asymmetry of more than 50% in all states; may be focal; may be totally suppressed in the focal area or hemisphere.
5. Positive sharp transients, including central (rolandic) positive sharp waves, if abundant and persistent (infrequent transients may not be significant).
6. Diffuse delta activity, with minimal intermixed theta activity, awake and asleep, and nonreactive to stimulation.

Further details on neonatal background abnormalities are given by Ellingson (21), Engel (23), Tharp (71), and Werner et al. (76).

Ictal abnormalities are those associated with clinical seizures. Lombroso (45) classifies neonatal seizures to include:

1. Focal clonic seizures (e.g., jerking of one arm, one leg, or one side of the face).
2. Multifocal clonic seizures (e.g., shifting or multiple focal seizures).
3. Minimal or subtle seizures (e.g., abnormal eye movements, abnormal leg movements, brief tremors, unusual posturing, apnea).
4. Tonic seizures (e.g., focal or generalized posturing, including apnea).
5. Myoclonic attacks (must be distinguished from startle reflex).

If a seizure occurs during the EEG recording, the technologist should make running notations on the record. If a seizure occurs before or after the actual recording, and it is observed by the technologist, a complete description should be attached to the record. The time before or after the recording must also be noted.

Focal ictal EEG patterns (those seen during a seizure) include:

1. High voltage focal sharp waves; may be hypersynchronous, asymmetrical, 5- to 10-Hz activity.
2. Hypersynchronous rhythmic activity, with an onset usually faster than 12 Hz, gradually slowing to 8 Hz, then to 5 Hz, and ending at 3 Hz to 0.5 Hz. This is a paroxysmal change emerging from background activity that is usually abnormal (slower low voltage).
3. Multifocal spikes or sharp activity emerging from a (usually) low voltage background or occurring during burst-suppression activity.
4. Polyphasic, sharp, PLED-like low frequency discharges, about 1 Hz, seen against a low voltage background.

Activity identical to ictal discharges may also occur in the absence of an observable seizure. Such discharges are also clearly abnormal.

There also may be abnormality in organization of the infant's states and in maturation (45,59):

1. No recognizable states occur or there is no cycling of either the state or the EEG. If persistent in serial records (2 weeks), this is very abnormal.
2. A normal, full-term infant, 7 to 12 days after birth, should spend about 50% of the time in REM sleep. A large deviation from this ratio may be abnormal.
3. Abnormal maturation of sleep cycles and EEG patterns. In the first week, a full-term infant's non-REM EEG pattern is primarily tracé alternant with little continuous slow wave activity. By 4 weeks, continuous slow-wave sleep is dominant. Poor concordance of age, state, and EEG is abnormal. By 8 weeks of age, REM sleep should not be greater than 25%.

Further, persistence of delta brushes after 40 weeks CA is abnormal. If spikes and frontal sharp waves are abundant at 40 weeks of age, or persist beyond 40 weeks, they are abnormal.

EEG ACTIVITY OF UNCERTAIN SIGNIFICANCE IN NEONATES

As is apparent from the foregoing review of neonatal EEG activities, particularly those in premature infants, many morphologically unique types of activity can mimic specific abnormalities in children and adults. Often it is the abundance of a particular activity, or its coincidence with a specific behavioral state (e.g., a seizure) that defines it as clearly abnormal. In general, if a record only looks "immature" it probably is not abnormal. It always is necessary to establish "immaturity" by the use of serial records at several points on the age scale, i.e., at weekly or bi-weekly intervals. Single records which do not meet rigid criteria of specific abnormality had best be regarded as of "uncertain significance."

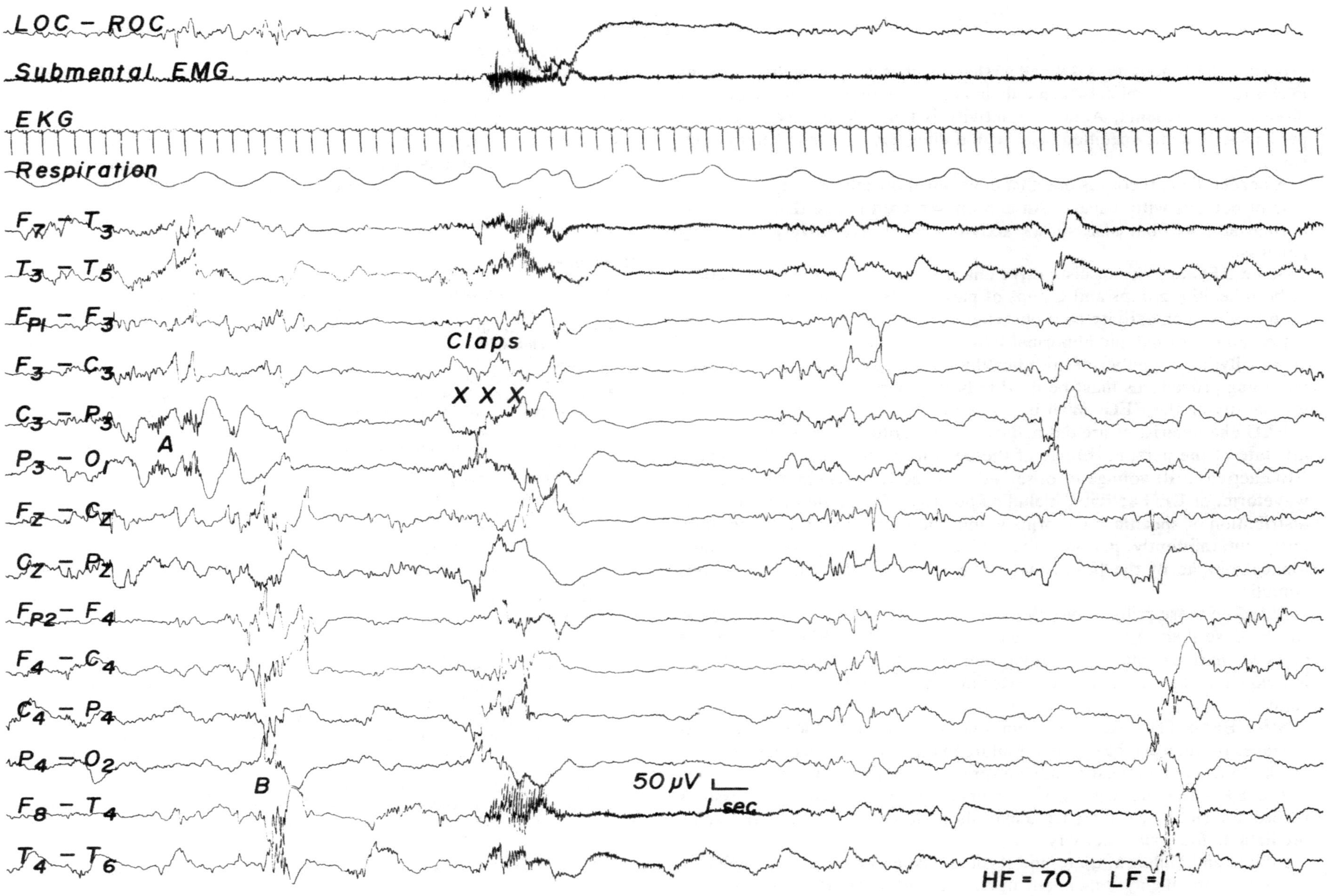

FIG. 14.62. Attenuation of background activity by auditory stimulation during tracé alternant in a premature infant (37 weeks gestational age, 38 weeks conceptional age). Note delta brushes at *A* and *B*. HF = 70 Hz; LF = 1 Hz.

SUMMARY

Normal EEG activity is defined as that which is seen in healthy persons in contrast to that which is seen only in persons with neurological or other disease, i.e., patients. Abnormal activity is that which appears only in persons with some specified disease and does not appear in healthy persons.

A normal EEG record is one that does not show any activity characteristic of persons with disease. An abnormal record is one that may show normal activity, but also shows activity that is exclusively shown by patients.

Some EEG activity of distinctive character may appear in the records of both healthy groups and groups of patients. If sufficiently common in each group, such activity is of uncertain clinical significance. The proper definition of normal and abnormal EEG activity depends on the study of an equally large number of both healthy persons and patients. The same recording procedures must be used in both groups and the same criteria for classifying the EEGs must be employed.

EEG characteristics are defined by several criteria, some of which are (a) state of the person, (b) age of the person, (c) frequency of observed EEG activity, (d) voltage of observed EEG activity, (e) morphology, or waveform, of EEG activity, including polarity, (f) amount of activity, (g) distribution of specific waveforms within the EEG record, e.g., continuously, intermittently, periodically, (h) location of activity within the anatomical outline of the brain, and (i) reactivity of the EEG to various stimuli.

Based on these criteria (at times in close coordination), normal activity can be described in the waking and sleeping states. Although there are many similarities within a healthy group, there also is variability between individuals. The variability is greater in the waking than in the sleeping state.

Sleep EEGs differ markedly from waking EEGs, and at least five levels or stages of sleep can be defined. Failure to recognize change in state from awake to asleep can lead to misinterpretation of the EEG.

The EEG changes with age. In comparison with a younger person's record, the elderly person's EEG may show slower activity and also some predictable focal slow activity.

Infants and children, up to and through adolescence, present EEG records that are highly dependent upon age and state. It is necessary to define the age of the newborn infant, either full-term or premature, in terms of time since conception (in weeks). Minute-by-minute change in state must be known to meaningfully describe and classify EEG activity. EEG characteristics change quite rapidly in premature infants. Many normal characteristics of this age range are abnormal in older infants and children. Many normal EEG characteristics of children, as related to state, are abnormal in older children and adults. Salient features of these changes, viewed as maturational processes, are discussed in detail in this chapter.

References

1. Aird, R. B., and Gastaut, Y. (1959): Occipital and posterior electroencephalographic rhythms. *Electroencephalogr. Clin. Neurophysiol.* 11:637–656.
2. American EEG Society (1980): 6. Minimal technical standards for pediatric electroencephalography. In: *Guidelines in EEG—1980.* American EEG Society, Tucker, Georgia.
3. Anders, T., Emde, R., and Parmelee, A., editors (1971): *A Manual of Standardized Terminology, Techniques and Criteria for Scoring States of Sleep and Wakefulness in Newborn Infants.* UCLA Brain Information Service, NINDS Neurological Information Network, Los Angeles.
4. Aserinski, E., and Kleitman, N. (1955): Two types of ocular motility occurring in sleep. *J. Appl. Physiol.,* 8:1–10.
5. Berger, H. (1930): Über das Elektrenkephalogramm des Menschen. Zweite Mitteilung. *J. Psychol. Neurol.,* 40:160–179.
6. Blume, W. T. (1982): *Atlas of Pediatric Electroencephalography.* Raven Press, New York.
7. Busse, E. W., Barnes, R. H., Silverman, A. J., Shy, G. M., Thales, M., and Frost, L. I. (1954): Studies in the process of aging: Factors that influence the psyche of elderly persons. *Am. J. Psychiatry,* 110:897–903.
8. Busse, E. W., and Obrist, W. D. (1965): Pre-senescent electroencephalographic changes in normal subjects. *J. Gerontol.,* 20:315–320.
9. Chatrian, G. E. (1976): The mu rhythm. In: *Handbook of Electroencephalography and Clinical Neurophysiology,* Vol. 6, Part A, edited by G. E. Chatrian and G. C. Lairy, pp. 6A46–6A78. Elsevier, Amsterdam.
10. Chatrian, G. E., Bergamini, L., Dondey, M., Klass, D. W., Lennox-Buchthal, M., and Petersén, I. (1974): A glossary of terms most commonly used by clinical electroencephalographers. *Electroencephalogr. Clin. Neurophysiol.,* 37:538–548.
11. Chatrian, G. C., and Lairy, G. C., editors (1976): *Handbook of Electroencephalography and Clinical Neurophysiology,* Vol. 6, Part A (The EEG of the Waking Adult). Elsevier, Amsterdam, 342 pp.
12. Cobb, W. A. (1950): Intracranial tumours. In: *Electroencephalography, A Symposium on its Various Aspects,* edited by D. Hill and G. Parr, pp. 273–301. Macdonald, London.
13. Cobb, W. A. (1963): The normal adult E.E.G. In: *Electroencephalography: A Symposium on its Various Aspects,* 2nd ed., edited by D. Hill and G. Parr, pp. 232–249. McDonald, London.
14. Davis, H., and Davis, P. A. (1936): Action potentials of the brain in normal persons and in normal states of cerebral activity. *Arch. Neurol. Psychiatry,* 36:1214–1224.

15. Davis, P. A. (1941): The electroencephalogram in old age. *Dis. Nerv. Syst.*, 49:186–194.
16. Dawson, G. D., and Walter, W. G (1944): The scope and limitations of visual and automatic analysis of the EEG. *J. Neurol. Neurosurg. Psychiatry*, 7:119–133.
17. Dement, W., and Kleitman, N. (1957): Cyclic variations of EEG during sleep and their relation to eye movements, body motility and dreaming. *Electroencephalogr. Clin. Neurophysiol.*, 9:673–690.
18. Eeg-Olofsson, O. (1971): The development of the electroencephalogram in normal children from the age of 1 through 15 years. 14 and 6 Hz positive spike phenomenon. *Neuropaediatrie*, 2:405–427.
19. Eeg-Olofsson, O. (1971): The development of the electroencephalogram in normal adolescents from the age of 16 through 21 years. *Neuropaediatrie*, 3:11–45.
20. Eeg-Olofsson, O., Petersén, I., andSelldén, U. (1971): The development of the electroencephalogram in normal children from the age of 1 through 15 years. Paroxysmal activity. *Neuropaediatrie*, 2:375–404.
21. Ellingson, R. J. (1979): EEGs of premature and full-term newborns. in: *Current Practice of Clinical Electroencephalography*, edited by D. W. Klass and D. D. Daly, pp. 149–177. Raven Press, New York.
22. Ellingson, R. J., and Peters, J. F. (1980): Development of EEG and daytime sleep patterns in normal full-term infants during the first 3 months of life: Longitudinal observations. *Electroencephalogr. Clin. Neurophysiol.*, 49:112–124.
23. Engel, R. C. H. (1975): *Abnormal Electroencephalograms in the Neonatal Period*. Charles C Thomas, Springfield, Illinois.
24. Frost, J. D., Jr., Carrie, J. R. G., Borda, R. P., and Kellaway, P. (1973): The effects of Dalmane (flurazepam hydrochloride) on human EEG characteristics. *Electroencephalogr. Clin. Neurophysiol.*, 34;171–175.
25. Gastaut, H., Terzian, H., and Gastaut, Y. (1952): Étude d'une activité électroencéphalographique méconnue: "le rythme rolandique en arceau." *Marseille Med.*, 89:296–310.
26. Gastaut, H. (1952): Étude électrocorticographique de la réactivité des rythmes rolandiques. *Rev. Neurol.* (Paris), 87:176–182.
27. Gastaut, Y. (1951): Un signe électroencéphalographique peu connu: les pointes occipital survenant pendant l'ouverture des yeux. *Rev. Neurol.* (Paris), 84:640–643.
28. Gibbs, F. A., and Gibbs, E. L. (1950): *Atlas of Electroencephalography, Vol. 1: Methodology and Controls*. Addison-Wesley, Reading, Massachusetts.
29. Gibbs, F. A. and Gibbs, E. L. (1952) *Atlas of Electroencephalography. Vol. 2: Epilepsy*. Addison-Wesley, Reading Massachusetts.
30. Gibbs, F. A., and Gibbs, E. L. (1964): *Atlas of Electroencephalography, Vol. 3: Neurological and Psychiatric Disorders*. Addison-Wesley, Reading, Massachusetts.
31. Gibbs, F. A., Gibbs, E. L., and Lennox, W. C., (1943): Electroencephalographic classification of epileptic patients and control subjects. *Arch. Neurol. Psychiatry*, 50:111–128.
32. Gibbs, F. A., and Knott, J. R. (1949): Growth of the electrical activity of the cortex. *Electroencephalogr. Clin. Neurophysiol.*, 1:223–229.
33. Hanley, J. W. (1981): A step-by-step approach to neonatal EEG. *Am. J. EEG Technol.*, 21:1–13.
34. Hughes, J. R. (1980): Two forms of 6/sec spike and wave complex. *Electroencephalogr. Clin. Neurophysiol.*, 48:535–550.
35. Hughes, J. R., Means, E. D., and Stell, B. S. (1965): A controlled study of the behavior disorders associated with the positive spike phenomenon. *Electroencephalogr. Clin. Neurophysiol.*, 18:466–483.
36. Jasper, H., and Andrews, H. L. (1938): Brain potentials and voluntary muscle activity in man. *J. Neurophysiol.*, 1:87–100.
37. Jasper, H. H., and Kershman, J. (1949): Classification of EEG in epilepsy. *Electroencephalogr. Clin. Neurophysiol.* (Suppl. 2):, 123–131.
38. Kellaway, P. (1978): An orderly approach to visual analysis: Parameters of the normal EEG in adults and children. In: *Current Practice of Clinical Electroencephalography*, edited by D. W. Klass and D. D. Daly, pp. 69–148. Raven Press, New York.
39. Kiloh, L. C., McComas, A. J., and Osselton, J. W. (1972): *Clinical Electroencephalography*, 3rd ed. Butterworths, London.
40. Kooi, K. A., Güvener, A. M., Tupper, C. J., and Bagchi, B. K. (1964): Electroencephalographic patterns in the temporal regions in normal adults. *Neurology* (Minneap.), 14:1029–1034.
41. Kuhlo, W. (1976): The beta rhythms. In: *Handbook of Electroencephalography and Clinical Neurophysiology*, Vol. 6, Part A, edited by G. E. Chatrian and G. C. Lairy, pp. 6A29–6A46. Elsevier, Amsterdam.
42. Lebel, M., and Reiher, J. (1976): Wicket spikes: A previously undescribed EEG pattern. *Electroencephalogr. Clin. Neurophysiol.*, 41:548 (abstr.).
43. Lindsley, D. B. (1939): A longitudinal study of the occipital alpha rhythm in normal children: Frequency and amplitude standards. *J. Genet. Psychol.*, 55:197–213.
44. Lipman, L. J., and Hughes, J. R. (1968): Rhythmic mid-temporal discharges. *Electroencephalogr. Clin. Neurophysiol.*, 27:43–47.
45. Lombroso, C. T. (1982) Neonatal electroencephalography. In: *Electroencephalography—Basic Principles, Clinical Applications and Related Fields*, edited by E. Niedermeyer and F. Lopes de Silva, pp. 599–637. Urban and Schwarzenberg, Baltimore.
46. Lombroso, C. T., Schwartz, I. H., Clark, D. M., Muench, H., and Barry, J. (1966): Ctenoids in healthy youths: Controlled study of 14- and 6-per-second positive spiking. *Neurology* (Minneap.), 16:1152–1158.
47. Loomis, A. L., Harvey, E. N., and Hobart, G. A. (1935): Potential rhythms of the cerebral cortex during sleep. *Science*, 81:597–598.
48. Loomis, A. L., Harvey, E. N., and Hobart, G. A. (1937): Cerebral states during sleep, as studied by human brain potentials. *J. Exp. Psychol.*, 21:127–144.
49. Maulsby, R. L. (1971): An illustration of emotionally evoked theta rhythm in infancy: Hedonic hypersynchrony. *Electroencephalogr. Clin. Neurophysiol.*, 31:157–165.
50. Maulsby, R. L. (1979): EEG patterns of uncertain diagnostic significance. In: *Current Practice of Clinical Electroencephalography*, edited by D. W. Klass and D. D. Daly, pp. 411–419. Raven Press, New York.
51. McGregor, P. A., Weitzman, E. D., and Pollak, C. P. (1978): Polysomnographic recording technique used for the diagnosis of sleep disorders in a sleep disorders center. *Am. J. EEG Technol.*, 18:107–132.
52. Milstein, V., and Small, J. G. (1971): Psychological correlates of 14 & 6 positive spikes, 6/sec. spike-wave, and small sharp spike transients. *Clin. Electroencephalogr.*, 2:206–212.
53. Niedermeyer, E. (1982): Maturation of the EEG: Development of waking and sleep patterns. In: *Electroencephalography—Basic Principles, Clinical Applications and Related Fields*, edited by E. Niedermeyer and F. Lopes de Silva, pp. 107–130. Urban and Schwarzenberg, Baltimore.
54. Niedermeyer, E. (1982): Abnormal EEG patterns (epileptic and paroxysmal). In: *Electroencephalography—Basic Principles, Clinical Applications and Related Fields*, edited by E. Niedermeyer and F. Lopes de Silva, pp. 155–177. Urban and Schwarzenberg, Baltimore.
55. Obrist, W. D. (1976): Problems of aging. In: *Handbook of Electroencephalography and Clinical Neurophysiology*, Vol. 6, Part A, edited by G. E. Chatrian and G. C. Lairy, pp. 6A275–6A342. Elsevier, Amsterdam.
56. Obrist, W. D., Henry, C. E., and Justiss, W. A. (1966): Longitudinal changes in the

senescent EEG: A 15-year study. In: *Proceedings of the 7th International Congress of Gerontology,* pp. 35–38. International Association of Gerontology, Vienna.

57. Pedley, T. A. (1980): Interictal epileptiform discharges: Discriminating characteristics and clinical correlations. *Am. J. EEG Technol.,* 20:101–119.
58. Pedley, T. A. (1980): EEG patterns that mimic epileptiform discharges but have no association with seizures. In: *Current Clinical Neurophysiology: Update on EEG and Evoked Potentials,* edited by C. E. Henry, pp. 306–336. Elsevier/North-Holland, New York.
59. Pedley, T. A., Lombroso, C. T., and Hanley, J. W. (1981): Introduction to neonatal electroencephalography: Interpretation. *Am. J. EEG Technol.,* 21:15–29.
60. Petersén, I., and Eeg-Olofsson, O. (1971): The development of the electroencephalogram in normal children from the age of 1 through 15 years. Non-paroxysmal activity. *Neuropaediatrie,* 2:247–304.
61. Rechtschaffen, A., and Kales, A., editors (1968): *A Manual of Standardized Terminology, Techniques and Scoring System for Sleep Stages of Human Subjects.* National Institutes of Health Publication No. 204, U.S. Government Printing Office, Washington, D.C.
62. Reiher, J. and Lebel, M. (1977): Wicket spikes: Clinical correlates of a previously undescribed EEG pattern. *J. Can. Sci. Neurol.,* 4:39–47.
63. Ross, J. J., Johnson, L. C., and Walter, R. D. (1966): Spike and wave discharges during stages of sleep. *Arch. Neurol.,* 14:399–407.
64. Sato, S., Dreifuss, F. E., and Penry, J. K. (1973): The effect of sleep on spike-wave discharges in absence seizures. *Neurology* (Minneap.), 23:1335–1345.
65. Sharbrough, F. W. (1981): Non-specific abnormal EEG patterns. In: *Electroencephalography—Basic Principles, Clinical Applications and Related Fields,* edited by E. Niedermeyer and F. Lopes de Silva, pp. 135–154. Urban and Schwarzenberg, Baltimore.
66. Simonova, O., Roth, B., and Stein, J. (1967): EEG studies of healthy population—normal rhythms of resting recording. *Acta Univ. Carol.* [*Med.*] (Praha), 13:543–551.
67. Smith, J. R. (1939): The "occipital" and "pre-central" alpha rhythms during the first two years. *J. Psychol.,* 7:223–226.
68. Spehlmann, R. (1981): *EEG Primer,* pp. 147–157. Elsevier/North-Holland, Amsterdam.
69. Spire, J. P. C. (1981): Polysomnography: Technical aspects. In: *Current Neurophysiology: Update on EEG and Evoked Potentials,* edited by C. E. Henry, pp. 375–418. Elsevier/North-Holland, New York.
70. Tharp, B. R. (1966): The 6-per-second spike and wave complex. *Arch. Neurol.,* 15:533–537.
71. Tharp, B. R. (1980): Neonatal and pediatric electroencephalography. In: *Electrodiagnosis in Clinical Neurology,* edited by M. J. Aminoff, pp. 67–117. Churchill Livingstone, New York.
72. Travis, L. E. (1937): Brain potentials and the temporal course of consciousness. *J. Exp. Psychol.,* 21:302–309.
73. Vogel, F., and Götze, W. (1962): Statistische Betrachtungen über die β-Wellen im EEG des Menschen. *Dtsch. Z. Nervenheilk.,* 184:112–136.
74. Walter, W. G. (1950): Normal rhythms—their development, distribution and significance. In: *Electroencephalography: A symposium on its various aspects,* edited by D. Hill and G. Parr. pp. 203–227. Macdonald, London.
75. Walter, W. G., and Dovey, V. J. (1944): Electroencephalography in cases of sub-cortical tumour. *J. Neurol. Neurosurg. Psychiatry,* 7:57–65.
76. Werner, S. S., Stockard, J. E., and Bickford, R. G. (1977): *Atlas of Neonatal Electroencephalography.* Raven Press, New York.
77. Westmoreland, B. F., and Sharbrough, F. W. (1975): Posterior slow wave transients associated with eye blinks in children. *Am. J. EEG Technol.,* 15:14–19.
78. White, J. C., Langston, J. W., and Pedley, T. A. (1977): Benign epileptiform transients of sleep: Clarification of the small sharp spike controversy. *Neurology* (Minneap.), 27:1061–1068.

Chapter 15

Commonly Used Activation Procedures

Many patients with known neurological signs and symptoms will have an abnormal EEG, but some will not. In these latter patients, several procedures may be used to activate (i.e., induce) EEG abnormalities that may provide useful diagnostic information.

Every EEG technologist should have a thorough knowledge of the more commonly used activation procedures, the EEG abnormalities they elicit, and the indications and contraindications for their use, as well as the significance of the EEG changes that occur.

HYPERVENTILATION

Hyperventilation is a routine procedure in most laboratories. Its greatest effectiveness is in evoking the EEG correlates of clinical absence (petit mal) seizures; it also may induce a clinical absence seizure. On rare occasions, a generalized tonic–clonic (grand mal) seizure may occur as a result of hyperventilation.

There are only a few contraindications to hyperventilation. Policies regarding the use of this procedure should be established by the medical director of the laboratory. A few of the contraindications are:

1. recent cardiac illness,
2. a recent stroke,
3. distressed breathing,
4. extreme hypertension,
5. subarachnoid hemorrhage.

Hyperventilation is accomplished by instructing the patient to breathe deeply (emphasis on full expiration, emptying the lungs of all air) at a regular and rapid rate (18–24 respirations per min) for 3 to 5 min. However, the length of time hyperventilation is carried out can vary from a few seconds to 5 min depending on its effectiveness (e.g., the appearance of a burst of a 3-Hz spike-wave activity after 30 sec) and the patient's condition and tolerance for the procedure.

Physiologically, hyperventilation causes a decrease in the carbon dioxide level in the blood, which results in constriction of cerebral arteries and arterioles. This constriction leads to a change in the brain's metabolism; it is this which brings about the EEG changes.

The manner in which the patient is directed to hyperventilate often determines the effectiveness of the procedure. A monotonous "Keep your eyes closed, breathe deeply until I tell you to stop," is not a particularly effective method. Instead, instruct the patient in this manner: "Please keep your eyes closed, open your mouth, and when I tell you to begin, breathe deeply through your mouth, completely emptying your lungs after every breath. Keep this up until I tell you to stop." A brief demonstration of the correct procedure by the technologist will enhance the desired effect. With coaxing and demonstration, even young children often will hyperventilate enthusiastically and effectively. The patient usually responds much more actively when the technologist paces the rate of breathing by counting. The patient should be observed closely for clinical changes as well as for cooperativeness in following directions. It may be necessary to remind the patient to continue the procedure at the proper rate until asked to stop.

The beginning of hyperventilation (usually abbreviated HV) must be marked clearly on the EEG record. A mark should be made every 30 sec during HV (e.g., "30," "60," or "90") and the termination also must be marked clearly. Some laboratories maintain a marked count for one or more minutes after cessation of HV. Notes written on the record during hyperventilation, relative to the patient's degree of cooperation and so on, often are helpful when the record is later reviewed. If there are apparent artifacts related to movement associated with deep breathing, pencil marks should be made directly on the record to indicate their coincidence with breathing (see Chapter 16). If the patient has an absence seizure, this should be noted and described on the record. For example: "Patient stopped HV and opened eyes. . .did not respond to calling name. . .closed eyes and resumed HV spontaneously."

The usual and normal response to hyperventilation is bilateral slow-wave activity (Fig. 15.1). This is fairly symmetrical, disappears within 30

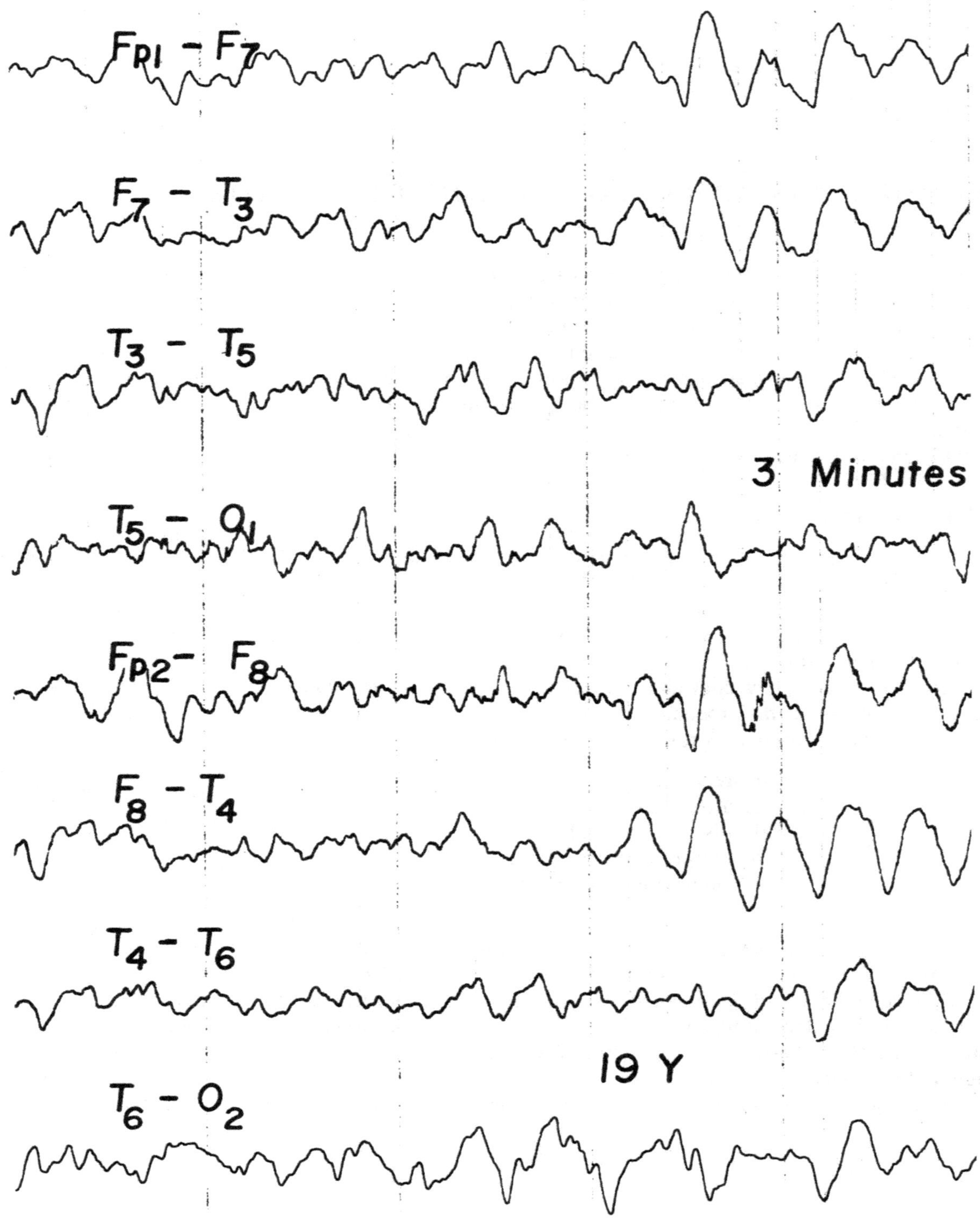
Fp1 - F7
F7 - T3
T3 - T5
3 Minutes
T5 - O1
Fp2 - F8
F8 - T4
T4 - T6
19 Y
T6 - O2

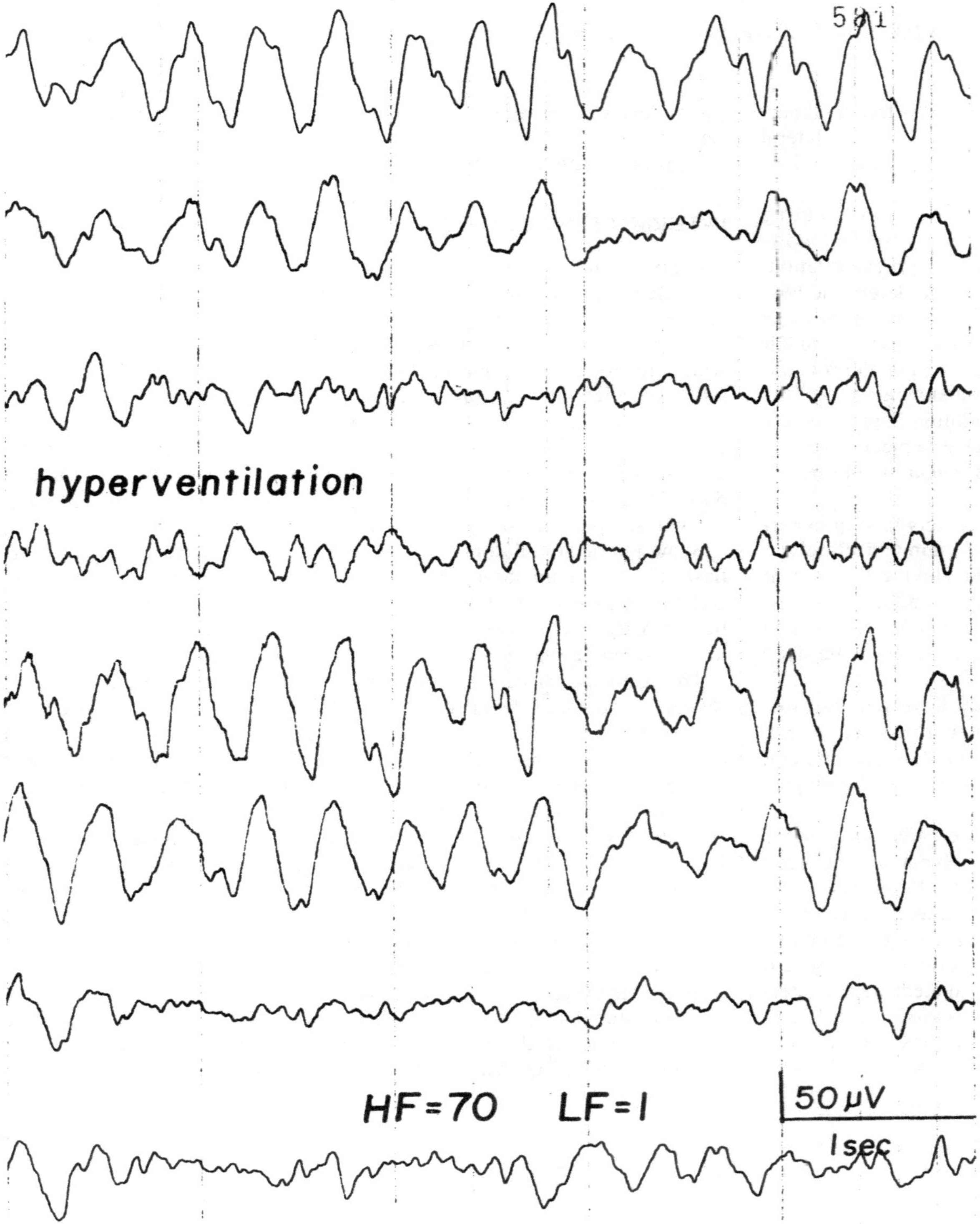

FIG. 15.1. Normal response to 3 min of hyperventilation in a 19-year-old subject.

to 60 sec following the cessation of hyperventilation, and is free of abnormal wave forms (e.g., has no definite spike components). The bilateral slow-wave response is seen more often in children than in adults. This response is often referred to as a "buildup."

A low blood sugar level enhances the buildup of slow waves during hyperventilation and may cause the persistence of slow activity following hyperventilation. When pronounced or prolonged hyperventilation-evoked slow activity is apparent, the technologist should determine how long it has been since the patient last ate and estimate the amount of sugar and carbohydrate ingested. If the patient had breakfast 3 hr earlier and if it consisted of a cup of black coffee and a piece of dry toast, in all probability a low blood sugar level has caused the prolonged slow activity. This can and should be checked by repeating hyperventilation approximately 15 min after giving the patient a glass of juice with sugar, a piece of candy, or a non-diet soft drink. If the patient has diabetes, sugar should be administered with caution.

On occasions, the patient may not hear the instructions to stop hyperventilation or may be unable to stop immediately on command. Rarely, a patient may involuntarily prolong hyperventilation. Having the patient rebreathe by holding a large paper bag over the mouth and nose may be beneficial. The technologist should observe a patient carefully at the end of the procedure to make certain that he does indeed discontinue deep breathing when so instructed.

Children with a history of absence seizures may have had seizures associated with running or excessive physical exertion. This suggests that the seizure was activated by hyperventilation as a result of exertion and that an absence seizure may be recorded during the hyperventilation procedure.

It may be useful to have the patient hyperventilate twice, or in some cases, even three times during the recording period. Hyperventilation on one montage may be more informative than on another. Reference to the patient's history may help in choosing an optimal montage. If focal brain disease is suspected, the focal area should be represented in the montage. In patients suspected of having absence seizures, a useful montage would be one that includes the frontal, temporal, and central electrodes bilaterally. Hyperventilation has been proven effective in evoking focal temporal slow activity. If a temporal spike focus already has been demonstrated, hyperventilation using a parasagittal montage only would be a poor choice; a montage including the temporal derivations would be preferred.

Hyperventilation occasionally helps the patient to relax.

INTERMITTENT PHOTIC STIMULATION

Photic stimulation is used routinely in most laboratories, although the incidence of photic-induced EEG abnormality is relatively low. However in some cases, it may prove to be of great value.

The light used for photic stimulation is produced by a stroboscope, which generates repetitive flashes of short duration (approximately 10 μsec) and high intensity (0.5 to 2 million foot candles). The flash rate or number of flashes per second can be varied, e.g., 1 to 60 per sec. The most commonly used frequencies are from 1 to 30 flashes per sec. Rates of 14 to 16 flashes per sec are most likely to elicit abnormalities. The usual procedure is to present a series of repetitive flashes at different frequencies for 5- to 10-sec periods, with an equal time between each series.

Some photic stimulators have a control that varies the intensity of the flash. If such a stimulator is being used, the technologist may start at the highest (or near the highest) level. If photic sensitivity is demonstrated, the intensity level can be lowered to establish an intensity threshold (the level just above that at which no reactivity is shown).

The lamp should be placed directly in front of the patient's eyes. Although no standard distance between the lamp and the eyes is used, 12 inches (30 cm) has been suggested (1,4). The intensity of the light at the eyes will decrease as a function of the square of the distance. It is important that the intensity be equal at all points in the visual field of each eye.

There are various methods used for photic stimulation. Some laboratories have the patient keep the eyes closed throughout the stimulation period. In others, the eyes are opened between flash groups and closed on command as the flash begins. Still others have the patient open and close the eyes during the period of the flash.

The color of the light may be an important variable. Red light usually is more effective in evoking abnormalities. Blue light is less effective. Some laboratories systematically vary colors in each examination.

Photic stimulators should provide a synchronous pulse to be delivered to one channel of the EEG instrument to record the incidence of the flashes on the EEG record. There may be a special channel available, called an event marker, that can be used to monitor the flashing light. If no marker channel is available, one of the recording channels may be used as a monitor. The marker should not be put in a channel recording the significant activity, e.g., the occipital area where driving responses are observed (Fig. 15.2). Certainly, the marker should not be superimposed on a focal abnormality.

Photic Responses

Photic Driving Response

The most common type of response occurs in the posterior head regions and is seen as a rhythm, the frequency of which is the same as the flash rate. This response is best developed in the range of 4 to 20 flashes per sec and usually is at or near alpha frequency. The responses may be harmonics of the flash frequency (usually two or three times the flash rate; subharmonics may appear, usually one-half the flash rate). This response is called photic driving or photic recruiting (Fig. 15.2). This response is normal. However, absence of a driving response is not abnormal.

Unilateral depression of photic driving (Fig 15.3) sometimes has been associated with focal pathology. However, normal individuals may present an asymmetric driving response and variability may exist from one day to another (*personal observation*). One must be certain that both left and right visual fields of each eye are equally illuminated (see placement of light, above) and that electrode placement is symmetrical.

Photoconvulsive Response

The EEG abnormality most commonly activated by photic stimulation is generalized spike-and-wave activity or multiple spike activity. This is known as a photoconvulsive response. The spike and/or spike-wave activity may be sustained and terminated with the end of flash interval, or the discharges may continue after the cessation of the flashes (Fig. 15.4). Unsustained photoconvulsive responses (Fig. 15.5) terminate during the flash period. A sustained photoconvulsive response is definitely abnormal and is of greater diagnostic value than a response that dies out while the flash continues (5).

Photomyoclonic Responses

Photomyoclonic responses are characterized by spikes of muscle origin (EMG). They are seen most predominantly in the frontal regions. They usually increase in amplitude (recruit) during photic stimulation and stop with the cessation of the flashes (Fig. 15.6). The EMG spikes are maximal around the eyes; the patient may have jerking movements of the head and face. Photomyoclonic responses have no clinical significance and are said to occur in 20% of normal subjects (1).

Further Comments

The technologist must be aware of the possibility of inducing a generalized tonic–clonic seizure by photic stimulation. If a photoconvulsive EEG response develops, stimulation should be stopped. It can be presented briefly two or three more times to verify the findings. Often it is useful to decrease the stimulus intensity to discover if there is a threshold for evoking this response. Occasionally the EEG of a patient may be activated by eye closure. The morphology is clearly abnormal (Fig. 15.7), with spikes and high voltage slow waves being present. This is readily detected when testing for reactivity of the alpha to eye opening.

SLEEP DEPRIVATION

Prolonged periods of sleep loss (24 to 36 hr of continuous waking time) may stress a potentially epileptogenic brain so that abnormalities will appear in the waking EEG. Thus, if a patient has been sleep-deprived, the initial part of the record must be in the awake state (3).

SLEEP

One of the most effective and simplest of all activating procedures is sleep (2,5,6,7). In one study of 1,620 patients (7), it was found that the sleep EEG was "crucial" in making the interpretation in 14.8% of the patients; in 24.6% of patients with all types of epilepsy, the sleep record was "crucial," but in only 1.3% of patients with tumors did it add significantly to the interpretation. Patients with complex partial seizures (temporal lobe epilepsy) in particular are likely to show abnormalities in sleep

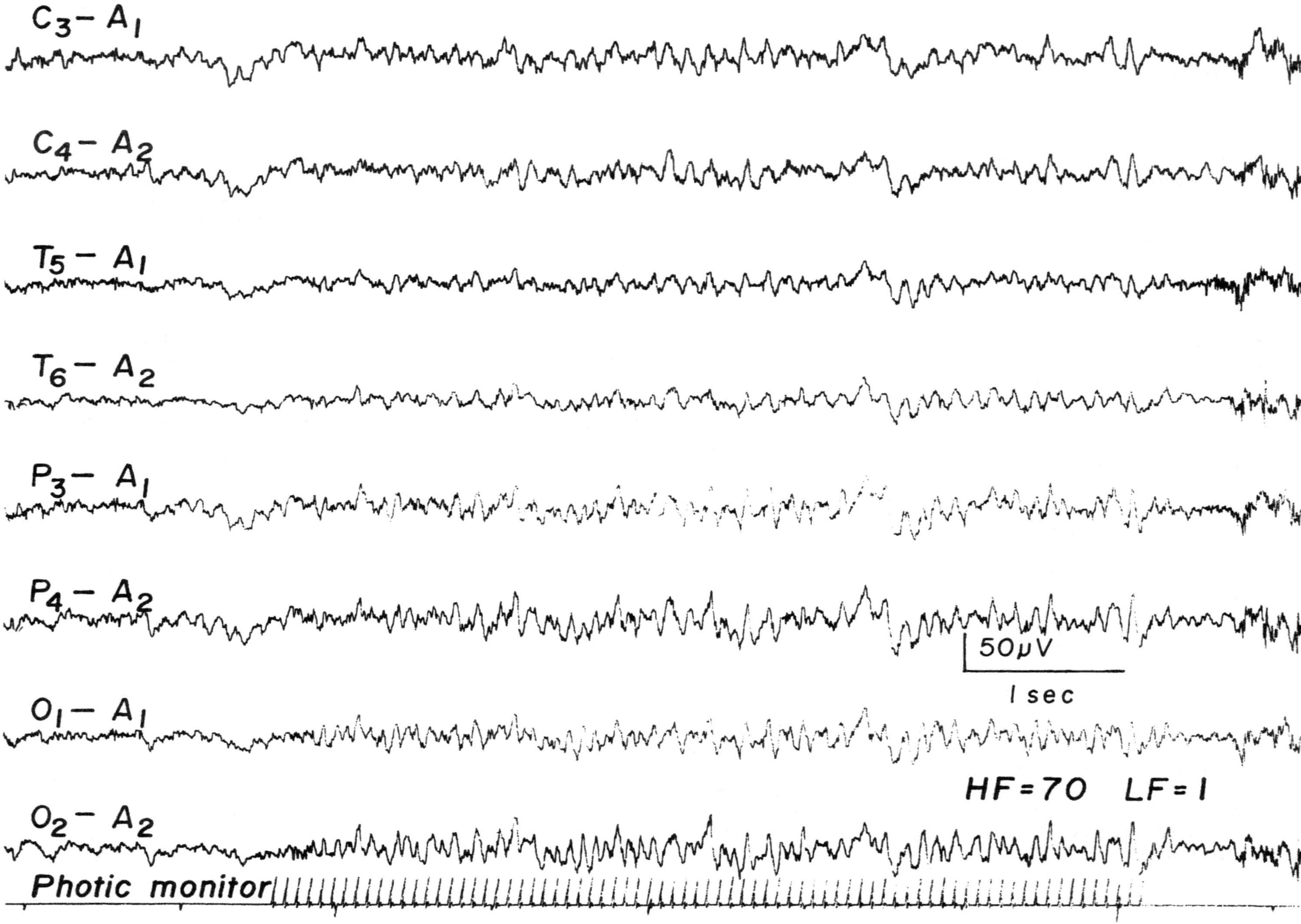

FIG. 15.2. Bilateral posterior photic driving with repetitive flash.

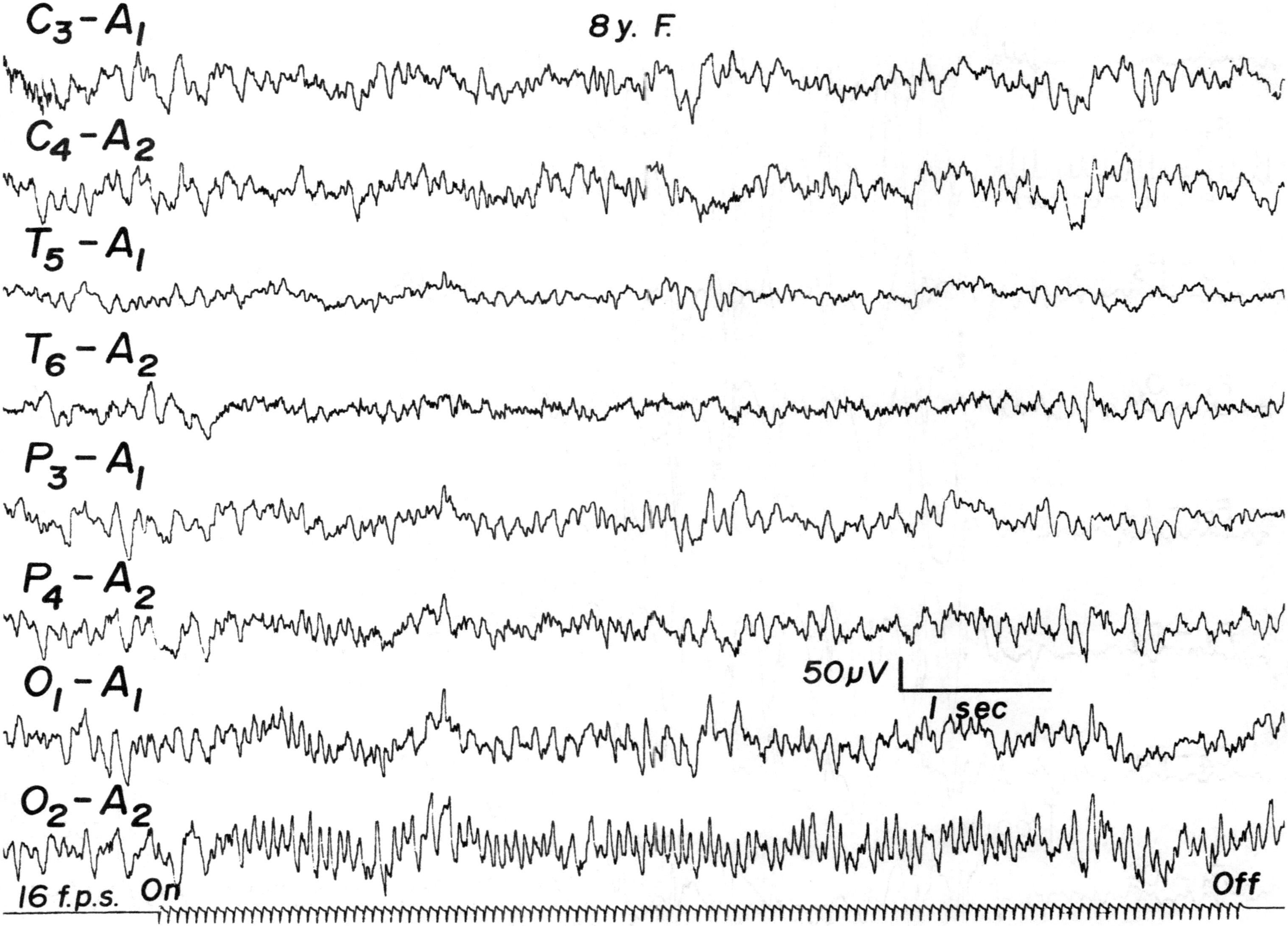

FIG. 15.3. Asymmetrical photic driving in patient without known pathological condition.

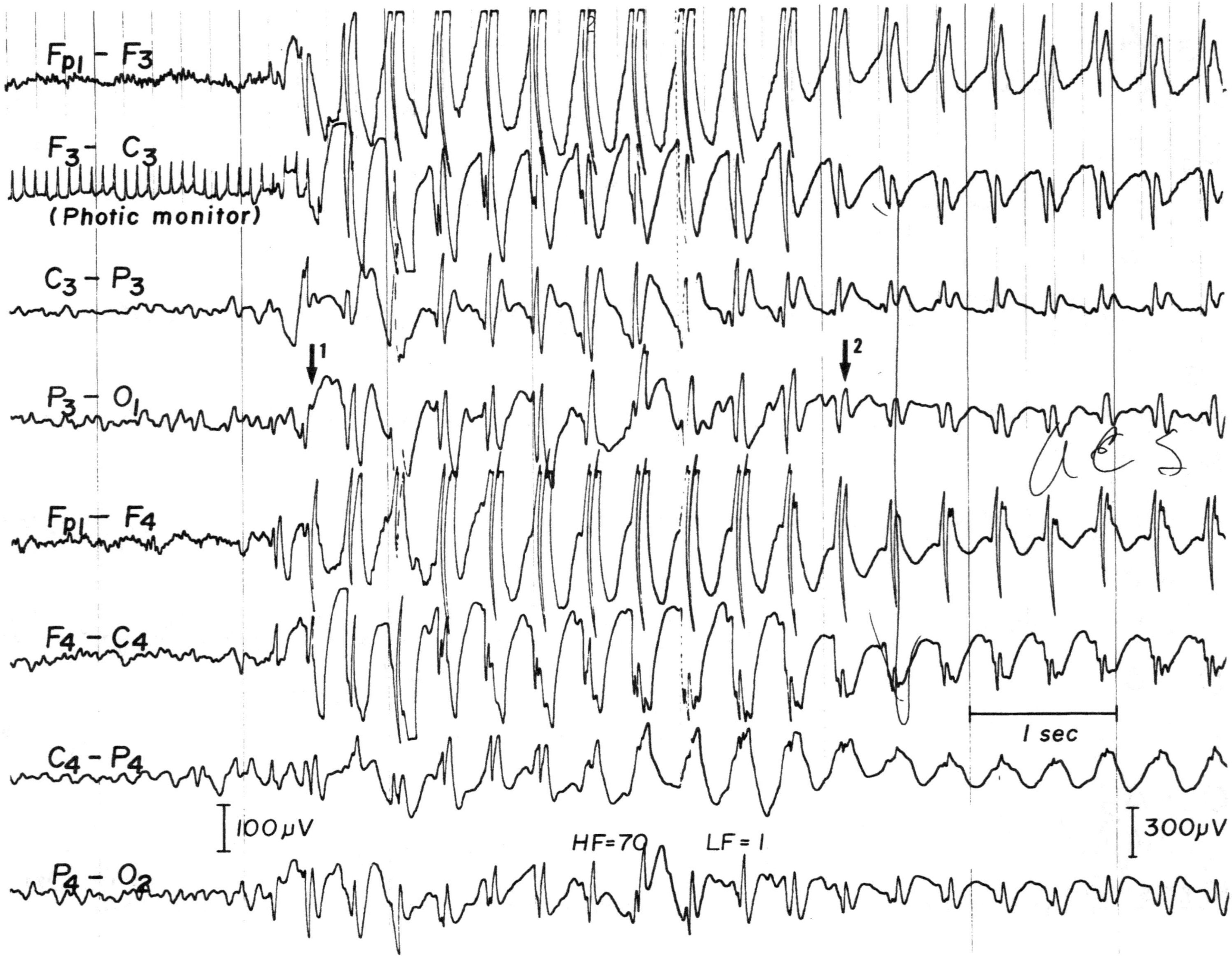

Fp1 - F3
F3 - C3
(Photic monitor)
C3 - P3
P3 - O1
Fp1 - F4
F4 - C4
C4 - P4
P4 - O2
1
2
100 μV
300 μV
1 sec
HF=70
LF = 1

(2). Sleep should be a routine procedure for patients who have or are suspected of having seizures of any type.

Activation procedures are carried out not only for the purpose of evoking a latent abnormality, but also for increasing a minimal abnormality. In many instances, EEG activity of an inconclusive type may appear during the waking record. During sleep, it may emerge clearly as abnormal activity.

It is highly desirable that every recording should include a period of spontaneous sleep. This is not always possible, but the technologist should be on the alert for the EEG signs of sleep onset and every effort should be made to allow the patient to continue into sleep at that time. Other activation procedures or sensory probing should not be carried out at the risk of interfering with spontaneous sleep. Hyperventilation and photic stimulation always can be carried out later, but the technologist is not in control of the patient's ability to go to sleep at a later time. It is extremely important that the technologist recognize the characteristics of light sleep and plan the examination strategy to use the sleep state, if indicated by the patient's medical history.

Drug-induced sleep may be requested by the referring physician, who should sign a written order for sedation. If sedation is used, the technologist always should check carefully to be certain that the patient does not plan to leave the laboratory unescorted (and perhaps drive home after the examination). The patient should have been instructed to have someone come with him to drive or accompany him home, but there is always the possibility that the patient, either by misunderstanding or otherwise, did not do this. If other arrangements cannot be made, the test should be rescheduled or an extended effort should be made to obtain spontaneous sleep.

The amount of sedation to be given to the patient will be prescribed by the medical director of the laboratory or by the patient's physician. The exact time at which it was given and the amount must be clearly written on the record. (In some states, it is illegal for any medications to be administered by a technologist; only a registered nurse or physician may do so.)

The montages selected for sleep activation should be chosen to display activity in areas in which abnormality may be expected and usually should include temporal derivations. The recording should be continuous from an initially awake record, into and during at least stage 2 sleep, during arousal, and for several minutes after awakening.

To regard sleep as "activation" may be questioned since it is a normal state. It is not a special procedure in the sense that some other activation procedures are regarded. However, it can be considered a "state related" procedure (1), and it does contrast findings of the waking EEG, at rest, with the EEG under another condition. If the initial waking EEG is abnormal and is consistent with the patient's medical history, a sleep record is sometimes regarded as unnecessary.

FIG. 15.4. Sustained photoconvulsive response to flash. Stimulation was terminated at ↓1. Sensitivity was reduced at ↓2, from 10 μV/mm to 30 μV/mm.

OTHER ACTIVATION PROCEDURES

Other types of activation procedures have been used, but not routinely. One procedure employs analeptic drugs such as pentylenetetrazol (Metrazol) which stimulate the central nervous system. This procedure may be of use in reproducing a patient's clinical seizure while recording the EEG at its onset. This method is considered to be most useful in patients with focal seizures who are candidates for surgical treatment. Its value is somewhat reduced because persons who do not have epilepsy can be triggered into having generalized tonic-clonic seizures, sometimes with relatively low doses of the drug. This procedure must be carried out by a qualified physician-electroencephalographer.

Patients with musicogenic epilepsy (seizures activated by particular types of music) may be tested if suitable audio equipment is available. A patient with a history of reading epilepsy (seizures occurring when reading) should have a period of reading included during the recording. The results of special types of activation cannot be predicted with certainty.

A note of caution: The use of some activation procedures, particularly hyperventilation and photic stimulation, may cause the patient to have a clinical seizure. These occasions are rare, but they do occur. The laboratory should be equipped to meet such an emergency, and the technologist should be knowledgeable about the management of a convulsing patient.

SUMMARY

Activation procedures use stimulation or changes in the patient's state to induce or to increase EEG abnormalities. One of the most commonly used methods of activation involves hyperventilation, which may evoke

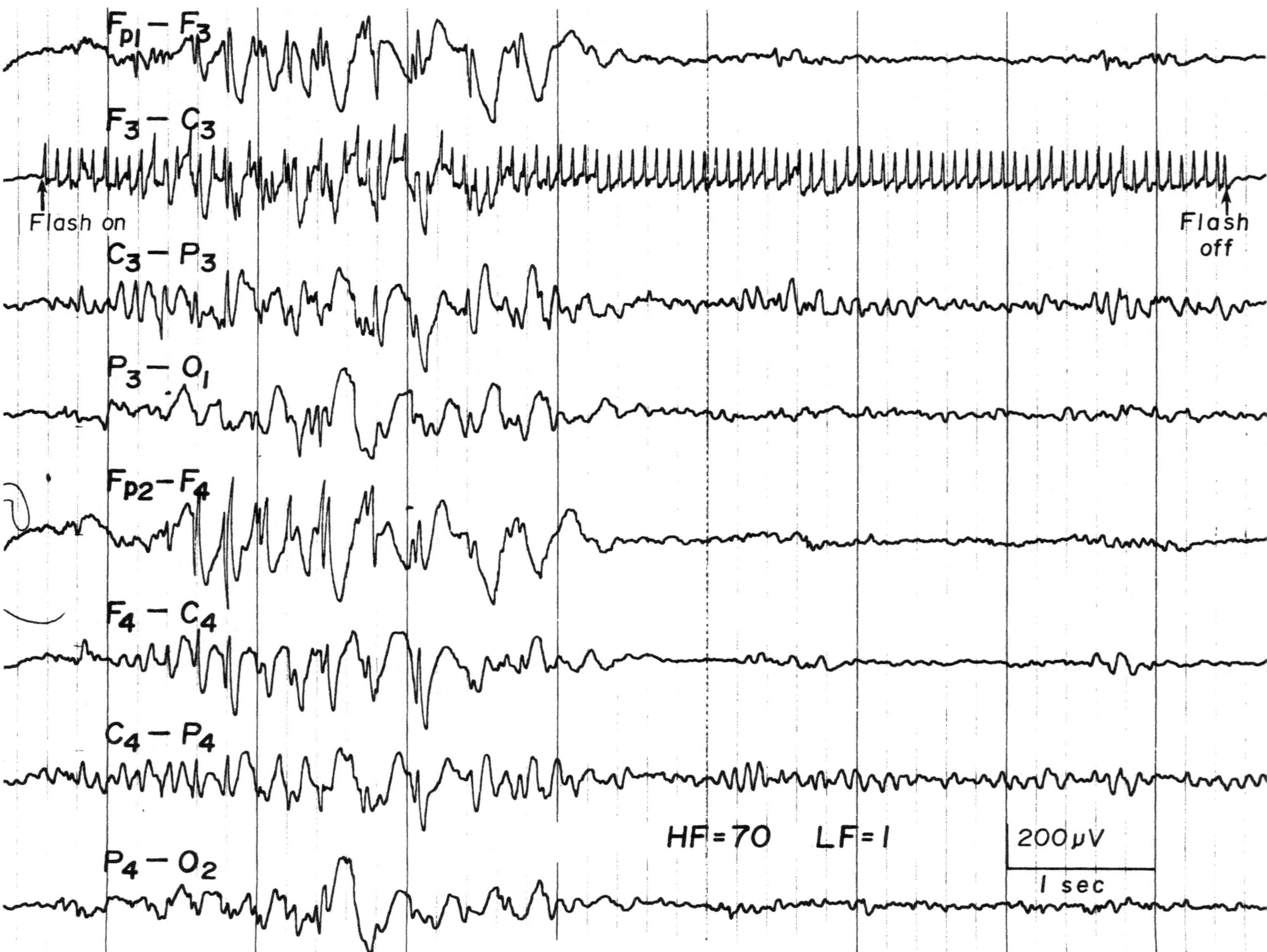

FIG. 15.5. Unsustained photoconvulsive response to flash.

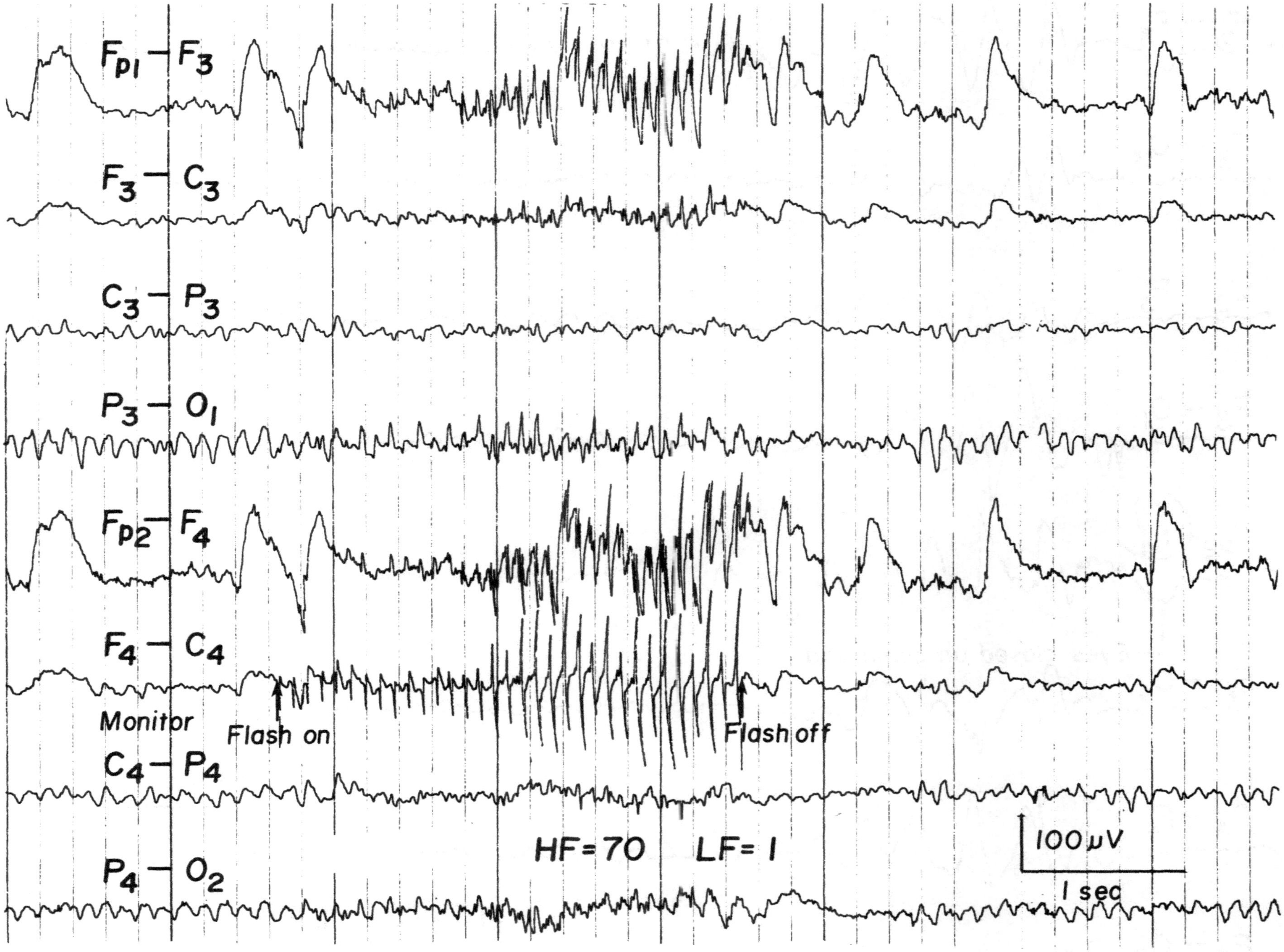

FIG. 15.6. Photomyoclonic response to photic stimulation. Frontal muscle response augments as flash continues.

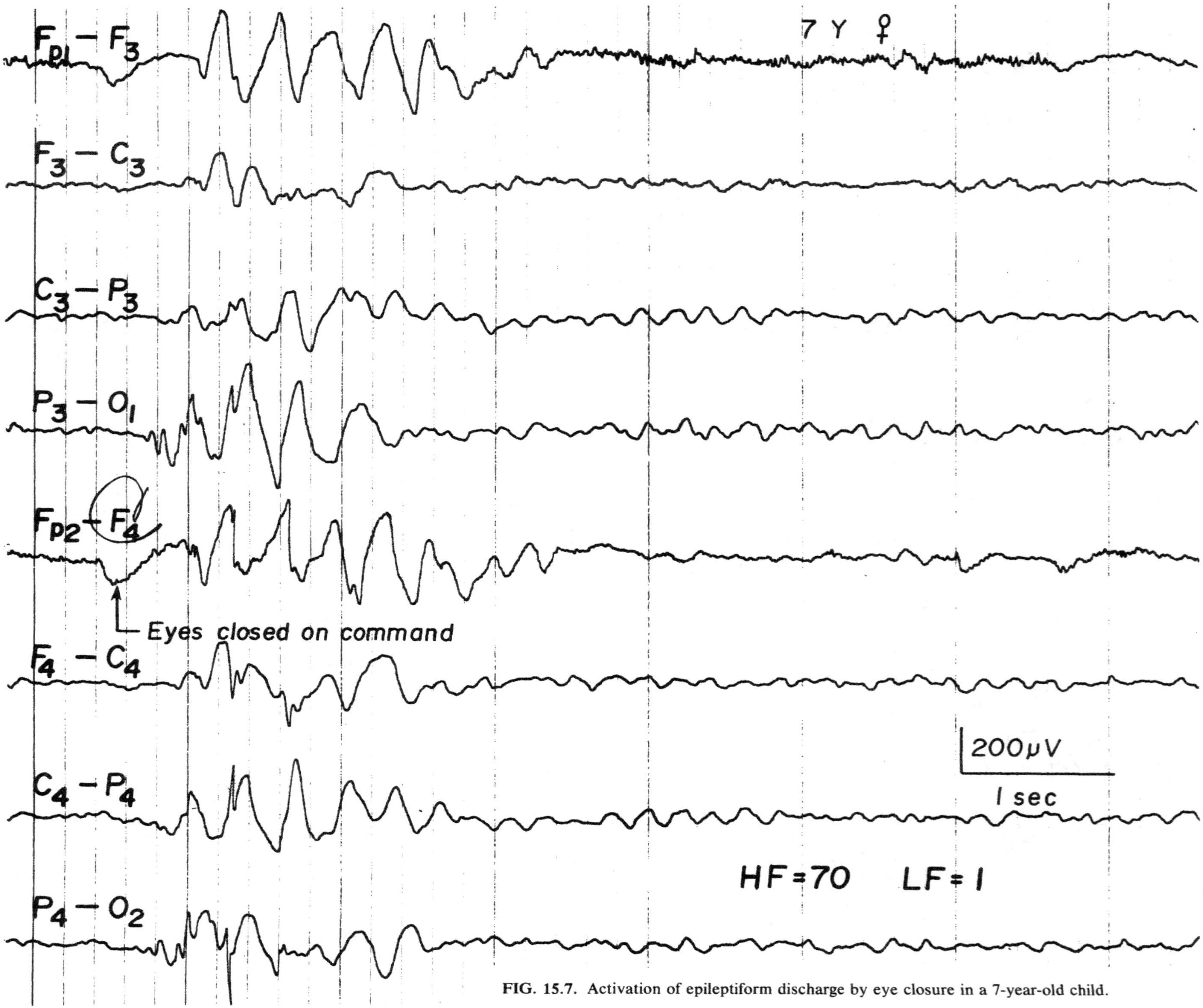

FIG. 15.7. Activation of epileptiform discharge by eye closure in a 7-year-old child.

distinctive patterns such as spike-wave discharges in some epileptic patients. Simple slow, rhythmic activity is a nonpathological response and is seen particularly in children.

Equally commonly used is repetitive photic stimulation. This procedure also may evoke distinctive activity. A benign type of activity is the photomyoclonic response, which is of muscle origin. Abnormal EEG responses are called photoconvulsive and consist of spikes or spike-wave discharges, or both. These may persist beyond the period of stimulation; if they do, they are more probably of diagnostic significance.

Sleep often is used as an activation method, based on an observed increase in EEG abnormality during sleep.

Sleep deprivation is another activation procedure, utilizing fatigue as a stress mechanism to evoke latent or minimal EEG abnormalities, usually in patients with epilepsy.

Other methods of activation include chemical stimulation from convulsant drugs. In some patients, particular stimulating conditions such as listening to music or reading may evoke seizures. Duplicating such conditions in the laboratory may evoke EEG abnormalities.

REFERENCES

1. Bickford, R. G. (1979): Activation procedures and special electrodes. In: *Current Practice of Clinical Electroencephalography,* edited by D. W. Klass and D. D. Daly, pp. 269–305. Raven Press, New York.
2. Gibbs, F. A., and Gibbs, E. L. (1952): *Atlas of Electroencephalography, Vol. II: Epilepsy,* p. 165. Addison-Wesley, Reading, Massachusetts.
3. Mattson, R. H., Pratt, K. L., and Calverley, J. R. (1965): Electroencephalograms of epileptics following sleep deprivation. *Arch. Neurol.,* 13:310–315.
4. Niedermeyer, E. and Lopes da Silva, F. (1982): *Electroencephalography: Basic Principles, Clinical Applications and Related Fields,* p. 180. Urban & Schwarzenberg, Baltimore.
5. Reilly, E. L., and Peters J. F. (1973): Relationship of some varieties of electroencephalographic photosensitivity to clinical convulsive disorders. *Neurology,* 23:1050–1057.
6. Sato, S., Dreifuss, F., and Penry, J. K. (1973): The effect of sleep on spike-wave discharges in absence seizures. *Neurology,* 23:1335–1345.
7. Silverman, D., and Morisaki, A. (1958): Re-evaluation of sleep electroencephalography. *Electroencephalogr. Clin. Neurophysiol.,* 10:425–431.

Chapter 16

Artifacts

The EEG record is presumed to represent only cerebral activity. In reality, it includes other electrical activity that is not of cerebral origin. The activity of the brain is the signal of primary concern, and any other activity that appears in the record will deteriorate the brain signal. These undesired activities are called *noise* or *artifact*. Their origins are multiple. Figure 16.1 lists the origins of artifacts, and diagrams their mixture with the EEG signal.

Physiological artifacts are electrical signals originating from the patient, but from sources other than the brain. These include muscle potentials, electrocardiographic potentials, potentials from the eyes (these may be corneoretinal and electroretinal), skin potentials, and glossokinetic potentials.

Nonphysiological artifacts may originate from electrodes or switch contacts of the EEG instrument or from external signals such as an electrocautery in the operating room, 60-Hz radiation from a nearby lamp, appliance, or power cord, and even radio frequency interference from nearby radio and television transmitters. Instrument noise is inherent internally in the active electronic circuits of the amplifying system and is an ever-constant factor. Its maximum allowable level is specified by the International EEG Federation (1).

At times it is difficult for even the most experienced technologist or electroencephalographer to distinguish between the fact, which is the EEG signal, and the artifact, which is the noise. Because artifacts may mimic abnormality, it is imperative that sources of noise be identified accurately. An artifact and its cause usually are obvious to the technologist at the time of the recording. But when the EEG is being interpreted (often long after the technologist has gone for the day), the record may take on an entirely different appearance, in a different setting, under a different pair of eyes. Therefore, it is essential that artifacts be clearly identified by the technologist and labeled during the recording.

PHYSIOLOGICAL ARTIFACTS

Muscle Artifact

One of the three most commonly encountered physiological artifacts is that generated by muscle. The patient may in all respects appear calm and relaxed, yet some electrode derivations may be more or less obscured by continuous electromyographic (EMG) activity with a voltage higher than the EEG (Fig. 16.2). This artifact occurs most commonly in the frontal and temporal areas, although it may occur in any derivation (4). It is especially prominent and appears to be generalized in referential recording when the ears, mandibles, or chin are used as the reference. Muscle activity is more often seen when the patient is awake, but it can continue in sleep.

Single motor units (Fig. 16.3) sometimes may be confused with cortical spikes. Motor unit discharges, however, have a shorter duration than scalp-recorded EEG spikes.

A form of artifact frequently associated with rapid lateral eye movements resembles spike activity (Fig. 16.4). It usually is restricted to electrodes F_7 and F_8. The origin is in the synchronous discharge of motor units in the external rectus muscle of the side to which the eye is moving. The moving of the eye usually can be identified by observation. If eye movement cannot be observed, monitoring should be carried out, as described later in this chapter.

Attempts to eliminate muscle artifact often are futile. Every effort should be made to make the patient more comfortable. Sometimes having the patient open his mouth slightly will decrease the amount of muscle artifact. Sometimes it is reduced after hyperventilation. If EMG persists, it often is best to do nothing, as constantly reminding the patient to relax can increase tension. With the passage of time, anxiety and tension tend to decrease and relaxation increases.

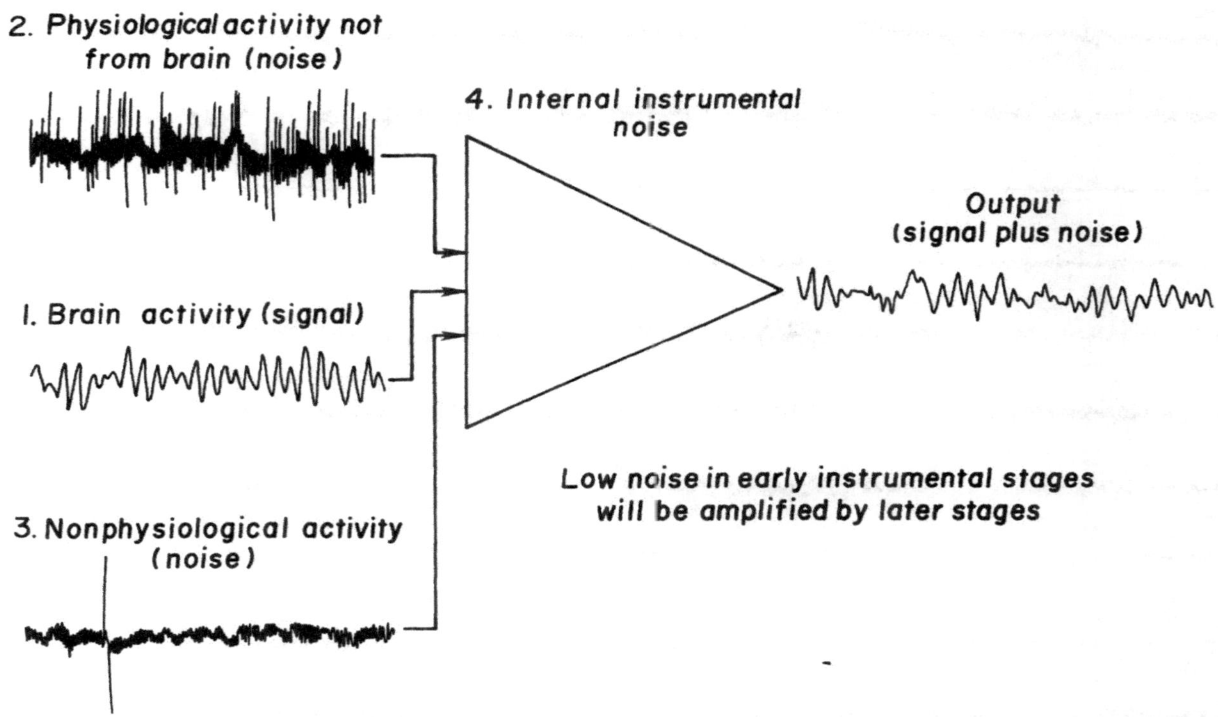

FIG. 16.1. EEG record is a combination of electrical activity of the brain and electrical activity from other sources, or noise (see text).

To attenuate muscle activity instrumentally when all else fails, the high frequency filters may be used. However, EMG activity, when heavily filtered, can simulate background beta activity, as shown in Fig. 16.5. An HF setting of 15 Hz should be used with discretion for a portion of the recording and only in extreme cases. Even greater confusion may result if 60-Hz filters are added to HF filters, since the roll-off characteristics of the HF filter change. Delta and theta activity, of course, will not be affected by changes in high frequency cut-off points. (Refer to Chapter 8.)

Electrocardiographic Artifact

Another common physiological artifact is that produced by the electrical activity of the heart (EKG or ECG), as shown in Fig. 16.6 (p. 286). Usually the EKG voltage at the scalp is small (1 to 2 μV) and is masked by most waking and sleeping EEG activity (usually 20-100 μV).

There is individual variability in the amount and persistence of EKG artifact. Its presence is related to the field of the heart potentials over the surface of the scalp. This in turn is related to the body's conduction pathway for the EKG to spread to the scalp. In general, short, stout persons who have a short and wide neck present the largest EKG artifacts in their EEGs. Because the artifact is related to the EKG field on the head, the voltage and apparent surface polarity will vary from derivation to derivation and, consequently, from montage to montage. It will be most obvious in referential montages using A_1 and A_2. When using a neck–chest reference, it almost always will be present to some degree. EKG artifact usually is recognizable by its rhythmicity. Sometimes components of EKG are mixed with EEG activity and may resemble sharp waves.

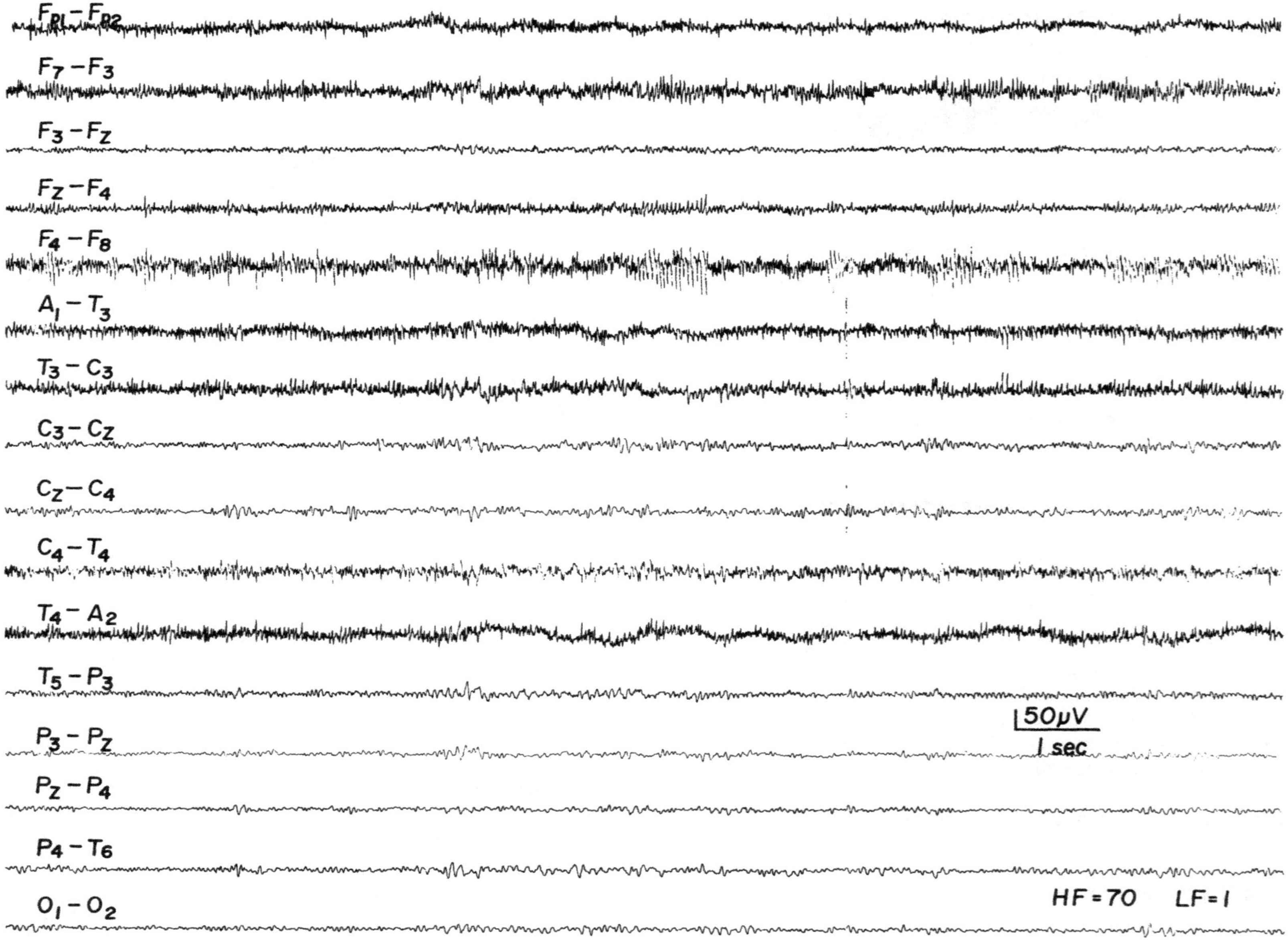

FIG. 16.2. EMG artifact distributed over scalp, with transverse bipolar montage. Highest voltage artifact is in anterior and lateral areas. Midline, central, parietal and occipital areas are relatively free of EMG activity.

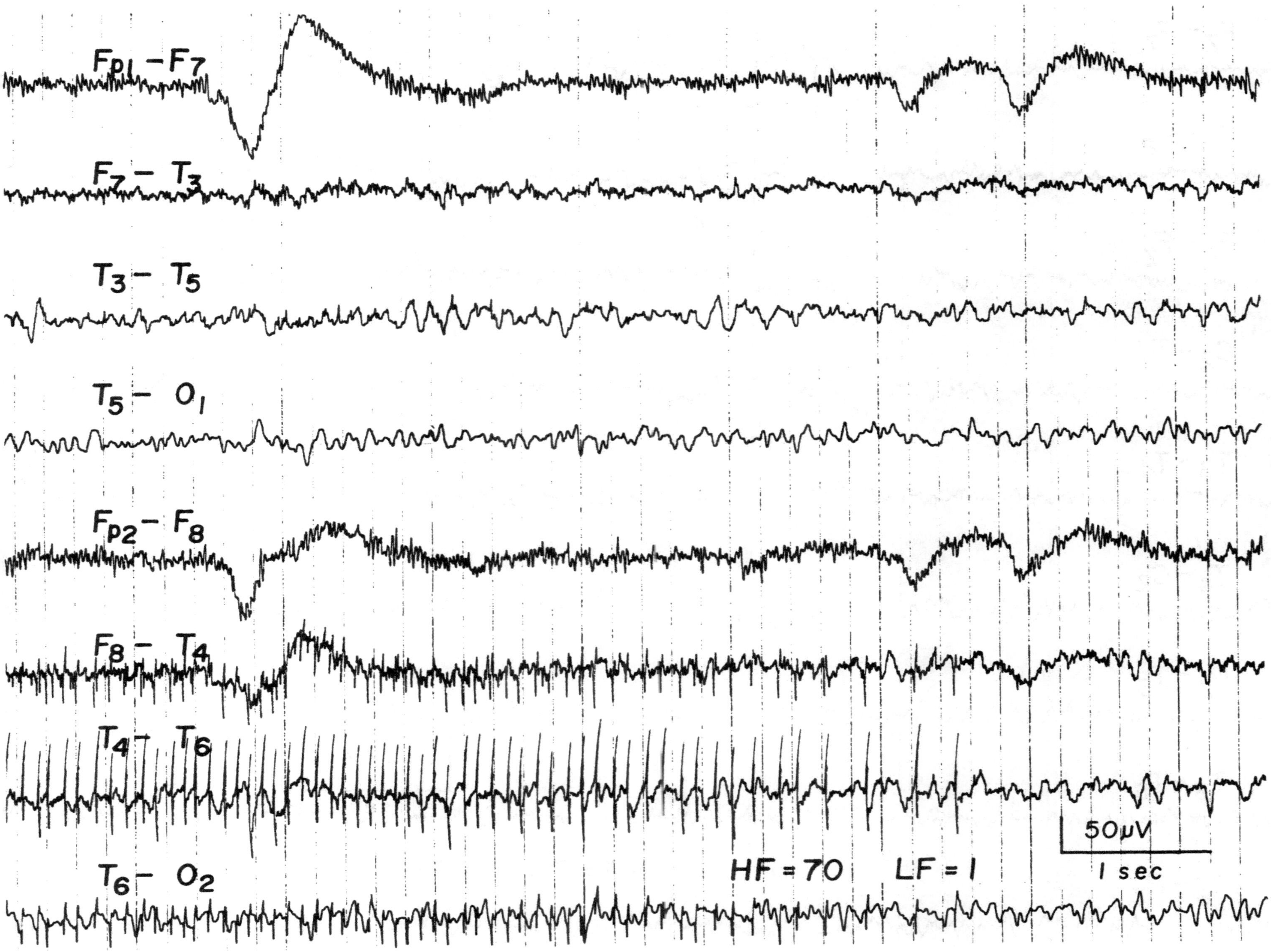

FIG. 16.3. Single motor units firing in right temporalis muscle.

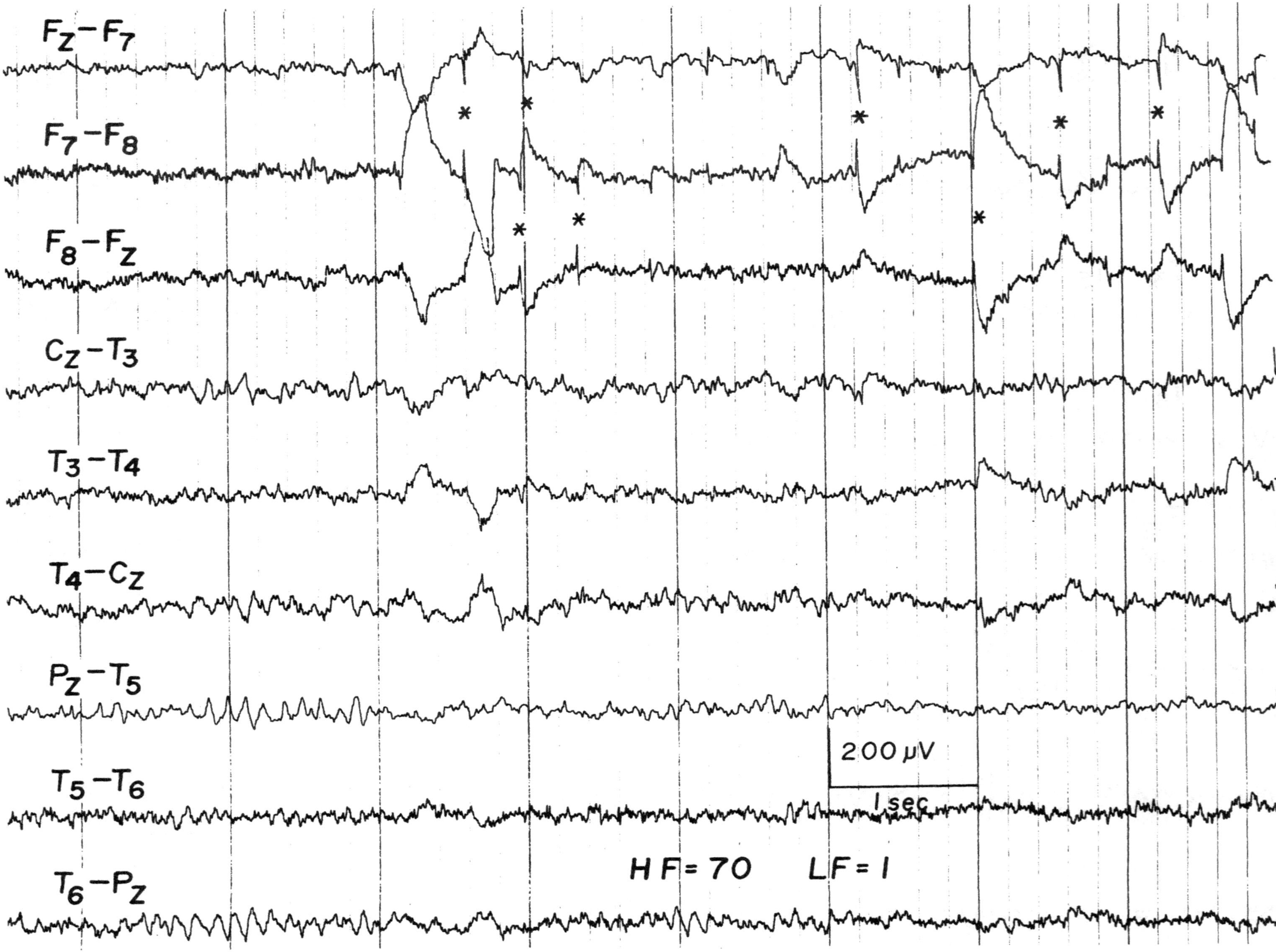

FIG. 16.4. Lateral rectus muscle discharge, appearing in derivations from F_7 and F_8 (marked *).

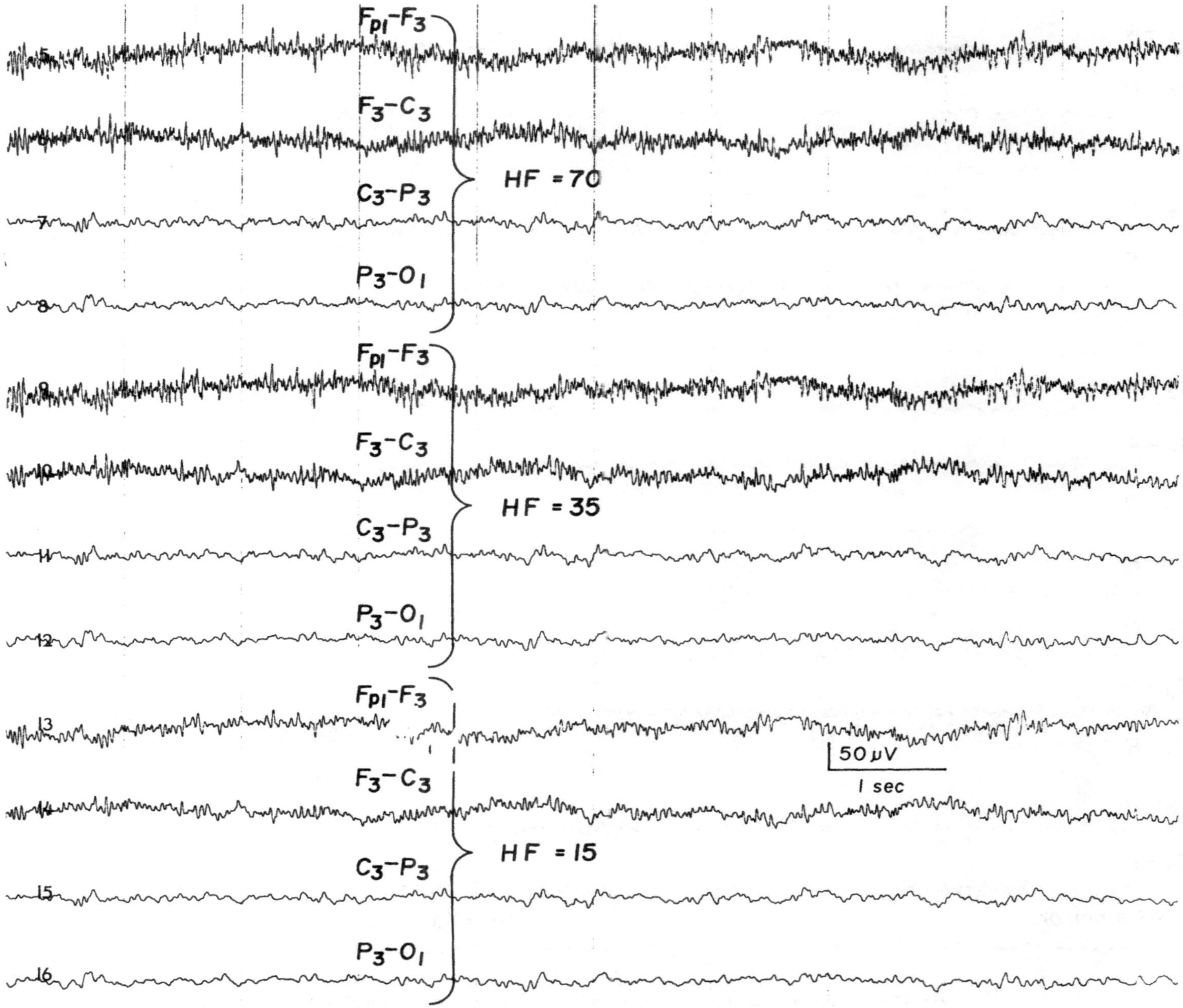

FIG. 16.5. Effects of high frequency filters on EMG activity. EEG is "lost in noise" with HF = 70 and HF = 35; with HF = 15, the EMG appears similar to background beta activity.

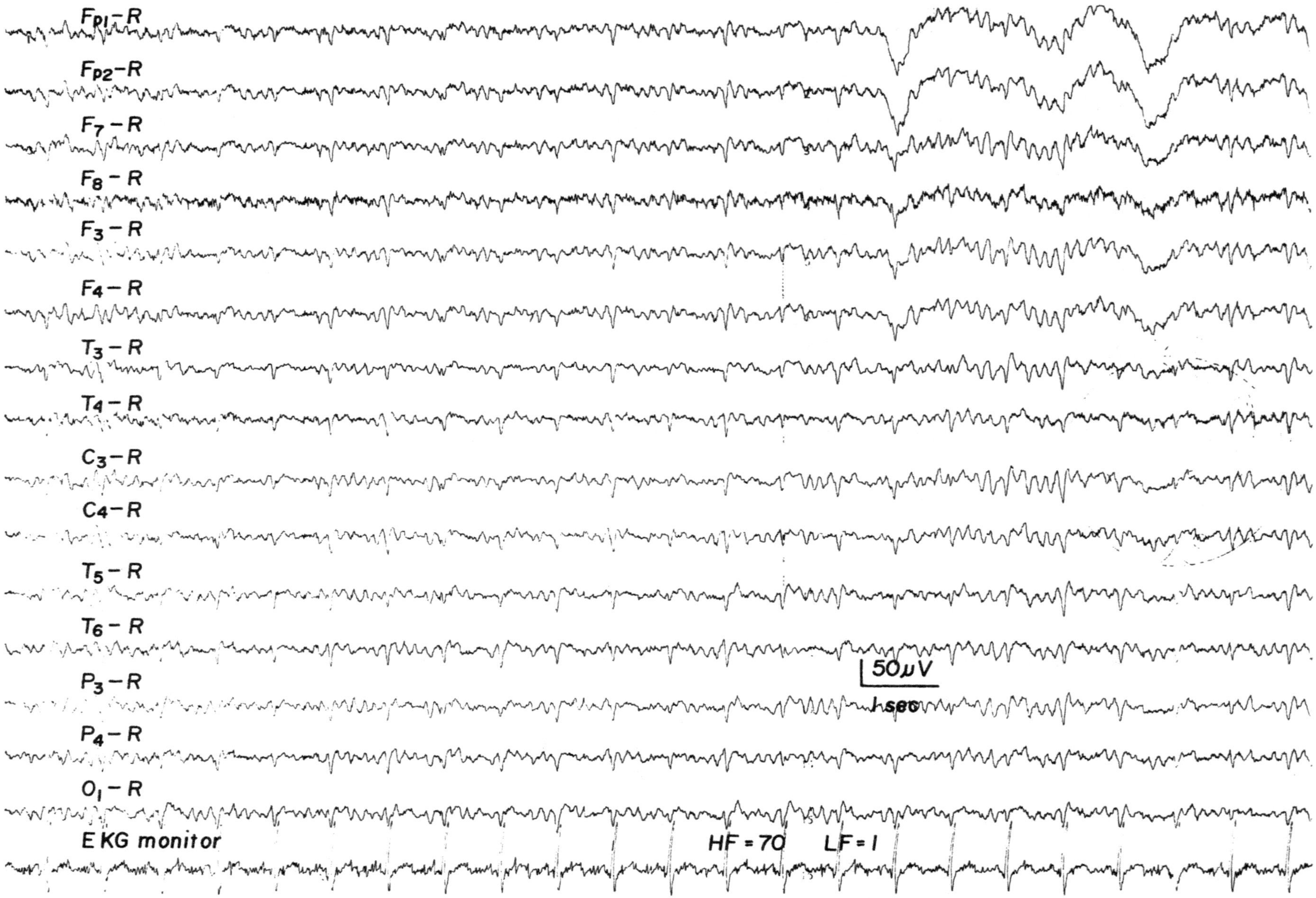

FIG. 16.6. EKG artifact. Referential recording using noncephalic (neck–chest) reference.

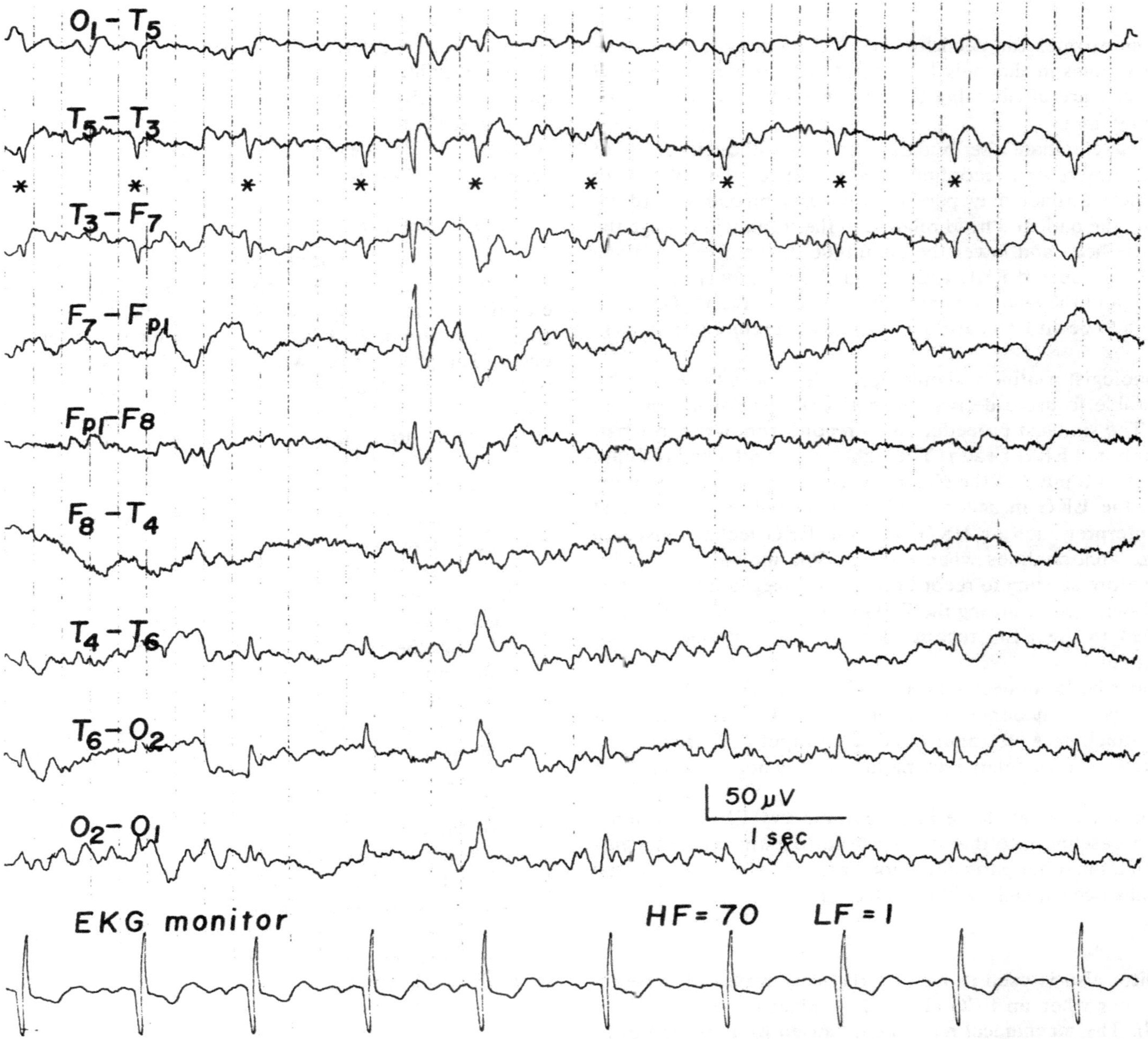

FIG. 16.7. EKG artifact and focal left temporal spike discriminated by use of EKG monitor. The artifacts are indicated by "*s". (See page 288.)

Figure 16.7 demonstrates the need for an EKG monitor to determine which of the sharp waves in channels 1 through 6 are attributable to EKG potentials and which are attributable to abnormal EEG activity in the patient's left frontal area.

There is no way to eliminate a serious EKG artifact, although the use of bipolar rather than referential recording usually reduces the voltage. In some persons, EKG artifact may persist even with bipolar recording. Sometimes turning the patient's head relative to the trunk will change the EKG field over the head and lower the amplitude of the artifact. When efforts to eliminate suspected EKG artifact fail, EKG activity should be directly monitored and the sharp component included in the EEG output then can be proven to be an EKG artifact or to be of cerebral origin, as in Fig. 16.7.

The EEG technologist routinely should apply electrodes to record the EKG. It is preferable to use a derivation that is conventionally used in EKG recording. The simplest procedure is to record from wrist to wrist. This is the conventional EKG Lead I. The right wrist is attached to Input 1 and the left wrist to Input 2 of the channel used to display the monitor. This will display the EKG in accord with its own polarity rule. Most physicians can interpret such an EKG, and the EEG technologist will learn to recognize abnormalities when present. The monitor electrodes can be attached before starting to record the EEG, plugged into the electrode board, and switched in during the EEG recording whenever necessary. EKG artifact in the EEG record then can be identified without disturbing the patient.

If EKG electrodes have not been placed in advance or if they have been detached by a restless or uncooperative patient, the EKG can sometimes be monitored by attaching A_2 to Input 1 and A_1 to Input 2 of one channel of the instrument. This is an emergency method and is not recommended for standard use.

A short portion of EKG should be included on every EEG recording. This establishes a baseline rate that can be used to estimate the occurrence of EKG artifact in other parts of the total record. Also, unsuspected cardiac arrhythmias occasionally will be detected.

Pulse Artifact

An EKG monitor also is used to identify the slow waves of pulse artifact, that can occur when an EEG electrode is placed over a pulsating vessel (Fig. 16.8). The mechanical movement caused by pulsation of an artery can cause a slow wave that sometimes simulates EEG activity. There is a direct relationship between the EKG and the pulse waves. The latter are slightly delayed, since the blood requires time to travel from the heart ("the EKG") to the blood vessel that pulsates.

Pulse artifact can occur in any lead. If the patient is lying on the involved electrode, the artifact sometimes may be eliminated by moving the head slightly. Relocation of the electrode may eliminate the artifact.

Pacemaker Artifact

Another artifact that is cardiac related (but is actually nonphysiological) is pacemaker artifact (Fig. 16.9). This is seen as a fast spike, which is the electrical stimulus delivered to the heart by an internal cardiac pacemaker. In Fig. 16.9 there is a 2.5-sec interval in which the spike does not occur. The patient from whom this activity was recorded had a demand pacemaker, which does not deliver a pulse unless it is necessary to cause the muscle to contract. If the demand is irregular, the artifact can be intermittent, although it still should be recognized.

Eye Movement

Eye movement is the basis of the third common physiological artifact. Eye movement can simulate a plausible EEG slow wave having frontal origin. The orbit of the eye is, effectively, a battery (Fig. 16.10), the front of the eye being electropositive and the back of the eye being electronegative. This potential is called the corneoretinal potential. Figure 16.10 shows the battery placed between the cornea and the retina. Actually, the source of the voltage probably is between the back and the front of the retinal surface.

If the eye moves, the field of this voltage will be distributed over the front of the head differently than when the eye was in its original position (7). Figure 16.11 is a schematic representation of the field of positivity around the eyes when their position is fixed in forward gaze. The center front of the eye is most positive, and the positivity decreases with distance. When the eye turns upward (Fig. 16.12A), areas above the eye become relatively more positive, but below the eye they become more negative. Downward movement (Fig. 16.12B) reverses this effect. Movement of the eye to the left (Fig. 16.12C) causes scalp areas to the left to become more positive, while those to the right become more negative, since the back of the eye is closer to them. Eye movement to the right causes scalp areas on the right to become more positive, while those over the left become more negative (Fig. 16.12D).

Understanding how the potential field changes relative to eye move-

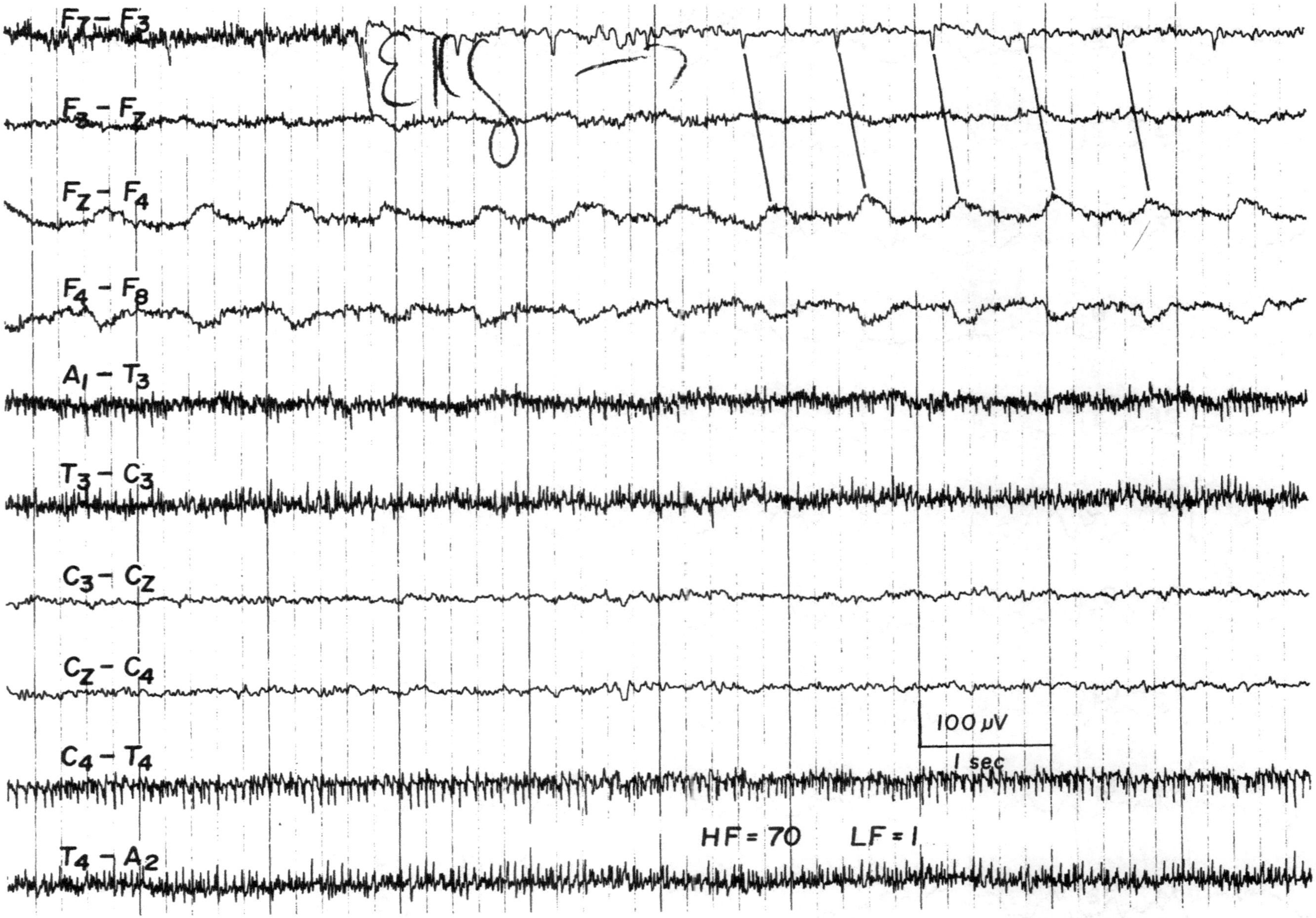

FIG. 16.8. Pulse artifact identified with EKG. Parallel lines indicate synchrony of heart contraction and pulse wave after delay of approximately 0.2 sec.

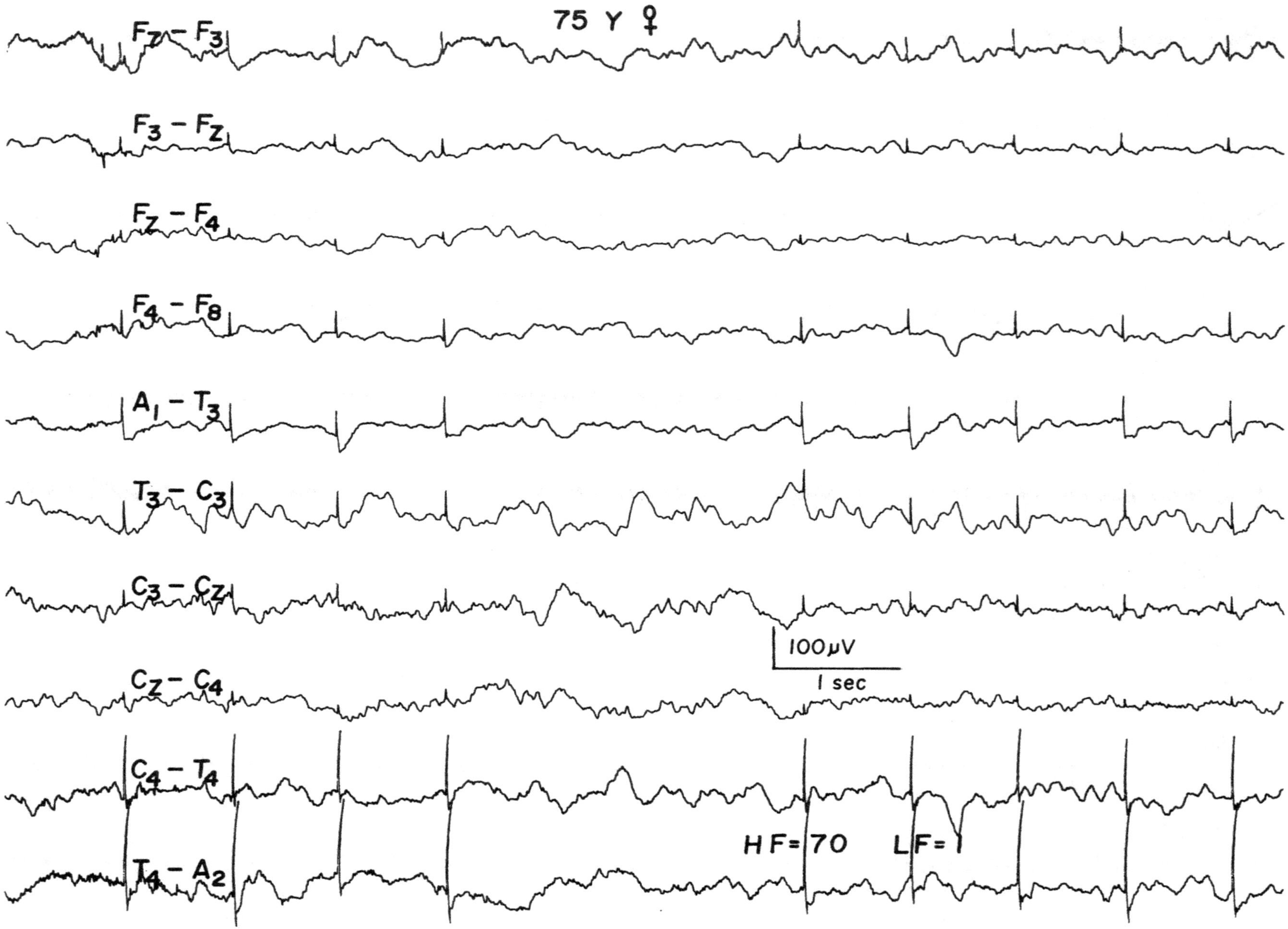

FIG. 16.9. Demand pacemaker artifact.

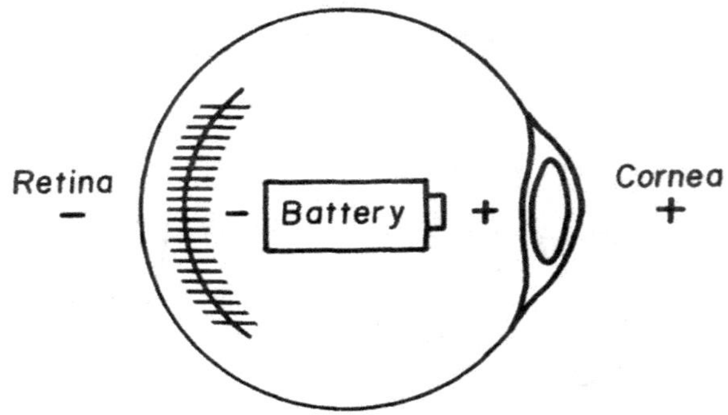

FIG. 16.10. Schematic representation of corneal–retinal potential.

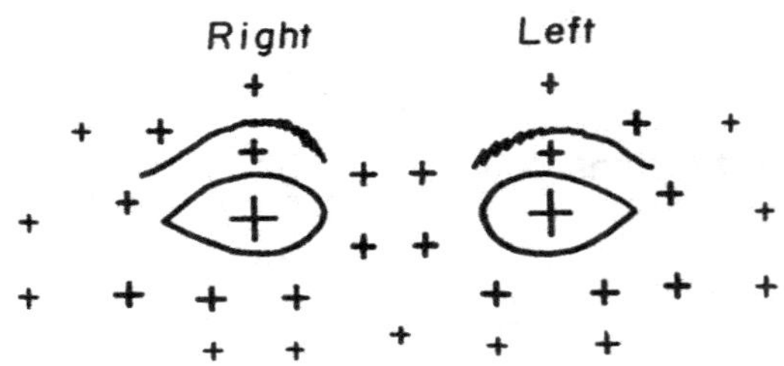

FIG. 16.11. Schematic representation of field of positivity around eye; polarity of eyes with position fixed forward.

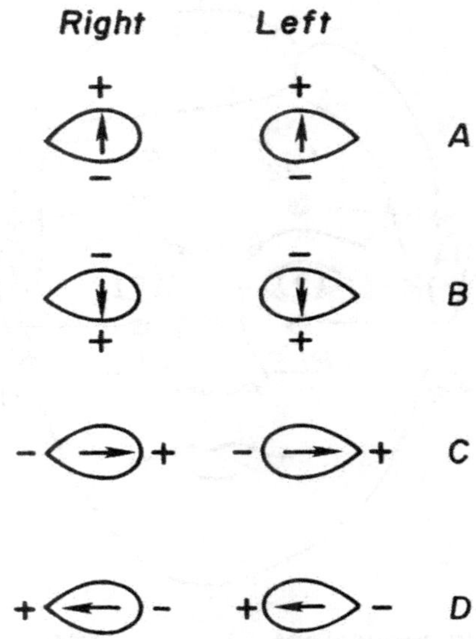

FIG. 16.12. Schematic of polarity changes in field with eye movement. A: up; B: down; C: left; and D: right.

ment, together with the rules of polarity, makes it possible to design a few basic montages that will differentiate true cerebral activity from eye movement. It is relatively easy to distinguish vertical eye movement from frontal slow activity. Standard EEG leads Fp_1 and Fp_2 are supraorbital leads. Additional leads are placed directly below the eyes, on the infraorbital ridge, left and right. The infraorbital electrodes are designated LLE (left) and RLE (right). Each of these four electrodes is referred to the ipsilateral ear, as shown in Fig. 16.13A. If anterior slow activity is caused by vertical eye movement, the activity from derivations above and below the eye will be out of phase (Fig. 16.13B). This is because Input 1 of the supraorbital channels is positive while the infraorbital Input 1 is negative, and vice versa. If the activity is of frontal cerebral origin, it will be in phase (Fig. 16.13C) because both the supra- and infraorbital channels have simultaneous positivity (or negativity) at Input 1.

A unilateral slow focus of cerebral origin (Fig. 16.14A) will produce unilateral in-phase activity (Fig. 16.14B). If there is unilateral eye movement due to absence of the eye or to unilateral paralysis of vertical gaze, the derivations above and below the intact eye will show out-of-phase activity, but no activity will be recorded from the abnormal eye. This effect also will occur if there is no corneoretinal potential due to retinal disease (10).

Another set of derivations is needed to identify the specific direction of movement of each eye (Fig. 16.15A). A pair of electrodes is placed diagonally in relation to each eye. One of each pair of electrodes is slightly below and lateral to the eye and the other electrode is above the eye and placed medially. The montage is designed to record from left to right as shown (Fig. 16.15A). With downward movement of the eyes, the direction of deflection will be downward on channel 1 and upward on channel 2 (Fig. 16.15B). With upward gaze (Fig. 16.15C), channel 1 will deflect upward and channel 2 will deflect downward. Eye movement to the left (Fig. 16.15D) will cause downward deflection in both channels. Movement to the right produces upward deflection in both channels (Fig.

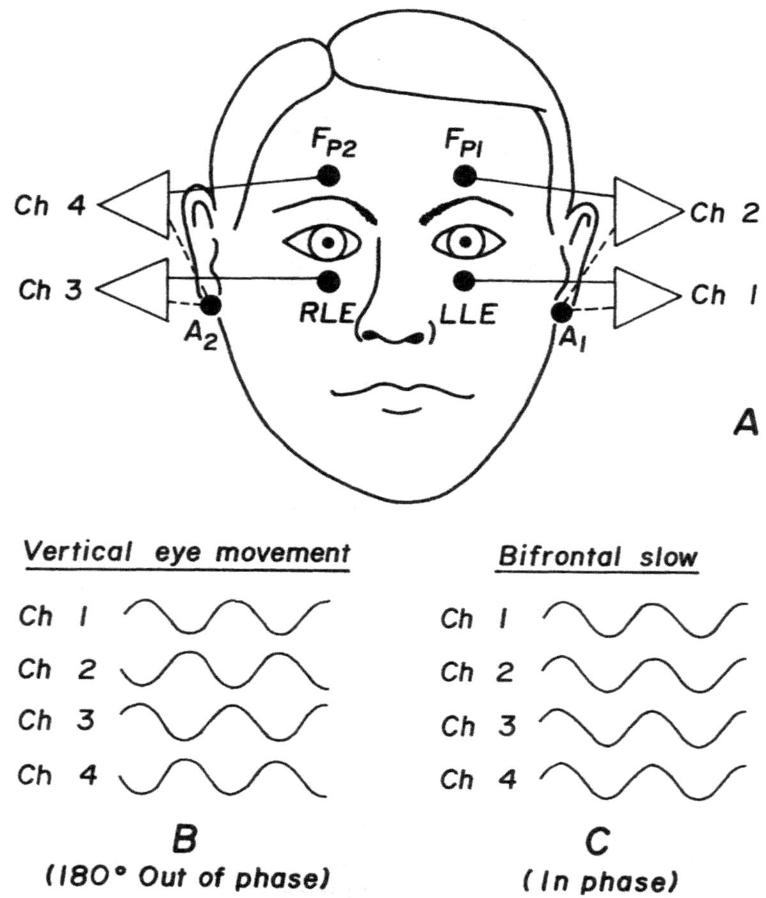

FIG. 16.13. Differentiation of vertical eye movement and bifrontal-polar slow activity. **A:** electrode locations; **B:** eye movement potentials; **C:** bilateral frontal slow activity. (See text.)

16.15E). Figure 16.16 shows these effects in an actual recording, which calibrates the procedure through voluntary eye movement in known directions.

Bipolar chains starting below the eye and proceeding upward and posteriorly (Fig. 16.17A) will *not* differentiate frontal polar slow activity from eye movement. In Fig. 16.17B, the effect of rhythmic vertical eye movement is established. However, suppose that there is rhythmic slow activity being generated bilaterally in the frontal polar areas (leads Fp_1 and Fp_2). This activity will appear in opposite phase in the LLE$-Fp_1$ and the Fp_1-F_3 derivations and similarly in the derivations from the right, as shown in Fig. 16.17C. Electrodes Fp_1 and Fp_2 will be alternately positive and negative due to the frontal slow activity, and phase reversal will occur. Such a montage can be confusing and lead to misinterpretation because a frontal focus will simulate eye movement and vice versa.

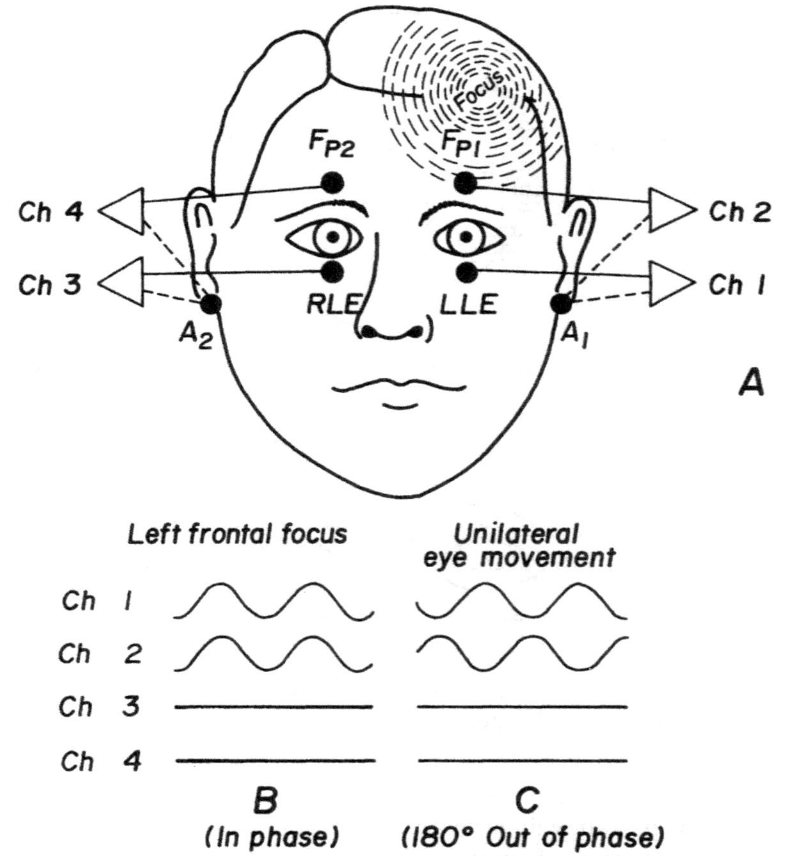

FIG. 16.14. A: Differentiation of unilateral eye movement and unilateral frontal polar slow activity. **B:** Left frontal slow focus. **C:** Unilateral movement, left eye. (Same derivations as Fig. 16.13.)

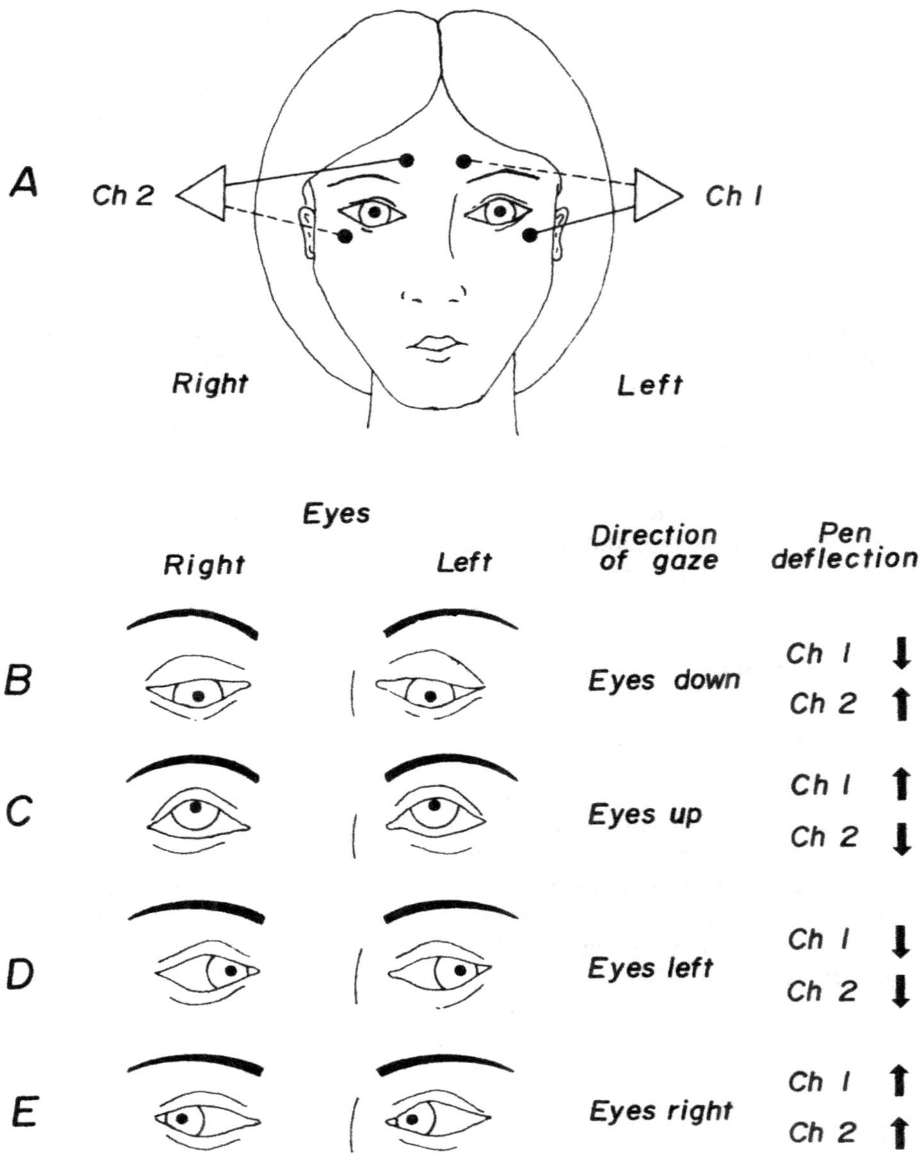

FIG. 16.15. Derivations for identifying specific directions of eye movement. **A:** Electrode locations and derivations. Direction of pen deflections is shown for eye movement: downward **(B)**; upward **(C)**; left **(D)**; and right **(E)**. (See text.)

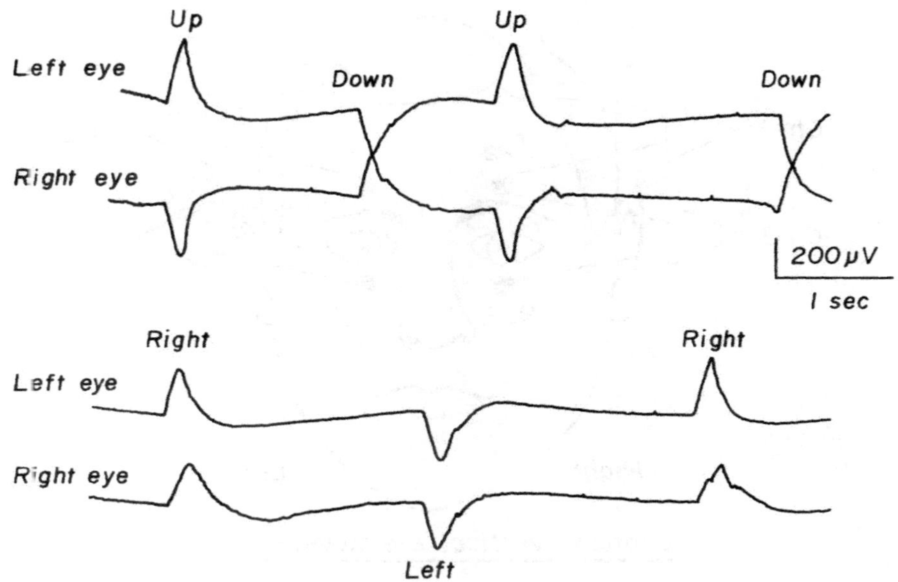

FIG. 16.16. Recording of corneoretinal potentials associated with change in direction of eye movement. (Refer to Fig. 16.15 for electrode locations and to text for details.)

Fluttering of the Eyelids

Fluttering of the eyelids may cause slow activity. Figure 16.18 shows eyes open for a period of 4 sec and an approximately 2-Hz wave is caused by blinking. After closure, the activity is much more rapid, but at varying rates that were observed by the technologist to correlate with small movements of the eyelids. This is a form of blepharospasm. Complete elimination of the slow activity will confirm its origin. The technologist should hold the patient's eyelids gently or tape cotton over them. The observations and the preventive steps should be noted on the record. *Pressure, no matter how light, should never be applied to the eyelids before inquiring whether the patient is or is not wearing contact lens.*

Fig. 16.18 also shows an example of the mixture of two artifacts: eye movement and EKG. The result is apparent sharp and slow activity in the anterior, particularly the frontal polar derivations.

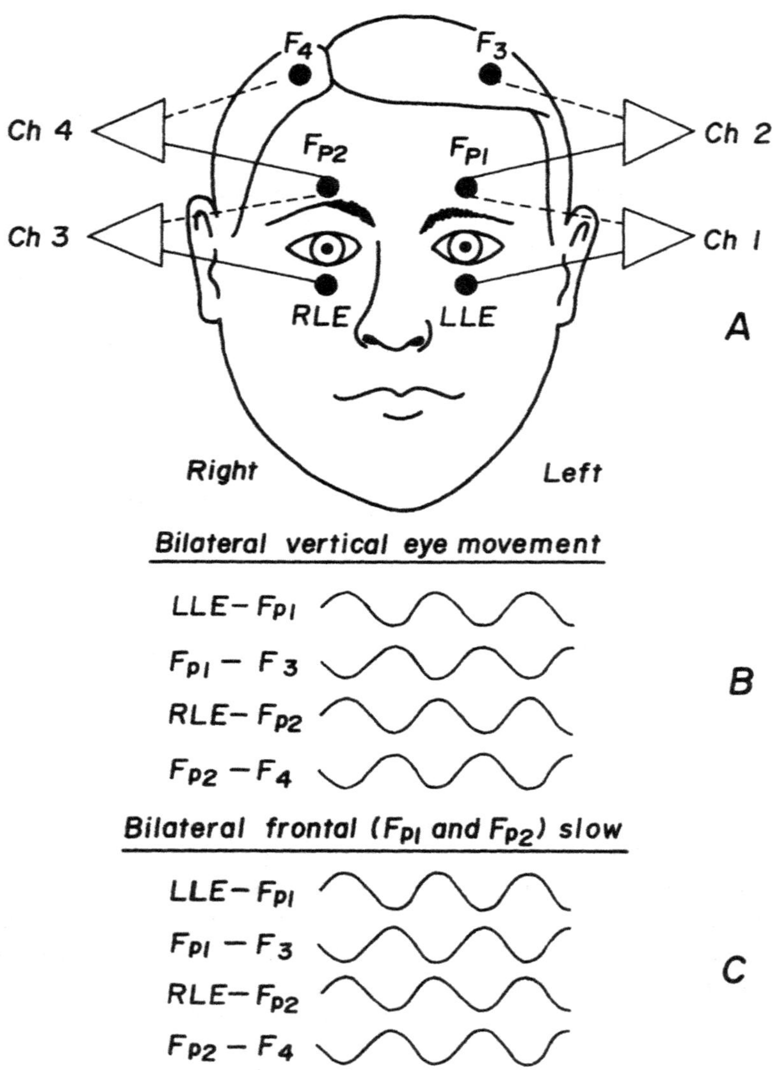

FIG. 16.17. Inability to differentiate frontal slow activity and rhythmic vertical eye movement and bipolar montages. **A:** Electrode locations and derivations. **B:** Phase reversal caused by rhythmic vertical eye movement. **C:** Phase reversal caused by bifrontal focal slow activity at F_{P1} and F_{P2}. (See text for details.)

Blinking and eyelid movements affect the EEG as noise in two ways. First, when the eyelid closes, there is an upward movement of the eyeball, which changes the field of the corneoretinal potential. Second, when the lid closes, there is a change in voltage outside the eye due to increased impedance, since the lid acts as a resistor.

The practice of recording eye movements from only one eye is not recommended. Confusion can arise when attempting to distinguish vertical eye movements from true frontal slow activity. Another reason to avoid the use of a unilateral monitor is because the potentials of the left and right eyes are not always equal. An eye in which vision has been lost may not produce artifact when there is observable eye movement (10). If a single monitor is by chance placed on the "blind eye," movement could occur without there being a potential to record.

An artificial eye has no corneoretinal potential, and movement of the normal eye leads to unilateral artifact. Such asymmetrical artifacts must be monitored for positive identification. A prosthetic eye made with metal is, however, capable of generating a slow potential when the eyelids are opened or closed (6), and this could lead to misinterpretation.

To verify activity recorded when using eye monitors, a calibration should be included before their use by asking the patient to "look up—look down" and to "look left—look right." The direction of the movements then should be indicated on the record. (Refer again to Fig. 16.16.)

Glossokinetic Potentials

The tongue, like the eye, is electrically charged (11). The tip of the tongue is more negative than the root. These charges act as a battery. Movement of one pole of the battery relative to the face will change the electrical field around the mouth and jaws. This field can sometimes spread to the upper part of the face (Fig. 16.19). These are called glossokinetic potentials and are a rather commonly overlooked form of noise or artifact in the EEG.

Movement of the tongue can cause single or rhythmic slow waves that are seen predominantly in the temporal regions, but also may be seen in other areas. These slow waves may be reproduced by asking the patient to say "lilt," "light," "long," or "large." The artifact may be monitored by placing an electrode on the cheek or lip near the mouth.

Chewing and sucking movements (Fig. 16.20) can cause a variety of artifacts including EMG potentials and slow activity, probably related to

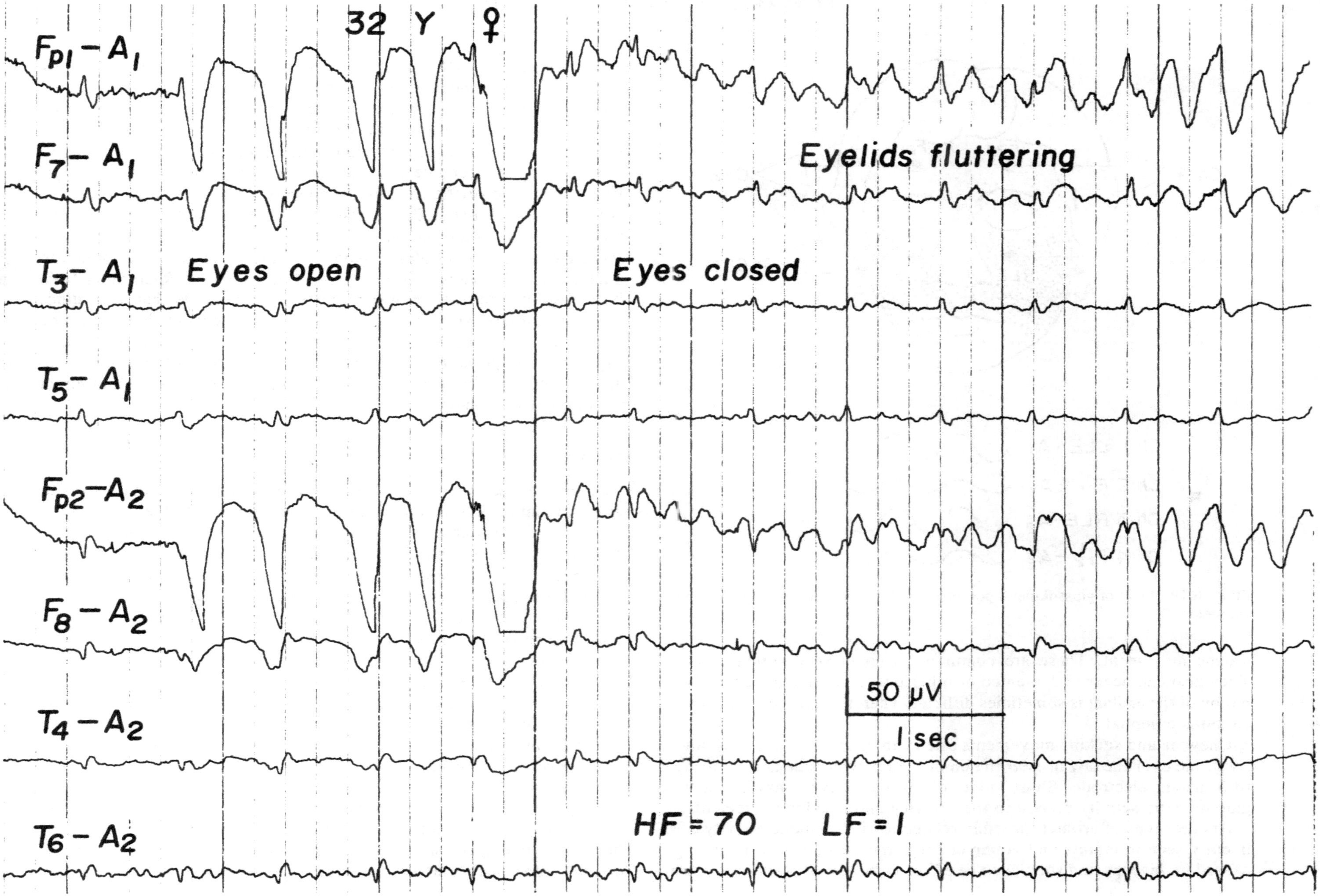

FIG. 16.18. Rhythmic activity in frontal leads related to blinking the eyes and fluttering of closed eyelids.

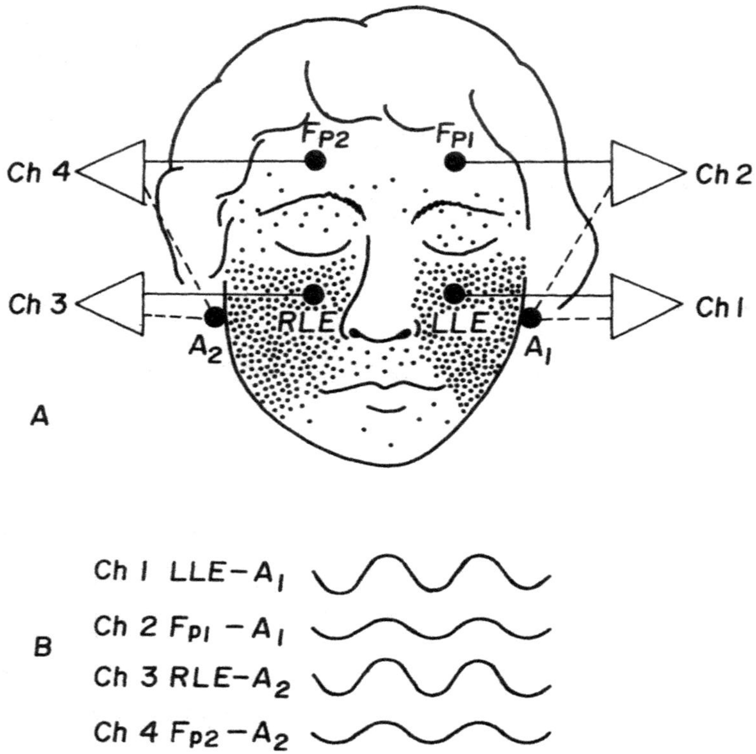

FIG. 16.19. Field of glossokinetic potentials and their relative amplitudes above and below the eye.

tongue movement. These are commonly seen in very young patients. They also can occur in demented or other uncooperative patients. Elimination of the artifact is sometimes difficult. Therefore, its definite identification is essential.

Chewing and sucking movements often can be monitored by placing an electrode over the jaw or near the lip of the involved side and referring it to a distant electrode. Short bursts of muscle activity may occur with glossokinetic activity related to the chewing and sucking movements.

Another type of artifact (possibly related to glossokinetic activity), frequently seen in infants and young children more often than in adults, is caused by hiccups and sobbing. The effect in the EEG sometimes resembles spike-wave or other transient discharge. The technologist should indicate the occurrence of this artifact by placing a distinctive mark and a notation on the record at the time of each sob or hiccup. In the event that a spike-wave or other transient discharge occurs when there is no hiccup or sob, the fact must be clearly noted on the record, i.e., "no sob." It then is possible to differentiate between the signal (the potential of cerebral origin) and the noise (the potentials of noncerebral origin). Positive identification that a signal is of EEG origin and not an artifact can significantly contribute to the interpretation of the EEG.

The electrical field of glossokinetic potentials may be large enough to reach infraorbital leads used in eye monitor montages. Recordings from the infraorbital derivations will be higher in amplitude than recordings from the supraorbital derivations and in phase. The technologist must be on the alert to detect such subtle differences. Verification of the true origin of the in-phase potentials must be carried out. If the origin is not glossokinetic, this must be firmly established by observation and direct monitoring from other facial areas.

Respiration

Respiration may cause two types of artifact. One may be in the form of fairly rhythmic, slow activity that is synchronous with the body movement related to respiration. The movement causes mechanically induced impedance changes in an electrode (Fig. 16.21). Respiration artifact may also appear as a slow or sharp wave occurring synchronously with inhalation and/or exhalation, involving only some electrodes, usually those on which the patient is lying. These artifacts sometimes may be eliminated by repositioning the patient's head.

Monitoring respiration is a simple procedure. With a pencil placed on the running record just ahead of the pens, the technologist observes the patient's respiration and makes an upward movement of the pencil to indicate inhalation and a downward return to indicate exhalation. The rate of respiration can be followed exactly. After observation and notation for a brief period, one can correlate the rate of respiration and slow activity in the EEG record.

A commercially available thermocouple can be placed under the nose and inputted on one channel of the EEG. This will detect respiration by the change in temperature of expired and inspired air. In infants, particularly neonates, such a monitor provides essential information for correla-

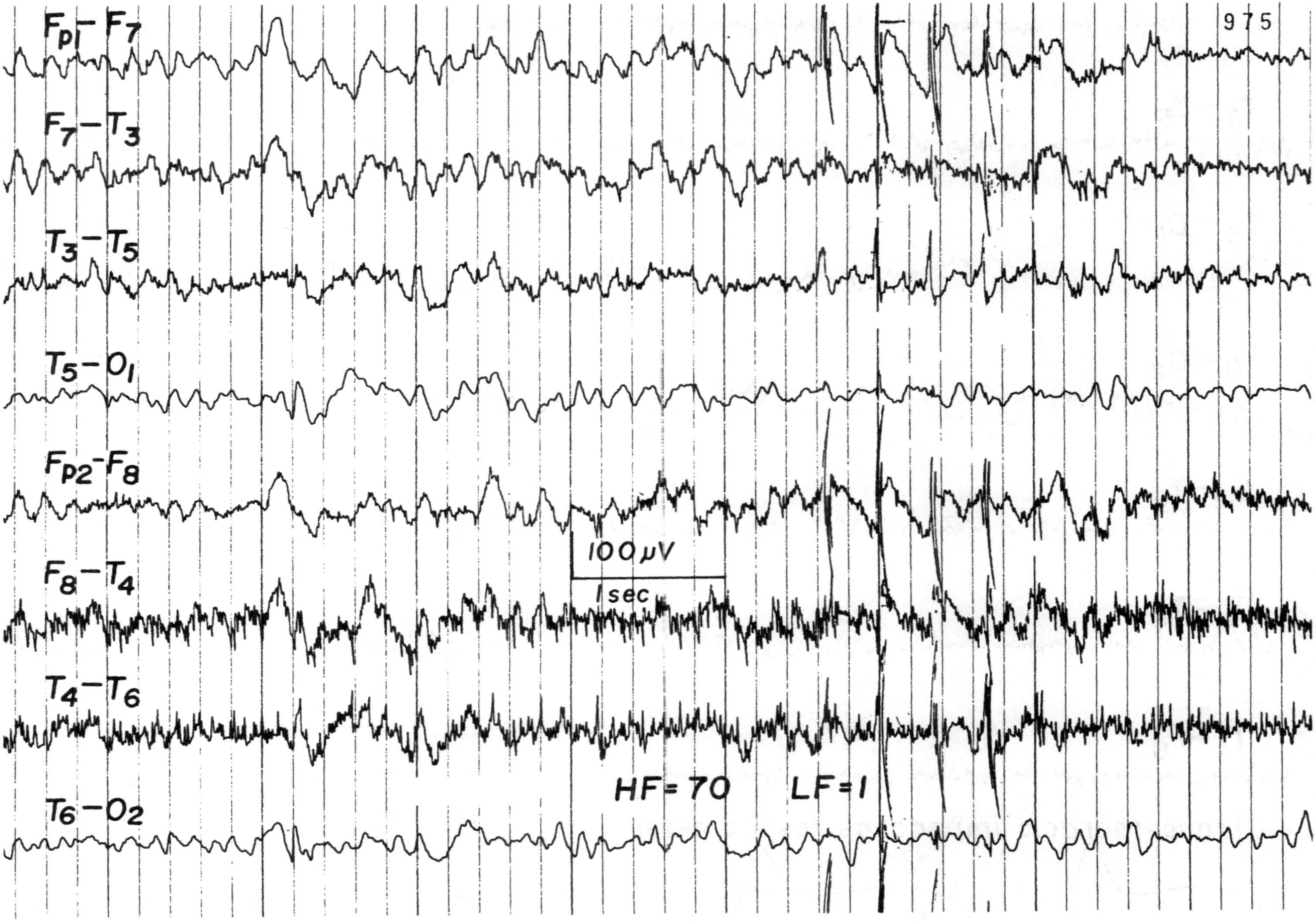

FIG. 16.20. Recording of glossokinetic potential noise in A–P bipolar temporal derivations related to chewing gum.

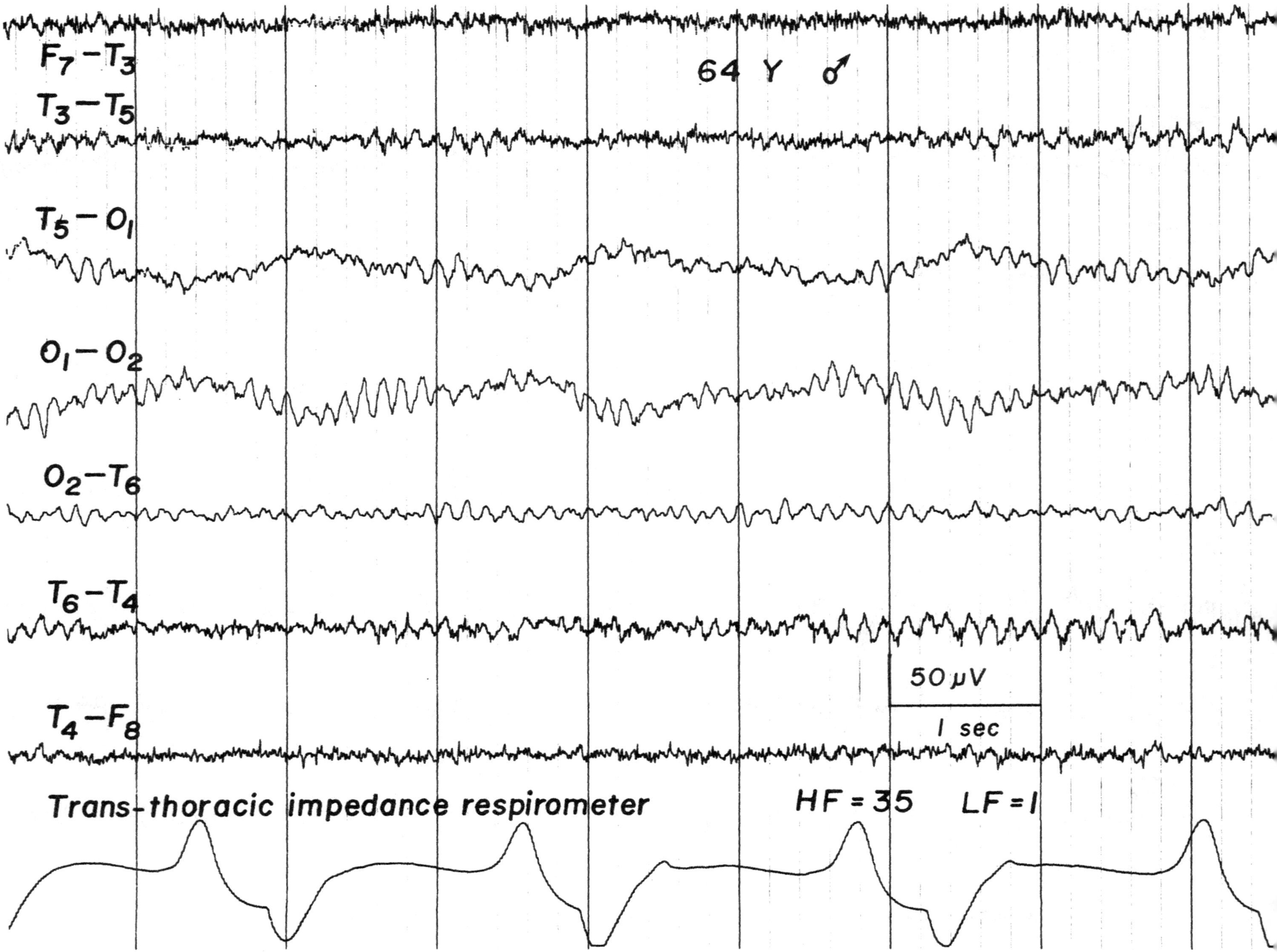
F7–T3
64 Y ♂
T3–T5
T5–O1
O1–O2
O2–T6
T6–T4
50 μV
1 sec
T4–F8
Trans-thoracic impedance respirometer
HF = 35 LF = 1

tion with the EEG data. There also are commercially available devices that measure impedance changes across the chest that occur with chest expansion and contraction during breathing (Fig. 16.21). Other readily available respirometers use a pneumograph.

A simple respirometer can be constructed in the laboratory. This uses an electrolyte-filled rubber tubing secured around the chest. Electrode wires at each end, inside the tubing, act as anode and cathode of a battery, together with the salt bridge between the wires. The voltage changes as the patient breathes. This device can be inputted to an EEG channel and respiratory movements will be recorded (3).

Artifact caused by artificially maintained respiration in the intensive or critical care unit can simulate EEG activity (Fig. 16.22). It can be identified by direct observation and notation on the record.

Tremor

It is difficult to obtain an artifact-free recording from a patient with a severe tremor, as occurs in Parkinson's disease, for example. A mixture of movement artifacts may be induced by the tremor and by muscle activity that occurs at 3 to 6 Hz. Figure 16.23 shows activity recorded from a patient with Parkinson's disease. The technologist observed that the tremor rate and the slow activity were correlated. The entire body was shaking, and there was pressure on and movement of the occipital electrodes that appeared as localized 4-Hz activity. If the tremor involves a limited region, e.g., an arm or a hand, it can be monitored by placing a pair of electrodes over the involved muscles and recording the associated EMG activity. Tremor can also be directly monitored by an accelerometer. This is an electromagnetic detector that records sudden movement and change in direction of movement.

The Electroretinogram

The electroretinogram (ERG) is a physiological artifact that is generated in the retina by light, as occurs during photic stimulation. The electrical activity may appear in derivations using the Fp_1 and Fp_2 electrodes. The ERG appears in synchrony with the flashes of light, and it is sometimes mistakenly called "frontal driving response." Its identity can be determined quickly by holding an opaque card over one eye and then over the other (Fig. 16.24). The artifact will disappear over the blocked eye if its source is in the retina. The flash also should be blocked from the Fp_1 and Fp_2 electrodes (but not the eyes) to see if the noise is being generated in the electrode (a photoelectric effect often related to high electrode impedance). If the artifact is unchanged when light does not strike the electrodes but does enter the eye, there is definite evidence of ERG artifact. A further positive identification of ERG usually can be made by recording from an electrode on or just above the infraorbital ridge or at the outer canthus to an ear reference.

Skin Potentials

Skin potentials cause low frequency artifact. Areas of the skin with many sweat glands are electrically negative with respect to an area less well supplied. The voltage difference may be as much as 50 mV (or up to 100 times the voltage of the EEG). The sweat glands generate electrical potentials when active. Secondarily, the production of sweat changes the concentration of electrolyte between the electrode and the skin, causing a battery effect which acts as a further source of slow artifact. There also are associated changes in skin resistance, and the interactive effects of these variables must be considered when considering the skin as a source of noise in the EEG (2).

The only method of reducing artifact associated with sweat gland activity is to reduce the cause of the sweating. Cooling the head, wiping the area with alcohol, and providing air conditioning to control the recording environment have been the time-honored procedures. Scratching the area under the electrode can reduce local skin potential, but the dangers of infection must be given full consideration (see Chapter 10).

NONPHYSIOLOGICAL ARTIFACTS

There are many nonphysiological artifacts. Indeed, any active EEG laboratory will probably discover a new artifact or a variation of an old one every few months.

FIG. 16.21. Slow activity at O_1 caused by respiration and head movement.

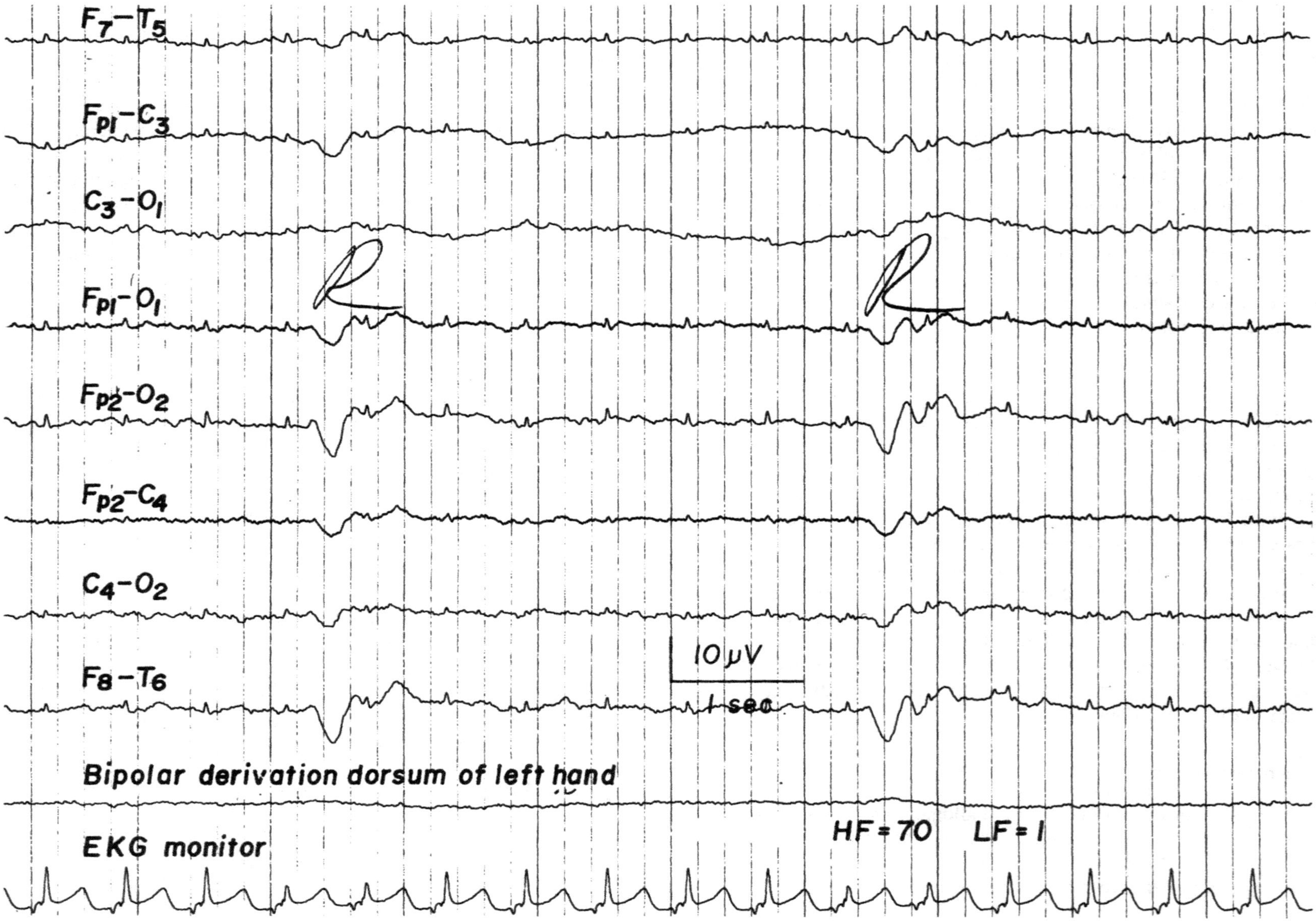

FIG. 16.22. Identification of periodic, slow transient as respiration artifact. Recorded as part of an evaluation to establish cerebral death. Technologist made direct observations of movements associated with artificial respiration and noted these on the record (R).

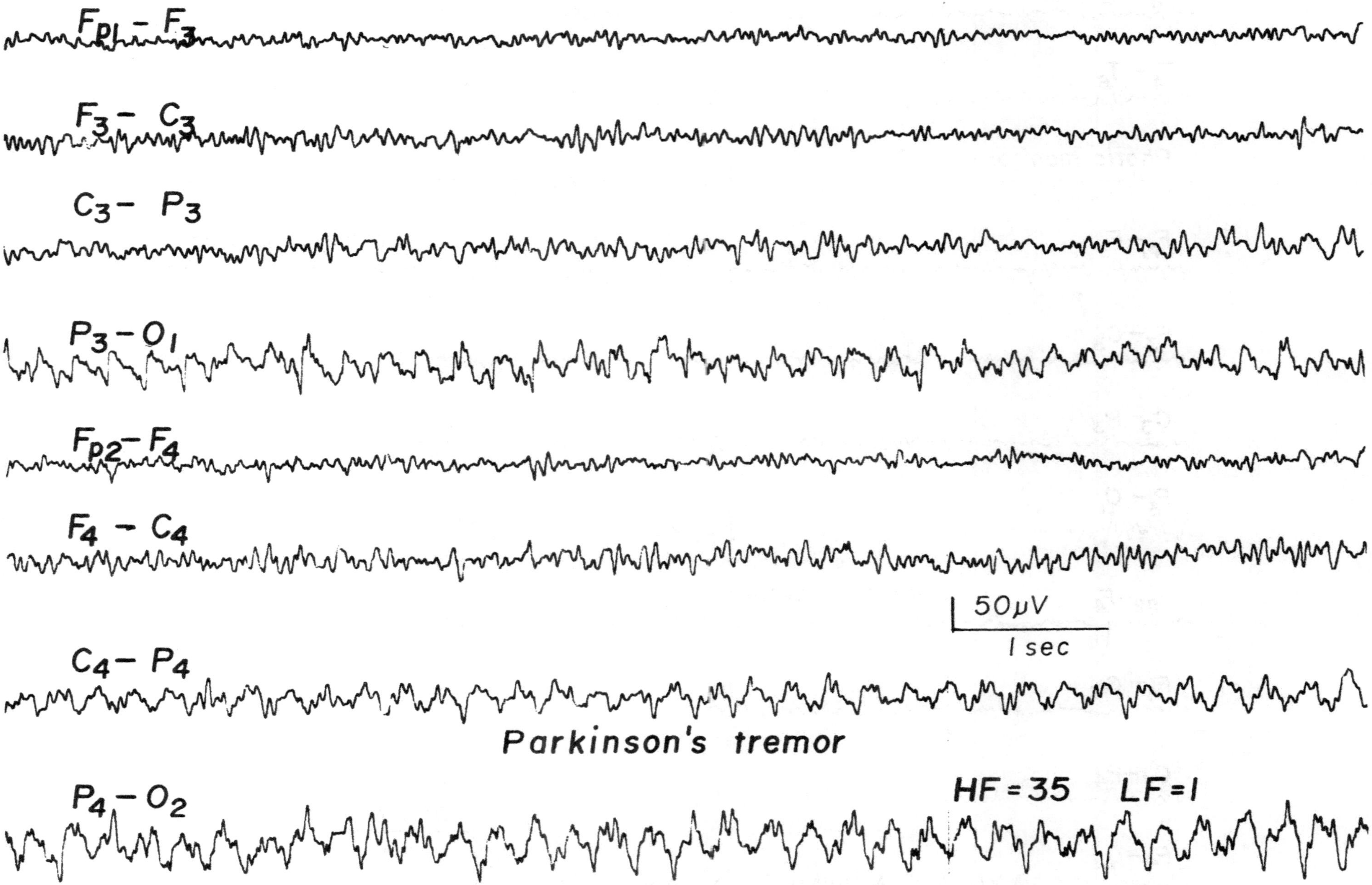

FIG. 16.23. Artifact related to movement recorded in a patient with Parkinson's disease.

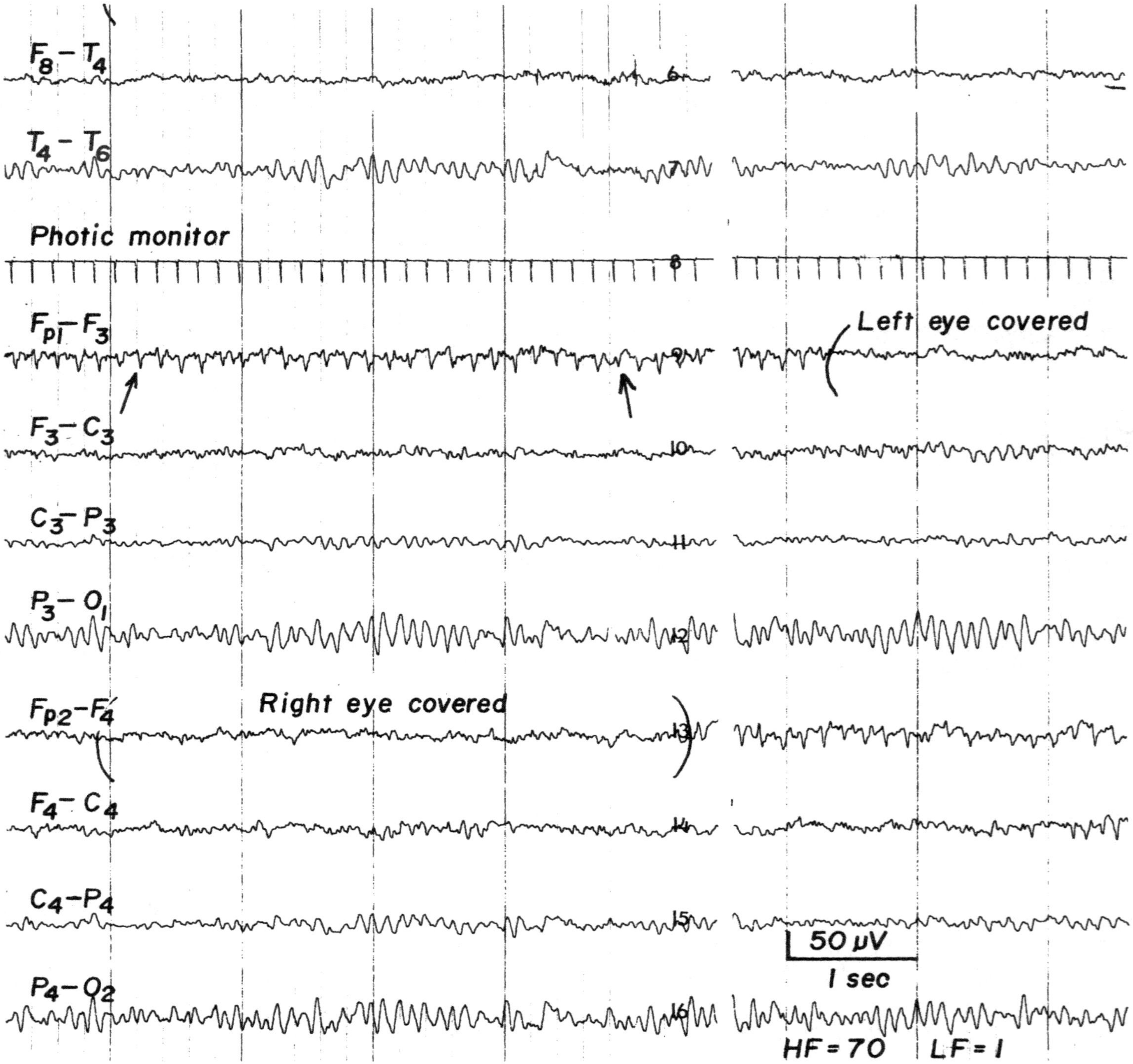

FIG. 16.24. Frontal artifact caused by electrical responses generated in the retina. Covering the eye eliminates the artifact (see text).

60-Hz Artifact

The greatest contributor to nonphysiological noise in the EEG derives from 60 Hz AC. There are two ways in which 60 Hz can produce interference in the EEG recording. The first is via electrostatic effects, caused by capacitance between 60 Hz conductors (the AC mains wiring) and other conductors that act as the second plate of a capacitor, e.g., EEG electrode wires, metal bed frames, the patient, the technologist, or any other conducting bodies in the vicinity. Any capacitively induced voltages that reach the inputs of the EEG amplifiers, if unequal at input 1 and input 2, will be amplified and appear at the output of the recording system as 60 Hz artifact. The artifact may be small and minimally disturbing, or it may be so large that it overwhelms and masks the EEG.

The second source of artifact attributable to 60 Hz is an electromagnetic effect, caused by electrical appliances such as transformers, motors, high-intensity lamps, power supplies in TV sets or in EEG-associated equipment. The electrical field generated in the offending device is inductively coupled to the electrode wires attached to the patient, which act as the secondary of a transformer. The resulting artifact usually is harmonically related to 60 Hz and appears as 120 Hz or as a complex waveform with a 60 Hz fundamental frequency.

Modern electrical building codes help in minimizing electrostatic interference since they require adequate grounding (earthing) of the 117-volt line and also require that all power wiring be enclosed in solid conduit (pipe) which is earthed. In older buildings, shielding the patient area with wire screening (an electrostatic shield) may be necessary, although in general it is not required.

Low voltage 60 Hz artifact sometimes is confused with EMG artifact, but its origin can be easily identified by its exact frequency and waveform. A precise identification of the artifact can be made by increasing paper speed to 60 mm/sec and counting the exact frequency of the interfering activity (1 cycle/mm). This is shown in Fig. 16.25, which also illustrates the relative degree of attenuation of 60 Hz by the use of HF 35 and HF 15 Hz filters.

A lamp or other electrical device in the vicinity of the patient may serve as the source of induced 60 Hz voltage in the EEG. When there is unexpected 60 Hz interference, the technologist should survey the environment for possible sources. Any lamps, heaters, electrical blankets, TV sets, etc. should be disconnected or moved. Sometimes the source may be part of the operating equipment: a portable air pump used to dry collodion, or a photic stimulator. These devices should, of course, be integrally shielded and grounded through their own power cords and returned to the same ground serving the EEG instrument. Sometimes the instrument's power cord is parallel to the electrode input cable, causing 60 Hz interference. The "cure" is to rearrange and separate the cables.

Electromagnetic interference may be reduced by minimizing loops in electrode wires. The leads may be twisted together, or bunched, to form a cable. Multiple grounds must be avoided. The source of the interference should either be switched off or removed as far as possible from the patient and the EEG instrument.

Interference, either electrostatic or electromagnetic, sometimes is caused by wiring or appliances in a room adjacent to the EEG patient recording area. The word "adjacent" does not only mean "next door." Interference can originate in rooms above and below the EEG area. A simple way to detect such interference is to place a 10 kΩ resistor (often called a "dummy patient") across the input to an EEG amplifier, by plugging it into two points on the electrode board and switching them into input 1 and input 2 of an amplifier-recorder channel. At a sensitivity of 2 to 5 μV/mm, there should be no 60 Hz visible at the output. In a "clean environment" increasing the sensitivity to 1 μV/mm should not alter this. If there is a substantial level of 60 Hz in the environment, 60 Hz artifact will appear. By moving the electrode board and the attached resistor around the recording area, the location of regions of minimal and maximal interference can be located (see also ref. 5., sec. IV). The patient should be placed in an area in which the density of 60 Hz is lowest. Sometimes orienting the head in a different direction minimizes density of 60 Hz at the electrodes. If density is high close to the wall, the source may be related either to wiring within the wall or to equipment on the other side of the wall. Quite often such extraneous equipment is in need of an adequate ground.

Sixty Hertz inteference may be picked up by the bed on which the patient reclines. This often occurs when recording EEGs in the intensive care unit. Grounding the bed *directly to the EEG instrument* usually clears up 60 Hz artifact introduced via capacitive sources. The use of the "dummy patient" will help identify the location and the sources of 60 Hz and to validate the "cure" for such artifacts.

Sixty Hertz artifact may be introduced via the technologist, nursing personnel, etc. Since induced voltage is present in them when they touch

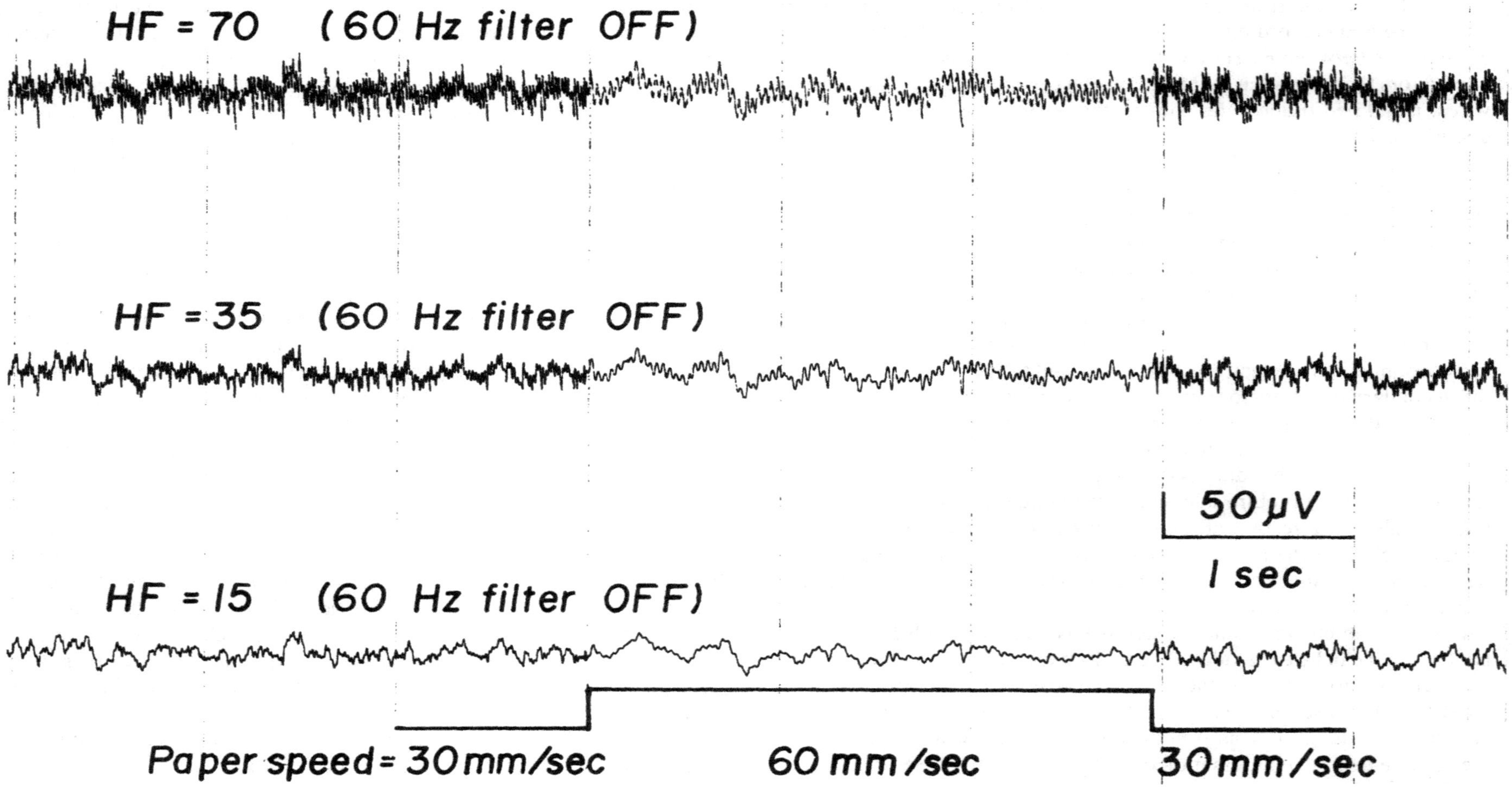

FIG. 16.25. Positive identification of 60-Hz artifact by recording at 60 mm/sec, which enhances perception of individual 60-Hz waves.

the patient, the voltage then is induced in the patient. As a matter of safety, the technologist should avoid touching the leads on a patient who has an indwelling cardiac catheter (Chapter 5).

"Clean" electrode technique is particularly important to minimizing 60 Hz artifact. Poorly applied electrodes which have high impedances increase 60 Hz interference. Unequal electrode impedances cause imbalance of induced 60 Hz voltages at the amplifier's inputs. The difference in 60 Hz voltage at input 1 and input 2 is amplified, together with the EEG signal. Lowering EEG electrode impedances and keeping them equal (or as nearly so as possible) will usually prevent this artifact from appearing.

Stress must also be placed on the necessity of having a low impedance and stable ground electrode on the patient. This should be returned directly to the EEG instrument ground. Exceptions to this are discussed in Chapter 6. (If there is another "ground" on a patient, no EEG ground should be used.)

While the use of 60 Hz "notch" filters will remove all except very high voltage interference (see Fig. 8.26), the artifact should be removed at its source and not by resorting to filters. An over-dependence on filters leads to poor technique.

Artifacts Originating in Electrodes

Many types of noise may be generated in the electrodes. A common artifact is electrode "pop" (Fig. 16.26). This may simulate a spike or sharp wave. It is caused by an electrically unstable electrode, by a drying electrolyte, or by slight mechanical instability that changes the area of electrode surface in contact with the skin. Corrective measures may require replacement of electrolyte, reapplication of the electrode, or sometimes application of a different electrode. On occasion, an electrode that has not been kept clean and has dried paste on it will develop pops and other electrical transients. Random, slow activity also may appear as the result of electrolyte instability.

Electrode artifacts of this type can simulate a developing focal discharge (Fig. 16.27). The necessity for having stable electrodes is imperative. The technologist must be able to discriminate true paroxysmal activity from artifact. Vital information will be lost if a recording is stopped to replace an electrode when a focal electrographic seizure is beginning. When an electrode fails, it should receive immediate attention and be reapplied, or, if necessary, replaced. However, if the patient is drowsy or asleep, it may sometimes be better to utilize an alternate montage than to disturb the patient.

Movement of the electrode wires between the electrode on the head and the electrode board can lead to electrostatic artifacts simulating slow activity. These occur at the frequency of the motion of the wires. Other objects moving in relation to the input electrode leads also can produce electrostatic effects by capacitive coupling. Plastic or rubber hose that swings near the electrode board may be a source.

Movement in the Environment

Movement of persons in the vicinity of the patient generates artifacts, usually of capacitive or electrostatic origin (Fig. 16.28). Notations of such movement should be placed on the record, and if possible, the movements should be prevented. In the operating room and intensive care units, this may not be possible, but notations should be made so that the origin of the movement is a matter of permanent record.

In the operating room, where EEG is frequently used as a monitor, movement of the patient by surgeons and movement of other personnel cannot be avoided. Again, notations must be made to verify the cause of changes in the record that are due, not to changes in the brain, but to changes in the environment.

Intravenous Drip

Another artifact (probably electrostatic) can be introduced by an intravenous drip (Fig. 16.29). With each drip, a transient occurs (8). The technologist should monitor the drip rate by placing check marks on the EEG to determine whether the effect is or is not present.

High Frequency Radiation

High frequency radiation from radio and television transmitters may overload EEG amplifiers and cause them to block. The pens may deflect upward or downward to full excursion and the EEG cannot be recorded (Fig. 16.30A). Problems of this type vary with respect to cause. They often occur in intensive care units where electronic devices using radio frequency carriers are connected to the patient. Hospital paging systems are a frequent source of this class of artifact. Consultation with the manufac-

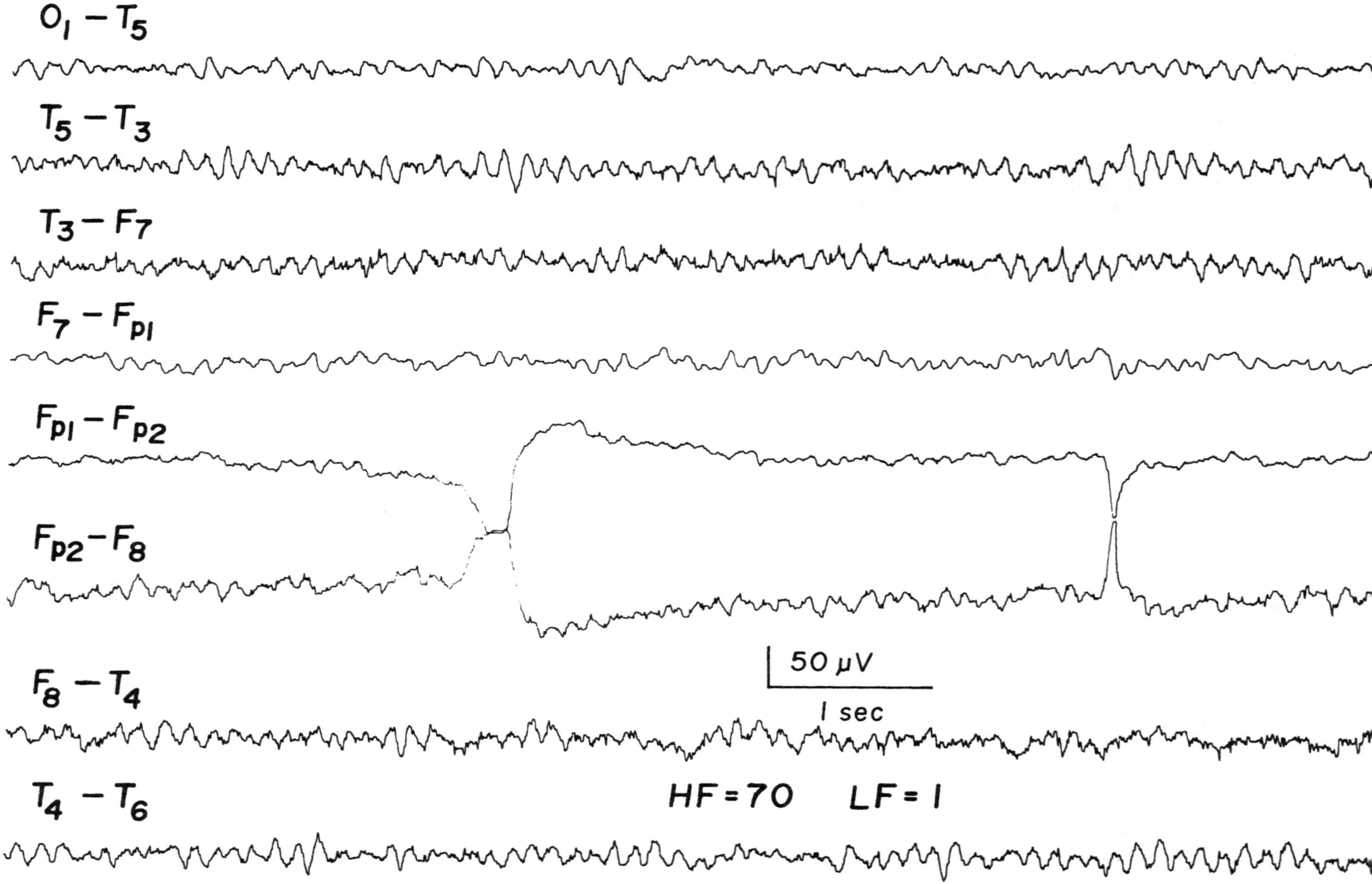

FIG. 16.26. Electrode noise seen as a pop localized at Fp_2.

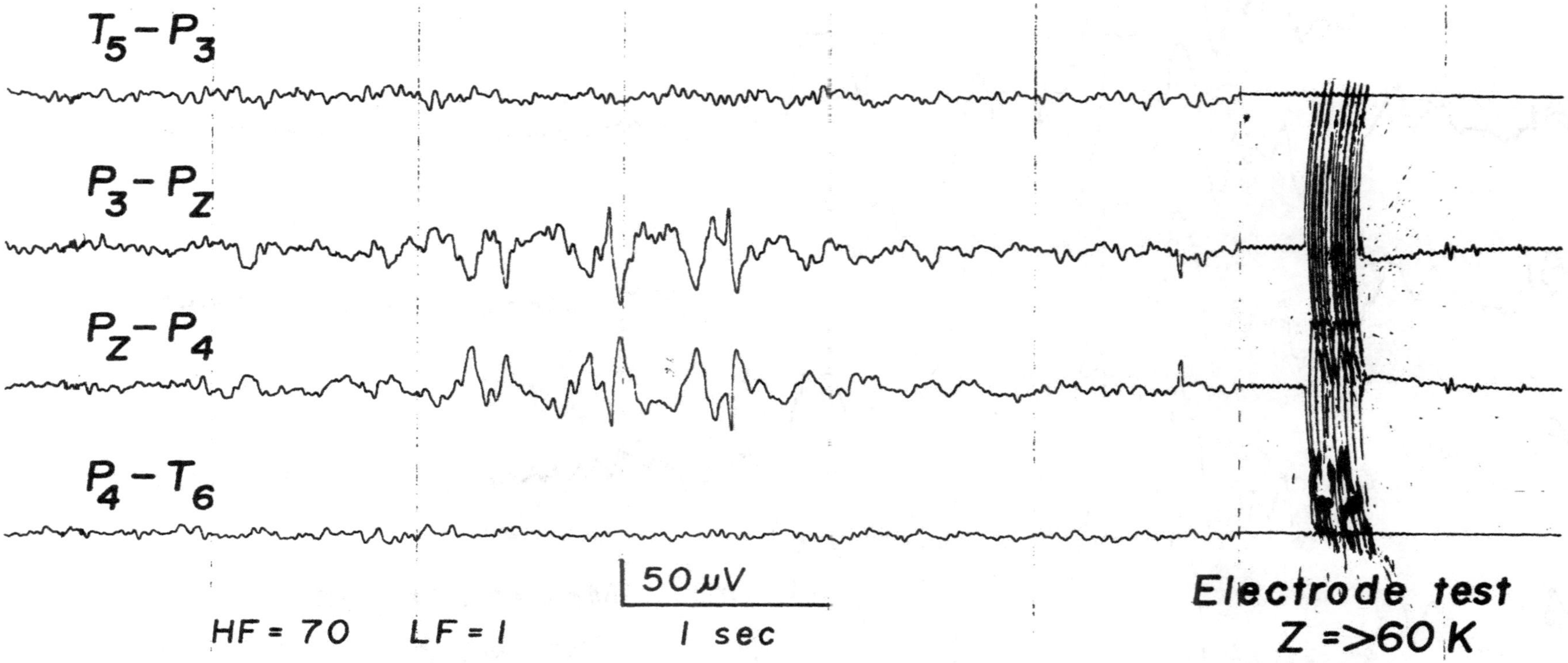

FIG. 16.27. Electrode noise simulating an epileptiform discharge at P_z. At the right of the record, the electrode test is used, and an impedance in excess of 60 kohms is indicated.

turer of the EEG instrument and with hospital biomedical engineers may be necessary to solve a specific problem.

Slow activity may appear in the EEG as a result of continuous or intermittent, relatively high intensity radio frequency carriers (Fig. 16.30B). Shielding may be necessary if the artifact cannot be reduced by other means. This should be a method of last resort, however, because of the expense involved.

Internal Noise

All amplifiers have internal noise. Internal noise is the result of electrons moving randomly in the various parts of the amplifier, as well as voltages created at all contact points in the circuit. With Inputs 1 and 2 interconnected through 5 kΩ and with a sensitivity setting of 1 μV/mm, there should be no transient deflections greater than 4 μV occurring more often than 1 per min and there should be none with an amplitude greater than 2 μV occurring more than 1 per sec (1).

Manufacturers choose components with low inherent noise for use in their EEG amplifiers and power supplies. The greatest source of noise is in the early stages of amplification since it will be amplified progressively in later stages. If components within an amplifier fail (capacitors, resistors, transistors, or in older instruments, tubes) there may be an increase in noise beyond tolerable limits.

If there is difficulty that seems attributable to the equipment, the man-

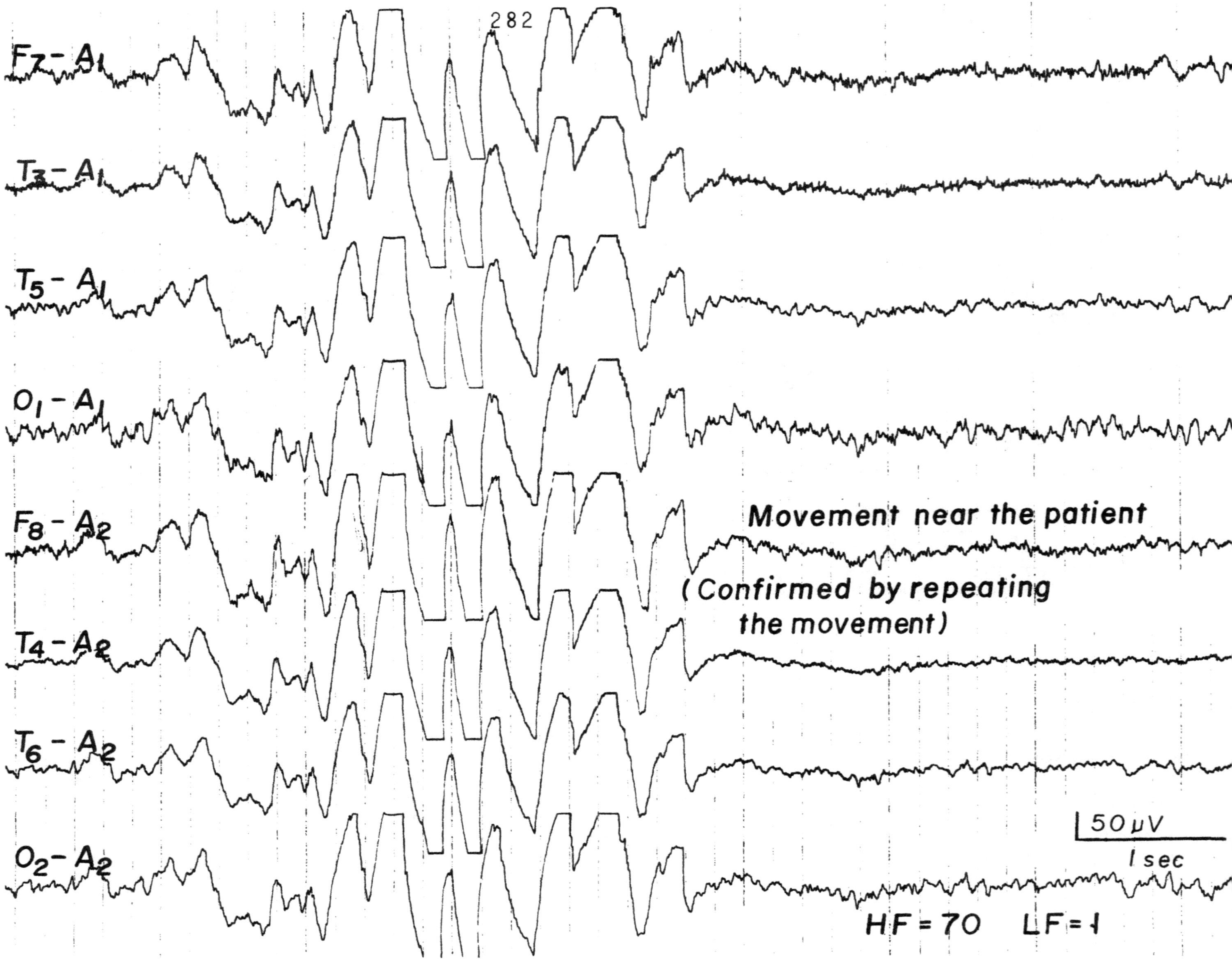
F7 - A1
T3 - A1
T5 - A1
O1 - A1
F8 - A2
T4 - A2
T6 - A2
O2 - A2
Movement near the patient
(Confirmed by repeating the movement)
50 μV
1 sec
HF = 70 LF = 1

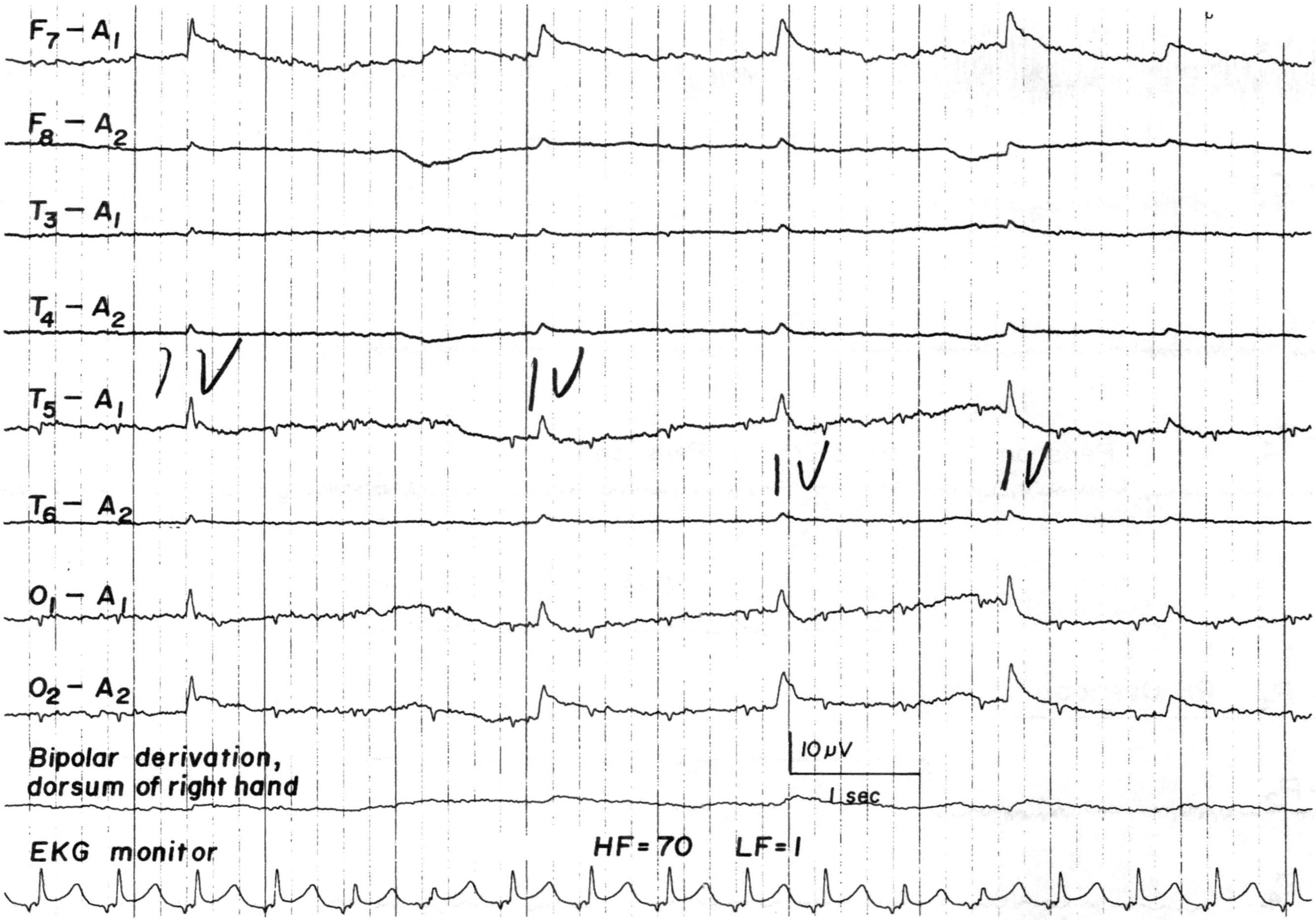

FIG. 16.29. Sharp transients induced by intravenous drip. Technologist's notation on record ("IV") correlates observed drip and the transient.

FIG. 16.28. Electrostatic artifact caused by movement of personnel near patient; confirmed by direct observation and by having the movement repeated and correlated with artifact noted.

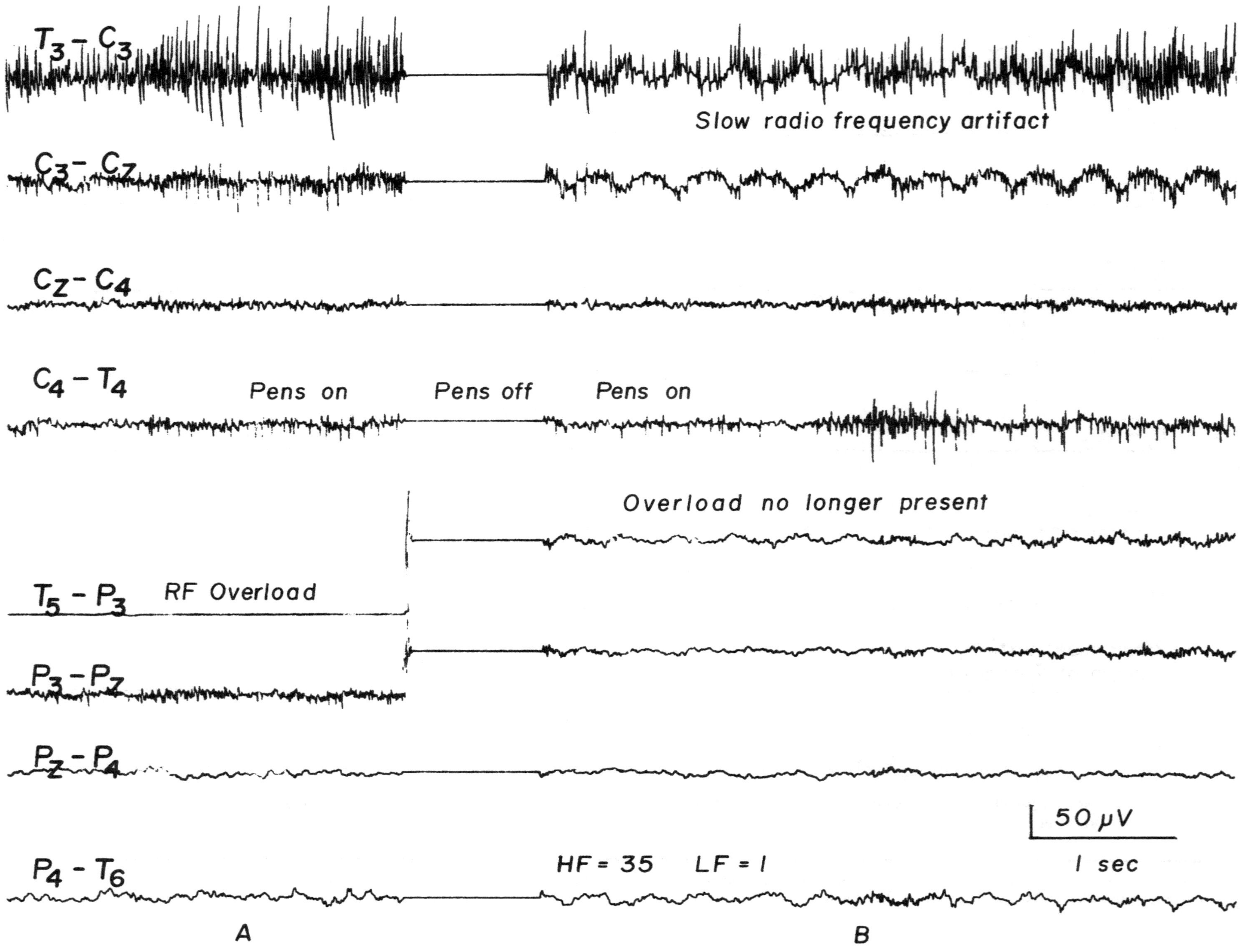

T3 - C3
Slow radio frequency artifact
C3 - CZ
CZ - C4
C4 - T4
Pens on
Pens off
Pens on
Overload no longer present
T5 - P3
RF Overload
P3 - PZ
PZ - P4
50 μV
HF = 35
LF = 1
1 sec
P4 - T6
A
B

ufacturer's instruction manual should cover the majority of problems. Thorough study of the manual before problems develop will speed their solution. It should be recognized that there are few universal rules for identifying instrument-generated artifacts because of differences in design between manufacturers.

It has been suggested (9) that every laboratory should compile an *Atlas of Artifacts*. The solutions should also be noted.

SUMMARY

Not all electrical activity recorded by an EEG instrument originates in the brain. The brain is the source of the EEG signal. The other sources give rise to noise that acts to obscure the signal. The noise is artifact. There are many artifacts. They may be physiological (generated in the patient, but in other than brain systems). They may be nonphysiological (generated by environmental sources or by the EEG instrument).

Physiological artifacts include electrical activities originating in muscle, heart, eye, tongue, and skin.

Nonphysiological artifacts include electromagnetic fields (may include 60 Hz), electrostatic fields (including 60 Hz), electrode noise (including movement, as with respiration), and internal instrument noise.

The EEG technologist must recognize artifacts, determine their sources, and, if possible, eliminate them. If not eliminated, they must be identified positively.

Written notations should be freely used to describe what the patient is and is not doing throughout the recording. This enables the interpreter, or any person who reviews the record at a later time, to have the advantage of the observations made by the technologist at the time of the recording.

REFERENCES

1. Barlow, J. S., Kamp, A., Morton, H. B., Ripoche, A., Shipton, H., and Tchavdarov, D. B. (1978): EEG instrumentation standards (revised 1977): Report of the Committee on EEG Instrumentation Standards of the International Federation of Societies for Electroencephalography and Clinical Neurophysiology. *Electroencephalogr. Clin. Neurophysiol.*, 45:144–147.
2. Geddes, L. A., and Baker, L. E. (1975): *Principles of Applied Biomedical Instrumentation*. John Wiley, New York, pp. 493–496.
3. Grice, S. T., and Jordan, J. E. (1978): The respirometer—a noncommercial respiratory transducer for the EEG laboratory. *Am. J. EEG Technol.*, 18:9–18.
4. Johnson, T. L., Feldman, R. G, and Sax, D. S. (1973): Reduction of muscle artifact in electroencephalographic recording. *Am. J. EEG Technol.*, 14:158–165.
5. MacGillivray, B. B., Binnie, C. D., and Osselton, J. W. (1974): Section IV. Artefacts, faults, and fault-finding. In: *Handbook of Electroencephalography and Clinical Neurophysiology, Vol. 3, Part C: Traditional Methods of Examination in Clinical EEG*, edited by B. B. MacGillivray, pp. 3C-88–3C-102. Elsevier, Amsterdam.
6. Matsuo, F., and Shaner, E. E. (1975): EEG artifact due to a metallic prosthetic eye. *Am. J. EEG Technol.*, 15:75–78.
7. Peters, J. R. (1967): Surface electrical fields generated by eye movements. *Am. J. EEG Technol.*, 7:27–40.
8. Redding, F. K., Wandel, V., and Nasser, C. (1968): Intravenous infusion drip artifacts. *Electroencephalogr. Clin. Neurophysiol.*, 26:318–320.
9. Saunders, M. G. (1979): Artifacts: Activity of noncerebral origin in the EEG. In: *Current Practice of Clinical Electroencephalography*. Edited by D. W. Klass and D. D. Daly pp. 37–67. Raven Press, New York.
10. Shaffer, M. A. (1970): Problem record of the month. No. 3: Asymmetrical eyeblink artifact. *Am. J. EEG Technol.*, 10:153–156.
11. Westmoreland, B. F., Espinosa, R. E., and Klass, D. W. (1973): Significant prosopoglossopharyngeal movements affecting the EEG. *Am. J. EEG Technol.*, 13:59–70.

FIG. 16.30. Artifacts caused by radio frequency interference. Continuous recording. **A**: Severe overload in channels 5 and 6 drives the amplifiers into nonlinearity beyond the dynamic range. **B**: Rhythmic, slow activity in channels 1, 2, 5, 6, 7, and 8, attributable to radio frequency interference. Eliminated by shielding.

Subject Index